Bayer-Symposium IX

Cardiovascular Effects of Dihydropyridine-Type Calcium Antagonists and Agonists

Edited by

A. Fleckenstein · C. Van Breemen

R. Groß · F. Hoffmeister

With 229 Figures and 50 Tables

Springer-Verlag

Berlin Heidelberg New York Tokyo

Bayer-Symposium IX
held at Boppard, Germany, October 3–6, 1984

Professor Dr. Dr. h.c. ALBRECHT FLECKENSTEIN
Physiologisches Institut der Universität Freiburg
Hermann-Herder-Straße 7, D-7800 Freiburg i. Br.

Professor CORNELIUS VAN BREEMEN, D.V.M., Ph.D.
University of Miami School of Medicine
Department of Pharmacology
P.O. Box 016189, Miami, FL 33101, USA

Professor Dr. RAINER GROSS
Bayer AG, Institut für Pharmakologie
Abteilung Herz-Kreislauf-Pharmakologie II
Postfach 101709, D-5600 Wuppertal 1

Professor Dr. FRIEDRICH HOFFMEISTER
Bayer AG, Institut für Pharmakologie
Postfach 101709, D-5600 Wuppertal 1

ISBN 3-540-15455-8 Springer-Verlag Berlin Heidelberg New York Tokyo
ISBN 0-387-15455-8 Springer-Verlag New York Heidelberg Berlin Tokyo

Library of Congress Cataloging-in-Publication Data. Bayer-Symposium (9th: 1984: Boppard, Germany) Cardiovascular effects of dihydropyridine-type calcium antagonists and agonists. "Bayer-Symposium IX held at Boppard, Germany, Oct. 3–6, 1984" – T.p. verso. Includes bibliographies and index. 1. Dihydropyridine – Derivatives – Testing – Congresses. 2. Cardiovascular system – Effects of drugs on – Evaluation – Congresses. 3. Calcium – Antagonists – Congresses. 4. Calcium – Agonists – Congresses. I. Fleckenstein, Albrecht. II. Title. [DNLM: 1. Blood Vessels – drug effects – congresses. 2. Calcium Channel Blockers – pharmacodynamics – congresses. 3. Calcium Channel Blockers – therapeutic use – congresses. 4. Myocardium – drug effects – congresses. 5. Pyridines – metabolism – congresses. W3 BA266 9th 1984c/QV 150 B358 1984c] RC684.D52B39 1984 615'.71 85-26242
ISBN 0-387-15455-8 (U.S.)

Typesetting, printing and bookbinding: Brühlsche Universitätsdruckerei, Giessen
2127/3130-543210

Contents

Session II: Molecular Interactions
Chairman: D.J. TRIGGLE

Session III: Myocardial Effects
Chairman: A. FLECKENSTEIN

Session VI: Hypertension
Chairman: F.R. Bühler

Session VII: Tissue Protection
Chairman: W.G. Nayler

List of Participants

BEVAN, J.A., Department of Pharmacology, The University of Vermont, College of Medicine, Given Building, Burlington, VT 05405, USA

VAN BREEMEN, C., Department of Pharmacology, University of Miami School of Medicine, P.O. Box 016189, Miami, FL 33101, USA

BROWN, D.A., MRC Neuropharmacology Group, Pharmacology Department, The School of Pharmacy, University of London, Brunswick Square, London WC1N 1AX, Great Britain

BÜHLER, F.R., Division of Cardiology, Department of Medicine, Kantonsspital Basel, CH-4031 Basel

CASTEELS, R., Laboratorium voor Fysiologie, Katholieke Universiteit Leuven, Campus Gasthuisberg, B-3000 Leuven

CAUVIN, C., Department of Pharmacology, University of Miami School of Medicine, P.O. Box 016189, Miami, FL 33101, USA

FLECKENSTEIN, A., Physiologisches Institut der Universität Freiburg, Hermann-Herder-Straße 7, D-7800 Freiburg i.Br.

FLECKENSTEIN-GRÜN, G.H., Physiologisches Institut der Universität Freiburg, Hermann-Herder-Straße 7, D-7800 Freiburg i.Br.

GLOSSMANN, H., Institut für Biochemische Pharmakologie, Peter-Mayr-Straße 1, A-6020 Innsbruck

GODFRAIND, T., Laboratoire de Pharmacodynamie Générale et de Pharmacologie, Université Catholique de Louvain, U.C.L. 7350, Avenue Emmanuel Mounier, 73, B-1200 Bruxelles

GROSS, R., Abteilung Herz-Kreislauf-Pharmakologie II, Institut für Pharmakologie, Bayer AG, Postfach 101709, D-5600 Wuppertal 1

HALL, C.E., The Department of Physiology and Biophysics, University of Texas Medical Branch, Galveston, TX 77550, USA

HARPER, A.M., Wellcome Surgical Institute, University of Glasgow, Garscube Estate, Bearsden Road, Glasgow G61 1QH, Great Britain

HESS, P., Department of Physiology, Yale University School of Medicine, P.O. Box 3333, New Haven, CT 06510, USA

HUGENHOLTZ, P.G., Thoraxcenter, University Hospital Rotterdam, Erasmus University, P.O. Box 1738, 3000 DR Rotterdam, The Netherlands

JANIS, R.A., Institute for Preclinical Pharmacology, Miles Laboratories Inc., P.O. Box 1956, New Haven, CT 06509, USA

KASS, R.S., Department of Physiology, University of Rochester, School of Medicine and Dentistry, 601 Elmwood Avenue, Rochester, NY 14642, USA

KAZDA, S., Abteilung Herz-Kreislauf-Pharmakologie I, Institut für Pharmakologie, Bayer AG, Postfach 101709, D-5600 Wuppertal 1

LEONETTI, G., Istituto di Clinica Medica IV, Università di Milano e Centro di Fisiologia Clinica e Ipertensione, Ospedale Maggiore di Milano, Via Francesco Sforza 35, I-20122 Milano

LICHTLEN, P.R., Department für Innere Medizin, Abteilung für Kardiologie, Medizinische Hochschule Hannover, Konstanty-Gutschow-Straße 8, D-3000 Hannover 61

DE MEY, J.G., Department of Physiology and Medicine, University of Antwerp, Groenenborgerlaan 171, B-2020 Antwerp

MEYER, H., Chemical Research Laboratories, Bayer AG, Postfach 101709, D-5600 Wuppertal 1

NAYLER, W.G., Department of Medicine, University of Melbourne, Austin Hospital, Heidelberg, Victoria 3084, Australia

SCHWARTZ, A., Departments of Pharmacology and Cell Biophysics, University of Cincinnati College of Medicine, 231 Bethesda Avenue, Cincinnati, OH 45267, USA

Steen, P.A., Department of Anesthesiology, Ullevål Hospital, University of Oslo, N-Oslo 1

Taira, N., Department of Pharmacology, Tohoku University School of Medicine, Sendai, 980, Japan

Towart, R., Research Department, Miles Laboratories Ltd., Stoke Court, Stoke Poges, Slough SL2 4LY, Great Britain

Triggle, D.J., Department of Biochemical Pharmacology, School of Pharmacy, State University of New York at Buffalo, Buffalo, NY 14260, USA

Warltier, D.C., Departments of Pharmacology, Toxicology and Medicine, Division of Cardiology, The Medical College of Wisconsin, 8701 Watertown Plank Road, Milwaukee, WI 53226, USA

Wier, W.G., Department of Physiology, University of Maryland School of Medicine, 655 West Baltimore Street, Baltimore, MD 21201, USA

Welcome

R. Krebs

It is the first time so far as I can see that we have the Ca agonists included in a meeting and from that you can conclude that beyond the Ca antagonists some new results are coming along with this exciting type of new drugs. Discussing Ca agonistic drugs opens the window for new indications – even those not covered by present drugs. Let us hope that we go for a developement of Ca agonistic drugs in a few years as intensively as we did and still do with the Ca antagonists.

With the Ca antagonists you know that we have some new drugs under registration for various indications. Therefore, one should believe we are almost close to the management comfort part of the R&D S-curve. That is the part where you get some results from the money you put on research. In new research areas it is quite different – the lack of results does not allow you to check whether the money is well spent, a situation which causes an uncomfortable feeling for general and research management. But we need to set up even more new research areas in order to guarantee future growth of the company. The reasons for this are the following:

1. Product cycles are becoming shorter
2. The innovation potential is decreasing
3. Maturation of a new area consumes more and more time – it now is approximately 15 years in pharmaceutical research
4. The actual patent life is shortened by prolongation of development time
5. Price control in many countries reduces the pay back of money invested in research.

This all together will have a serious impact on future pharmaceutical research and consequently on the discovery of new drugs.

In actual fact the number of new chemical entities is decreasing over the last years. However, at the same time the R&D budgets are increasing since 1967 by an annual rate of approx. 15% – a rather dramatic increase. Consequently more money is spent for less drugs. Where is the money going to? Very simple, there is a process of shifting larger parts of the budget from basic research to development areas – i.e. toxicology, kinetics and clinical research.

New guidelines and drug laws were established in order to improve safety of drugs. This trend is reflected by a simple example: In 1938 Adrenaline – a really different drug – was registered on the basis of 27 pages. In the early 80's our penicilline Mezlocillin needed more than 600,000 pages. Does this really improve safety? Is it possible for any agency to carefully go through a submission like the last one? Or do we fight a sham fight for more safety? The money we loose by any questionable work is lacking for basic research. In actual fact the part of total R&D budget spent for basic research is now below 30%. This development would be no matter of concern if safety would be really increased.

Opening this symposium I hope very much for interesting presentations and stimulating discussions. The latter certainly will continue during the social part which I consider to be an important part of such a meeting.

Bayer-Symposium IX
Cardiovascular Effects of Dihydropyridine-Type
Calcium Antagonists and Agonists, 3–31

Calcium Antagonists and Calcium Agonists: Fundamental Criteria and Classification

A. FLECKENSTEIN

Introduction

Excitation-contraction coupling is a Ca^{++}-dependent chain reaction that begins with superficial membrane depolarization and finishes with intracellular contractile tension development. The elucidation of the intermediate and the final links of this chain, i.e. of the interaction of Ca^{++} ions with intracellular organelles and with the protein constituents of the contractile system, has progressed tremendously during the past 3 decades. The name of Setsuro Ebashi [1] may be quoted here as being representative for many investigators who have decisively contributed to the striking achievements on this field of muscle research. Conversely, our own work delt with the initial events in excitation-contraction coupling, namely the transmembrane cation fluxes, particularly across the stimulated myocardial fibre membranes. The present article covers new developments that allow a reliable identification and classification of the drugs which inhibit or promote the Ca^{++} currents specifically, i.e. without concomitant influences on Na^{+}- or Mg^{++}-dependent sarcolemma membrane effects.

I. Selective Inhibition by Calcium Antagonists of Myocardial Contractility

It has been proposed by Reuter and Beeler [20] that there are two special transmembrane carrier systems in atrial and ventricular myocardium: A so-called fast channel for Na^{+} entry that initiates the cardiac fibre action potentials, and a separate slow channel for Ca^{++} ions that activate the contractile machinery. In fact, drugs which predominantly reduce Na^{+} conductivity, such as local anesthetic substances and antiarrhythmic agents of the quinidine-lidocaine type, preferentially inhibit myocardial excitability. Conversely, as first demonstrated in our

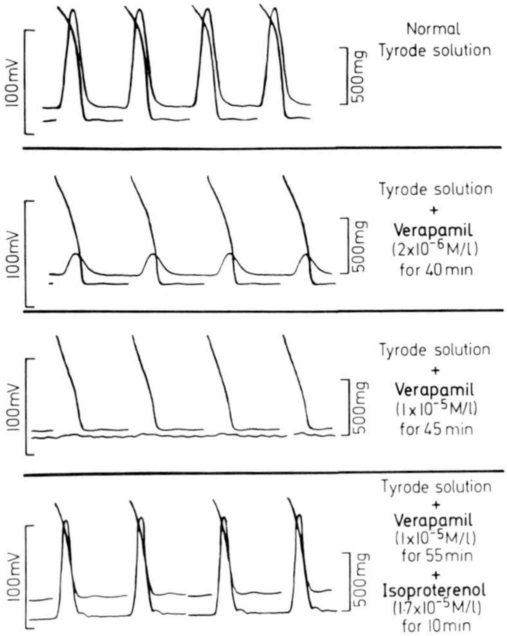

Fig. 1. Selective loss of cardiac contractility under the influence of a high overdose of verapamil, and the reversal of this effect by isoproterenol. Experiments on an electrically driven (2 shocks/sec) isolated papillary muscle of a guinea-pig in Tyrode solution with 2 mM Ca^{++}. From Fleckenstein (1968) Verh Dtsch Ges Kreisl-Forsch 34:15–34; Proc V, Eur Congr Cardiol, Athens, Sept. 1968, pp 255–269

laboratory[1] with verapamil and D 600, the possibility exists to block selectively the transmembrane inward Ca^{++} current so that myocardial contractility is exclusively abolished without any appreciable influence on the Na^+-dependent action potential parameters (see Fig. 1). Therefore, in 1967–69 Fleckenstein and coworkers [2–6] introduced the new name "competitive Ca^{++} antagonist" in order to distinguish clearly this novel principle of cardiac inhibition from other interventions as for instance β-receptor blockade. Figures 2 and 3 represent further observations with the Ca^{++} antagonists nifedipine and diltiazem, added to an ordinary Tyrode's solution with 2 mM $CaCl_2$. While, in Figs. 1–3, Ca^{++}-dependent isometric tension development was totally suppressed by suitable doses of these drugs, resting potential as well as Na^+-dependent upstroke velocity and overshoot of the action potential remained practically unchanged. There was only an abbreviation of the plateau after the transmembrane Ca^{++} conductivity had been blocked, since Ca^{++} ions normally contribute to the maintenance of depolarization during the late phase of action potential. Naturally, this electrogenic Ca^{++} effect also disappears when the inward Ca^{++} current ceases. All Ca^{++} antagonist actions on myocardial tension development can easily be neutralized by measures that are capable of increasing the availability of free Ca^{++} to the contractile system. Thus simple elevation of the extracellular Ca^{++} concentration as well as administration of β-adrenergic catecholamines (or cardiac glycosides)restore myo-

---

1 A detailed report on the discovery of Ca^{++} antagonism as a new pharmacodynamic principle has recently been given in a monograph by Fleckenstein: Calcium Antagonism in Heart and Smooth Muscle – Experimental Facts and Therapeutic Prospects, John Wiley, New York

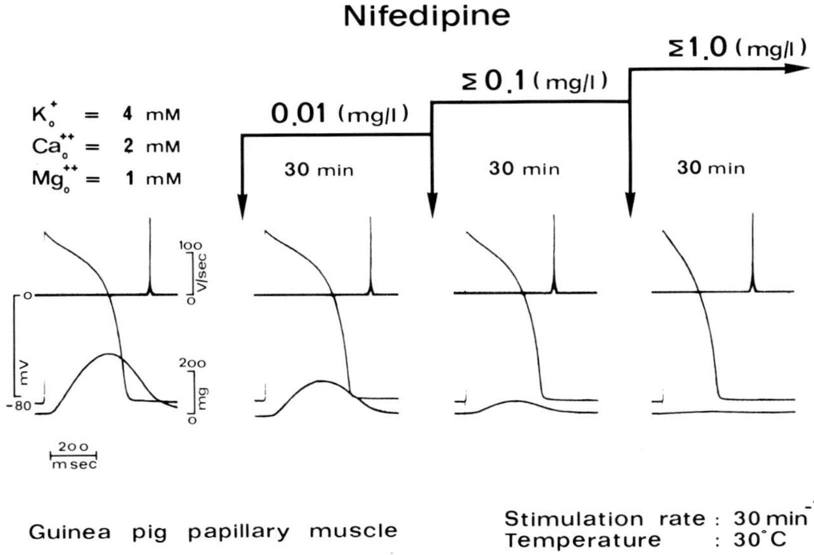

Fig. 2. Complete excitation-contraction uncoupling of a guinea-pig papillary muscle by a stepwise increase of the nifedipine concentration from 0.01 to 0.1 and finally 1 mg/l. The uptroke velocity of the action potentials (dV/dt max = 175 V/s), indicating the fast Na^+ influx, did not change at all (see upper curve). Only the plateau of action potential was abbreviated. See Fleckenstein [5]

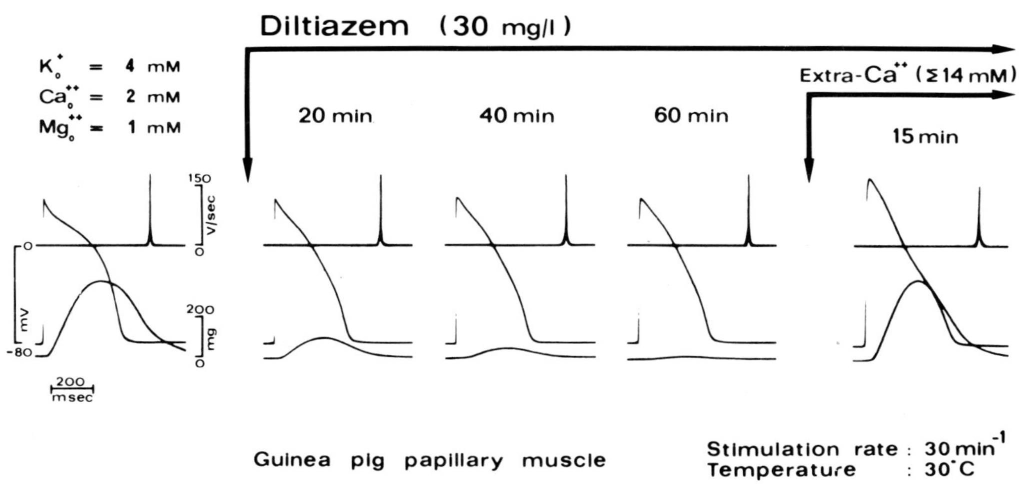

Fig. 3. Selective suppression by diltiazem of contractility of a guinea-pig papillary muscle without reduction of resting potential and of velocity of rise (dV/dt max) of action potential. At the end of experiment, restitution of contractility is attained by elevation of Ca^{++} concentration of the diltiazem-containing Tyrode solution from 2 to 14 mM. From Fleckenstein [5]

Table 1. *Group A*: Calcium antagonists of outstanding specificity. Criteria: Inhibition by 90 to 100% of slow inward Ca^{2+}-current *without* concomitant influence on transmembrane Na^+ conductivity

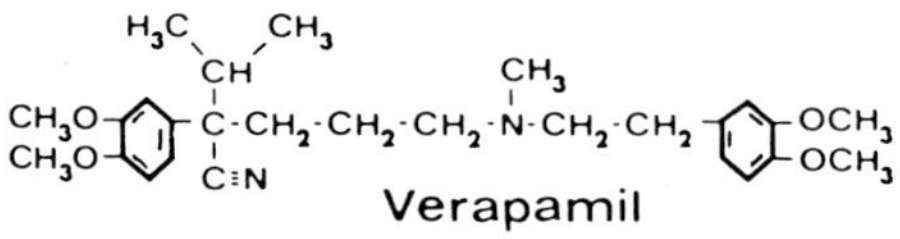 Verapamil (Mol. wt. 454.59)	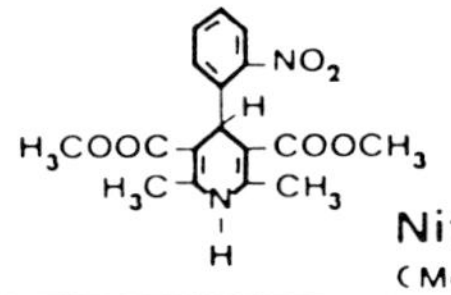 Nifedipine (Mol. wt. 346.34)
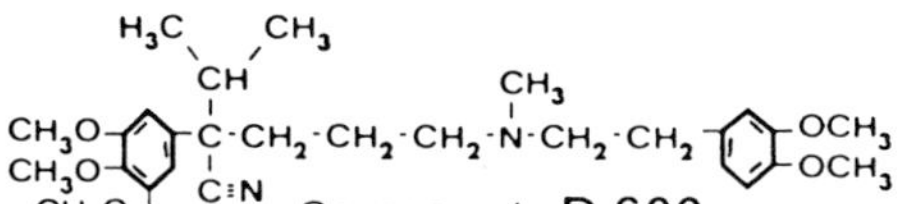 Compound D 600 (Gallopamil, Mol. wt. 485.59)	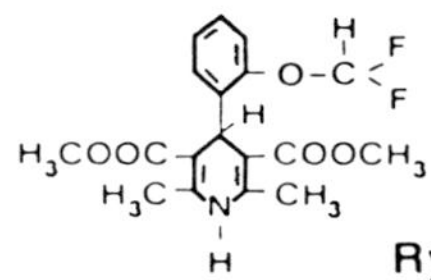 Ryosidine (Mol wt. 367.35)
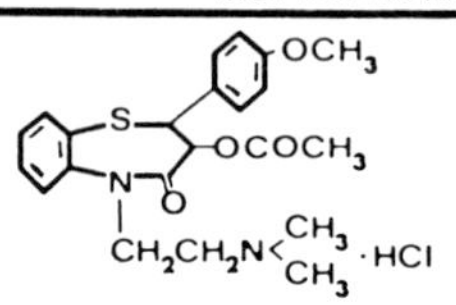 Diltiazem (Mol. wt. 414.52)	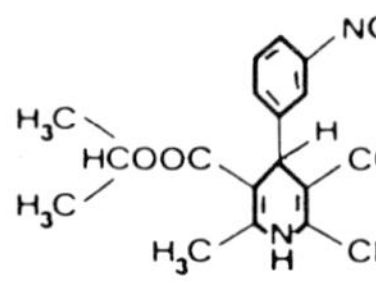 Nimodipine (Mol. wt. 418.45)
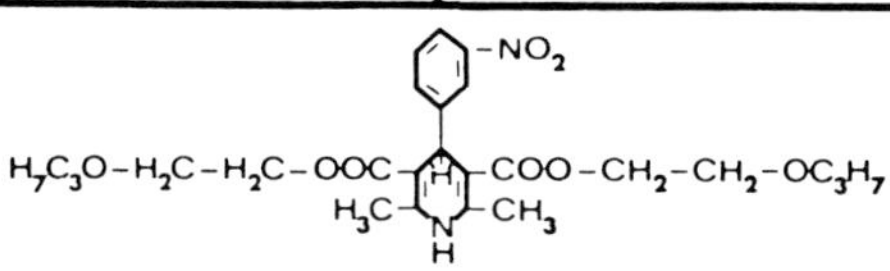 Niludipine (Mol. wt. 490.55)	

cardial contractility, even in the presence of the Ca^{++} antagonists (see Figs. 1 and 3). Separate measurements of the individual transmembrane Ca^{++} and Na^+ currents with voltage clamp techniques, and extensive studies of the inhibitory influence of Ca^{++} antagonists on myocardial radiocalcium uptake have further substantiated these observations (see the reviews by Fleckenstein [2–5]).

Table 1 represents a compilation of the top Ca^{++} antagonists that were identified first in our institute, namely verapamil, D 600, nifedipine, nimodipine, niludipine, and ryosisidine. Diltiazem, which is, according to our tests, another Ca^{++} antagonist of outstanding specificity, originates from Japan. It was launched as a Ca^{++} antagonist by Dr. Nakajima and his colleagues in 1975 [18]. We should like to designate the compounds listed in Table 1, as Ca^{++} antagonists of group A. All these drugs are capable of inhibiting excitation-contraction coupling of the mammalian ventricular myocardium by 90 to 100% before the fast Na^+ influx, during the rising phase of action potential, is also affected. Moreover, the drugs of group A do not interfere with electrogenic Mg^{++} effects. Table 2 contains substances, classified by us as Ca^{++} antagonists of group B, namely prenylamine, fendiline, terodiline, perhexiline, and caroverine. These Ca^{++} antagonists are somewhat less potent and specific. This means that under their influence, a concomitant inhibition of the Na^+-dependent excitatory process can be seen, when Ca^{++}-dependent contractile tension development of isolated papillary muscle

Table 2. *Group B*: Calcium antagonists of satisfactory specificity. Criteria: Inhibition by 50 to 70% of slow inward Ca^{2+}-current *before* fast Na^{+}-influx is also affected

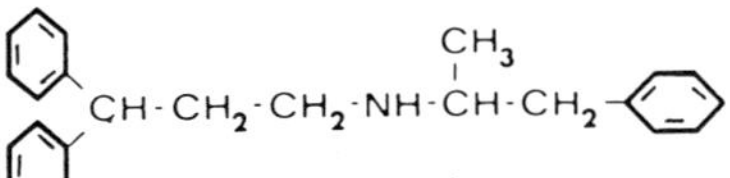

Prenylamine
(Mol. wt. 329.46)

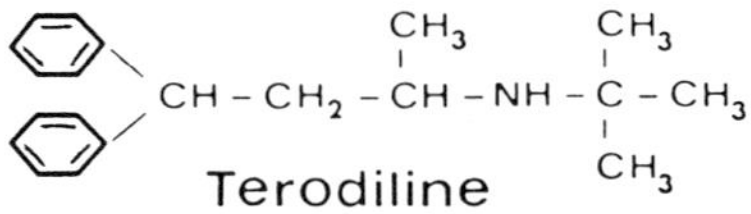

Terodiline
(Mol. wt. 281.0)

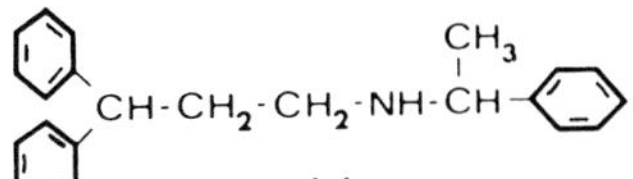

Fendiline
(Mol. wt. 315.46)

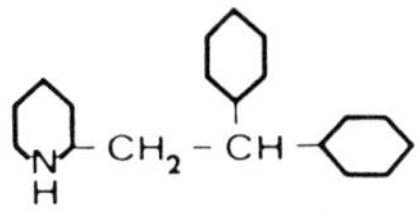

Perhexiline
(Mol. wt. 277.50)

Caroverine
(Mol. wt. 366.49)

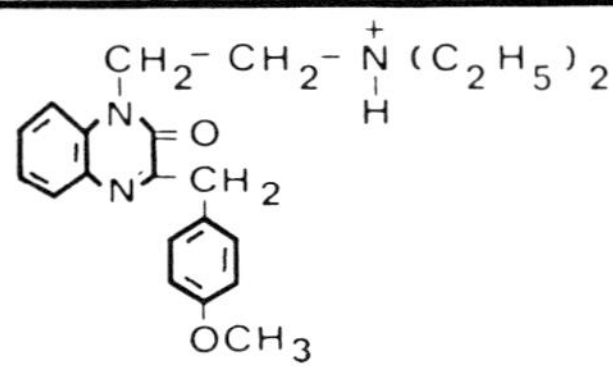

has been reduced by 50 to 70%. However, such serious degrees of contractile depression can never be observed in vivo as long as the drug concentrations remain in the therapeutic dosage range. There are some indications that cinnarizine and flunarizine also belong to group B. However, the poor water solubility of these drugs did not allow us a satisfactory electrophysiological analysis on isolated myocardial tissue.

We are actually facing a Ca^{++} antagonist boom. In fact, the new family of Ca^{++} antagonists is steadily growing, particularly with respect to many nifedipine derivatives (see Table 3). But among true Ca^{++} antagonists, there are also drugs that were claimed to be Ca^{++} antagonists without the necessary verification of their Ca^{++}-antagonistic specificity. This applies for instance to tiapamil and lidoflazine. Tiapamil exerts both Na^{+}- and Ca^{++}-antagonistic effects to an equal extent. Lidoflazine inhibits the Na^{+}-dependent action potential parameters even more than Ca^{++}-dependent contractility. There are also many other drugs with Ca^{++}-antagonistic side effects: Certain β-blocking agents, barbituric acid derivatives and a considerable number of antidysrhythmic drugs with a negative inotropic influence. As proposed by Fleckenstein several years ago, the name of a Ca^{++} antagonist or Ca^{++} entry inhibitor should only be accredited to such drugs which possess, in all their actions, a clear Ca^{++}-antagonistic specificity. Specificity means that the Ca^{++}-antagonistic effects are so predominant, that other pharmacodynamic properties, at least in a reasonable dosage range, are more or less negligible. If one follows this definition, the designation "Ca^{++} antagonist" has to be reserved for such drugs that fit into group A or B. For this classification, electrophysiological data obtained on cardiac fibres are indispens-

Table 3. 1,4-Dihydropyridine compounds which share their fundamental Ca^{++}-antagonistic properties with the prototypical substance nifedipine

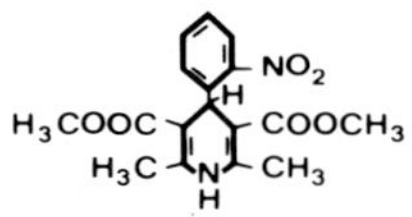 **Nifedipine*** (MW 346.34)	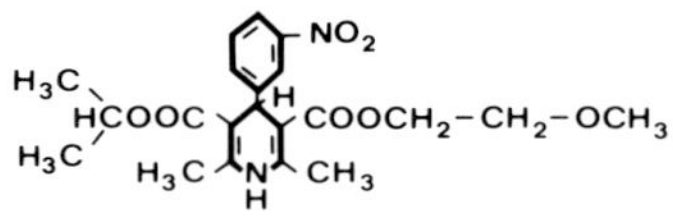 **Nimodipine** (MW 418.45)	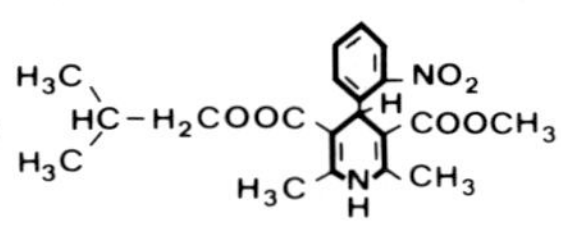 **Nisoldipine** (MW 388.42)
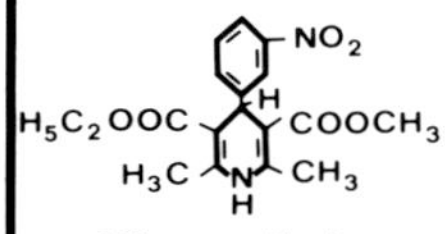 **Nitrendipine** (MW 360.37)	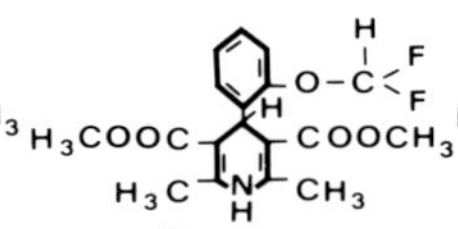 **Ryosidine** (MW 367.35)	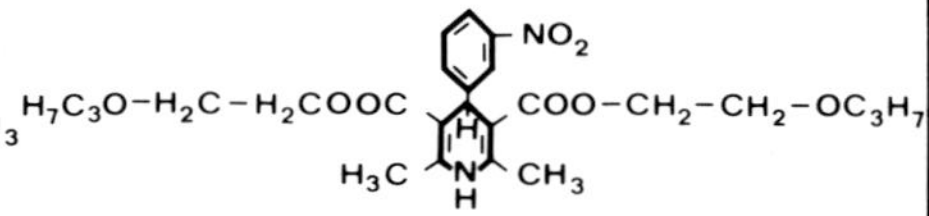 **Niludipine** (MW 490.55)
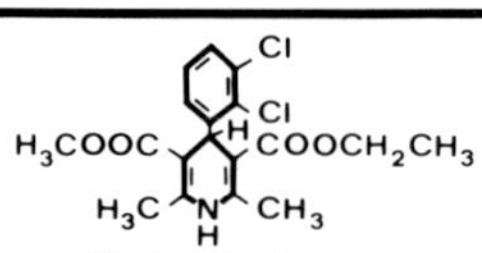 **Felodipine** (MW 384.26)	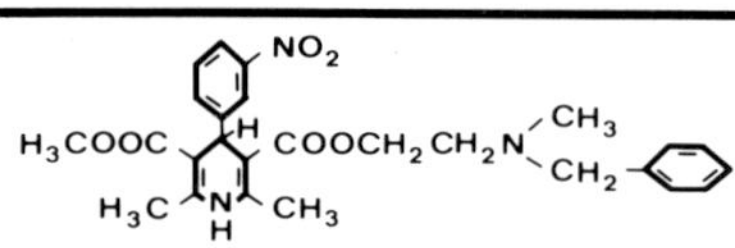 **Nicardipine** (MW 515.99)	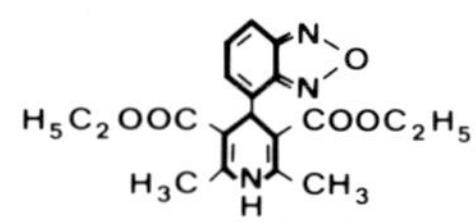 **PY-108-068** (MW 371.40)

* Nifedipine was identified as a highly potent and selective calcium antagonist by Fleckenstein in 1969/70. First communication in 1970 by Fleckenstein [2]. A detailed description of the Ca^{++}-antagonistic heart effects of nifedipine was given by Fleckenstein, Tritthart, Döring and Byon (1972): Bay a 1040, a highly potent Ca^{++}-antagonistic inhibitor of excitation-contraction coupling in mammalian myocardium (in German), Arzneimittelforsch (Drug Res) 22:22–33. The first detailed report on the Ca^{++}-antagonistic vascular effects of nifedipine was published by Grün and Fleckenstein (1972): Excitation-contraction uncoupling of vascular smooth muscle as the fundamental principle of coronary dilation by 4-(2′-Nitrophenyl)-2,6-dimethyl-1,4, dihydropyridine-3,5-dicarbonsäure-dimethylester (Bay a 1040, nifedipine). (In German) Arzneimittelforsch (Drug Res) 22:334–344

able. It is to be remembered that the smooth muscle membranes, whether of visceral or vascular origin, are not provided with a TTX-sensitive fast Na^+-carrier system. Therefore, vascular smooth muscle does not allow a visualization or quantitative differentiation of the particular Na^+- and Ca^{++}-antagonistic drug effects. Or in other words: A judgment on the *primary specificity criterium* of a Ca^{++}-antagonistic agent, i.e. *preferential suppression of the transmembrane* Ca^{++} *influx without a major inhibitory effect on* Na^+ conductance, can *not* be derived from smooth muscle experiments. In fact, specific Ca^{++} antagonists are indistinguishable, with respect to their actions on isolated smooth muscle preparations, from those compounds which impede transmembrane Ca^{++} entry merely as a side effect. In keeping with this, the concept of specific Ca^{++} antagonism was originally established in our laboratory on the basis of electrophysiological studies on mammalian myocardium.

Moreover, vasular smooth muscle cells do not allow a separate assessment of Ca^{++}-antagonistic drug actions from inhibitory effects on Mg^{++}-induced membrane phenomena (see Sect. III of the present article). However, this discrimination between divalent Ca^{++} and Mg^{++} ions constitutes the *second fundamental criterium* for the distinction of the top Ca^{++} antagonists of group A from those of group B which exhibit a somewhat lower specificity. Thus, again, pertinent studies on myocardial fibres are indispensable.

Needless to say: The designation of a drug as a highly specific Ca^{++} antagonist of group A is – to some extent – a mark of quality. These compounds of group A represented by verapamil and gallopamil (D 600), nifedipine, and other 1,4-dihydropyridines (see Table 3) as well as diltiazem, fulfill the ultimate expectations on Ca^{++}-antagonistic specificity. Interestingly enough, this classification, originally based on our rather sophisticated studies on myocardial transmembrane cation movement, has also obtained, subsequently, *practical significance* in cardiovascular therapy. As a matter of fact, even on purely empirical grounds, clinical interest centers more and more on the drugs of group A. Due to their selective Ca^{++}-antagonistic impact first evidenced on heart muscle, these agents of group A also proved to be the most powerful drugs in the treatment of vascular disorders such as Ca^{++}-dependent spastic coronary constriction or excessive height of systemic vascular tone in hypertensive crises and essential hypertension. Also in cerebral vessels (A. basilaris of pigs), the specific Ca^{++} antagonists of group A exert outstanding inhibitory effects on voltage-dependent Ca^{++} uptake of K^+-depolarized preparations. For instance, the cerebral vascular relaxing potency of the 1,4-dihydropyridine Ca^{++} antagonists nifedipine, nitrendipine, nimodipine, nisoldipine, and felodipine surpass that of flunarizine by roughly 1,000 to 10,000 times (see the chapter of Fleckenstein-Grün, Makita, Byon and Fleckenstein on pp. 290–305 in this book).

II. Linear Correlation between Inhibition by Calcium Antagonists of Transmembrane Calcium Influx and Decrease in Myocardial Tension Development

We have made in recent years a careful study of the quantitative correlation between the changes in Ca^{++} influx and myocardial tension development [3, 5, 7, 29]. For these investigations isolated cat and guinea-pig papillary muscles were used, in which the fast Na^+ transport system had previously been blocked. For instance, if the cardiac fibre membrane potential is reduced to -45 mV, the fast inward Na^+ current becomes inactivated, whereas the slow Ca^{++} channel continues to respond to electric stimulation. The simplest method of producing this critical degree of depolarization, consists of giving additional KCl (19 mM) into the experimental Tyrode's solution [12]. Such predepolarized myocardial fibres are still capable of conducting propagated impulses. However in this situation, not only contractile performance, but also bioelectric activity depends on the slow inward Ca^{++} current. Such Ca^{++}-mediated action potentials of partially depolarized myocardial fibres are highly sensitive to changes in the extracellular Ca^{++} concentration: Hence upstroke velocity, height and duration of the Ca^{++}-carried action potentials decrease rapidly in a Ca^{++}-deficient medium. In the experiment of Fig. 4, bioelectric activity totally disappeared together with the contractile function within 12 min after the Ca^{++} concentration had been reduced from

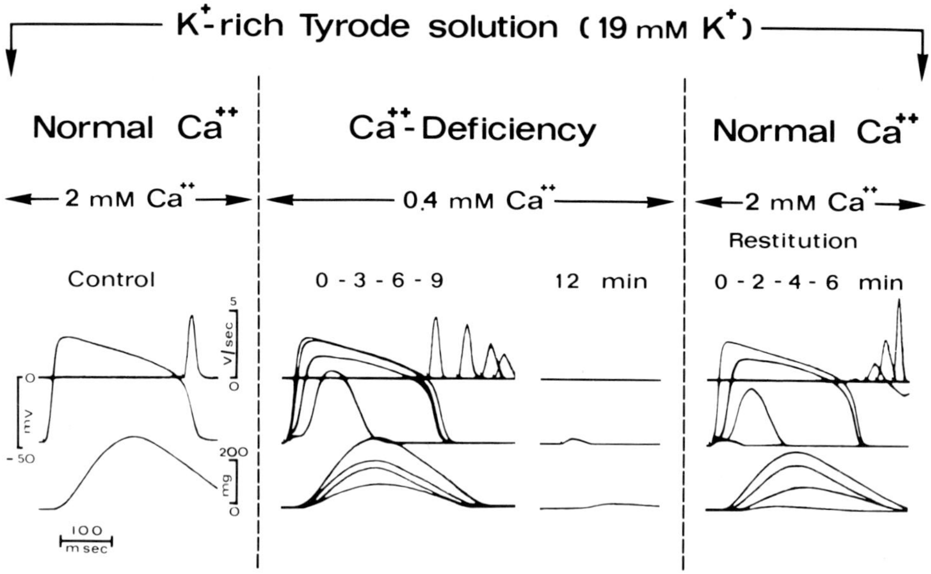

Fig. 4. Parallel suppression of Ca^{++}-dependent electric excitability and contractility of a partially depolarized guinea-pig papillary muscle in a K-rich (19 mM) Tyrode solution by lowering the Ca^{++} content from 2 to 0,4 mM. The upstroke velocity (=dV/dt max) of the single-fibre action potentials is directly registered in the upper line. Underneath, the superimposed traces of the action potentials and the corresponding mechanograms visualize the progressive decay of the bioelectric and contractile function at time intervals of 3, 6, 9, and 12 min after the muscle has been transferred into the solution with low Ca^{++} concentration. Following readmission of 2 mM Ca^{++} at the °end of the experiment, there was a full recovery of all bioelectric and mechanical parameters to their original heights (=100%) within 6 min. The bioelectric activity was recorded during 70 min with an inserted microelectrode on one single myocardial fibre

2 mM to 0.4 mM. However, the Ca^{++}-dependent action potentials and contractile force recovered within 6 min following return into the original medium with 2 mM Ca^{++}.

Figures 5 and 6 show how perfectly the Ca^{++} antagonists mimic the effects of simple Ca^{++} withdrawal on such partially depolarized guinea-pig papillary muscles. As can be easily seen from the superimposed traces (registered with a storage oscilloscope), the papillary muscles (treated in Fig. 5 with 0.2 mg nifedipine/1; 0.4 mg D 600/l, or 2 mg verapamil/l) behaved in the presence of a nor-

Fig. 5. Parallel suppression by Ca^{++} antagonists of the Ca^{++}-dependent bioelectric and mechanical activities of partially depolarized guinea-pig papillary muscles in a K-rich (19 mM) Tyrode solution with normal Ca^{++} content (2 mM). Three identical experiments with nifedipine (0.2 mg/l) D 600 (0.4 mg/l), and verapamil (2 mg/l). In each experiment the upper registration curve demonstrates the gradual reduction of upstroke velocity (dV/dt max) during an observation period of 20 to 40 min following the addition of the drugs. The superimposed records underneath show the corresponding decrease of height and duration of the Ca^{++}-dependent action potentials and of the isometric mechanograms. Finally, the cardiodepressant effects of the Ca^{++} antagonists were overcome by raising the Ca^{++} content of the K^{+}-rich Tyrode solutions from 2 to 6 or 8 mM. The bioelectric records of each experiment were derived from microelectrode insertions on one and the same myocardial fibre lasting for 70 to 120 min. From Fleckenstein [3]

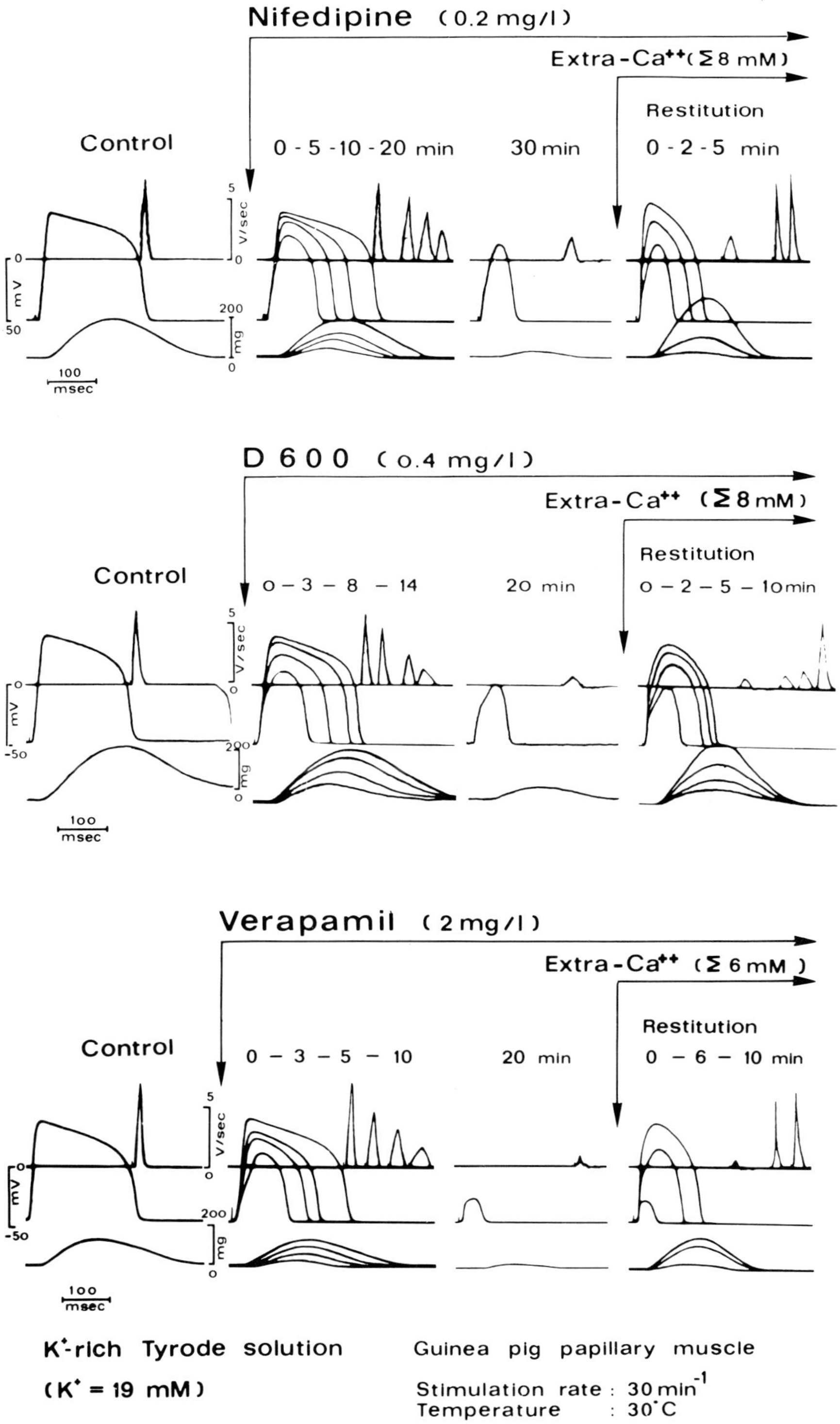
Nifedipine (0.2 mg/l)
Extra-Ca++ (Σ8 mM)
Restitution
Control
0 - 5 - 10 - 20 min
30 min
0 - 2 - 5 min
V/sec
mV
mg
100 msec
D 600 (0.4 mg/l)
Extra-Ca++ (Σ8 mM)
Restitution
Control
0 – 3 – 8 – 14
20 min
0 – 2 – 5 – 10 min
Verapamil (2 mg/l)
Extra-Ca++ (Σ6 mM)
Restitution
Control
0 – 3 – 5 – 10
20 min
0 – 6 – 10 min
K+-rich Tyrode solution
(K+ = 19 mM)
Guinea pig papillary muscle
Stimulation rate : 30 min-1
Temperature : 30°C

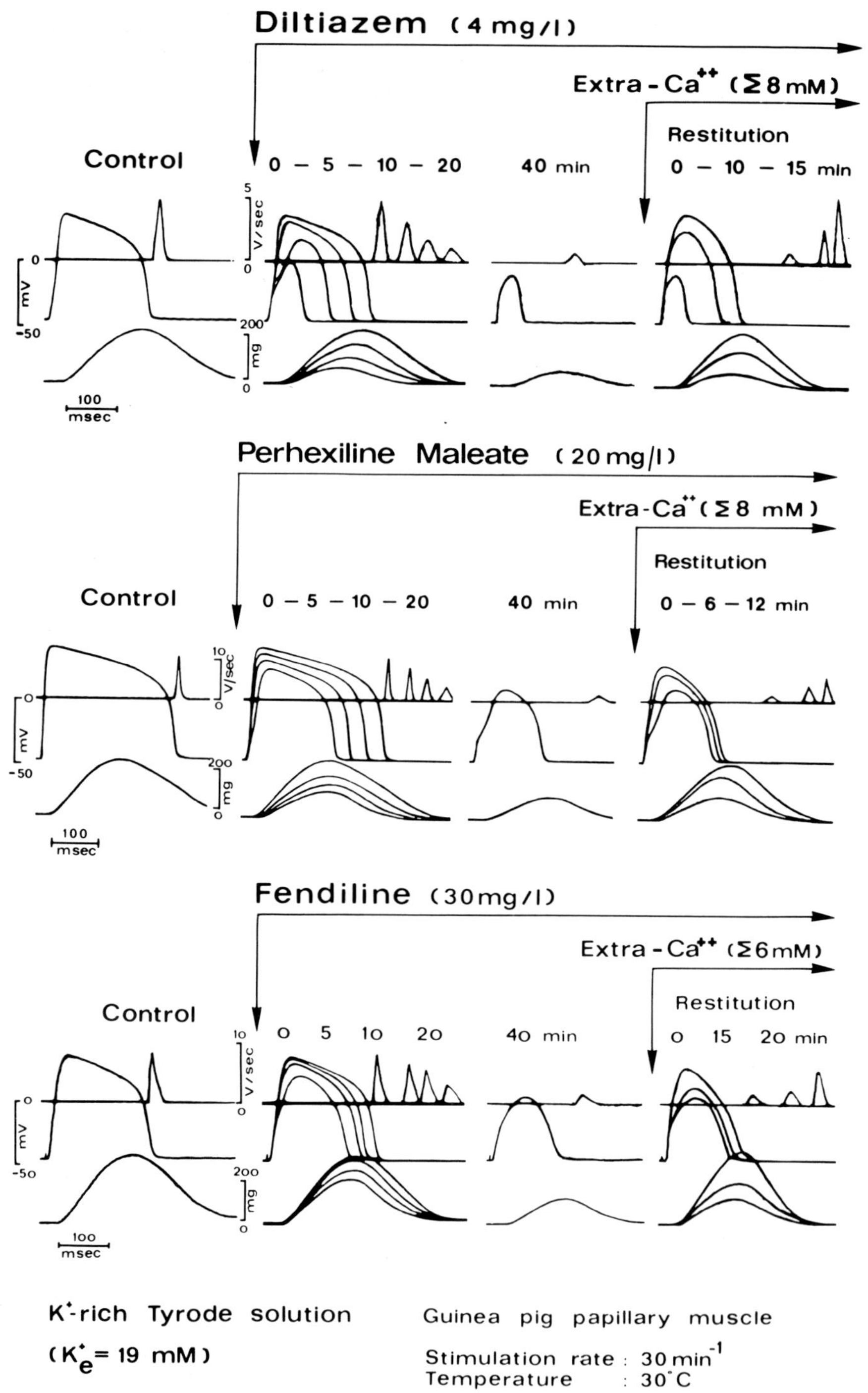

Fig. 6. Same as Fig. 5, however with the use of diltiazem (4 mg/l), perhexiline maleate (20 mg/l), and fendiline (30 mg/l)

mal 2 mM Ca^{++} concentration as if they were exposed to a Ca^{++}-deficient medium. Obviously, in all these cases, the time course of inhibition of the Ca^{++}-mediated action potentials coincides with the development of contractile incompetence. At the end of the experiment, the Ca^{++} antagonists were neutralized by increasing the Ca^{++} concentration up to 6 or 8 mM. Consequently, the bioelectric membrane activity of the partially depolarized myocardium recovered again more or less in parallel with the mechanical performance. Figure 6 represents identical experiments with the use of the Ca^{++} antagonists diltiazem, perhexiline maleate, and fendiline (for more details see the earlier publications from our laboratory summarized by Fleckenstein [5]).

Partially depolarized ventricular myocardium offers unique possibilities of testing in this way the quantitative correlation between transmembrane Ca^{++} influx, as indicated by the bioelectric parameters of the Ca^{++}-mediated action potentials, and the mechanical responses. For instances, the upstroke velocity (dV/dt max) of Ca^{++}-mediated action potentials indicates the intensity of transsarcolemmal Ca^{++} influx through the slow channels, whereas the duration of the Ca^{++}-mediated action potentials reflects the length of time of Ca^{++} entry: In fact, contractile tension changes in parallel with these bioelectric parameters [3, 5]. As an example, the areas of the Ca^{++}-dependent isometric mechanograms, representing tension-time, as the most appropriate parameter of contractile performance, are plotted in Fig. 7 against the areas of the Ca^{++}-mediated action potentials

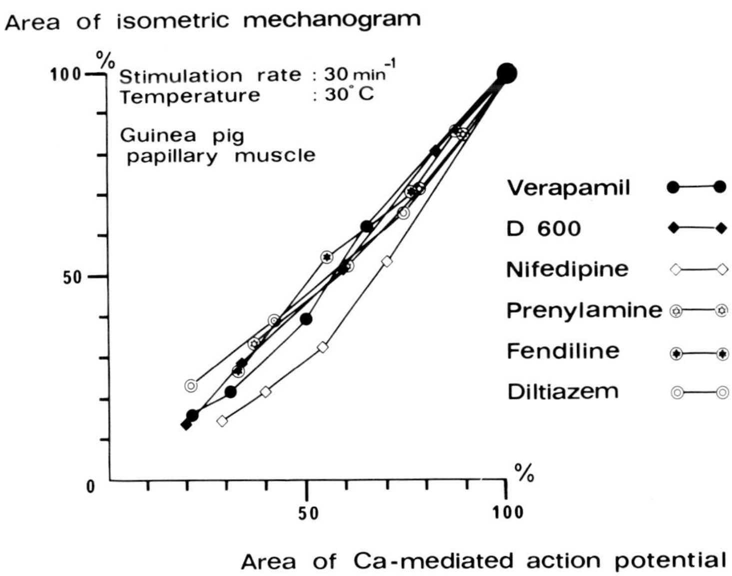

Fig. 7. Linear relationship between the decrease of the area of the isometric mechanograms and the reduction of the area of the Ca^{++}-mediated action potentials under the influence of various Ca^{++} antagonists. The control data (=100%) were obtained on partially depolarized guinea-pig papillary muscles after incubation in a K^+-rich (19 mM) Ca^{++}-containing (2 mM) Tyrode solution for 30 min. Then, each Ca^{++} antagonist was applied in different effective concentrations for 20 to 40 min until the definite changes on the Ca^{++}-dependent action potentials and mechanograms were measured. From Fleckenstein [3, 5]

tential curves. It is evident from this graph that there is a perfect linearity between the magnitude of the Ca^{++}-dependent bioelectric and mechanical responses. Hence the conclusion is justified that the various Ca^{++} antagonists, tested in the present study on partially depolarized myocardium, act uniformely in that they inhibit contractile tension development always to the same extent as they are capable of restricting the slow transsarcolemmal inward Ca^{++} current which is responsible, in this situation, for both the bioelectric and the mechanical events.

As it is evident from the pioneering work of Cornelius van Breemen and his group and of George Weiss and his associates [35] on various types of vascular smooth muscle, the quantitative correlation between transmembrane Ca^{++} uptake and contractile performance is in such cells more complex than in cardiac tissue: If vascular smooth muscle is stimulated by depolarization, a transmembrane Ca^{++} influx is elicited which passes through the so-called "voltage-dependent" channels, and determines the strength of contraction quantitatively as in myocardial fibres (Fig. 8). Accordingly, Ca^{++} antagonists inhibit this type of contractile activation pari passu with the decrease in Ca^{++} uptake. On the other hand, contractile responses which are due to a non-electric "receptor-operated"

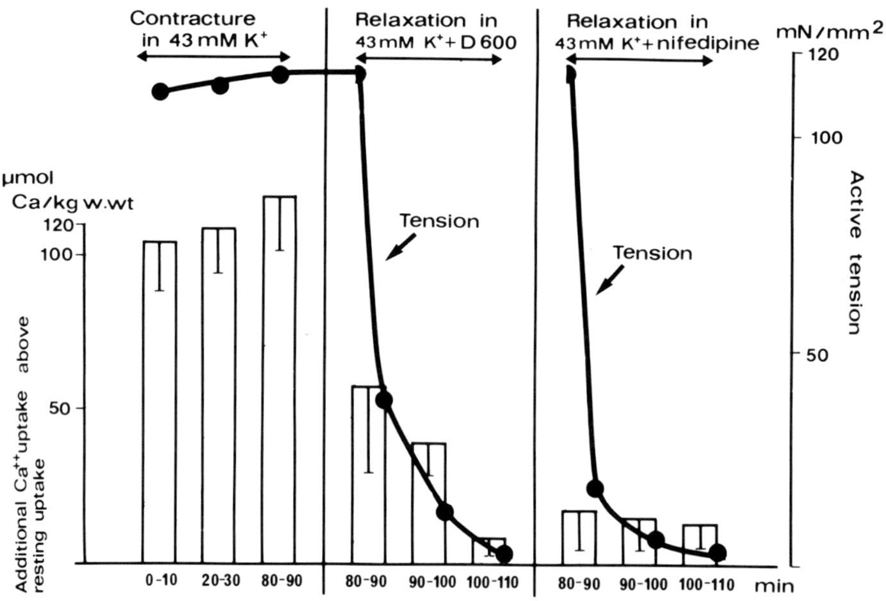

Fig. 8. Extra-uptake of labelled Ca^{++} into K^{+}-depolarized pig coronary artery strips (a) during long-term contractures over 80 min, and (b) during subsequent relaxation brought about by administration of the Ca^{++} antagonists gallopamil (D 600) and nifedipine. During the first 10 min, there is a steep rise in height of contracture, while a plateau is reached after 80 min. In parallel with this increase in tension development, the Ca^{++} uptake rates grow. Conversely, after addition of the Ca^{++} antagonists, the rates of transmembrane Ca^{++} incorporation decline almost to resting level within 30 min, while active tension falls to the base-line. Before and after administration of the Ca^{++} antagonists, the net uptakes of ^{45}Ca were determined at different intervals, each time during a 10 min period. The radioactivity measurements between the 80th and the 90th min were carried out both in the presence and absence of the Ca^{++} antagonists. From Fleckenstein-Grün (to be published)

release of Ca^{++} from cellular stores, are more resistant to Ca^{++} antagonists. Recent observations of our laboratory indicate that this receptor-operated Ca^{++} release is a Ca^{++}-triggered process which does not require a major transmembrane Ca^{++} supply, but nevertheless ceases as soon as Ca^{++}-antagonistic drugs completely block Ca^{++} entry. (For details see the chapters of Van Breemen et al., pp. 58–71, and of Fleckenstein-Grün et al., pp. 290–305 in this book.)

III. Distinction Between Calcium Antagonists of Group A and Group B by Means of Their Different Influences on Ca^{++}- and Mg^{++}-Induced Bioelectric Membrane Effects

In the course of our studies on partially depolarized guinea-pig papillary muscles, it turned out that, after suppression of fast-channel-mediated Na^{+} conductivity, action potentials could still be produced not only with Ca^{++}, but also with Mg^{++} ions, supposedly acting as substitutive transmembrane electric charge carriers [26]. However, these Mg^{++}-mediated action potentials of partially depolarized myocardium exhibited bioelectric features and drug susceptibilities that were totally different from those of the Ca^{++}-mediated action potentials. Thus Mg^{++} -carried action potentials, in comparison with those mediated by Ca^{++}, are characterized (a) by a definitely higher upstroke velocity, (b) by a shorter duration, and (c) by the fact that they never elicit a contractile response (see Fig. 9 upper part). Naturally, in this situation, the question arose, how specifically Ca^{++} antagonists can discriminate between the electrogenic Ca^{++} and Mg^{++} effects. The answer that we have obtained was clear: The highly specific Ca^{++} antagonists of group A (verapamil, D 600, diltiazem, nifedipine, and its derivatives niludipine and nimodipine) selectively suppress the slow Ca^{++} current, but do not inhibit the Mg^{++}-induced action potentials. In contrast, all Ca^{++} antagonists of group B (prenylamine, fendiline, terodiline, perhexiline, and caroverine) affect both the electrogenic Ca^{++} *and* Mg^{++} actions since the latter drugs are lacking a discriminating power toward these two divalent cations.

The particular influences of a drug on the Ca^{++} or Mg^{++} conductivities can even be studied in one single experiment using "mixed" Ca^{++}/Mg^{++}-mediated action potentials (see Fig. 9 lower part). These "mixed" action potentials appear regularly upon stimulation of partially depolarized papillary muscles in a K^{+}-rich Tyrode's solution with 19 mM K^{+}, 2 mM Ca^{++}, and 14 mM Mg^{++}. These action potentials are two-phasic, in that they consists (a) of a rapid Mg^{++}-dependent upstroke phase which manifests itself in the differentiation curve as a sharp peak No. 1, and (b) of a second blunt peak No. 2 which represents the electrogenic slow Ca^{++} inflow. Figures 10 and 11 demonstrate that nifedipine, gallopamil (D 600), verapamil and diltiazem (as the most important representatives of the Ca^{++} antagonists of group A) abolish selectively the Ca^{++}-dependent peak No. 2, together with contractility, but do not impair the Mg^{++}-dependent peak No. 1 [5, 7, 26]. Conversely, perhexiline and fendiline, similar to all other Ca^{++} antagonists of group B, also suppress the Mg^{++}-dependent peak No. 1, indistinctively from the Ca^{++}-dependent peak No. 2 (see Fig. 12).

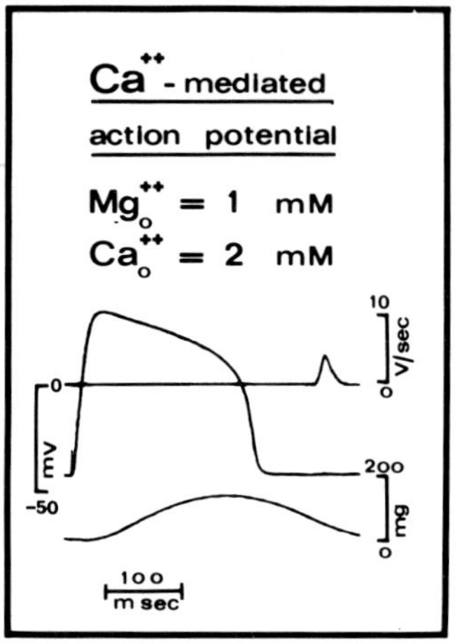

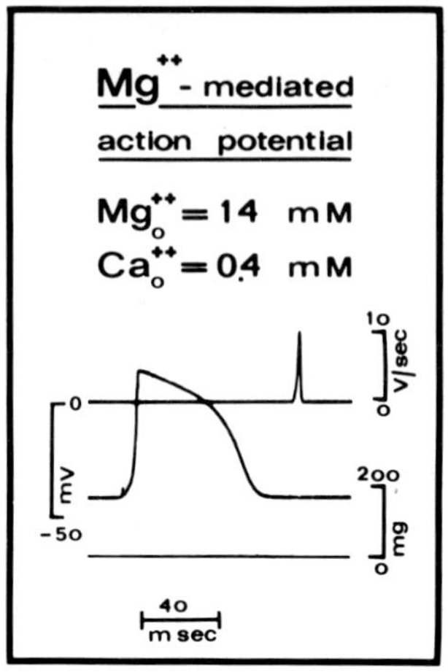

	Ca - mediated action potential	Mg - mediated action potentials		
	2 mM Ca_o	14 mM Mg_o	24 mM Mg_o	34 mM Mg_o
Upstroke velocity (V/sec)	6.5 ± 0.4	21.2 ± 3.5	33.7 ± 4.2	45.5 ± 4.7
Overshoot (mV)	35.3 ± 2.7	11.2 ± 2.6	22.8 ± 3.4	30.4 ± 5.3
Duration of action potential 50% Repolarisation (msec)	196.2 ± 12.6	63.6 ± 3.8	68.2 ± 4.5	75.3 ± 5.1
Duration of action potential 90% Repolarisation (msec)	218.7 ± 15.7	68.5 ± 4.7	77.8 ± 5.3	83.5 ± 5.6
Isometric tension (mg / mg muscle)	188.9 ± 13.2	no mechanical activity		

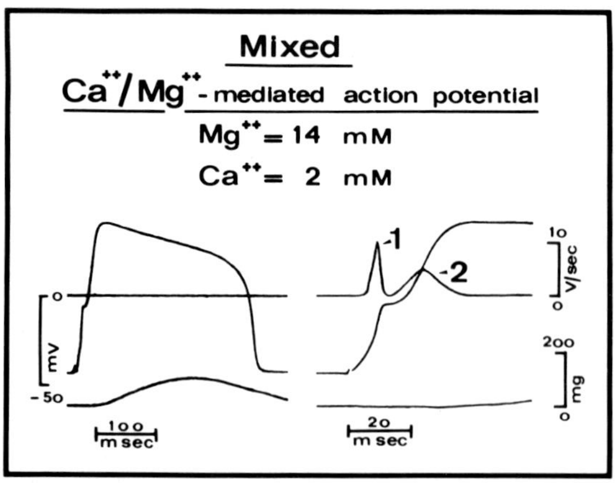

Fig. 9. Electrogenic Ca^{++} and Mg^{++} effects on partially depolarized ventricular myocardium. From Späh and Fleckenstein [26]

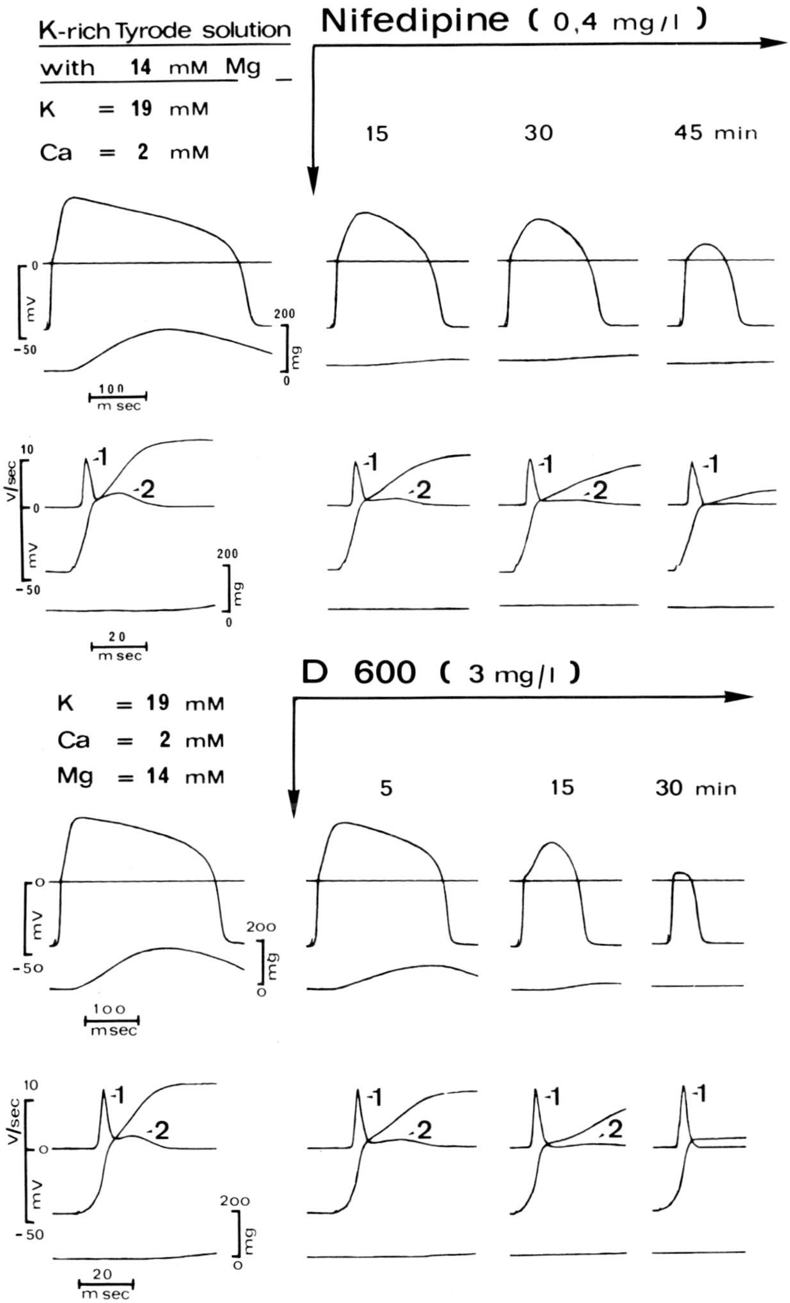

Fig. 10. Selective disappearance of the Ca^{++}-dependent peak No. 2 of upstroke velocity (dV/dt max) of a mixed Mg^{++}/Ca^{++}-carried action potential under the influence of the powerful Ca^{++} antagonists nifedipine and D 600. No effect of nifedipine and D 600 on the Mg^{++}-dependent peak No. 1. After 30 to 45 min, the remaining bioelectric activity is exclusively mediated by Mg^{++} ions. Experiments on isolated guinea-pig papillary muscles. Stimulation rate, 30/min; temperature, 30 °C. From Späh and Fleckenstein [26]

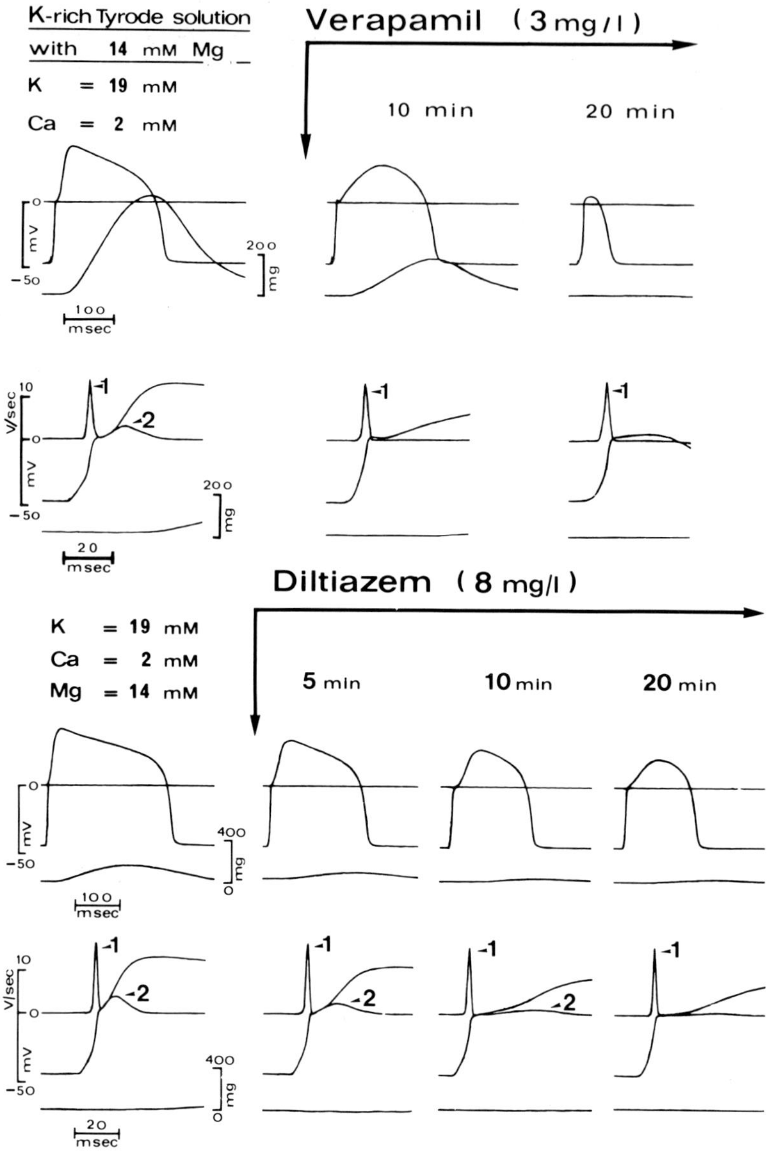

Fig. 11. Selective suppression of the Ca^{++}-dependent peak No. 2, of upstroke velocity (dV/dt max) of mixed Mg^{++}/Ca^{++}-carried action potentials by verapamil and diltiazem. No influence on the Mg^{++}-peak No. 1. Experimental procedure as in Fig. 10. From Späh and Fleckenstein [26] and Fleckenstein and Späh [7]

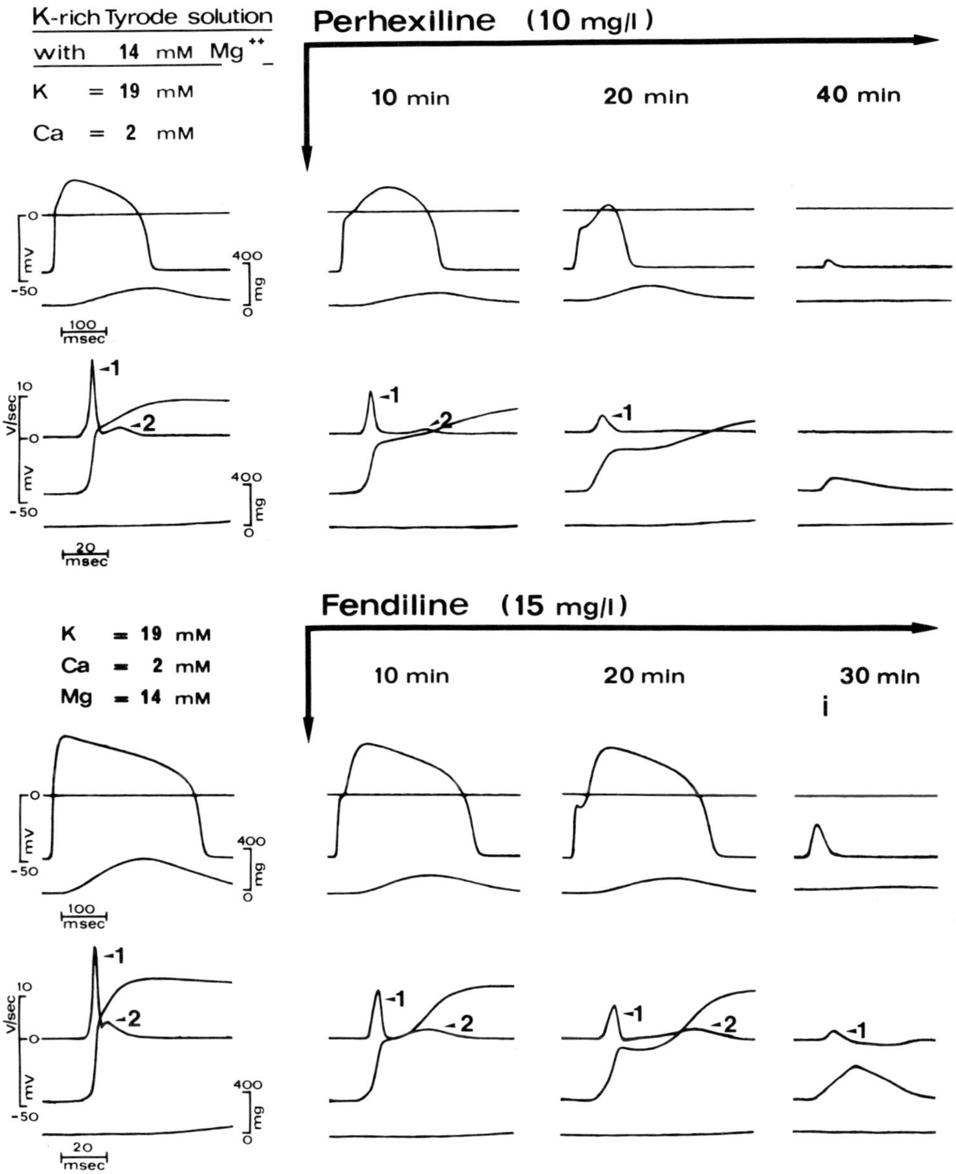

Fig. 12. The Ca^{++} antagonists of group B do not discriminate between divalent Ca^{++} and Mg^{++} ions. Therefore, perhexiline (maleate) and fendiline inhibit simultaneously both the Mg^{++}-dependent peak No. 1 and the Ca^{++}-dependent peak No. 2, of the mixed Mg^{++}/Ca^{++}-carried action potentials. Experimental procedures as in Figs. 10 and 11. From Fleckenstein and Späh [7]

IV. Neutralization of the Inhibitory Actions of Calcium Antagonists on Transsarcolemmal Calcium Influx and Contractility by Calcium Entry Promotion

As we have shown 20 years ago, it is characteristic of a Ca^{++}-antagonistic inhibitor of myocardial excitation-contraction coupling that its negative-inotropic effect is easily overcome by any drug or procedure which restores the Ca^{++} supply to the contractile system. Thus even in the presence of Ca^{++} antagonists, contractile force is brought back by the following experimental measures:

1) Elevation of Ca^{++} concentration in the extracellular fluid.
2) Increase in availability of intracellular activator Ca^{++} following a reduction in Ca^{++} extrusion (cardiac glycosides) or due to intracellular Ca^{++} release from the sarcoplasmic reticulum (caffeine, theophylline).
3) Facilitation of Ca^{++} entry by sympathetic neurotransmitters and other agents which raise the Ca^{++} conductance of the slow channels.

Needless to say: Under physiological conditions the latter possibility, i.e. facilitation of the slow-channel-mediated Ca^{++} influx, is of primary importance. Overwhelming evidence has accumulated in recent years indicating that cyclic AMP plays a key-role in potentiating the Ca^{++} current through these gates. For instance cyclic AMP is produced (a) following stimulation of adrenergic β-receptors or histaminergic H_2-receptors, (b) following receptor-independent activation of adenylate cyclase with forskolin, or (c) following administration of cyclic AMP (see Table 4). Then, in the further sequence of events, a membrane-located phos-

Table 4

Stimulation of β-receptors [9, 10, 28, 30, 32–34]	Stimulation of H_2-receptors [9, 11, 13, 14, 19]	Stimulation of adenylate cyclase by forskolin [11, 17, 23, 25, 27]	Administration of dibutyryl cAMP [9, 15, 16, 24]
↓	↓	↓	↓

Formation of cyclic AMP

↓

Phosphorylation of sarcolemmal proteins by a membrane-located phosphokinase

↓

Increase in Ca^{++}-binding capacity of membrane proteins in sarcolemma and slow channels

↓

Increase in transmembrane Ca^{++} supply to contractile system = positive inotropism

Table 5. Positive inotropism by new "calcium-agonists" without involvement of cyclic AMP.[a] Fundamental mechanism: Facilitation of Ca^{++} entry by operating at the same sarcolemmal receptor groups that otherwise would produce slow channel blockade under the influence of Ca^{++}-antagonistic 1,4-dihydropyridine derivatives (nifedipine etc.)

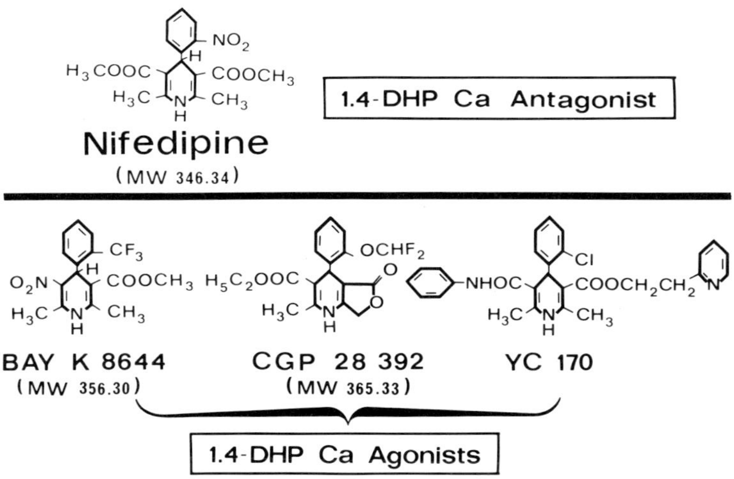

[a] The fact that stimulation of Ca^{++} influx by Bay K 8644 and CGP 28392 takes place in a cAMP-independent way, was reported by Kokubun and Reuter (1984), who studied these drug effects on cultured cardiac cells from neonatal rats [8]. Fleckenstein (1984) also stressed this peculiarity of a cAMP-independent Ca^{++} entry promotion. On uterine smooth muscle too, Bay K 8644 was lacking any promoter effect on cAMP formation (personal communication by Dr. H. Metzger, Pharmacological Research Laboratories, Hoechst AG, Frankfurt)

phokinase seems to use the cyclic AMP for phosphorylation of sarcolemmal membrane proteins [36]. The appearance of new additional phosphate groups in the superficial layers of the sarcolemma membrane and the slow channels leads – in all probability – to an increase in Ca^{++} binding capacity and transmembrane Ca^{++} conductivity. Thereby, the supply of activator Ca^{++} from extracellular sources (and in consequence, the Ca^{++}-triggered Ca^{++} release from intracellular stores) is potentiated so that positive-inotropic effects are elicited.

However, as summarized in Table 5, there is still another pathway of transmembrane inward Ca^{++} fluxes which does *not* involve the usual mediation by cyclic AMP. This cAMP-independent Ca^{++} transport mechanism is activated by the new 1,4-dihydropyridine derivatives that are acting as "calcium agonists". They are operating at the same receptor groups as the original Ca^{++}-antagonistic substance nifedipine does, but instead of blocking Ca^{++} entry in the usual manner, the new Ca^{++} agonists intensify Ca^{++} inflow dramatically. The most potent Ca^{++} agonist listed in Table 5 is Bay K 8644. Its fundamental action, i.e. potentiation of contractile force, has been first described by Schramm et al. [21, 22].

V. Experimental Differentiation Between cAMP-Mediated and cAMP-Independent Ca^{++} Entry Promotion on the Basis of Divergent Influences on Electrogenic Membrane Effects of Mg^{++} Ions

Interestingly, the fundamental differences between the two types of Ca^{++} entry promoters, operating with or without intermediate formation of cyclic AMP, manifest themself also in other respects: So we were able to demonstrate on partially depolarized myocardial fibres that the influence of the two types of Ca^{++} entry promoters on Mg^{++}-mediated or mixed Mg^{++}/Ca^{++}-induced action potentials is totally divergent [31]: As we have demonstrated in previous investigations, Mg^{++}-mediated action potentials are always depressed or extinguished in partially depolarized myocardium by those agents which stimulate Ca^{++} entry via formation of cyclic AMP [5, 7, 25–27]. This means that, always when the slow Ca^{++} current rises above normal (following β- or H_2-receptor stimulation or administration of forskolin or dibutyryl cyclic AMP), a reciprocal inhibition of the electrogenic Mg^{++} effects takes place. On the other hand, there is a rapid recovery of the Mg^{++}-mediated bioelectric membrane activity if these agents are washed off or neutralized by β-receptor blockade (pindolol) or H_2-receptor blockade with burimamide, metiamide and cimetidine (examples are given in Fig. 13). Analogous observations were made in our studies on mixed Mg^{++}/Ca^{++}-mediated action potentials: Under these particular conditions too, all agents which possess – as a common denominator – the ability to produce cyclic AMP, influence the Mg^{++}-dependent peak No. 1 in the differentiation curve (dV/dt max) *reciprocally* to the Ca^{++}-dependent peak No. 2: Whereas the sharp Mg^{++} peak No. 1 progressively declines, the blunt peak No. 2, mirroring the transmembrane inward Ca^{++} current, largely grows together with the isometric mechanogramm (see Figs. 14–16). In other words: All these observations indicate that cyclic AMP potentiates the transsarcolemmal influx of Ca^{++} ions at the expense of Mg^{++}. Conversely, when the intensified formation of cyclic AMP comes to an end, the high Ca^{++} fluxes return to normal, while the bioelectric Mg^{++} effects reappear.

In sharp contrast, the potentiation of the transsarcolemmal inward Ca^{++} current by the new Ca^{++} agonists, particularly Bay K 8644 is not accompanied by any decrease in height or duration of the Mg^{++}-mediated action potentials (Fig. 17). Similarly, under the influence of Bay K 8644, there is also no change of the Mg^{++}-dependent part No. 1 of the mixed Mg^{++}/Ca^{++} action potentials, even if the Ca^{++}-dependent part No. 2 reaches a maximum (see Fig. 18). It is evident from these observations that the 1,4-dihydropyridine compounds, whether

Fig. 13. Suppression of Mg^{++}-mediated action potentials by β-receptor stimulation with noradrenaline (*upper experiment*), with isoproterenol (*middle experiment*), or histamine (*lower experiment*). Restoration of the Mg^{++}-mediated action potentials by washout or β-receptor blockade with pindolol. Parallel changes of upstroke velocity (dV/dt max) in the upper tracing of each experiment. Guinea-pig papillary muscles; stimulation rate, 30/min; temperature, 30 °C. From Späh and Fleckenstein [26], Fleckenstein [5]

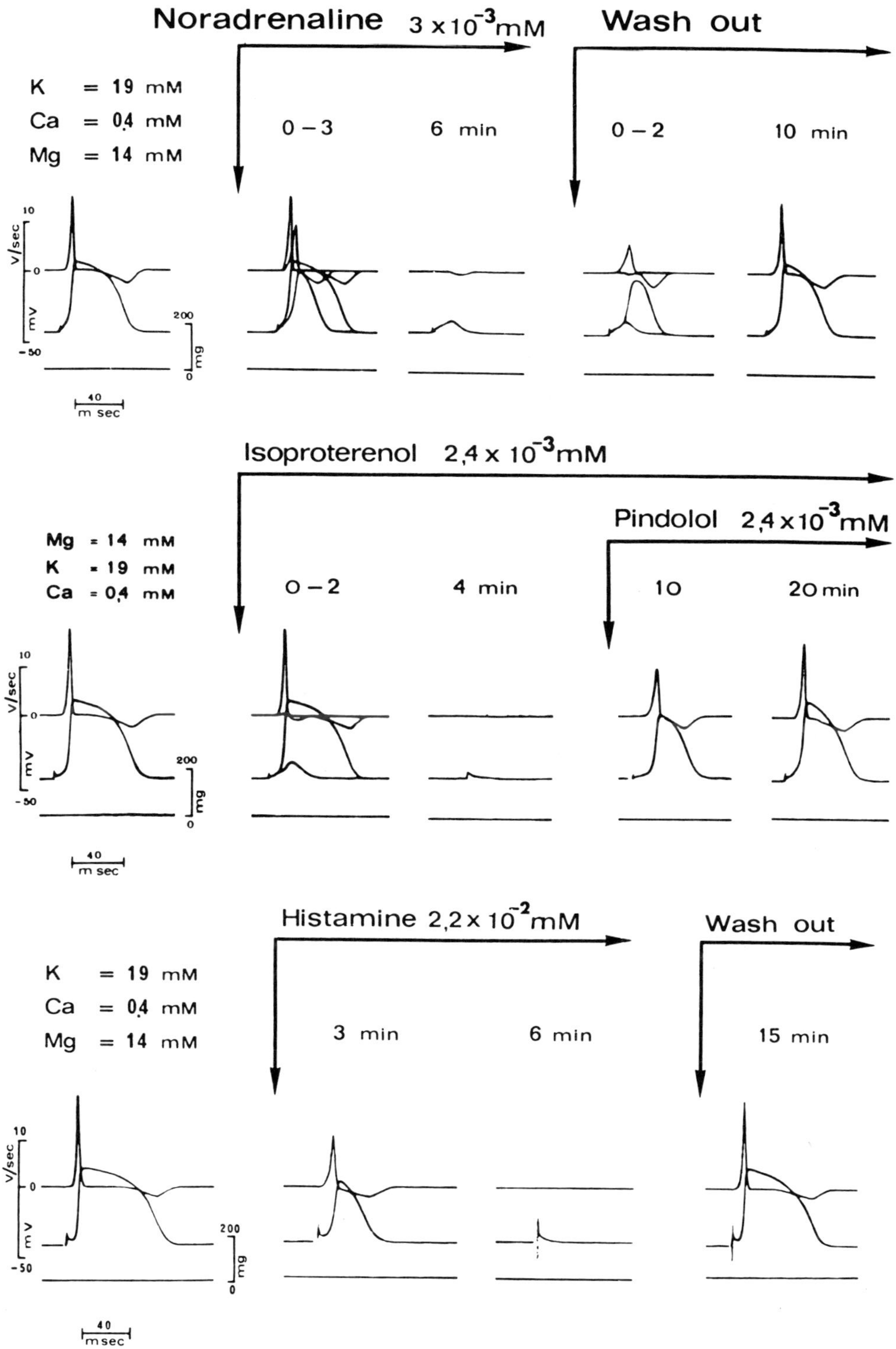
Noradrenaline 3 x 10⁻³ mM
Wash out
K = 19 mM
Ca = 0.4 mM
Mg = 14 mM
0 – 3
6 min
0 – 2
10 min
10
V/sec
0
mV
-50
200
mg
0
40
m sec
Isoproterenol 2,4 x 10⁻³ mM
Pindolol 2,4 x 10⁻³ mM
Mg = 14 mM
K = 19 mM
Ca = 0,4 mM
0 – 2
4 min
10
20 min
Histamine 2,2 x 10⁻² mM
Wash out
K = 19 mM
Ca = 0.4 mM
Mg = 14 mM
3 min
6 min
15 min

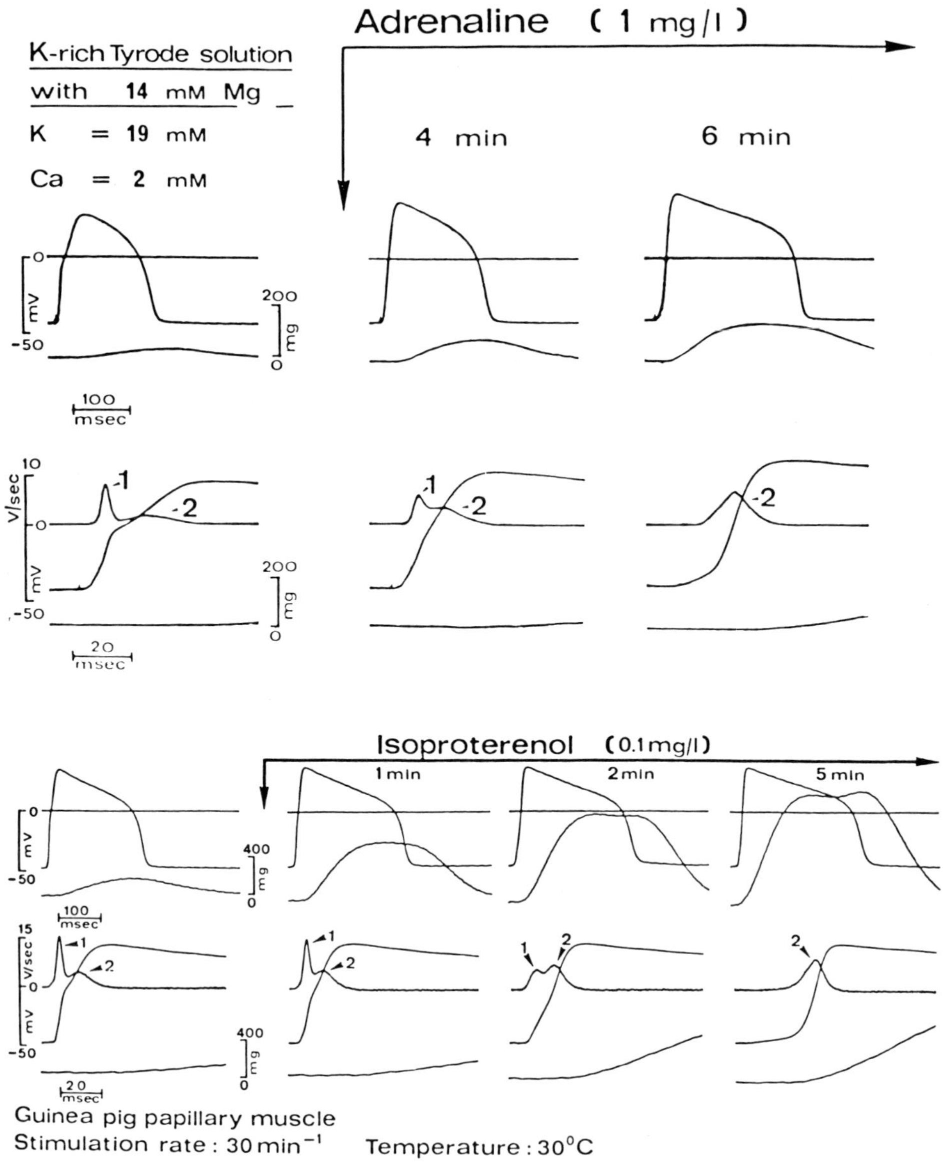

Fig. 14. Reciprocal effects of adrenergic β-receptor stimulation with adrenaline or isoproterenol on the Mg^{++}- and Ca^{++}-mediated bioelectric membrane activities: Suppression of the Mg^{++}-dependent peak No. 1 of upstroke velocity (dV/dt max) of mixed Mg^{++}/Ca^{++}-mediated action potentials simultaneously with a maximum reinforcement of the Ca^{++}-dependent peak No. 2. Isometric tension grows with decrease of the Mg^{++} peak, and with potentiation of the Ca^{++} peak which reflects the raise in slow-channel-mediated Ca^{++} influx

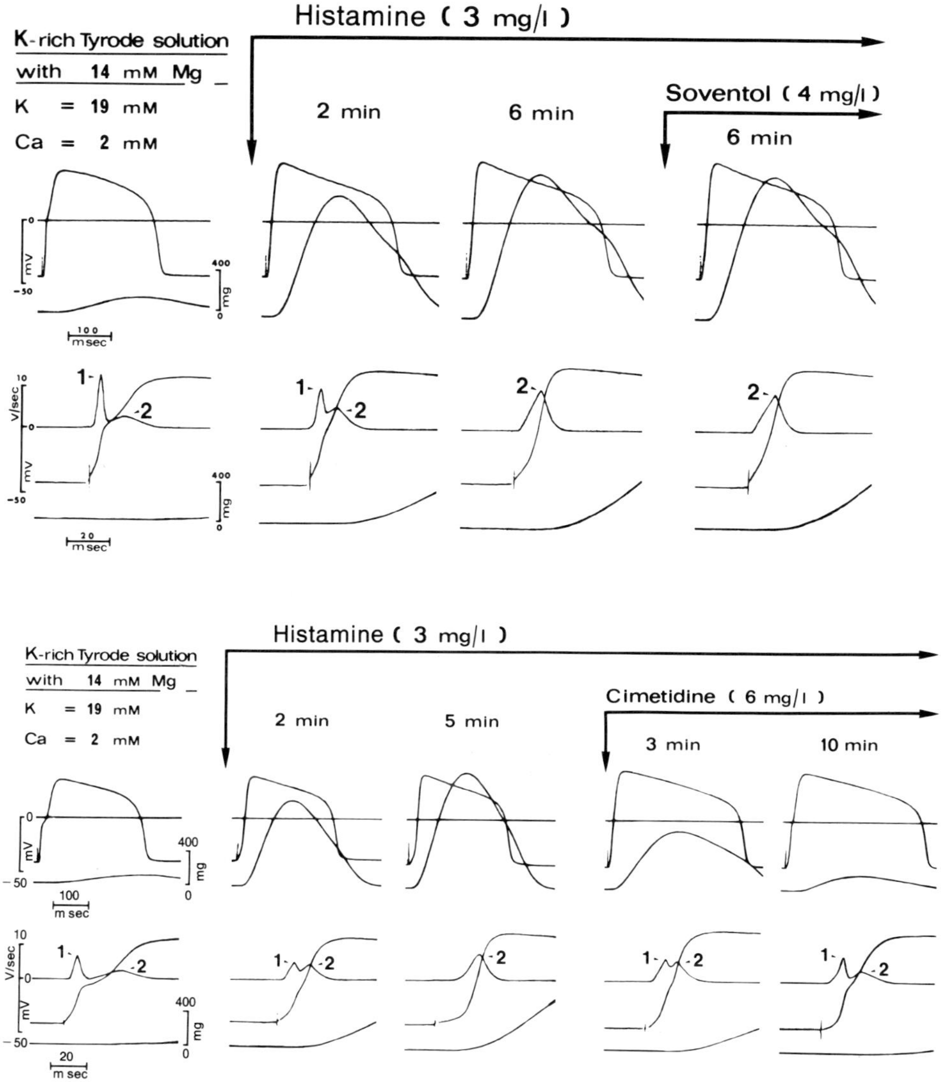

Fig. 15. Only H_2-receptor stimulation leads to intermediate formation of cyclic AMP, and accordingly, exerts the same reciprocal influence on the Mg^{++}- and Ca^{++}-dependent parts of "mixed" action potentials as β-receptor stimulation does. Therefore, only H_2-receptor blockade with cimetidine (*lower experiment*) neutralizes the histamine effects on the Mg^{++} and Ca^{++} peaks. On the other hand, H_1-receptor stimulation does not lead to an increase in cyclic AMP level. Thus it is irrelevant whether the H_1-receptor blocking agent bamipine (Soventol) is adminstered or not (*upper experiment*)

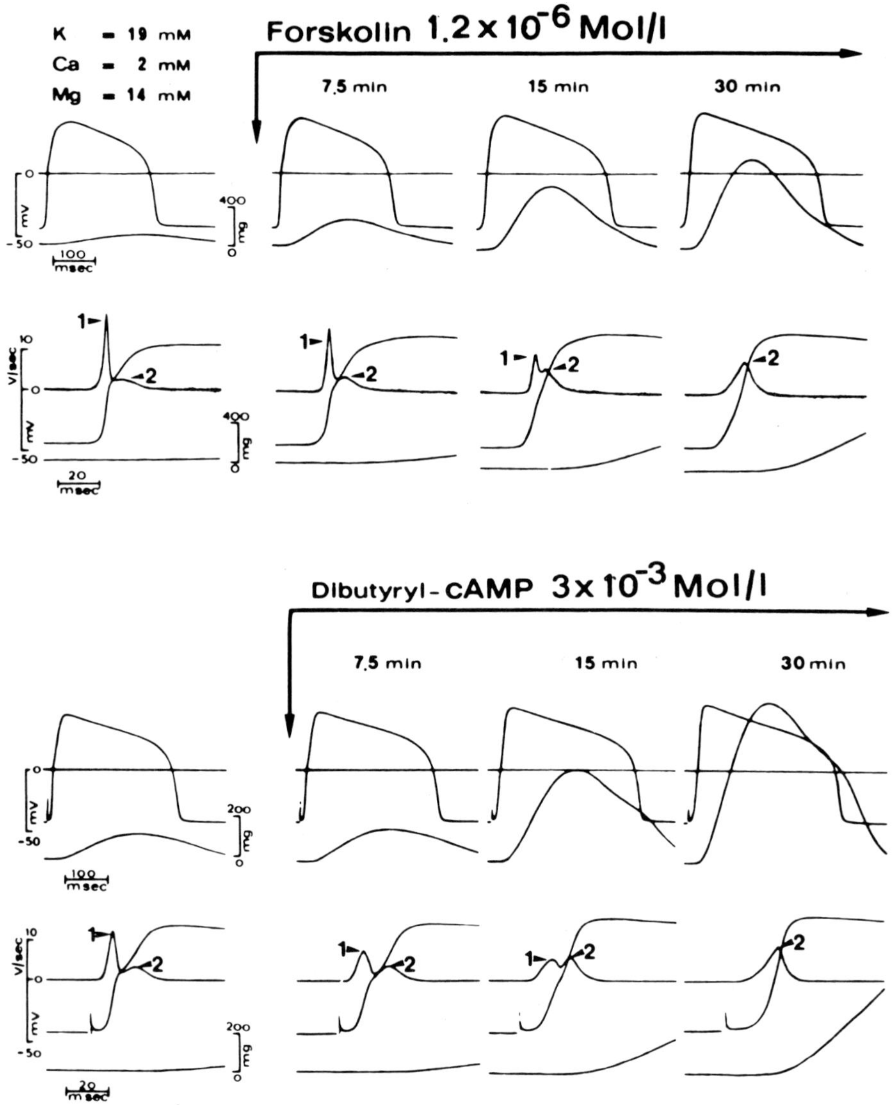

Fig. 16. Reciprocal influence on the Mg^{++}- and Ca^{++}-dependent peaks of mixed action potentials following intermediate formation of cyclic AMP by activation of adenylate cyclase with forskolin (*upper experiment*) or by administration of dibutyryl cyclic AMP as precursor (*lower experiment*). Same methods as in Figs. 10 and 11

they are acting as inhibitors (nifedipine) or promoters (Bay K 8644) of transsarcolemmal Ca^{++} influx, modulate the passage of Ca^{++} ions through the slow channels *selectively*, i.e. without repercussions on Mg^{++}-induced membrane phenomena. In this respect, the 1,4-dihydropyridines keep a unique position.

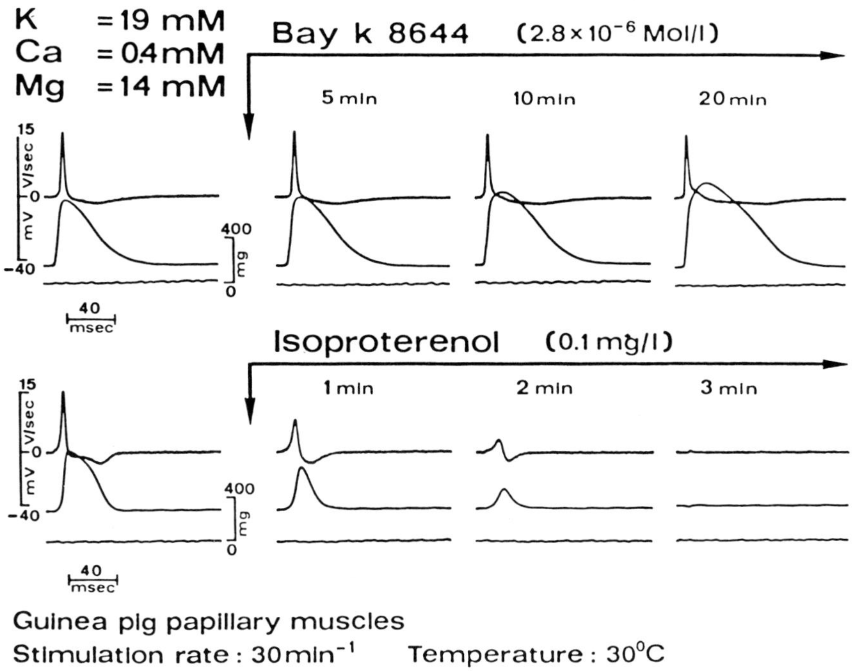

Fig. 17. *Upper experiment:* Lack of any inhibitory influence of the Ca^{++} agonist Bay K 8644 on Mg^{++}-induced action potentials of partially depolarized guinea pig papillary muscle kept in a K^{+}-rich, Ca^{++}-deficient, high-Mg^{++}-containing Tyrode's solution (19 mM K^{+}; 0,4 mM Ca^{++}; 14 mM Mg^{++}). The curves represent (from top to bottom) simultaneous records of (a) upstroke velocity (dV/dt max, expressed as V/s); (b) tracings of Mg^{++}-induced action potentials; (c) mechanogramms, showing absence of contractile responses. *Lower experiment:* In sharp contrast isoproterenol, by virtue of formation of cyclic AMP does suppress such Mg^{++}-induced action potentials under otherwise identical conditions (see also Fig. 13). Obviously, isoproterenol shares this suppressive influence on electrogenic Mg^{++} effects with all producers of cyclic AMP (other β-adrenergic stimulants, histamine, forskolin, dibutyryl cyclic AMP)

Conclusions and Summary

The present investigations justify the following conclusions:

1) Only such drugs ought to be classified as *Ca^{++} antagonists of group A* which exhibit an outstanding Ca^{++}-antagonistic specificity. The experimental criteria are: High-grade blockade of slow-channel-mediated transmembrane Ca^{++} entry by 90 to 100% without a concomitant inhibition of the fast Na^{+} current or of electrogenic Mg^{++} effects in partially depolarized myocardium. These high specificity requirements are hithertoo only fulfilled by verapamil, gallopamil (D 600), diltiazem, and nifedipine, as well as by a considerable number of other Ca^{++}-antagonistic 1,4-dihydropyridine derivatives. These top Ca^{++} antagonists are also most effective in the therapy of many vascular disorders, produced by excessive Ca^{++}-induced vascular smooth muscle activity, such as coronary, pulmonal, cerebral, renal or intestinal artery spasms. Moreover, the drugs of group A

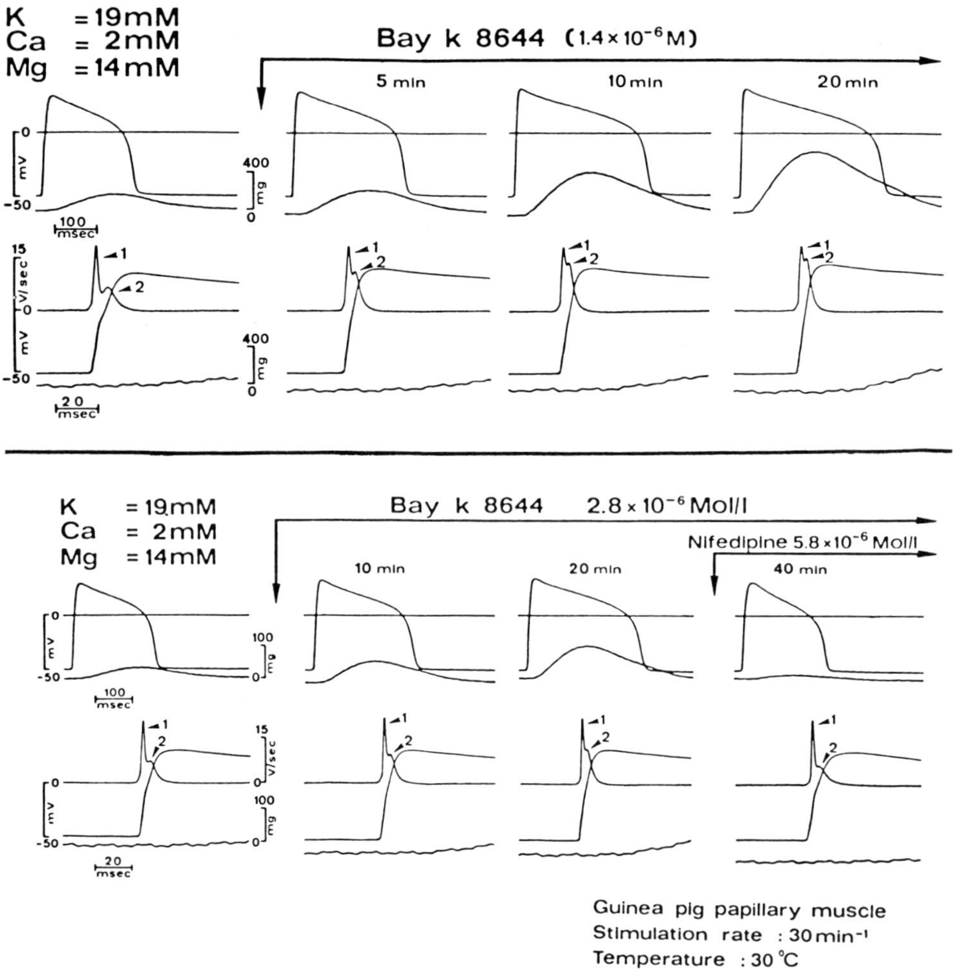

Fig. 18. Absence of any inhibitory action of the Ca^{++} agonist Bay K 8644 on the Mg^{++}-dependent component of mixed Ca^{++}/Mg^{++}-mediated action potentials of partially depolarized myocardium. The curves represent (from top to bottom) simultaneous records of (a) mixed Ca^{++}/Mg^{++}-mediated action potentials; (b) mechanogramms; (c) differentiation curves of the mixed Ca^{++}/Mg^{++}-mediated action potentials with the rapid Mg^{++}-dependent peak No. 1 and the slow Ca^{++}-influx-dependent peak No. 2; (d) high-speed records of upstroke of the mixed action potentials; (e) high-speed records of the rising phase of the mechanogramms. The Ca^{++} agonist Bay K 8644 potentiates Ca^{++} influx *selectively* as indicated by (1) prolongation of action potential plateau; (2) increase in height and duration of the contractile responses; (3) amplification of the Ca^{++}-dependent peak No. 2 of the mixed action potentials; (4) lack of influence of Bay K 8644 on the sharp initial Mg^{++}-dependent peak No. 1 in the differentiation curve of the mixed action potentials. At the end of the lower experiment nifedipine was added to the Bay K 8644-containing solution. As expected, the Ca^{++} antagonist nifedipine totally neutralized the Ca^{++} agonist Bay K 8644. However, while the Ca^{++}-dependent peak No. 2 returned to its initial height upon the administration of nifedipine, the Mg^{++}-dependent peak No. 1 remained again unaffected

are the only Ca^{++} antagonists which exert so powerful inhibitory effects on hypercontractured systemic resistance vessels that they are appropriate for the normalization of blood pressure in hypertensive crises and essential hypertension.

2) The *Ca^{++} antagonists of group B* (prenylamine, fendiline, perhexiline, terodiline, caroverine), in conformity with the drugs of group A, also inhibit the slow channel-mediated Ca^{++} influx into excited myocardial fibres distinctly more than the Na^{+}-dependent action potential parameters. However, a somewhat lower specificity manifests itself in two respects:

a) The Ca^{++} antagonists of group B interfere additionally with the fast inward Na^{+} current if the Ca^{++} influx is inhibited by 50 to 70%, and

b) The Ca^{++} antagonists of group B are unable to discriminate between the electrogenic Ca^{++} and Mg^{++} effects on partially depolarized myocardial fibres.

Thus the classification of Ca^{++} antagonists into group A or B must primarily be based upon electrophysiological tests on myocardial fibres: Vascular smooth musculature does not possess separate channels for Na^{+} and Ca^{++} that would allow an individual assessment of the specific Ca^{++}-antagonistic drug actions independently from Na^{+}-antagonistic effects.

3) The negative-inotropic actions of Ca^{++} antagonists can be neutralized best with the help of Ca^{++} entry promoters. There are two principal possibilities of facilitation of transmembrane Ca^{++} supply:

a) *Production of cyclic AMP* following stimulation of adrenergic β-receptors or histaminergic H_2-receptors, direct activation of adenylate cyclase with forskolin or administration of dibutyryl cyclic AMP. This type of enhancement of transmembrane Ca^{++} supply is always accompanied, in partially depolarized myocardium, by a reciprocal suppression of Mg^{++}-induced electrogenic membrane effects.

b) *Direct increase in the Ca^{++} transport capacity* of the slow channels – probably by prolongation of the "open state" (Kokubun and Reuter [8]) without intermediate formation of cyclic AMP. This type of potentiation of the inward Ca^{++} current is brought about by the new 1,4-dihydropyridine Ca^{++} agonists, particularly Bay K 8644. In contrast with cAMP-mediated promotion of Ca^{++} influx, the new Ca^{++} agonists enhance the transsarcolemmal Ca^{++} supply *exclusively*, that is to say: In this case, the inward Ca^{++} current grows whereas there is *no* concomitant change in the Mg^{++}-induced bioelectric responses.

Thus the 1,4-dihydropyridine compounds possess a highly specific and selective Ca^{++} channel affinity, irrespective of whether they are acting as Ca^{++} entry inhibitors or promoters.

References

1. Ebashi S (1980) Regulation of muscle contraction. The Croonian Lecture 1979: Proc R Soc Lond [Biol] 207:259–286
2. Fleckenstein A (1970/71) Specific inhibitors and promotors of calcium action in the excitation-contraction coupling of heart muscle and their role in the production or prevention of myocardial lesions. In: Harris P, Opie L (eds) Calcium and the heart. Proc of the Meeting of the Europ Section of the Internat Study Group for Research in Cardiac Metabolism, London, Sept. 6, 1970. Academic Press, London New York, pp 135–188

3. Fleckenstein A (1981) Fundamental actions of calcium antagonists on myocardial and cardiac pacemaker cell membranes. In Weiss GB (ed) New perspectives on calcium antagonists. Clin Physiol Series, Amer Physiol Soc, pp 59–81
4. Fleckenstein A (1983) History of calcium antagonists. In: Schwartz A, Taira N (eds) In: Calcium channel-blocking drugs: A novel intervention for the treatment of cardiac disease. Monograph No. 95 of the Amer. Heart Association, Circ. Research, Part II, Vol. 52, No. 2, pp 3–16
5. Fleckenstein A (1983) Calcium antagonism in heart and smooth muscle – Experimental facts and therapeutic prospects. Wiley, New York Chichester Brisbane Toronto Singapore
6. Fleckenstein A, Kammermeier H, Döring HJ, Freund HJ (1967) Zum Wirkungsmechanismus neuartiger Koronardilatatoren mit gleichzeitig Sauerstoff-einsparenden Myokard-Effekten, Prenylamin und Iproveratril. Z Kreislaufforsch 56:716–744, 839–853
7. Fleckenstein A, Späh F (1981/82) Excitation-contraction uncoupling in cardiac muscle. Yoshida H, Hagihara Y, Ebashi S (eds) Advances in pharmacology and therapeutics II, vol 3, Cardio-renal and cell pharmacology, 8th Internat. Congress of Pharmaocology, Tokyo, 1981. Pergamon Press, Oxford New York, pp 97–110
8. Kokubun S, Reuter H (1984) Dihydropyridine derivatives prolong the open state of Ca channels in cultured cardiac cells. Proc Natl Acad Sci 81:4824–4827
9. Kukovetz WR, Pöch G (1970) Cardiostimulatory effects of cyclic 3′,5′-adenosine monophosphate and its acylated derivatives. Naunyn-Schmiedebergs Arch Exp Pathol Pharmakol 266:236–254
10. Kukovetz WR, Pöch G, Wurm A (1973) Effects of catecholamines, histamine and oxyfedrine on isotonic contraction and cyclic AMP in the guinea-pig heart. Naunyn-Schmiedebergs Arch Exp Pathol Pharmakol 278:403–424
11. Lindner E, Dohadwalla AN, Bhattacharya BK (1978) Positive inotropic and blood pressure lowering activity of a diterpene derivative isolated from Coleus forskohli: forskolin. Arnzneim. Forsch (Drug Res) 28:84–89
12. Mascher D (1970) Electrical and mechanical responses from ventricular fibres after inactivation of the sodium carrying system. Pflügers Arch 317:359–372
13. McNeill JH, Muschek LD (1972) Histamine effects on cardiac contractility, phosphorylase and adenyl cyclase. J Mol Cell Cardiol 4:611–624
14. McNeill JH, Verma SC (1974) Blockade by burimamide of the effects of histamine and histamine analogs on cardiac contractibility, phosphorylase activation and cyclic adenosine monophosphate. J Pharmacol Exp Ther 188:180–188
15. Meinertz T, Nawrath H, Scholz H (1973) Dibutyryl cyclic AMP and adrenaline increase contractile force and ^{45}Ca uptake in mammalian cardiac muscle. Naunyn-Schmiedebergs Arch Exp Pathol Pharmakol 277:107–112
16. Meinertz T, Nawrath H, Scholz H (1973) Stimulatory effects of DB-c-AMP and adrenaline on myocardial contraction and ^{45}Ca exchange. Experiments at reduced calcium concentration and low frequencies of stimulation. Naunyn-Schmiedebergs Arch Exp Pathol Pharmakol 279:327–338
17. Metzger H, Lindner E (1981) The positive inotropic-acting forskolin, a potent adenylate cyclase activator. Arnzeim-Forsch (Drug Res) 31:1248–1250
18. Nakajima H, Hoshiyama M, Yamashita K, Kiyomoto A (1975) Effect of diltiazem on electrical and mechanical activity of isolated cardiac ventricular muscle of guinea pig. Jpn J Pharmacol 25:383–392
19. Reinhardt D, Schmidt U, Brodde OE, Schümann HJ (1977) H_1- and H_2-receptor mediated responses to histamine on contractility and cyclic AMP of atrial and papillary muscles from guinea-pig hearts. Agents and Actions 7:1–12
20. Reuter H, Beeler GW (1969) Calcium current and activiation of contraction in ventricular myocardial fibers. Science 162:399–401
21. Schramm M, Thomas G, Towart R, Franckowiak G (1983) Activation of calcium channels by novel 1,4-dihydropyridines. A new mechanism for positive inotropics or smooth muscle stimulants. Arzneim-Forsch 33:1268–1272
22. Schramm M, Thomas G, Towart R, Franckowiak G (1983) Novel dihydropyridines with positive inotropic actions through activation of Ca^{2+} channels. Nature 303:535–537

23. Seamon KB, Daly JW (1981) Forskolin: a unique diterpene activator of cyclic AMP-generating systems. J Cyclic Nucleotide Res 7:201–204
24. Skelton CL, Levey GS, Epstein SE (1970) Positive inotropic effects of dibutyryl cyclic adenosine 3′,5′-monophosphate. Circ Res 26:35–43
25. Späh F (1984) Forskolin, a new positive inotropic agent, and its influence on myocardial electrogenic cation movements. J Cardiovasc Pharmacol 6:99–106
26. Späh F, Fleckenstein A (1979) Evidence of a new, preferentially Mg-carrying, transport system besides the fast Na and the slow Ca channels in the excited myocardial sarcolemma membrane. J Mol Cell Cardiol 11:1109–1127
27. Späh F, Fleckenstein A (1984) Influence of forskolin, a direct promoter of the formation of cAMP in heart muscle, on Na-, Ca-, and Mg-dependent myocardial membrane phenomena. Frühjahrstagung der Deutsch Physiol Gesell, Dortmund, März 1984, Pflügers Arch Ges Physiol Suppl to Vol 400, R 6
28. Sutherland EW, Robison GA, Butcher RW (1968) Some aspects on the biological role of adenosine 3′,5′-monophosphate (cyclic AMP). Circulation 37:279–306
29. Tritthart H, Volkmann R, Weiss R, Fleckenstein A (1973) Calcium-mediated action potentials in mammalian myocardium: Alteration of membrane response as induced by changes of Ca or by promoters and inhibitors of transmembrane Ca inflow. Naunyn Schmiedebergs Arch Pharmakol 280:239–252
30. Tsien RW, Giles W, Greengard P (1972) Cyclic AMP mediates the effects of adrenaline on cardiac Purkinje fibers. Nature New Biol 240:181–183
31. Wagner WL, Fleckenstein A (1984) Electric and mechanical effects of Bay K 8644, a new positive inotropic dihydropyridine calcium agonist, on mammalian ventricular myocardium. 60. Meeting der Deutschen Physiologischen Gesell. (Fall Meeting), Okt. 1984 in Dortmund, Pflügers Arch, Suppl to Vol 402, R 22, 77
32. Watanabe AM, Besch Jr HR (1974a) Cyclic adenosine monphosphate modulation of slow calcium influx channels in guine-pig hearts. Circ Res 35:316–324
33. Watanabe AM, Besch Jr HR (1974b) Subcellular myocardial effects of verapamil and D 600: comparison with propranolol. J Pharmacol Exp Ther 191:241–251
34. Watanabe AM, Besch Jr HR (1975) The relationship between adenosine 3′,5′-monophosphate levels and systolic transmembrane calcium flux. In: Fleckenstein A, Dhalla NS (eds) Basic functions of cations in myocardial activity. Recent advances in studies on cardiac structure and metabolism, vol 5. University Park Press, Baltimore London Tokyo, pp 95–102
35. Weiss GB (1977) Calcium and contractility in vascular smooth muscle. In: Narahashi T, Bianchi CP (eds) Advances in general and cellular pharmacology, vol 2. Plenum Press, pp 71–154
36. Wollenberger A (1975) The role of cyclic AMP in the adrenergic control of the heart. In: Nayler WG (ed) Contraction and relaxation in the myocardium. Academic Press, New York, pp 113–190

Session I: Ca-Channels

Chairman: C. Van Breemen

Bayer-Symposium IX
Cardiovascular Effects of Dihydropyridine-Type
Calcium Antagonists and Agonists, 34–55

Mechanism of Calcium Channel Modulation by Dihydropyridine Agonists and Antagonists

P. HESS, J. B. LANSMAN, and R. W. TSIEN

Abstract

Single cardiac Ca channels exhibit three modes of gating, expressed as current records with brief openings occurring in bursts (mode 1), records with long-lasting openings and very brief closings that appear only rarely (mode 2), and records that lack openings because of channel unavailability (mode 0). The dihydropyridine Ca agonist Bay K 8644 enhances Ca channel current by promoting mode 2, while the Ca antagonists nitrendipine and nimodipine reduce the current by favoring mode 0.

Introduction

Dihydropyridines such as nifedipine and nitrendipine are among the newest and most interesting of the many agents that modify Ca channel activity in excitable cells [36, 43]. As therapeutic agents, they have already gained wide use in the treatment of cardiovascular disorders [11, 12, 40, 41]; as specific ligands, they open the way toward eventual biochemical purification and reconstitution of Ca channels [9, 15, 30, 46]. Questions about their mechanism of action have grown with the discovery of "Ca agonists" such as Bay K 8644 and CGP 28392 [39, 42]. These "Ca agonists" increase cardiac contractility and divalent cation influx [4, 8, 14, 17, 18, 24, 33, 37, 39, 42] even though they are dihydropyridines, very similar in structure to nifedipine and other "Ca antagonists". It is challenging to ask how such closely related compounds can produce effects that seem so diametrically opposite. Here we report analysis of Ca agonist and Ca antagonist effects on Ca channel activity of single heart cells and single Ca channels. We find that Bay K 8644 increases the chances that the channel will show a mode of gating marked by long opening and brief closing events. The same type of gating can be seen occasionally in the absence of drug. On the other hand, nitrendipine and nimodipine exert their Ca antagonist effect by increasing the proportion of sweeps in which the channel fails to open. The results provide an explanation for partial agonist or antagonist actions of dihydropyridines; in particular, we find that nitrendipine's effects include a Ca agonist component.

Methods

Single ventricular cells were obtained from guinea pig or frog hearts by enzymatic dispersion as previously described [3, 23]. Whole cell membrane current recordings were made under voltage clamp conditions with the suction pipette method of Lee at al. [25] (guinea pig) or the patch clamp method of Hamill et al. [16] (frog).

Recordings of unitary Ca channel activity were made from cell-attached patches on guinea pig ventricular cells (see [6, 7]) with patch pipettes containing 110 mM $BaCl_2$, 10 mM glucose, and 10 mM Hepes (titrated with Ba(OH) to pH 7.5). The cells were bathed in a solution containing 10 mM KCl, 140 mM NaCl, 1 $MgCl_2$, 10 mM glucose and 10 mM Hepes (titrated with NaOH to pH 7.5). In some of the experiments, the external solution also contained 0.5 mM EGTA. Current signals were filtered with an eight-pole Bessel filter with a cut-off frequency (3 db) of 1 kHz and sampled at 5 kHz. Automated analysis of the digitized signals was carried out on a PDP-11/23 minicomputer with procedures similar to those previously described [6, 7]. Opening and closing events were counted when the current crossed the midline between the open and closed current level and for an event to be counted it hat to last for at least two sampling points. Open or closed periods that lasted up until the end of the depolarizing pules were disregarded. With the exception of Figs. 9 and 10, all results shwon were obtained from patches containing only one channel, as judged by the absence of multiple conductance levels. All experiments were carried out at room temperature (22 °C).

Results

Effects of Dihydropyridines on Ca Channel Current in Single Cells

Figure 1 shows a comparison of the effects of a Ca-channel agonist (Bay K 8644) and an antagonist (nitrendipine) on the whole cell Ca-currents recorded from a single guinea pig myocyte. The two drugs clearly have opposite effects on the amplitude of the peak current but interestingly they both accelerate the rate of decay of the current. As shown in Fig. 1 c, that effect of the two drugs can be addititve: As previously described [26], nitrendipine reduces the peak current and speeds up its rate of decay (Fig. 1 b). Subsequent addition of Bay K 8644 partially reverses the effect of Nitrendipine on the amplitude of the peak current but it further accelerates its rate of decay. Bay K 8644 strongly enhanced peak Ca channel current in both guinea pig and frog ventricular cells. With 10 mM external Ca, and test depolarizations from −60 mV to +10 or +20 mV, 1 μM Bay K 8644 increased

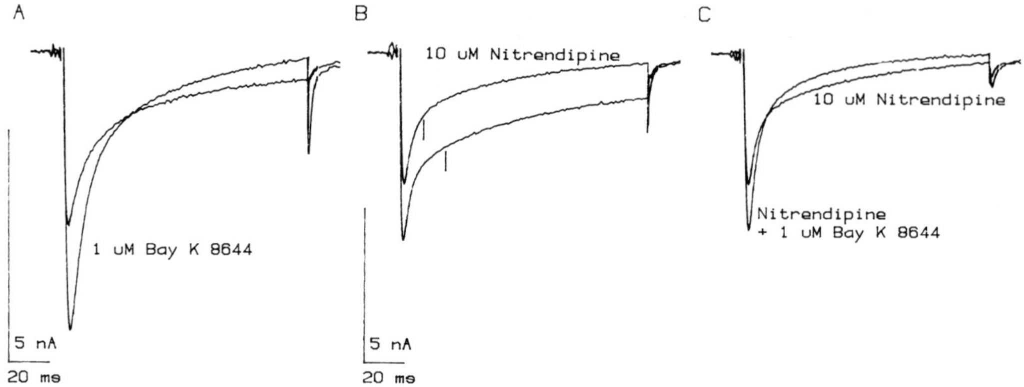

Fig. 1. Comparison of the effects of Bay K 8644 and Nitrendipine on whole cell Ca currents. Single guinea pig ventricular myocytes voltage clamped and internally dialysed with a suction pipette [25]. Each panel shows net currents after subtraction of linear leak and capacity currents evoked by voltage clamp depolarizations from a holding potential of -60 m*v* to $+20$ m*v*. **A** Superimposed current records in the absence (smaller peak current, slower decay) and presence of 1μM Bay K 8644. Cell 201 I. **B** Superimposed current records in the absence (larger current) and presence of 10 μM Nitrendipine. Vertical marks indicate the time at which the current has decayed to half its peak level. Cell 203 B. **C** Same cell as in **B**. Superimposed records of the current in the presence of 10 μM Nitrendipine (smaller peak current, slower decay) and after addition of 1 μM Bay K 8644. External solution contained (mM) 10 $CaCl_2$, 85 Cs-aspartate, 2.85 $MgCl_2$, 5 glucose, and 10 Hepes titrated with CsOH to pH 7.4. Internal dialysate contained (mM) 75.5 Cs-aspartate, 75.5 Cs-phosphate, 5 glucose, and 10 Hepes titrated with CsOH to pH 7.0

the peak inward current by $3.0+0.3$ fold (s.e.m.) in guinea pig myocytes ($n=6$) and $4.05+0.52$ fold in frog ventricular cells ($n=7$). 10 μM drug gave no greater enhancement than 1 μM; half-maximal effects were obtained at between 30–100 nM drug. At maximally effective doses, Bay K 8644 increased whole cell Ca channel current within seconds, and in all cases the enhancement was sustained.

The Ca agonist altered the voltage- and time-dependence of Ca channel currents carried by either Ca^{2+} or Ba^{2+}. The analysis of Ba current is somewhat simpler because of the absence of Ca-induced Ca channel inactivation (e.g. [28]). Figure 2 illustrates the effect of Bay K 8644 (5 μM) on Ba current in a whole-cell suction pipette recording from a guinea pig myocyte. The agonist-induced enhancement of peak current was largest at weak depolarizations (where the current was small in the absence of drug) and became progressively smaller with increasing depolarization. For example, the enhancement was ~1-fold at -31 mV (a) and only ~1.8-fold near $+80$ mV (e,e′). As the current-voltage relationship indicates, the current through the Ca channel reversed near $+50$ mV (due to a balance of Ba influx and Cs efflux [27]) and the reversal potential remained unchanged with agonist.

The time-dependence of Ba current through Ca channels was changed by the agonist in a similar way to that of the Ca current shown in Fig. 1: In the presence of Bay K 8644, the current signal reached its peak value sooner, and showed a greater tendency to decay. As the depolarizing pulse grew stronger, the enhance-

the absence of drug (a) as in previous studies [7, 35]. The test depolarization was kept small enough to give large, easily resolved unitary currents. Exposure of the cell to Bay K 8644 did not detectably alter the amplitude of the unitary event, but it produced a striking change in the pattern of channel opening (b). In many of the sweeps, the channel spent the majority of its time open, rather than closed; channel openings were very much prolonged; channel closings were abbreviated. As a result of these effects, the average current signal in the presence of agonist (d) was about 11-fold greater than its amplitude before drug (c). This response was typical of results from 5 patches, and it agrees fairly well with the whole-cell response at comparably weak depolarizations (Fig. 2a) in the degree of enhancement and in the absence of a drug-promoted relaxation of inward current.

When the agonist effect was large at a maximally effective drug concentration as in Fig. 3b, a substantial fraction of sweeps still contained no detectable openings or only rapidly flickering openings like those found in the absence of drug. Such sweeps are easily differentiated from sweeps with long openings and short closings. The combination of both types of behavior provides an interesting clue to the agonist's mechansim of action.

Sweep-to-sweep variations are illustrated for the same experiment by plots of the probability of channel openness (p) for each sweep (Fig. 4a, b). The value of p was obtained by integrating over a period when the current signal was steady (see legend for Fig. 4). In the control run (a), p was less than 0.20 in all but one of the sweeps. After exposure to Bay K 8644 (b), changes in p were immediate and well-maintained throughout the 15 min exposure to the drug. These date are represented as histograms of p values in panels c and d. In the presence of the agonist (d), the distribution of p values is strikingly bimodal: over the range between $p = 0.5$ and $p = 1.0$ a new group of p values appears; however, between $p = 0$ and $p = 0.5$, the distribution remains similar to that in the absence of drug (c).

Separate Analysis of Sweeps with Low p and High p

Taking advantage of the bimodal distribution of p values, we separated records taken in the presence of Bay K 8644 into two groups of records for analysis of the kinetics of opening and closing; "low p" sweeps with $p < 0.3$ (Fig. 5, middle column), and "high p" sweeps with $p > 0.65$ (right column). The kinetic behavior in the absence of drug is shown in the left column. Comparison of the left and middle columns confirms the impression that the behavior of low p sweeps in the present of agonist is very similar to that in the absence of drug. Both of these open time histograms are fitted by a single, rapidly decaying exponential ($T \sim 0.5$–0.6 ms). Both of the shut time distributions are well-fitted by the sum of two exponentials as described elsewhere [6, 7]. The mean latency-to-first opening is similar in both cases (21 ms control, 19 ms for low p sweeps in Bay K 8644). The percentage of sweeps with no openings is also very similar ($132/420 = 31\%$ in control and $42/127 = 33\%$ for the low p sweeps after agonist).

The behavior of the high p sweeps is strikingly different. The open time histogram shows a predominance of long openings (mean value ~ 20 ms), as expected from the records illustrated in Fig. 4. The distribution fits a single exponen-

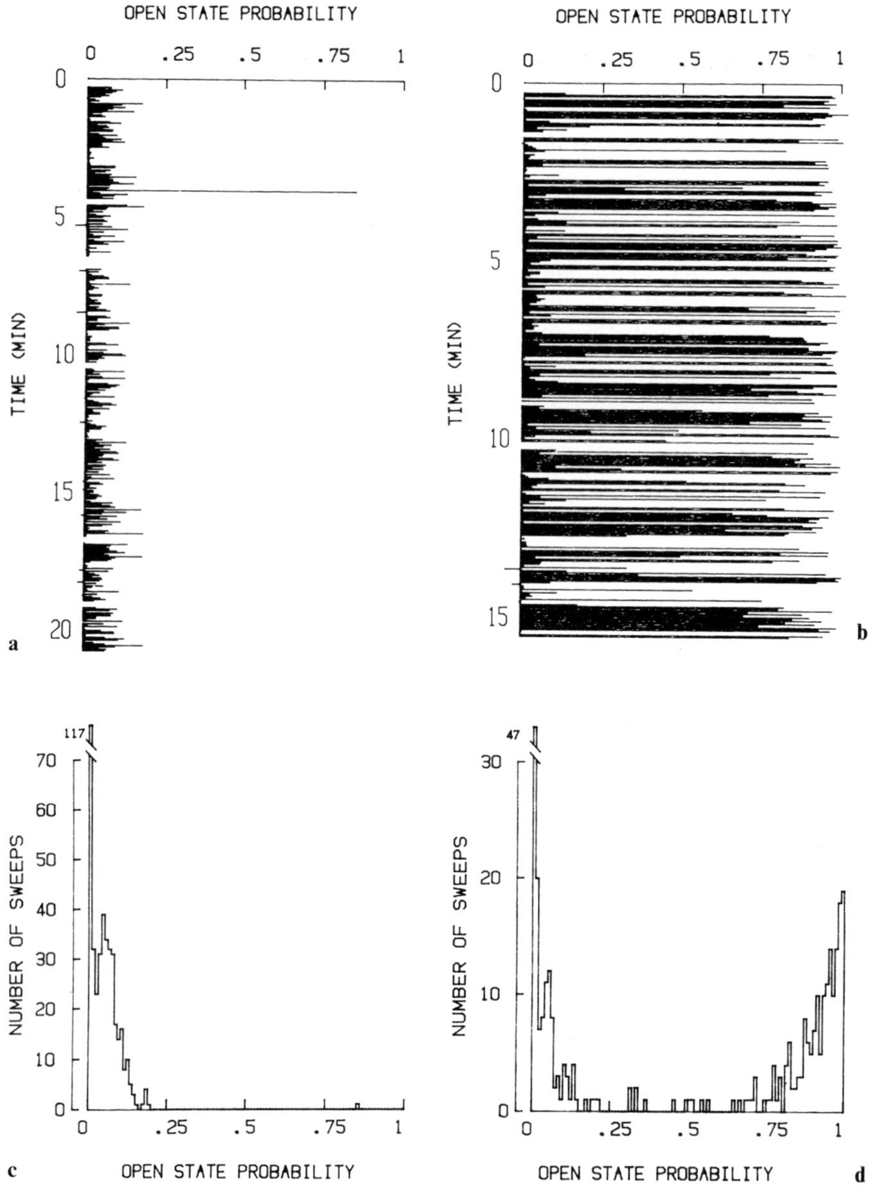

Fig. 4. Influence of Bay K 8644 on probability of channel openness (p) during individual sweeps. Control (*left*), 5 μM Bay K 8644 (*right*). **a, b** p plotted against time. Gaps along time axis indicate sweeps used to measure leak conductance or sweeps marred by noise interference. **c, d** Histograms of p values for the runs shown in **a, b**. Each bin is 0.008 wide. For each sweep, steady-state values of p were determined as p = <I>/i, where i is the unitary current, and <I> is the steady-state value of current, averaged over a period from 22 ms after the depolarizing step until the end of the pulse. Sweeps with no detectable opening ("nulls") have near-zero values of p, and show up in the first few bins. For example, in panel **c**, bins 1 to 5 contain 108, 18, 4, 1, and 1 nulls respectively; if the null sweeps had been excluded from the histogram in **c**, the distribution of p values would rise to a single peak and fall smoothly. Same patch as in Fig. 3. From [18]

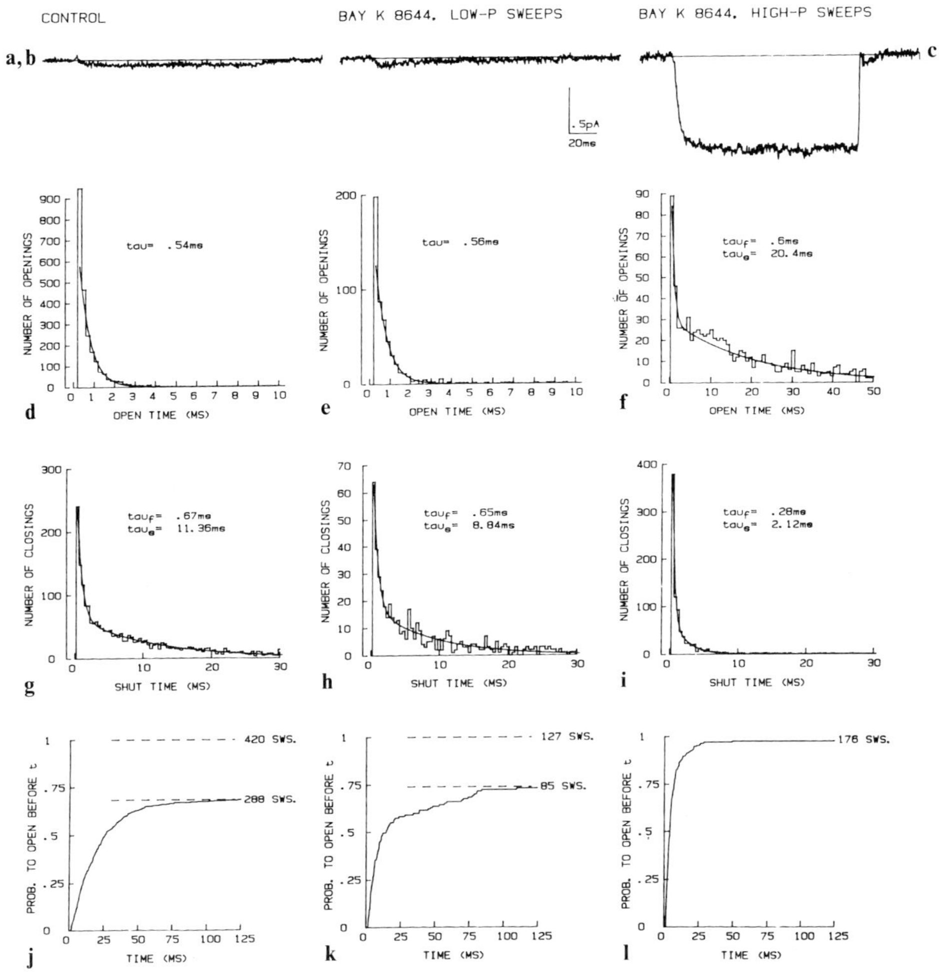

Fig. 5. Effect of Bay K 8644 on Ca channel kinetics. *Left column*: Analysis of all sweeps from the control run; *middle column*: all sweeps from agonist run with $p<0.3$; *right column*: all sweeps from agonist run with $p>0.65$. The rows show averaged current records (*first row*), distributions of open times (*second row*), closed times between openings (*third row*), and cumulative distributions of the latency to first opening (*fourth row*). Smooth curves in panels **d** and **e** are single exponentials (the fits ignore the first bin of the histogram data). Smooth curves in panels **f–i** are sums of two exponentials. Fits were obtained by minimizing chi-square, with the use of a computer program kindly provided by Dr. R. S. Kass. Same patch as in Fig. 3. From [18]

tial reasonably well, except for a surplus of brief openings in the first few bins, which may reflect imperfect exclusion of the low p behavior with its much greater density of open events per unit time. The shut time distribution is fitted by the sum of two exponentials, as in the other two cases, but the mean closed time is much briefer. Likewise, the cumulative histogram of latency-to-first opening is biased toward shorter times. The combination of longer openings and shorter closings accounts for the extremely high values of p.

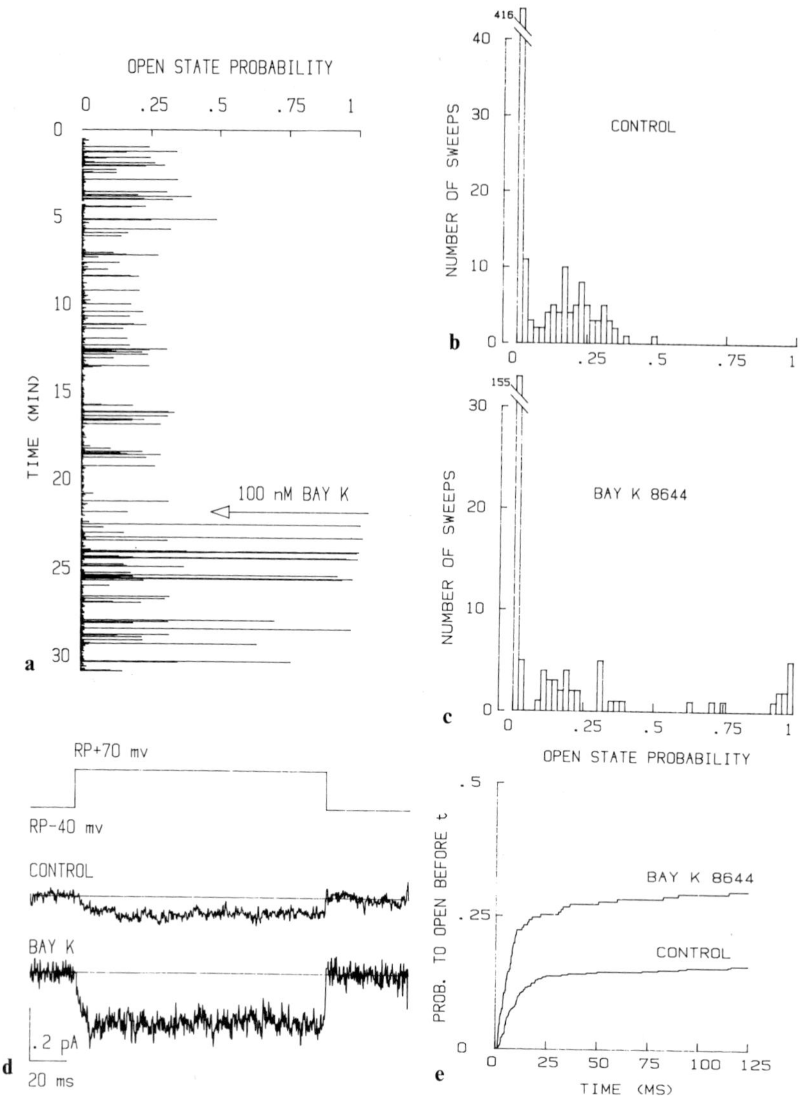

Fig. 6. Effect of 100 nM Bay K 8644 on a single Ca channel. Cell-attached patch recording with 110 mM Ba in the pipette as in Figs. 3–5. **a** Channel openness in each sweep plotted as a function of time. **b, c** Histograms of channel openness in the absence and presence of Bay K 8644. **d** Averaged currents of all the records with and without the drug. Voltage protocol shown above the traces. Estimated resting potential (RP) = −60 mv. **e** Superimposed cumulative distributions of the latency to first opening. Cell 6 D

The results from this patch were representative of a total of 3 experiments with 5–10 μM Bay K 8644. As shown in Fig. 6, 100 nM drug caused the averaged current to increase by only a factor of 2–3 (Fig. 6 d). The proportion of high p sweeps was clearly lower than with maximally effective doses of drug (compare Figs. 4 and 6), whereas the p-values and mean open time within the high p sweeps were similar at the two drug concentrations. Therefore we conclude that the concentration dependent increase of the averaged current results from a concentration dependent increase of the proportion of high p sweeps. At both drug concentrations the increased proportion of high p sweeps in the presence of Bay K 8644 was paralleled by a decrease of the proportion of sweeps with no detectable openings (see e.g. the cumulative distribution of latencies to first opening in Fig. 6e, which reaches a significantly lower level in the absence of drug).

Multiple Modes of Channel Gating and Agonist and Antagonist Effects

All of the analysis is consistent with the idea that the Ca channel switches between different modes of channel gating. Figure 7 presents our working hypothesis. We use the terms mode 0, mode 1, and mode 2 to refer to the three distinct patterns of gating.

Mode 1 is characterized by brief (~1 ms) openings occuring in rapid bursts. The most obvious form of gating in the absence of drug, it has been the main focus

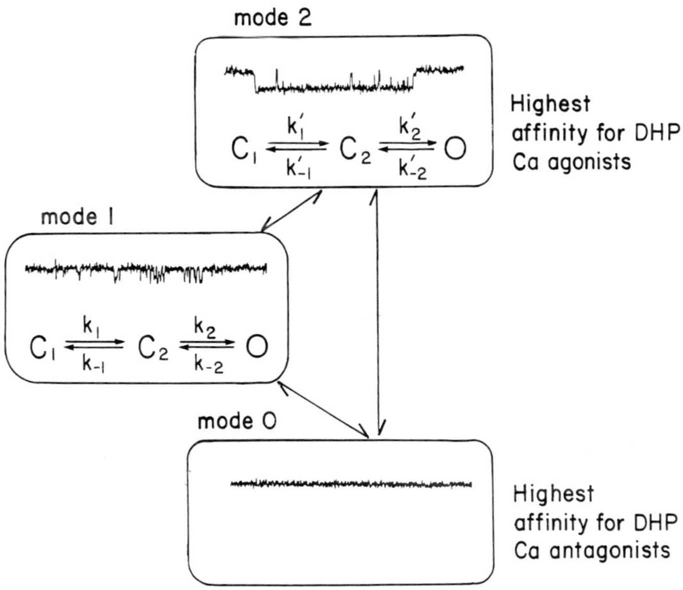

Fig. 7. Hypothetical modes of Ca channel gating (see text). In the absence of drug, transitions between modes are assumed to be much slower than gating reactions within modes; details of inter-mode connections are left unspecified and require further study. At the test potentials studied, mode 1 and mode 2 are distinguished by qualitatively different patterns of opening and closing. This is put in terms of a kinetic model for Ca channel gating with two closed (C1, C2) and one open (0) state: rate constants for transitions between the states are assigned different values depending upon the mode. No gating reactions are depicted form mode 0 because it represents conditions in which the channel is unavailable for opening at the test depolarization. Since voltage-dependent inactivation is one factor that biases the channel toward mode 0, the rate constants for transitions to and from mode 0 are presumably voltage-dependent. The voltage-dependence of transitions between mode 1 and mode 2 are not known. From [18]

of single-channel recordings up to now [6, 7]. The probability of openness in this mode is relatively low at membrane potentials where the unitary current is easily resolved, although it must be remembered that p can approach levels as high as 0.7 at stronger depolarizations [7, 35]. The observed distributions of open and shut times have been interpreted in terms of two closed states (C1, C2) and one open state (0) (see [6, 7, 10]).

Mode 2 can be distinguished by relatively long-lasting channel openings (~20 ms) and typically brief closings. Probability of channel openness is typically high (>0.7) even at relatively negative test potentials. The distributions of open and closed times in Fig. 5, right column are compatible with a C1-C2-O scheme, with very different values of rate constants than those appropriate for mode 1.

Although mode 2 behavior is most easily studied after administration of Ca agonist, it can also be seen in the absence of drug. For example, Fig. 4a showed a sweep with a p value of ~0.85; this sweep had openings lasting 3.6, 9.5, 10.8, 3.2, 0.6, and 77.5 ms, typical of what we define as mode 2. The sweep was the only one out of 420 that clearly showed long openings. In a total of 11 patches with one or two channels, sweeps with long openings and unusually high p typically appeared at a rate of about 1%, with a wide range (0.4 to 11%). Figure 8 illustrates the behavior of the patch with the highest incidence of sweeps showing intrinsic mode 2 behavior. Two main points can be made. First, sweeps with high p appear significantly clustered in time (Fig. 8a, see figure legend). Second, sweeps with high p in the absence of agonist show a pattern of channel opening and closing (Fig. 8c) very similar to that found in the presence of agonist (Fig. 3b). For example, in the experiment illustrated in Fig. 8 the mean open time in the high p sweeps was 16.4 ms, close to the ~20 ms time constant of the slow exponential in Fig. 5f.

Similarly good agreement was found in other experiments: average values for the mean open time of high p sweeps were 19.0 in control (93 sweeps, 7 cells) and 18.2 in the presence of Bay K 8644 (338 sweeps, 4 cells).

Mode 0 refers to a condition or conditions where the channel is unavailable for opening. It is expressed by sweeps showing no openings, in excess of those empty sweeps expected from the C1-C2-O kinetics of mode 1. Voltage-dependent inactivation is one factor that increases the proportion of time a channel spends in mode 0 (see [7, 35]). However, we found an excess of null sweeps even at negative holding potentials where voltage-dependent inactivation of averaged current records was maximally removed.

The distinction between mode 0 and mode 1 can be indicated in at least two ways. The cumulative histogram of first latency (Fig. 5j) levels off at about 70%. This runs contrary to a simple C1-C2-O model, which predicts that the saturating level should be 100% (sooner or later, the channel should reach the open state for long enough for an event to be detected). Instead, the data seem consistent with the idea that the channel was simply unavailable for opening at the test potential 30% of the time.

Another way of distinguishing mode 0 from mode 1 relies on the histogram of p values, as in Figs. 4c and 6b,c for example. The first two bins of the histogram largely represent sweeps for which no openings could be detected. When these sweeps are disregarded, the remaining distribution rises smoothly to a peak

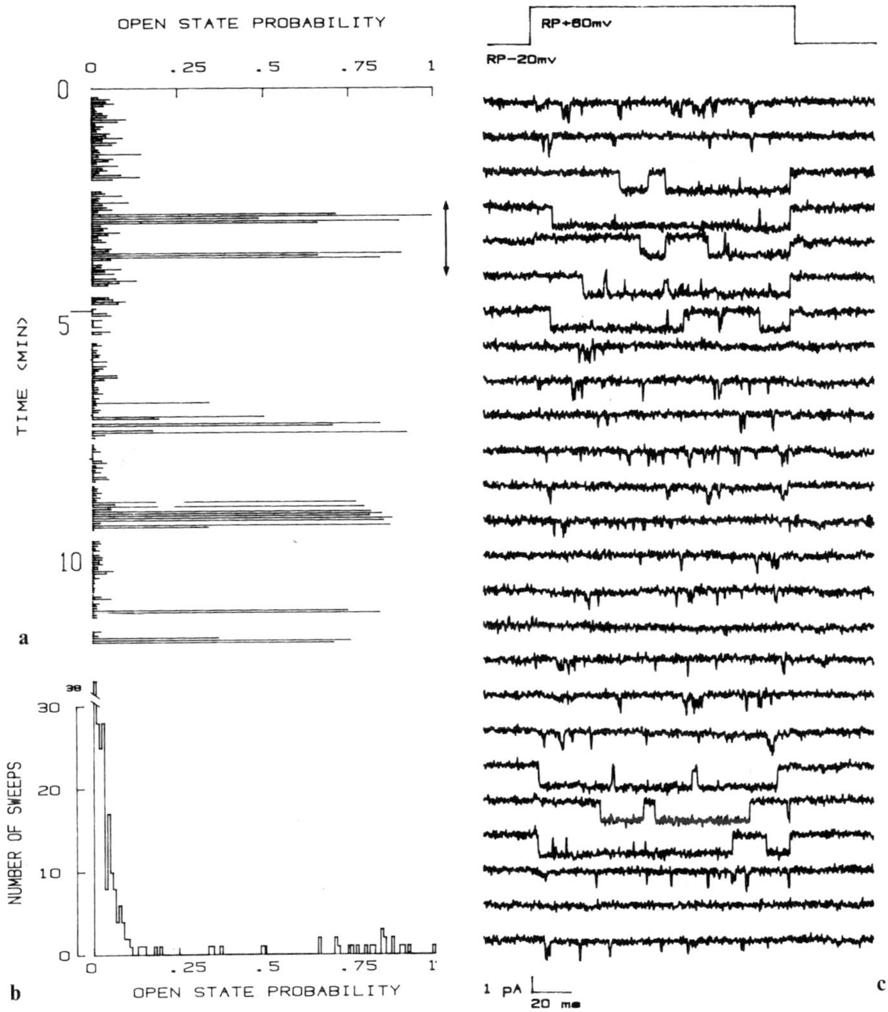

Fig. 8. Spontaneous appearance of sweeps with long-lasting openings and high p in the absence of drug. Cell-attached patch, experimental conditions as in Fig. 3a. **a** Probability of channel openness during 250 sweeps at 0.33 Hz. Gaps correspond to measurements of leak current with weak depolarizing pulses. **b** Histogram of p values for the set of sweeps shown in **a**. In 31 sweeps, no openings were detected by the analysis program. **c** Representative current records associated with the depolarizing pulse shown above. 25 records taken sequentially during the period marked in **a**, illustrating the tendency for mode 2 activity to occur in clusters of consecutive sweeps. The incidence of high p sweeps following immediately after a previous high p sweep was (11/21) = 52%., significantly higher than the overall incidence of high p sweeps, (21/198) = 11% (chi= square: $p < 0.0001$). The incidence of a null sweep following a null sweep was (8/29) = 29%, significantly higher than the overall incidence of null sweeps (30/198) = 15% (chi-square: $p < 0.05$). In the presence of Bay K 8644, sweeps with high p values also tended to follow each other. Cell 5F. From [18]

at the fifth bin and then falls smoothly, as might be expected for a single type of gating behavior, namely mode 1.

By either of these criteria, the vast majority of patches in our experiments show an appreciable number of null sweeps in excess of those expected from C1-C2-O kinetics. A similar excess has been observed by other investigators (e.g. [5, 34]). Like sweeps showing mode 2 behavior, null sweeps show a tendency to follow each other (see Fig. 8 legend).

Mechanism of Current Inhibition by Dihydropyridine Antagonists: Nimodipine

The fact that Bay K 8644 exerts its effect by changing the gating pattern of the Ca channel suggests that a similar mechanism on channel gating rather than a "plugging" of the channel might also explain the actions of the dihydropyridine antagonists. We propose that these drugs reduce Ca channel current by preferentially stabilizing the channel in its mode 0. Our results obtained on two patches with nimodipine are consistent with that idea and an example is illustrated in Figs. 9 and 10: The most dramatic effect of the drug on the single channel records is that the proportion of sweeps with no detectable openings (mode 0) is greatly increased. The opening and closing events in the other sweeps look indistinguishable from control except for the fact that the openings tend to preferentially occur near the beginning of the pulse. This uneven distribution of activity during the pulse leads to the decay of the averaged current shown in Fig. 9 b. When such an accelerated rate of decline was first observed with global current recordings [26, 38], it was attributed to open channel block [26]. We now favor the interpretation that the faster decay results from antagonist-promoted inactivation (transitions from mode 1 to mode 0, see discussion). The lack of effect of nimodipine on the gating kinetics within mode 1 is illustrated in Fig. 10. Both open and closed time distributions in the presence of the drug (Fig. 10 b) are similar to those in control (Fig. 10 a). However, as expected if the channel spends more time in mode 0, the cumulative histogram of the latency to first event (in this case corrected for the presence of two channels in that patch, see [1]) levels off at a clearly lower level, which simply reflects the fact that in an increased proportion of sweeps no openings were detected.

Mechanism of Partial Agonists and Antagonists: Nitrendipine

The identification of different modes of Ca channel gating leads naturally to the hypothesis that the dihydropyridine (DHP) Ca agonists and antagonists exert their effects by stabilizing the channel in one of its gating modes (Fig. 7). Within a mode, the kinetics of gating transitions need not be different when DHP occupies its binding site. Pure agonist effects arise when mode 2 is specifically favored, and pure antagonist effects result when mode 0 is preferentially stabilized; these extremes encompass a wide range of intermediate possibilities for "partial agonist" or "partial antagonist" effects when in addition to one favored mode another one is also stabilized. An example of such partial agonist action in the case of an antagonist is shown in Figs. 11 and 12 for nitrendipine.

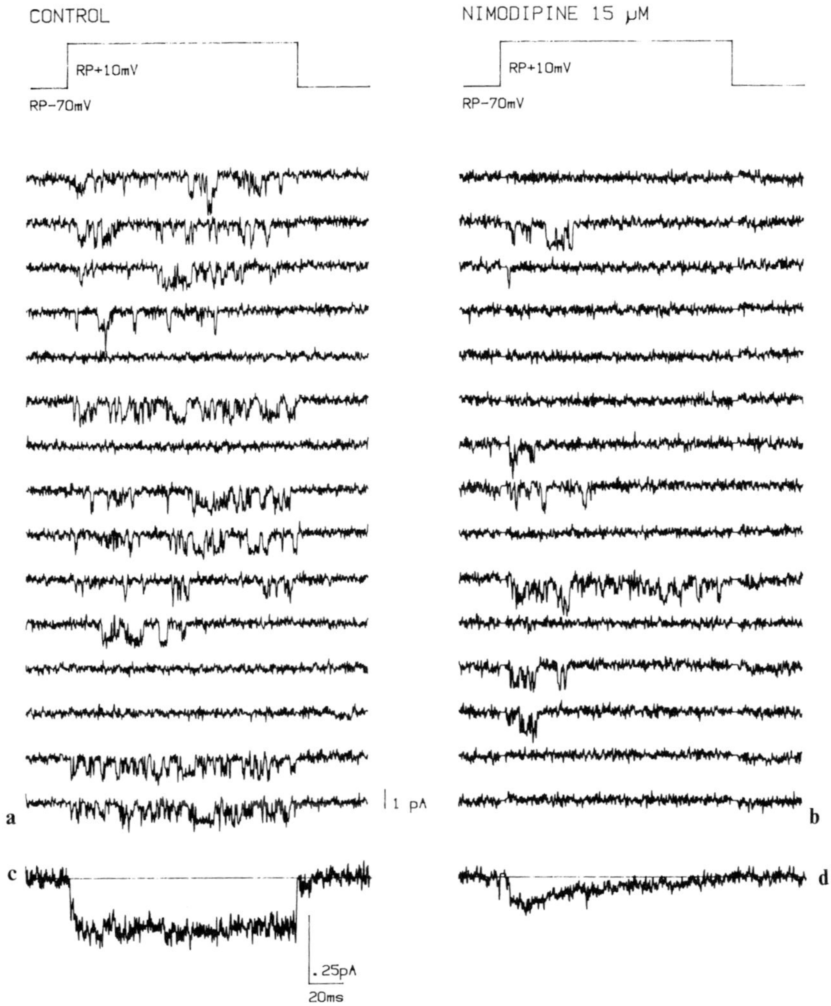

Fig. 9. Effect of nimodipine on single channel activity. Cell-attached patch, experimental conditions as in Fig. 3. The patch contained two Ca channels as judged from the appearance of 2 conductance levels. **a, b** Representative groups of sweeps in the absence (**a**) and presence (**b**) of 15 μM nimodipine. Voltage clamp protocol shown above the current records. **c, d** Averaged currents from all sweeps in runs **a** (368 sweeps) and **b** (337 Sweeps). Cell G 18 A

Although nitrendipine is generally assumend to be pure antagonist, we found that its net inhibitory effect is the resultant of agonist as well as antagonist components. Figure 11 illustrates the response of a single Ca channel to 5 μM nitrendipine, a partially inhibitory dose in the presence of the 110 mM Ba [26]. As panels a and c indicate, the control run included a large number of empty sweeps, as well as sweeps with bursts of flickery openings (mode 1), and sweeps with long openings (mode 2), some lasting beyond the repolarizing step (not shown). Nitrendipine altered channel activity in several ways (panels b, d). It reduced the

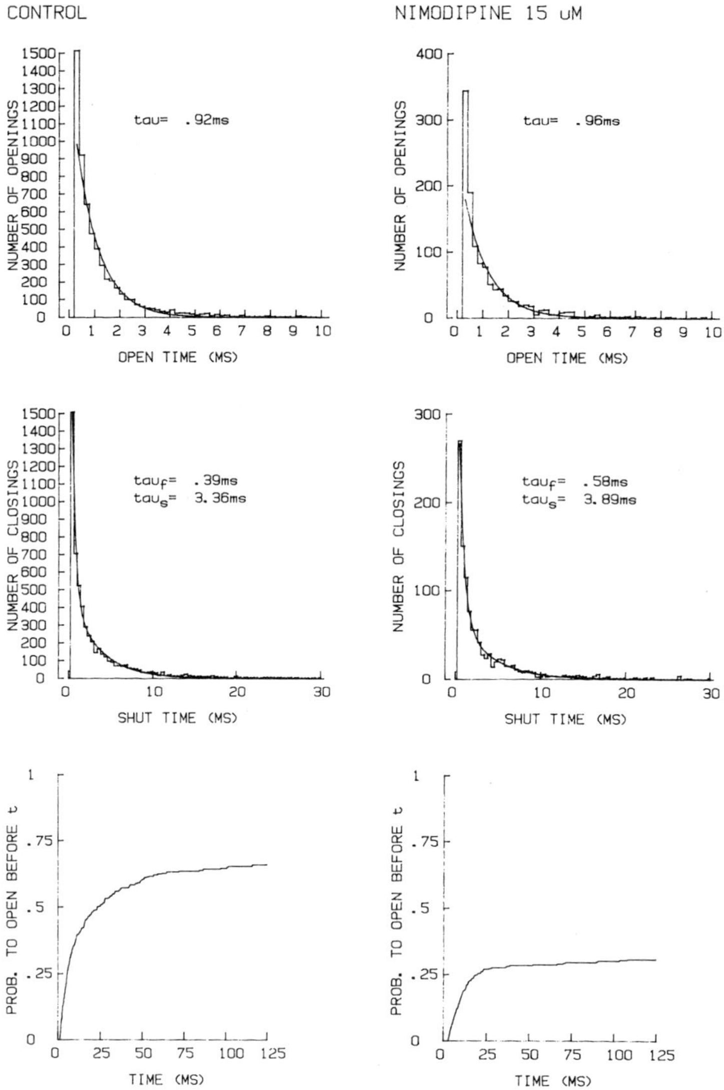

Fig. 10. Effects of nimodipine on Ca channel kinetics. Same patch as for Fig. 9. *Top row*: Open time distributions in the absence (*left*) and presence of 15 μM nimodipine, fitted by a single exponential. *Middle row*: Close time distributions fitted by the sum of two exponentials. *Bottom row*: Cumulative distribution of latency to first opening. The cumulative histogram of first latency was corrected for the presence of two channels (see [1])

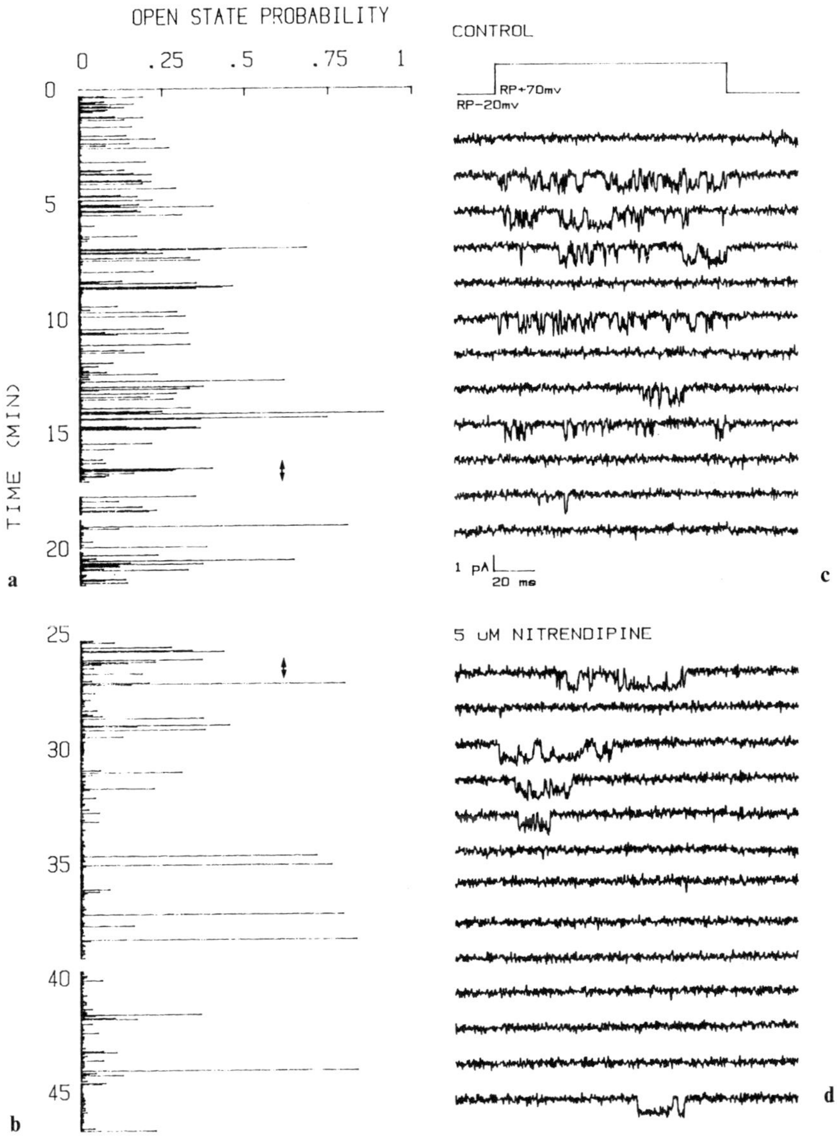

Fig. 11. Effect of nitrendipine on the activity of a single Ca channel. **a, b** p values for consecutive sweeps plotted against time, in the absence of drug (**a**), and in the presence of 5 μM nitrendipine (**b**). **c, d** Representative groups of consecutive sweeps taken over the periods in **a** and **b**. Cell 16E

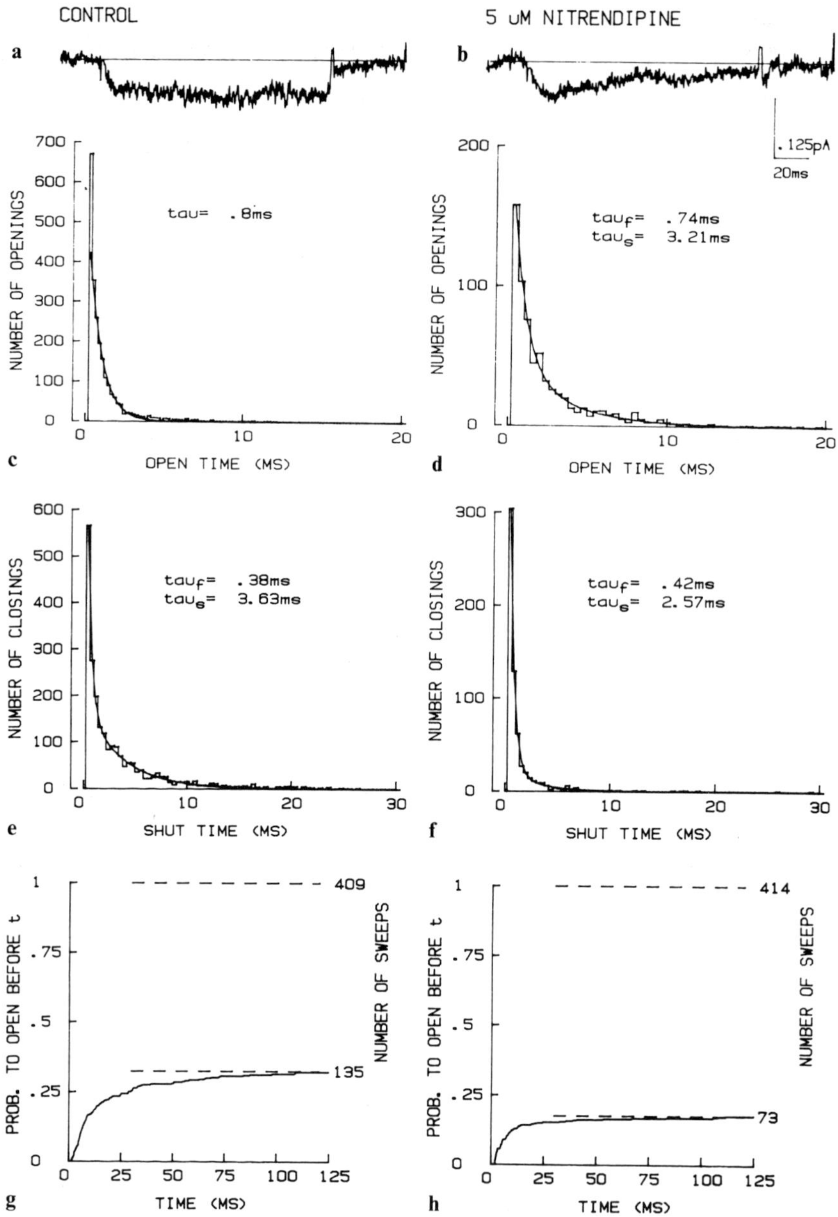

Fig. 12. Effects of nitrendipine on Ca channel kinetics. **a, b** Averaged currents from run **a** and run **b** in Fig. 11. **c** Distribution of open times in the absence of drug, fitted by a single exponential. **d** Distribution of open times in nitrendipine, fitted by the sum of two exponentials. **e, f** Distributions of closed times in the absence and presence of nitrendipine. **g, h** cumulative distribution of latency to first opening

proportion of sweeps with detectable openings: sweeps with brief, flickery openings occured less frequently and empty sweeps appeared more often. When a more complete reduction of inward current was obtained at 10 μM nitrendipine in other experiments, the proportion of empty sweeps approached 100%. These effects are similar to those seen with nimodipine (Fig. 9) and we attribute them to stabilization of mode 0, in line with a pure antagonist action.

Other aspects of the nitrendipine response were rather surprising. (a) the percentage of sweeps with $p > 0.5$ was not decreased; (b) a larger percentage of sweeps contained long openings (Fig. 11 d), and the distribution of open times was prolonged (Fig. 12 d), (c) closed times were abbreviated (Fig. 12 e, f), (d) latencies-to-first opening were shortened (Fig. 12 g, h). In all of these respects, nitrendipine shows "agonist" behavior like Bay K 8644.

The distribution of open times in nitrendipine (Fig. 12 d) consisted of a fast exponential component as in control ($T \sim 0.75$ ms), plus an additional slow component. The time constant of the slow component (3.2 ms) falls short of the ~20 ms time constants characteristic of mode 2 activity in control and with Bay K 8644. The cause for this discrepancy is not clear. We cannot exclude the possibility that nitrendipine not only influences the proportion of sweeps the channel spends in mode 2, but also affects the kinetics of opening and closing within mode 2. Another explanation is that openings of nitrendipine-bound channels are cut short by an accelerated inactivation reaction (transition from mode 2 to mode 10), which acts in parallel with the closing reaction within mode 2 (O–C2) and thereby increase the overall closing rate above its normal value.

At the time of peak inward current, the agonist-like effects largely counteracted the increase in the number of empty sweeps; consequently, the peak amplitude of the mean current signal was decreased very little by nitrendipine (Fig. 12 b). The overall inhibitory action of nitrendipine is more obvious toward the end of the depolarization since the average current decays more quickly in the presence of the drug. Individual records show a corresponding tendency for openings to occur toward the beginning of the pulse and not toward the end.

Even though in the two patches studied, nimodipine had a "pure" antagonist effect (Figs. 9 and 10), we at present cannot yet conclude with certainty that it is a purer antagonist than nitrendipine. It is likely that the balance of which gating mode is preferentially stabilized depends not only on the drug but can also be influenced by experimental conditions such as the holding potential and possibly other as yet unknown factors (see next paragraph and discussion).

Classification of Other Dihydropyridines as Partial Agonists or Antagonists

Nitrendipine is not exceptional in its mixed effects [44]. For example, nifedipine is used widely as an inhibitory agent, but it can increase cardiac contractility at low doses [21, 39], see also A. Schwartz et al., this volume). The drug CGP 28 392 has agonist effects on contractile activity and Ch channel current in heart and smooth muscle [24, 42] and Ca fluxes in cultured cells [14], but its presence partially occludes the stimulatory effect of Bay K 8644 [14]. Bay K 8644 itself it probably not a pure agonist since like the antagonists is speeds the rate of decay of the macroscopic Ca channel currents (Figs. 1 and 2). Sanguinetti and Kass ([37] and this volume) have reported that this drug increases Ca channel current in Purkinje fibers when the holding potential is negative, but reduces it when the holding potential is positive to −40 mV. We have seen similar effects of holding potential on the effects of Bay K 8644 in single ventricular cells.

Discussion

Although this work began with an analysis of the effects of Ca agonists and antagonists, the experiments led us to some unexpected conclusions about the fundamental properties of Ca channels. We believe that the strikingly long openings seen with Bay K 8644 are not a new form of gating, but an intrinsic form of gating (mode 2) whose likelihood is merely enhanced by the drug. Without the agonist-promoted activity as a guide, the intrinsic mode 2 activity might be overlooked, since it appears only rarely in most experiments, and contributes only a small number of events per sweep to histograms of open or closed times. But once attention is focussed on the mode 2 pattern of long openings and short closings, even single sweeps of this type of activity can be easily picked out. The distinction between mode 2 and mode 1 is particularly clearcut at weak depolarizations where the open probability in mode 1 is low.

Our results provide an attractive explanation for how structurally similar dihydropyridines can exert seemingly opposite effects on Ca influx. They argue against the idea that the inhibitory action of nitrendipine and other Ca antagonists reflects a physical plugging of the Ca channel pore. A simple binding and plugging hypothesis seems highly unlikely [22] since a nitrendipine molecule cannot plug the channel and show agonist-like activity at the same time. Recently, two binding sites with different affinities for DHP drugs have been described in radioligand binding studies and interpreted as evidence for separate receptors for agonist and antagonist DHP effects ([45], see also A. Schwartz et al., this volume). However, our model of different drug affinities of the DHP receptor with different conformations (gating modes) of the channel would explain the results of these binding studies without the necessity of two physically distinct receptors. Bean [2] and Kass and Sanguinetti (this volume) have shown that such a modulated receptor hypothesis, analogous to that for the action of local anasthetics on the Na channel [20], can indeed quantitatively account for the apparent discrepancies between (high affinity) radioligand binding and (low affinity) pharmacological effects.

Our results point to modulation of gating as the mechanism of DHP agonist or antagonist action. In fact, the changes in gating revealed by the single channel analysis fit very nicely with a large number of earlier observations in single cell or multicellular cardiac preparations.

(a) Previous experiments suggested that Ca antagonists act at a different site than Cd^{2+} and other inorganic ions [26], just as expected if inorganic ions interfere with the ion transfer process [19, 29], while dihydropyridine Ca antagonists influence gating.

(b) When inward and outward currents are enhanced by Bay K 8644 (Fig. 2) or inhibited by nitrendipine [26], the Ca channel reversal potential remains unchanged; this is also expected if the dihydropyridines influence the open probability without affecting the process of ion transfer and selectivity itself.

(c) Bay K 8644 speeds activation of Ca channel current following a sudden depolarization, and slows deactivation of tail current following a sudden repolarization (Fig. 2), while Ca antagonists leave activation and deactivation kinetics little changed. According to the hypothesis, the lack of symmetry is not surprising since agonist and antagonist effects are not diametrically opposed: agonist enhances mode 2 at the expense of mode 1, while antagonists accentuate mode 0 at the expense of mode 1.

(d) While enhancement of Ca channel activity by Bay K 8644 is much larger at negative test potentials than at strongly positive ones (Fig. 2; [8]), the inhibitory effect of antagonist is not strongly dependent on test depolarization level [26]. The striking voltage-dependence of agonist enhancement is consistent with the different behavior of modes 1 and 2. The agonist-induced enhancement is large at weak depolarization where p(mode 2)/p(mode 1) is $>>1$, and smaller at strongly positive potentials where p(mode 1) approaches 0.5–0.7 and where the ratio cannot exceed 1.4–2.0.

(e) A number of investigators have already pointed out synergistic effects of Ca antagonists and Ca channel inactivation, and parallels to interactions between local anesthetics and Na channel inactivation. For example, steady depolarizations that inactivate Ca channels strongly promote the inhibitory effect of DHP antagonists [2, 37]. Also, nitrendipine and nisoldipine slow the recovery of channel availability following a pulse [26, 38]. Our single channel recordings are consistent with the idea that inactivation and DHP Ca antagonists reinforce each other: like voltage-dependent inactivation [7, 35], the inhibitory effect of nitrendipine and nimodipine on single channel activity consists of a decrease in the availability of the channel, expressed as a change in the percentage of empty sweeps. Cavalie, Pelzer and Trautwein [34] have shown that D 600 also exerts its inhibitory action primarily through an increase of the percentage of null sweeps. However, they find that in addition to this effect D 600 also shortens open times and lengthens closed times on a millisecond timescale.

(f) The decay of Ca channel current is speeded by nitrendipine in both whole cell and unitary current recordings (Figs. 1 and 12; [26]). We interpret the acceleration as an indication that drug-bound channels undergo a more rapid transition to mode 0, as expected if drug binding stabilizes mode 0. A similar acceleration is seen with Bay K 8644 at stronger test depolarizations (Figs. 1 and 2), and is tentatively attributed to the drug's partial antagonist action.

Our hypothesis provides a simple explanation of partial agonist or partial antagonist effects, and a framework for classifying the 500 or more dihydropyridine compounds that remain less well studied than nifedipine or nitrendipine. It will be interesting to see if any of these molecules behaves as a pure agonist or antagonist, exclusively stabilizing mode 2 or mode 0. The range of possibilities is not limited to a one-dimensional scale between agonism and antagonism, since stabilization of three modes needs to be taken into account. In addition to the ideal agonist and ideal antagonist, one might imagine a compound that exclusively stabilizes mode 1, and thereby opposes effects of both agonists and antagonists.

The mechanism of transitions between modes is not known. The clustering of mode 2 activity indicates that switching can be relatively slow and raises the question of whether the transition between modes is an expression of a covalent modification of the channel protein. For the moment, we can only say that the modulatory process is probably not cyclic AMP-dependent protein phosphorylation, since the effect of agonist is quite different than that produced by elevation of cyclic AMP with isoprenalin [5, 35] or 8-bromo cyclic AMP [6]. Unlike Bay K 8644, isoprenaline slows both the activation and inactivation of Ba currents through Ca channels [3, 5] but it does not by itself slow significantly the decay of inward tails [3]; it does not induce mode 2 activity, but it modifies the rate constants within mode 1 [5, 6, 35]. Isoprenaline-induced increases in the number of functional channels [3] might be accounted for by a recruitment of channels from mode 0 to mode 1.

Like the cardiac cells described here, sensory neurons from chick dorsal root ganglion and neuroblastoma cells show a mixture of modes 0, 1 and 2, and an enhancement of mode 2 behavior with Bay K 8644 [13, 31, 32]. The apparently widespread existence of the gating modes and their positive response to Ca agonist gives new reason to wonder whether dihydropyridines have endogenous counterpart(s) that up- or down-modulate Ca channels (cf. [39]).

Acknowledgments. We thank Drs. R.W. Aldrich, C.J. Cohen, A.P. Fox, R.A. Janis, M.C. Nowycky, and Dr. A. Scriabine for helpful discussions, and the USPHS and the Miles Institute for support.
Part of this work has recently been published as an article in Nature [18]. Material from this article is reproduced with permission of Macmillan Journals, Ltd.

References

1. Aldrich RW, Corey DP, Stevens CF (1983) Nature 306:436–441
2. Bean BP (1984) Proc Natl Acad Sci 81:6388–6392
3. Bean BP, Nowycky MC, Tsien RW (1984) Nature 307:371–375
4. Brown AM, Kunze DL, Yatani A (1984) Nature 311:570–572
5. Brum G, Osterrieder W, Trautwein W (1984) Pfluegers Arch 401:111–118
6. Cachelin AB, dePeyer JE, Kokubun S, Reuter H (1983) Nature 304:462–464
7. Cavalie A, Ochi R, Pelzer D, Trautwein W (1983) Pfluegers Arch 398:284–297
8. Cohen CJ, Chung M (1984) Biophys J 45:394a
9. Curtis BM, Catterall WA (1983) J Biol Chem 258:7280–7283
10. Fenwick EM, Mary A, Neher E (1982) J Physiol, Lond 331:599–635
11. Flaim SF, Zelis R (1982) Calcium blockers. Urban & Schwarzenberg, Baltimore
12. Fleckenstein A (1983) Calcium antagonism in heart and smooth muscle. Wiley, New York
13. Fox AP, Hess P, Lansman JB, Nowycky MC, Tsien RW (1984) J Physiol 353:75P
14. Freedman SB, Miller RJ (1984) Proc Natl Acad Sci (to be published)
15. Glossmann H, Ferry DR (1983) Naunyn-Schmiedeberg's Arch Pharmacol 323:279–291
16. Hamill O, Marty A, Neher E, Sakmann B, Sigworth FJ (1981) Pfluegers Arch 391:85–100
17. Hess P, Lansman JB, Tsien RW (1984) Biophys J 45:394a
18. Hess P, Lansman JB, Tsien RW (1984) Nature 311:538–544
19. Hess P, Lansman JB, Tsien RW (1985) J Physiol 358:61P
20. Hille B (1977) J Gen Physiol 69:497–515

21. Himori N, Ono H, Taira N (1976) Japan J Pharmacol 26:427–435
22. Janis RA, Sarmiento JG, Maurer SC, Bolger GT, Triggle DJ (submitted for publication) J Pharm Exp Ther
23. Kao RL, Christman EW, Luh SL, Krauhs JM, Tyers GFO, Williams EH (1980) Arch Biochem Biophys 203:587–599
24. Kokubun S, Reuter H (1984) Proc Natl Acad Sci 81:4824–4827
25. Lee KS, Akaike N, Brown AM (1980) J Neurosci Methods 2:51–78
26. Lee KS, Tsien RW (1983) Nature 302:790–794
27. Lee KS, Tsien RW (1984) J Physiol 354:253–272
28. Marban E, Tsien RW (1981) Biophys J. 33:143a
29. Nelson MT (1984) Biophys J 45:395a
30. Norman RI, Borsotto M, Fosset M, Lazdunski M (1983) Biochem Biophys Res Comm 11:878–883
31. Nowycky MC, Fox AP, Tsien RW (1985) Proc Natl Acad Sci 82:2178–2182
32. Nowycky MC, Fox AP, Tsien RW (1984) Soc Neurosci Abs 10:526
33. Ochi R, Hino N, Niimi Y (1984) Proc Jap Acad Ser B 60:153–156
34. Cavalie A, Pelzer D, Trautwein W (1985) J Physiol 358:59P
35. Reuter H, Stevens CF, Tsien RW, Yellen G (1982) Nature 297:501–504
36. Reuter H (1983) Nature 301:569–574
37. Sanguinetti MC, Kass RS (1984) Biophys J 45:394a
38. Sanguinetti MC, Kass RS (1984) Circ Res 55:336–348
39. Schramm M, Thomas G, Towart R, Franckowiak G (1983) Nature 303:535–537
40. Schwartz A, Taira N (eds) (1983) Symposium on calcium channel blocking drugs: a novel intervention for the treatment of cardiac disease. Circ Res 52 (suppl, part II): 1–181
41. Scriabine A (ed) (1984) Nitrendipine. Urban & Schwarzenberg, Baltimore
42. Truog AG, Brunner H, Criscione L, Fallert M, Kuhnis H, Meier M, Roog H (1984) In: Rubin PR, Weiss GB, Putney Jr JW (eds) Calcium in biological systems. Plenum Press, New York (to be published)
43. Tsien RW (1983) Ann Rev Physiol 45:341–358
44. Vaghy PL, Grupp IL, Grupp G, Schwartz A (1984) Circ Res (to be published)
45. Vaghy PL, Grupp IL, Grupp G, Balwierczak JL, Williams JS, Schwartz A (1984) Eur J Pharm 102:373–374
46. Venter JC, Fraser CM, Schaber JS, Jung CY, Bolger G, Triggle DJ (1983) J Biol Chem 258:9344–9348

Discussion

(pp. 34–55)

Fleckenstein: It is very interesting that in these new experiments nitrendipine has exceptional actions in that it is only a weak blocker of the Ca^{2+}-channel and this corresponds with our observations on the isoproterenol stimulated Ca^{2+} influx. In the myocardium it was only weakly or even not at all influenced by nitrendipine. It has not strong cardiac inhibitory effects, but it has a very strong relaxing action on the peripheral resistance vessels. This is one reason for choicing nitrendipine as an antihypertensive drug. Regarding Mg^{2+} influx we agree completely: We believe that this Mg^{2+}-influx is mediated probably by an other carrier system. When we only block the Ca^{2+}-influx with a true Ca^{2+}-antagonist we don't inhibit the electrochemical Mg^{2+} effect. This is clear evidence that other carrier systems are involved. The experiments with beta-stimulators are also in favour of the idea that Ca^{2+} and Mg^{2+} use different channels. If Ca^{2+} is accumulated in the superficial layer of the sacrolemmal membrane, $Mg+2^{+}$ is displaced by the accumulated Ca^{2+} and cannot come in contact with the superficial layers of the sacrolemmal membrane. This may be the explanation of the reciprocal influence of beta-receptor stimulations on Ca^{2+} and Mg^{2+}.

Hess: I agree that we don't think that $Mg^{2}+$ goes through the Ca^{2+} channel. It is slightly more complicated because Mg^{2+} is a blocker of Ca^{2+} channels and its blocking actions are voltage dependent: at negative voltages Mg^{2+} blocks Ca^{2+} channels much better than it does at positive voltages. Those experiments were chosen to show the partial agonist effect of nitrendipine but our number of observations on both nimodipine and nitrendipine is too small for us to be able to say that one drug is like this, or one drug is like that. I have chosen them to make a certain point about the possibility for mixed effects, not to say that we know that nimodipine is a more pure antagonist than nitrendipine.

Kass: The peaks of the current voltage curves appear to be shifted in the hyperpolarising direction. Do you think that the open-channel probability for the activation curve is shifted in that direction as well?

Hess: Yes, that is one way to put it. Of course, if we say that the main effect of Bay K 8644 is to shift the channel from mode 1 to mode 2 behaviour, then, as it has been reported for the Ca^{2+}-channel that the open probability in mode 1 can be quite at positive potentials (it can go up high to 0.6–0.7), there we only have room for a 30% increase. At negative potentials, however, you have a lot of room and that is what we think is the basis for the large effect at negative potentials. Because normally the open probability there is very small, you can increase it tremendously by the long mode 2 openings.

Bayer-Symposium IX
Cardiovascular Effects of Dihydropyridine-Type
Calcium Antagonists and Agonists, 58–71

Ca Entry into Vascular Smooth Muscle

C. VAN BREEMEN, K. HWANG, R. LOUTZENHISER, S. LUKEMAN, and H. YAMAMOTO

Introduction

This paper is intended as a brief review of our work on the mechanisms whereby Ca enters into the myoplasm of vascular smooth muscle cells. We propose that there are two components to this Ca entry process. The first is the permeation of Ca ions through the proteolipid plasmalemma mediated by a resting Ca leak and several excitable channels. The second component is the diffusion through a narrow space near the inner surface of the membrane which contains a regulated Ca^{2+} buffer. The evidence for the resting Ca^{2+} leak and the excitable Ca^{2+} channels as well as that for the regulated buffer was derived from correlations between ^{45}Ca influxes and force development in the rabbit aorta.

Methods

The assumptions underlying the measurement of ^{45}Ca influx will be discussed rather than the detailed protocols which are given elsewhere [3, 31]. In principle, Ca influx is measured by exposing the isolated arterial rings to ^{45}Ca labeled bathing solution for such a short time (in this study 90 seconds) that the uptake of ^{45}Ca by the cells is not significantly complicated by its backflux into the extracellular space. However, the problem with Ca flux measurements in isolated tissues has always been that the ^{45}Ca accumulated in the extracellular space, both as free ions and the ionically bound species, exceeds that taken up by the cells by roughly a factor of 10 [30]. This problem can be overcome by washing the preparation in an ice cold physiological salt solution for a period of time which allows removal of extracellular ^{45}Ca and leaves a representative sample of ^{45}Ca within the cells. The rationale for this cold wash is based on the assumption that the diffusion of Ca through the extracellular space and the dissociation of Ca from the extracellular binding sites will be slowed much less by the 37° temperature reduction than will the active Ca extrusion across the plasmalemma. Due to the thickness of the rabbit aortic preparation, the experimental validation of these assumptions is complicated by the slowness of ^{45}Ca loss from the extracellular space. The criteria which are necessary to be met for successfully quenching the intracellular label by cold washing, are better tested in monolayers of cultured rat aortic smooth muscle cells (see [32] for culture methods). Figure 1 shows the washout of ^{45}Ca into ice cold Ca free PSS containing 2 mM EGTA from a rat aortic primary culture which was previously labeled for 90 min. The initial washout of ^{45}Ca is rapid and after ten min the loss of ^{45}Ca becomes monoexponential indicating that after 10 min Ca is lost from a single compartment with at $t_{1/2}$ of 75 min.

The most probable explanation for this observation is that the initial rapid ^{45}Ca washout is derived from extracellular label, and that the slow component constitutes cellular ^{45}Ca loss. This is further supported by the recent study of Scheid and Fay [25] who found a very similar ^{45}Ca washout pattern for isolated toad stomach smooth muscle cells at room temperature. In addition, they were able to show that the Ca content of the slow component could be increased by high K^+ exposure which is known to stimulate cellular Ca uptake, while the fast component was insensitive to high K^+ application during prior ^{45}Ca labeling. The single exponential ^{45}Ca washout from the cultured cells at 0 °C implies that at this temperature the cell membrane is the rate limiting barrier for loss of exchangeable Ca stored in the various cellular compartments such as the cytoplasm,

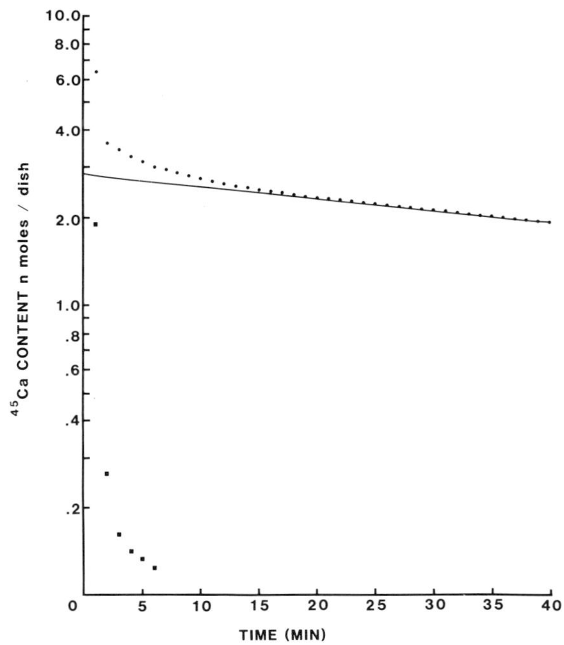

Fig. 1. Monolayers of cultured rat aortic smooth muscle cells were incubated in ^{45}Ca labeled PSS (in mM: NaCl 140; KCl 5; $CaCl_2$ 1.5; $MgCl_2$ 1; HEPES buffer 5, dextrose 10, pH 7.2, bubbled with 100% O_2, T=37 °C) for 2.5 h. They were subsequently rinsed with ice cold PSS without Ca and with 2 mM EGTA added and then washed out in the same solution for 40 min changing the solution at 1 min intervals. The decline of ^{45}Ca averaged from 4 experiments is given in the *upper curve*. The lower *square dots* mark the loss of ^{45}Ca from dishes devoid of cells

sarcoplasmic reticulum (SR) and mitochondria. Sampling during this slow phase of washout will thus provide a representative sample of cellular ^{45}Ca.

In the cultured cells a 10 min cold wash suffices to quench the cellular label such that the representative sample only slightly underestimates the true cellular label. Due to the much greater thickness of the rabbit aortic rings removal of extracellular ^{45}Ca requires 45 minute cold wash such that the representative measured cellular label underestimates the true cellular ^{45}Ca content by approximately one third (the slow component of ^{45}Ca washout from the aorta in the cold has a halftime between 90–120 min.

The third assumption of limited backflux during the ^{45}Ca influx measurement can easily be satisfied if the ^{45}Ca uptake is limited to 10% or less of the equilibrium ^{45}Ca uptake value. Under these conditions, it can be calculated that the contribution of even a complete inhibition of Ca extrusion during the course of the experiment would lead to an overestimation of the stimulated influx measurement of about 6%. Since we have never measured any effect on Ca extrusion which is even close to total inhibition, we may safely assume that the error of our influx measurements due to the possible perturbation of Ca efflux is less than the biological variation of our experiments.

The high reproducibility of the aortic ^{45}Ca measurements and the fact that as many as 40 tissue samples can be obtained from each rabbit aorta, make this preparation the most convenient for the analysis of Ca influx across arterial smooth muscle cell membrane.

Other advantages of the ^{45}Ca influx techniques in smooth muscles are that the fluxes can be measured under physiological conditions identical to those used for the measurement of force development and that we are able to measure the basal Ca leak was well as possible electrically silent Ca movement across the surface membrane.

The protocols for tension recordings and ^{45}Ca efflux have been described previously [3, 8].

Results and Discussion

Ca Entry and Blockade

According to Fleckenstein's original hypothesis, Ca antagonists inhibit cardiac and smooth muscle contractility by blocking Ca entry into the cells [9]. For smooth muscle, this mechanism of action was first validated by the demonstration that D 600 inhibited the ^{45}Ca uptake stimulated by high K^+ depolarization and spontaneous activity [18]. However, it did not inhibit the ^{45}Ca uptake associated with the resting state of the smooth muscle. These studies were confirmed for nifedipine, flunarizine and diltiazem [10, 11, 24, 31]. However, one uncertainty which remains in some of the above experiments, is that when ^{45}Ca uptake is measured over a relatively long time period (5 min or more) its accumulation is determined by both of Ca influx and Ca extrusion. This problem of interpretation can be circumvented by reducing the time period of influx such that the complication due to backflux was minimal as described in the methods section.

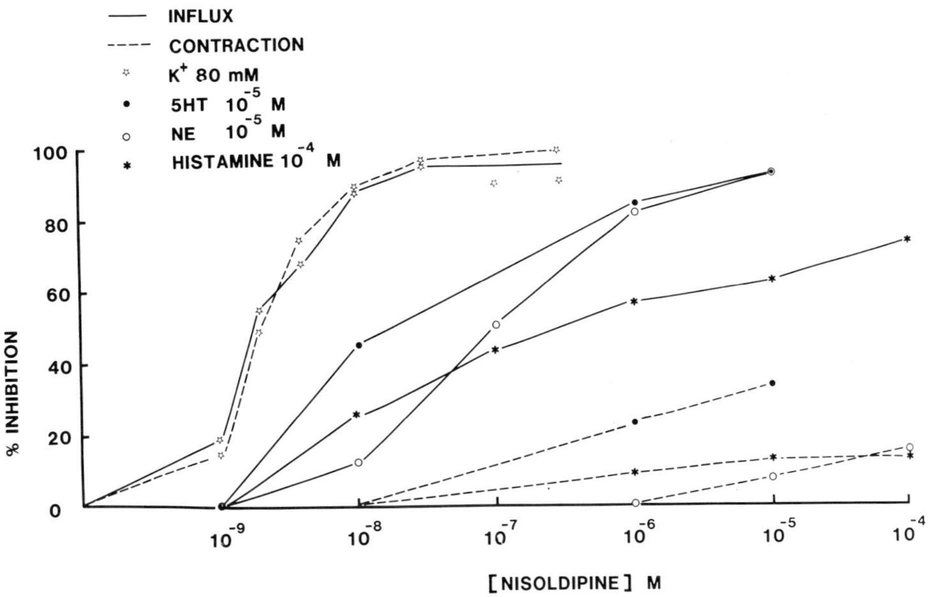

Fig. 2. Inhibition of ^{45}Ca influx and contractions stimulated by maximally effective doses of K^+, serotonin (*5HT*) norepinephrine (*NE*) and histamine by varying concentrations of nisoldipine. Each point is the average of at least 5 determinations. The standard errors are less than 10% of the mean. (High K solutions were prepared by isotonic replacement of KCl for NaCl)

Figure 2 shows the results of one set of such experiments performed on the rabbit aorta. The curves on the left show the percentile inhibition of both high K^+ induced force development and stimulated ^{45}Ca influx as a function of nisoldipine concentration (the values for ^{45}Ca influx seen during rest which were not affected by nisoldipine were subtracted from the measurements of ^{45}Ca influx seen during stimulation). The parallel inhibition of stimulated ^{45}Ca influx and force development argues for the tenet that the two phenomenon are causally linked. Actions of nisoldipine at sites distal to the Ca channels such as Ca release, Ca uptake by the SR, myofilament regulation, and Ca extrusion would obviously disrupt the parallel relationship seen for nisoldipine inhibition of ^{45}Ca influx and contraction. The hypothesis that pharmacologically relevant concentrations of the dihydropyridine Ca antagonists act solely by Ca entry blockade is further reinforced by the curves on the right of figure 2. Norepinephrine, serotonin and histamine are pharmacological agonists which activate vascular smooth muscle by stimulating Ca entry and, in addition, activating intracellular Ca release. When the Ca entry is inhibited by nisoldipine as indicated by the solid dose response curves, the tension is not inhibited to the same extent as indicated by the much flatter dotted D-R curves for inhibition of contraction. This is due, as we have confirmed in more direct experiments, to the fact that nisoldipine does not inhibit the release of intracellular Ca by these agonists. It is also clear from figure 2, that the Ca influxes stimulated by norepinephrine, serotonin and histamine are much less sensitive to nisoldipine than is the Ca influx stimulated by high

K^+ depolarization. NE, histamine and serotonin stimulated ^{45}Ca influxes are not additive indicating that activation of different receptors may result in the opening of common ROCs. The disparate sensitivities of high K^+- and agonist-induced responses to antagonists holds true for all vascular smooth muscle investigated although in the resistance arteries the NE induced Ca influx is the more sensitive response [7]. In the rabbit aorta we have also found a difference in the patterns of Ca antagonist potencies for NE- and high K^+-induced ^{45}Ca fluxes. The potency of nisoldipine decreased fifty fold on increasing the NE concentration while no such effect was seen with high K^+ activation.

We have interpreted these differences in CAt potencies for blockade of the depolarization- and the agonists stimulated Ca entry as evidence for the presence of two separate excitable Ca channels [29]. Bolton simultaneously and independently arrived at the same conclusion [5]. There are several other lines of evidence which support the concept of separate potential sensitive channels (PSCs) and receptor operated channels (ROCs) in smoth muscle. Both the high K^+ stimulated ^{45}Ca influx and the Ca agonist Bay K 8644 stimulated ^{45}Ca influx are additive to the norepinephrine stimulated ^{45}Ca influx, but maximal K^+ and BAy K 8644 responses are not additive to each other [33]. These results indicate that Bay K 8644 opens up the PSCs and not the ROCs and, in addition, satisfy another criterium of separate channels in that the two channels can simultaneously be maintained in the open state. The only other way that such additivity could be interpreted on the basis of a single Ca channel is that depolarization (or Bay K 8644) and norepinephrine would open up Ca channels in such a way that the maximal open probability of each separate stimulation would not exceed .5 and that the opening probability when both stimuli are present simultaneously would be close to 1. However, this interpretation becomes unlikely in the light of experiments of Hess et al. who showed that the opening probability of cardiac Ca channels in the presence of Bay K 8644 was already close to one [13].

Another line of evidence for the existance of separate receptor and potential activated Ca channels in vascular smooth muscle is that they appear to be differently regulated by physiological mechanisms. Thus Meisheri and van Breemen [20] reported that increases of cyclic AMP mediated by β-stimulation, phosphordiasterase inhibition and application of dibutyryl cyclic AMP all favored inhibition of the potential sensitive Ca channels, over inhibition of receptor operated Ca channels. We (Lukeman and van Breemen, unpublished results) later demonstrated that large increases in cyclic AMP by the agent forskolin were also able to inhibit the ROCs. The ROCs activated by NE appear to allow entry of Na^+ as well as Ca^{2+} since NE stimulated Na^+ influx has the same sensitivity to diltiazem as the ^{45}Ca influx [2].

On the other hand, the two channels may make use of some molecular components which are similar. Figure 3 demonstrates that the calmodulin inhibitor trifluorpyrazine inhibits ^{45}Ca influx stimulated by 10^{-5} M NE and 80 mM K^+ with the same potency. We (Lukeman and van Breemen, unpublished results) found this to be true for several other calmodulin inhibitors and noticed a close correlation between the potency of Ca influx inhibition and the inhibition of other calmodulin dependent processes. It may therefore be possible that both the PSCs and ROCs utilize calmodulin or a calmodulin-like molecular component in the

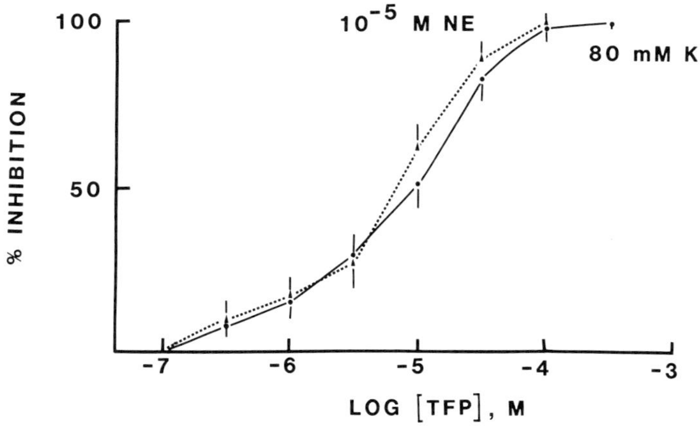

Fig. 3. Inhibition of ^{45}Ca stimulated by maximally effective doses of NE and K^+ by varying concentrations of trifluropyrazine (*TFP*). Each point is the average of at least four determinations and verticle bars equal the SEMs

gated Ca transport process. One possible function for such a calmodulin like component could be that of the high affinity Ca transport sites recently proposed by Hess and Tsien to be the essential aspect of the two sites Ca channel transport mechanism [12].

It may be concluded from the above section that Ca entry through the vascular smooth muscle plasmalemma is mediated by at least 3 different transport mechanisms: 1) A Ca^{2+} leak resistant to organic calcium antagonists but sensitive to lanthanum and some other polyvalent cations 2) A Ca channel activated by depolarization which probably is similar to those observed in cardiac muscle and nerve. 3) A channel activated by NE which appears to allow entry to both Ca^{2+} and Na^+ [2] and which may be shared by other agonists. In addition to the above three Ca entry mechanisms it is conceivable that under certain conditions Ca ions may enter via the Na^+/Ca exchange carrier, which however is not very prominent in smooth muscle [1, 29], and other channels activated by stretching the muscle cells [4].

Regulated Intracellular Ca Buffering

In 1977, van Breemen reported that force development in vascular muscle was not only a function of the amount of Ca which entered the cells but also of the rate at which this Ca entry process occured [28]. Thus when a certain quantity of Ca was rapidly introduced into aortic smooth muscle cells for a short time it produced a much faster and larger contraction than when the same amount of Ca entered more slowly over a longer time interval. This effect suggested the hypothesis that as Ca^{2+} enters the cells the superficial SR removes a variable fraction of it from an area close to the inner surface of the plasma membrane [28]. Some recent data support this conclusion and in addition, show that this type of "buffer barrier" to Ca entry is regulated by neurotransmitters and autocoids.

Figure 4 shows the force development and ^{45}Ca influx induced by Bay K 8644 in solutions containing different K^+ concentrations. Although the left panel of figure 4 confirms the finding of Schramm et al. [25] that the aorta needs to be primed with a partial high K^+ induced depolarization in order to obtain a Bay K 8644 induced contractile response, the right panel indicates that this does not hold true for the Bay K 8644 stimulated Ca^{++} influx. Bay K 8644 stimulated a 60% maximal Ca influx at 0 mM or 5 mM K^+ even though little force development can be seen under these conditions. The influx indeed becomes larger at 15 mM K^+ and again smaller as the K^+ concentration is raised. This latter finding is due to the fact that in the aorta Bay K 8644 and high K^+ depolarization open the same potential sensitive Ca channels [33].

The small contractile effects of Bay K 8644 stimulated influx in PSS could be the result of an increased stimulation of Ca^{2+} extrusion such as to prevent intracellular Ca^{2+} accumulation or could be due to Ca^{2+} removal by an intracellular Ca buffer. To decide between these possibilities, we measured the net Ca accumulation resulting from Bay K 8644 simulation in PSS. Figure 5 shows that the Bay K 8644 stimulated Ca influx produces a large accumulation of intracellular Ca which can be reversed by the application of 50 mM caffeine and thus confirms the earlier conclusion that the Ca which entered the cells at a submaximal rate can be accumulated by superficial SR before it reaches the myofilaments in the deeper regions of the cell. In other words, a second barrier to Ca entry into the myoplasm is created by removing Ca, which has just entered through the plasmalemmal Ca^{2+} channels, through the active transport of the superficial SR and perhaps the Ca pumps in the caveolar portions of the plasmalemma.

We next asked how this superficial buffering activity is related to the rates of Ca influx and whether it is regulated by external messengers. Figure 6 shows the dependence of force developed during the opening of PSCs by Bay K 8644 and

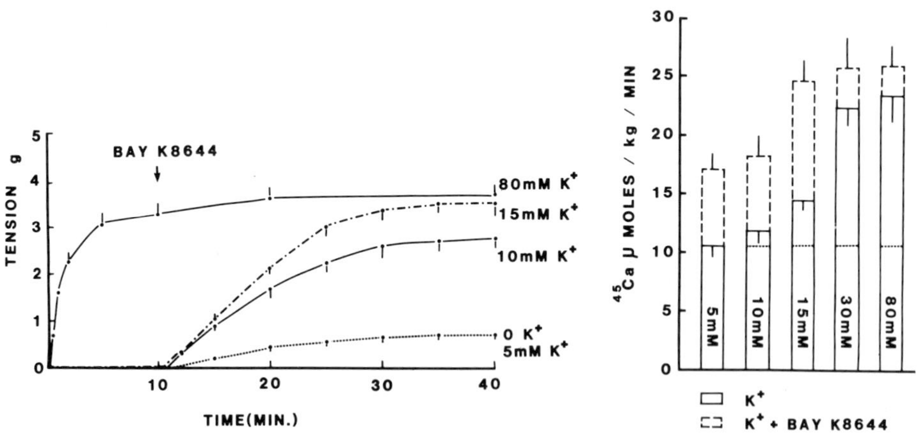

Fig. 4. *Left:* Force development induced by varing concentration of K^+ applied at t = 0 and the subsequent addition of 10^{-6} M Bay K 8644 at t = 10. *Right:* ^{45}Ca influx measured during the tonic phases of force development in the above solutions. The *solid line bars* indicate the ^{45}Ca influx in the solutions without Bay K 8644, while the dotted portions indicate the additional influx stimulated by Bay K 8644. *Verticle line bars* equal SEMs (n = 5)

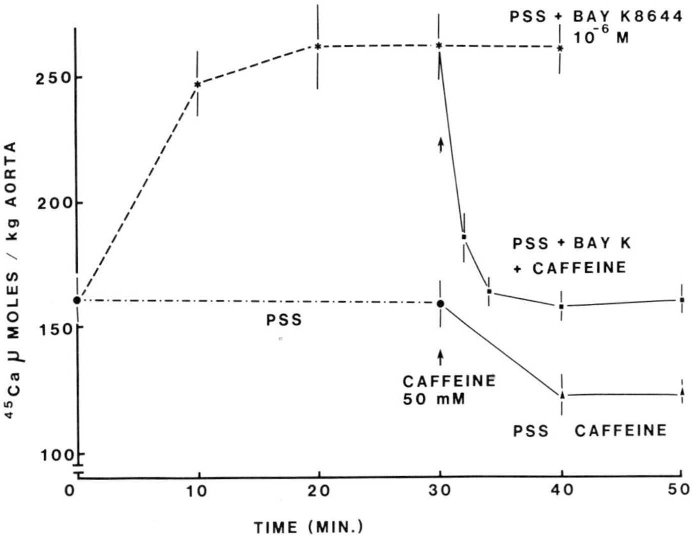

Fig. 5. The net Ca gain induced by Bay K 8644 addition to PSS measured by allowing the aortic rings to equilibrate in ^{45}Ca labeled PSS for three hours before adding Bay K at t=0. 50 mM caffeine was added at 30 minutes. The *lower curve* serves as a control without addition of Bay K 8644. Each point is the average of 4 determinations with the bars equalling 2 × SEM

high K^+ on the total Ca^{2+} influx (the data are taken from the experiments illustrated in Fig. 4). The resting Ca^{2+} influx is 11 μ moles kg^{-1} min^{-1} (0.02 pmoles cm^{-2} s^{-1} using an extracellular volume of 45% and a surface to volume ratio of 1.5 μm^{-1} [14]. The PSCs must increase the influx to 15 μmoles kg^{-1} min^{-1} before the threshold for contraction is reached. Further stimulation of Ca influx generates a very steep force activation curve which saturates at 24 μmuoles kg^{-1} min^{-1}. In Fig. 7 the developed force influx curves are generated in a different fashion. The rabbit aortic rings are fully activated by either 80 mM K^+ or 10^{-5} M NE whereupon the influx is reduced by either D 600 (10^{-8} – 10^{-4} M) or $LaCl_3$ ($2 \times 10^{-5} - 2 \times 10^{-3}$ M). In the case of stimulation by high K^+ depolarization and its calcium antagonist inhibition we again observe the effects of varying numbers of open PSCs on force development and find essentially the same curve as with high K and Bay K 8644 (Fig. 6). However when a maximal concentration of NE is used to activate Ca entry the threshold for myofilament activation is shifted to the much lower Ca influx of 7 μmoles kg^{-1} min^{-1}. In this set of preparations the resting influx was 14.8 μmoles/kg^{-1} min^{-1} and it can be seen that D 600 did not lower the Ca^{2+} influx below this value in the case of NE. However even after all the ROCs were blocked, NE caused a 50% of maximal tonic contraction which lasted long after the discharge of intracellularly stored Ca^{2+} was completed. This remaining contraction thus depends on Ca influx through the leak since inhibition of this fraction of Ca influx by La^{2+} abolishes the remaining tension. The 5 μmoles $Ca \cdot kg^{-1} \cdot min^{-1}$ ^{45}Ca influx remaining after maximal La^{3+} blockade may not deliver ionic Ca to the cytoplasm and perhaps represents internalization of "structural" Ca^{2+} during plasmalemmal turnover [25].

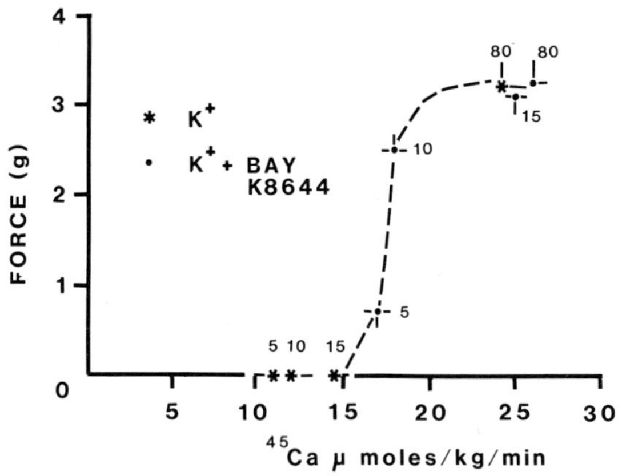

Fig. 6. Force development as a function of ^{45}Ca influx stimulated by high K^+, Bay K 8644 or combinations of the two. The data were obtained from the experiment illustrated in Fig. 4. *Bars* to one side of each point indicate SEMs

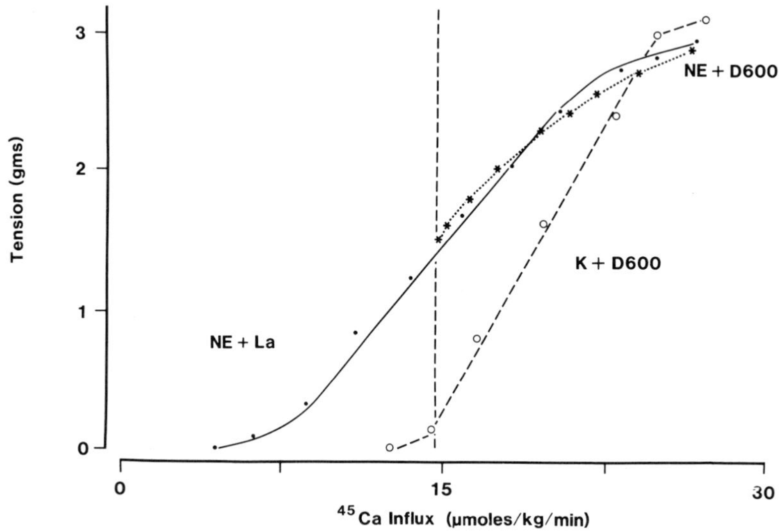

Fig. 7. Tonic tension as a function of ^{45}Ca influx simulated by 80 mM K^+ and gradually diminished by increasing doses of D 600, or by 10^{-5} M NE and gradually diminished by increasing doses of D 600 or La^{3+}

If we accept the assumption that the superficial SR is able to effectively buffer the Ca influx at values below the threshold for activation by depolarization then we may attribute the lowering of this threshold by NE to inhibition of the "buffer barrier". The lesser slope of the Ca influx-contraction curve in the presence of NE than during high K activation confirms our previous postulate that the "buffer barrier" is most effective at the lower values of Ca influx.

Figure 5 shows that caffeine releases the Ca taken up by the superficial buffer during stimulated Ca^{2+} influx. Since NE and caffeine release the same intracellular Ca store from the aorta [8, 15] it would follow that prior depletion of this store by NE would increase the effectiveness of the superficial buffer to sequester Ca during a subsequent period of stimulated Ca influx [16, 17].

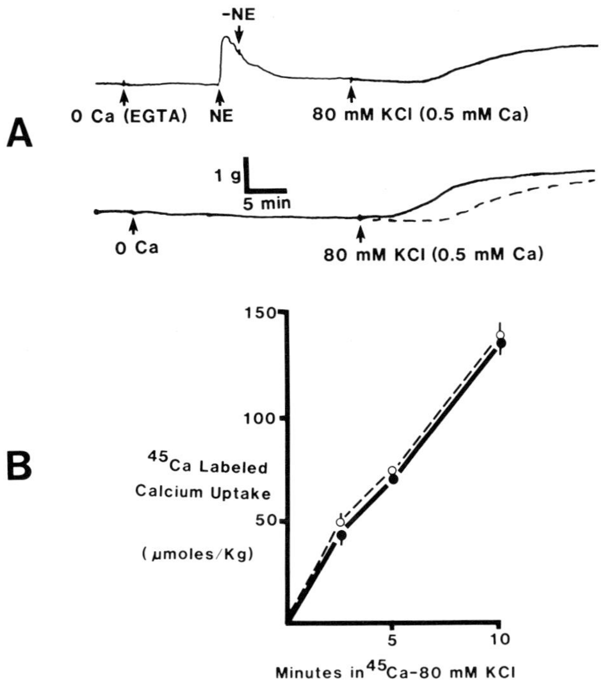

Fig. 8. A Isometric tension is recorded during intracellular Ca release by a 3 minute NE application in Ca Free PSS and the subsequent addition of 0.5 mM Ca in 80 mM K^+ PSS. The *lower tracing* shows the same high K^+ contracture without prior intracellular Ca release. **B** The ^{45}Ca uptakes during the high K applications in A are measured as a function of time in ^{45} Ca labelled 0.5 mM Ca, 80 mM K Cl PSS. The *dotted line* is with prior depletion of NE sensitive intracellular Ca and the *solid line* without such prior depletion of the intracellular Ca^{2+} store

Figure 8 shows an experiment of this nature. First Ca is removed and 2 mM EGTA added to lower the the $[Ca^{2+}]_e$ to 10^{-9} M. During this Ca free incubation, the agonist sensitive Ca store is discharged by a 2 min exposure to 10^{-5} M NE. After the NE is washed out, Ca influx is stimulated by 80 mM K PSS containing 0.5 mM Ca^{2+}. The upper record in Fig. 8 A shows that this pretreatment causes a long delay after stimulation followed by a slow contraction. The lower tracing of Fig. 8 A demonstrates a shorter delay and more rapid contraction if the agonist senistive Ca pool was not depleted. The difference between these two curves must be due to the increased Ca uptake by the superficial buffer since there is no difference in the rates of Ca entry into the cells as seen in Fig. 8 B. Figure 9 shows that NE does not exhibit the same delay in force development as high K^+ even after depletion of the agonist releasable pool. If the agonist releasable pool is not depleted, a biphasic contraction is seen upon simultaneous administration of NE and the repletion of Ca^{2+} to the external medium. A final piece of evidence supporting the concept that the "buffer barrier" is identical with the agonist releasable Ca pool is shown in Fig. 10. The inset shows the protocol used; first the agonist releasable pool is depleted by a short NE exposure in Ca free (2 mM EGTA)

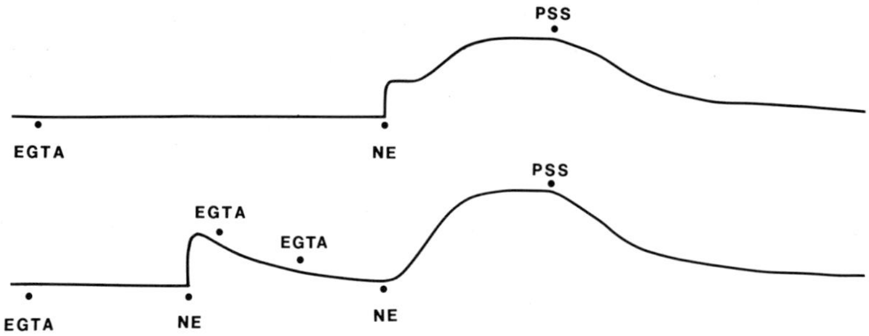

Fig. 9. Contractions induced by 10^{-5} mM NE in PSS following 15 minutes Ca free exposure with (*lower*) and without (*upper*) prior depletion of the NE sensitive intracellular Ca store

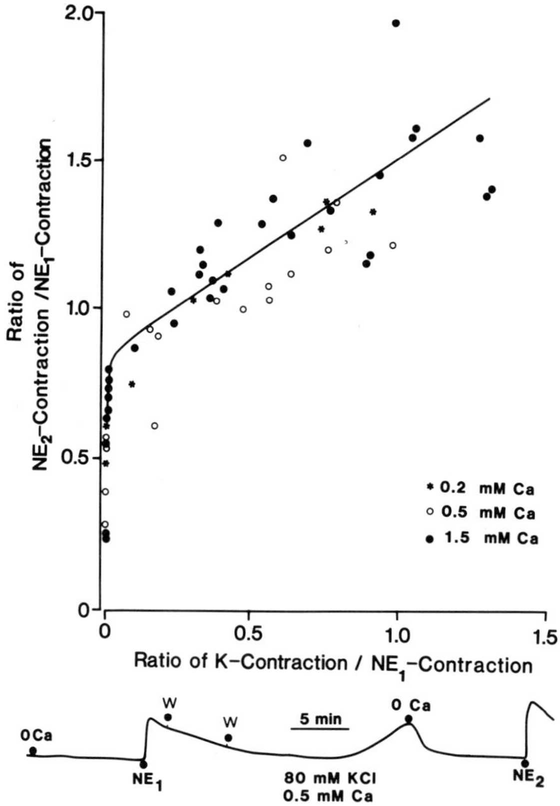

Fig. 10. The *inset* shows the protocol used; first the agonist releasable pool is depleted by a short NE exposure in Ca free (2 mM EGTA) PSS. The resulting contraction is arbitrarily set at 1 on the ordinate. The pool is then reloaded in a low Ca^{2+}, high K solution for varying times. The magnitude of the contraction seen during reloading relative to that of the first NE release contraction is indicated on the abcissa. Subsequent to the reloading of the agonist releasable pool with Ca^{2+} during high K^+ exposure the aortic ring is returned to Ca free PSS. After five minutes in this solution, NE is applied to test the extent to which the agonist releasable pool has refilled. The magnitude of this contraction relative to the initial reference Ca free NE contraction is given on the *ordinate*

PSS. The resulting contraction is arbitrarily set at 1 on the ordinate. The pool is then reloaded in a low Ca^{2+}, high K solution. The magnitude of the contraction seen during reloading relative to that of the first NE release contraction is indicated on the abcissa. Subsequent to the reloading of the agonist releasable pool with Ca^{2+} during high K^+ exposure the aortic ring is returned to Ca free PSS. After five minutes in this solution, NE is applied to test the extent to which the agonist releasable pool has refilled. The magnitude of this contraction relative to the initial reference Ca free NE contraction is given on the ordinate. The striking conclusion derived from this experiments is that the high K induced Ca influx does not lead to force development until the agonist releasable Ca pool is filled to its physiological level. Only after this threshold (where the test NE, Ca free contraction equals the reference NE, Ca free contraction), has been exceeded does the depolarization stimulated Ca^{2+} influx induce tension. These data strongly support the earlier hypothesis [28], that the superficial SR absorbs Ca which has just entered the cell. If the SR is depleted and the Ca entry rate is slow, then it can remove virtually all the Ca before it can bind to calmodulin to activate the myofilaments. A number of authors have argued that NE discharges Ca from the SR [5, 8, 15] and Somlyo and coworkers [6] have recently presented direct evidence, using electron probe analysis, that NE deminishes the Ca content of superficial SR in the portal vein. Synthesizing all this information we postulate the model depicted in Fig. 11.

At rest, Ca^{2+} permeates the plasmalemma at the rate which could lead to full myofilament activation within a period of minutes. The muscle remains in the relaxed state, however, because the Ca pump of the superficial SR removes the Ca from the peripheral cytoplasm. This process sets up a local Ca gradient near the inner membrane surface functioning as a barrier to Ca entry into the bulk of the myoplasm. Activator Ca^{2+} can pass this barrier under two conditions: 1) If the opening of Ca^{2+} channels increases Ca influx to above a certain threshold where it saturates the SR Ca pumps and passes through the superficial buffer barrier, and 2) when activation by NE or other agonists inhibits Ca accumulation by the superficial SR and thus abolishes the peripheral cytoplasmic Ca gradient.

There are several reports in the literature which may be related to the hypothesis of a "regulated buffer barrier". Popescue [23] has shown that oxytocin and prostaglandins can inhibit smooth muscle derived microsomal Ca pumps suggest-

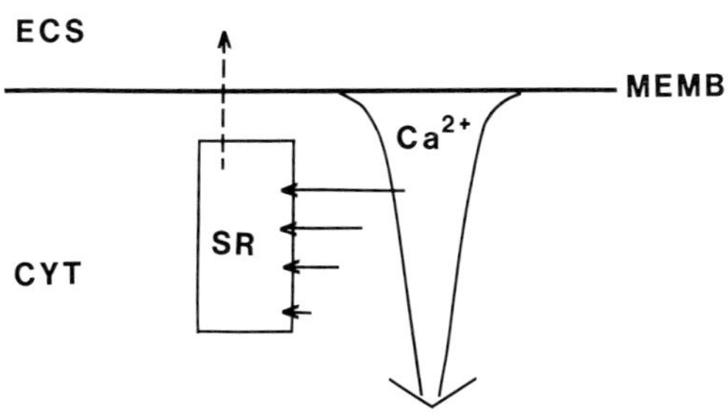

Fig. 11. The "regulated buffer barrier" is depicted in its simplest form. As Ca^{2+} enters the cell its concentration is diminished by active Ca^{2+} transport into the superficial SR thus creating a concentration gradient near the inner plasmalemmal surface. An unspecified transport system transfers SR Ca to the extracellular space (*ECS*). The buffering action of the superficial SR can be inhibited by neurotransmitters and antocoids

ing that a continual discharge of the SR by agonists may be due to inhibition of Ca uptake as well as stimulation of release. The abolition of the peripheral cytoplasmic Ca gradient by NE could also explain, at least partially, the finding by Morgan and Morgan [21] that NE causes more tension per unit of aquorin fluorescence than high K depolarization. In the latter case aquorin might yield an average signal from the peripheral Ca gradient and the bulk of free cytoplasmic Ca. This signal would be greater than during identical contractile activation by NE where the peripheral $[Ca^{2+}]$ would be equal to the bulk cytoplasmic $[Ca^{2+}]$.

In conclusion of this last section, we propose that the superficial SR functions as a "regulated buffer barrier" which modulates the entry of Ca from the extracellular space into the myoplasm of smooth muscle cells.

References

1. Aalkjaer C, Mulvany MJ (1984) Sodium metabolism of rat resistance vessels. J Physiol 343:105–116
2. Aaronson P, Jones A (1983) Effects of forskolin and diltiazem on polyionic fluxes in rabbit arterial smooth muscle. Fed Proc 42:399
3. Aaronson P, van Breemen CA (1981) Effects of sodium gradient manipulation upon cellular calcium ^{45}Ca fluxes and cellular sodium in the guinea-pig taenia coli: J Physiol 319:443–461
4. Bevan JA, Hwa JJ, Owen MP, Winquist RJ (1985) Calcium and myogenic or stretch-dependent vascular tone. In: Rubin RP, Weiss GB, Putney JW jr (eds) Calcium in biological systems. Plenum Press, London, pp 391–398
5. Bolton TB (1979) Mechanisms of action of transmitters and other substances on smooth muscle. Physiol Rev 3:606–718
6. Bond M, Kitazawa T, Somlyo AP, Somlyo AV (1984) Release and recycling of calcium by the sarcoplasmic reticulum in guinea-pig portal vein smooth muscle. J Physiol 355:677–695
7. Cauvin C, Saida K, van Breemen C (1984) Extracellular Ca dependence and diltiazem inhibition of contraction in rabbit conduit arteries and mesenteric resistance vessels. Blood Vessels, 21:23–31
8. Deth R, Casteels R (1977) A study of releasable Ca^{++} fractions in smooth muscle cells of the rabbit aorta. J Gen Physiol 69:401–416
9. Fleckenstein A (1983) Calcium antagonists in heart and smooth muscle. Wiley, New York
10. Godfraind T (1983) Actions of nifedipine on calcium fluxes and contraction in isolated rat arteries. J Pharmacol Exp Ther 224:443–450
11. Godfraind T, Dieu D (1981) The inhibition by flunarizine of the norepineprine-evoked contraction and calcium influx in rat aorta mesenteric arteries. J Pharmacol Exp Ther 217:510–515
12. Hess P, Tsien RW (1984) Mechanisms of ion permeation through calcium channels. Nature (London) 309:453–456
13. Hess P, Lansman, Tsien RW (1984) Different modes of Ca channel gating behavior favoured by dihydropyridine Ca agonists and antagonists. Nature 311:538–544
14. Jones AW (1981) Vascular smooth muscle and alterations during hypertension. In: Bulbring E, Brading AS, Jones AW, Tomita T (eds) Smooth muscle: An assessment of current knowledge. London, pp 397–429
15. Leijten P, van Breemen C (1984) The effects of caffeine on the noradrenaline-sensitive calcium store in the rabbit aorta. J Physiol 357:327–339
16. Loutzenhiser R, van Breemen C (1983) Mechanisms of stimulated Ca^{2+} influx and consequences of Ca^{2+} influx inhibitions. In: Merrill GF, Weiss HR, Scriabine A (eds) Symposium on Ca^{2+} entry blockers, adenosine and neurohumors. Urban & Schwarzenberg, München Wien Baltimore, pp 73–91

17. Loutzenhiser R, van Breemen C (1983) The influence of receptor occupation on Ca^{++} influx-mediated vascular smooth muscle contraction. Circ Res 52 (suppl I): 97–103
18. Mayer CJ, van Breemen C, Casteels R (1972) The action of lanthanum and D 600 on the calcium exchange in the smooth muscle cells of the guinea-pig taenia coli. Pflugers Arch 337:333–350
19. Meisheri K, Hwang O, van Breemen C (1981) Evidence for two separate Ca^{2+} influx pathways in smooth muscle plasmalemma. J Memb Biol 59:19–25
20. Meisheri K, van Breemen C (1982) Effects of β-adrenergic stimulation on calcium movements in rabbit aortic smooth muscle: Relationship with cyclic AMP. J Physiol 331:429–441
21. Morgan JP, Morgan KG (1984) Stimulus specific patterns of intra cellular calcium levels in smooth muscle of ferret protal vein. J Physiol 351:164–167
22. Petersen TT, Mulvany MJ (1984) Effect of sodium gradient on the rate of relaxation of rat mesenteric small arteries from potassium contractures. Blood Vessels 21:279–289
23. Popescu LM, Panoiu C, Foril CP, Hinescu M, Nutu O (to be published) Ca^{++}-pumping ATPase of the smooth muscle cell membrane jis a molecular target for hormones and drugs. In: Mirroneau J (ed) Calcium regulation in smooth muscles. INSERM Series, Proc of the Internat Symposium, Bordeaux, July 25–27, 1984
24. Rosenberger LB, Ticlen MK, Triggle DJ (1979) The effects of Ca^{2+}-antagonists on mechanical responses and Ca^{2+} movements in guinea pig ileal longitudinal smooth muscle. Can J Pharmacol 57:333–347
25. Scheid CR, Fay FS (1984) Transmembrane ^{45}Ca fluxes in isolated smooth muscle cells: basal Ca^{2+} fluxes. Am J Physiol 246:C422–C430
26. Schramm M, Thomas G, Towart R, Tranckowiak G (1983) Novel dihydropyridines with positive inotropic action through activation of Ca^{2+} channels. Nature 303:535
27. Somlyo AP, Somlyo AV (1968) Vascular smooth muscle I, normal structure pathology, biochemistry and biophysics. Pharmacol Ref 200:197–272
28. van Breemen (1977) Calcium requirement for activation of intact aortic smooth muscle. J Physiol 272:317–329
29. van Breemen C, Aaronson P, Loutzenhiser R (1979) Sodium-calcium interactions in mammalian smooth muscle. Pharmac Reviews 30:167–208
30. van Breemen C, Farinas BR, Gerba P, McNaughton ED (1972) Excitation-contraction coupling in rabbit aorta studied by the lanthanum method for measuring cellular calcium influx. Circ Res 30:44–54
31. van Breemen C, Hwang O, Meisheri, KD (1981) The mechanism of inhibitory action of diltiazem on vascular smooth muscle contractility. J Pharmacol Exp Ther 218:459–463
32. Yamamoto H, Kanaide H, Nakamura M (1983) Metabolism of glycosaminoglycons of cultured aortic smooth muscle cells altered during subculture. Br J Exp Path 64:156–165
33. Yamamoto H, Hwang O, van Breemen C (1984) Bay K 8644 differentiates between potential and receptor operated Ca^{2+} channels. Eur J Pharmacol 102:555–557

Discussion

(pp. 58–71)

Krebs: A basis for your conclusion is the specific release of Ca^{2+} from the sarcoplasmic reticulum by caffeine. Are there results showing that caffeine produces just a release of Ca^{2+} from its intracellular stores and not form its membranes binding sites?

Van Breemen: We have no evidence for that. It may also release calcium from the internal surface of the cells. However, in the partially skinned cells, where we have left the SR membranes intact, but the surface membrane is permeabilized, norepinephrine is not able to release any calcium anymore. In that situation we have seen mainly release from the SR. Of course, caffeine can release calcium from that system.

Schwartz: Is anything known about the presence of intracellular sites such as an endo- or sarcoplasmic reticulum in other vascular smooth muscle, particularly the coronaries? How would that influence your concept?

Van Breemen: Of course, the rabbit aorta is a very unimportant target of the calcium antagonists, so a lot of people are investigating coronary arteries, cerebral arteries etc. And there we have a great deal of species variability. The dog coronary arteries, in which the intracellular releasable calcium is almost absent are therefore very sensitive to the calcium antagonist, even if you stimulate them with norepinephrine. But some work by Ginsburg and Godfraind indicates that human coronary arteries have intracellular calcium that can be released by histamine and norepinephrine. Therefore it depends on the mode of activation: for example, electrical stimulation or ergonovine is mainly stimulating calcium entry, whereas histamine or norepinephrine will also cause a lot of calcium release.

Schramm: Dr. Fleckenstein explained that Bay K 8644 creates additional calcium leaks. It is difficult to understand it from the data shown by Dr. Hess. Does it create additional leaks?

Fleckenstein: I regret having used the work leak; calcium entry is activated.

Nayler: How much of passive calcium entry which is lanthanum sensitive is due to sodium-calcium exchange?

Van Breemen: In smooth muscle in general, there is much less sodium-calcium exchange than in heart. In the rabbit aorta it is almost absent.

Nayler: I am intrigued that you can put EDTA onto these membranes and they don't fall apart, because cardiac muscle does that. Do you know of any condition in which that passive leak can be greatly increased?

Van Breemen: I did not show you any measurements of the leak during the EGTA applications, which is of course an impossibility. But if we restore the calcium immediately after the EGTA treatment, for the minute following that, the leak is greatly enhanced, but then soon the membrane reseals and you get normal permeability back. This augmented leak is not very sensitive to calcium antagonists.

Kadowitz: Have you distinguished between alpha-1 and postsynaptic alpha-2 mechanisms with this norepinephrine-type activation or blockade?

Van Breemen: Yes, especially Dr. Cauvin in our laboratory has done a number of experiments on that, and we can say for sure that alpha-1 stimulation both releases calcium and opens up calcium channels. So the hypothesis that alpha-1 only releases Ca^{2+} and alpha-2 stimulation only opens channels is not correct.

Fleckenstein: I am very grateful for your clear statement. The main effect of all calcium antagonists including diltiazem is the inhibition of calcium entry. From our analyses we can conclude that there is no stimulation of calcium efflux by diltiazem as reported by Zellis and Flaim. These authors reported that there is an increase in oxygen uptake under the influence of diltiazem. If in our experiments the coronary artery relaxes under the influence of diltiazem, the oxygen consumption decreases, because the smooth muscle cell is inactivated by the calcium antagonist.

Bayer-Symposium IX
Cardiovascular Effects of Dihydropyridine-Type
Calcium Antagonists and Agonists, 74–87

Calcium Currents in Mammalian Central Neurones

D. A. Brown, R. J. Docherty, B. H. Gahwiler, and J. V. Halliwell

Introduction

Voltage-activated Ca-currents (I_{Ca}) are present in most neurones (Hagiwara and Byerly 1981; Kostyuk 1981). This article concerns the Ca-currents observed in mammalian central neurones. Their properties have been inferred from a variety of Ca-dependent voltage-transients (reviewed by Llinas and Walton 1980); and Ca-currents have been recorded directly in voltage-clamp experiments on spinal motoneurones (Schwindt and Crill 1980a, b), in hippocampal pyramidal cells (Johnston et al. 1980; Brown and Griffith 1983b; Halliwell 1983) and in olfactory cortex neurons (A. Constanti and M. Galvan, unpublished observations).

These Ca-currents probably subserve a variety of functions. *Firstly*, and ubiquitously, Ca-currents in axon terminals trigger the release of neurotransmitters and neurohormones. *Secondly*, all-or-none Ca-*spikes* may subserve a signalling function akin to the Na-spike, particularly in the long dendritic trees of neurones such as cerebellar Purkinjie cells (Llinas and Sugimori 1980) and hippocampal pyramidal cells (Wong et al. 1979; Benardo et al. 1982). (One might speculate that the advantage of a Ca-spike for this purpose could be its slower conduction velocity, allowing more effective integration of dendritic synaptic stimulation – rather akin to the function of the Ca-spike in cardiac conducting tissue.) *Thirdly*, Ca-currents appear to exert an important influence on the individual "behaviour" patterns of different neurone types. This influence may be exerted *directly*, through the depolarizing effect of the inward Ca-current in (e.g.) initiating pacemaker depolarizations required for repetitive firing (e.g. Llinas and Yarom 1981) or slow depolarizing envelopes yielding (burst) firing (e.g. Schwartzkroin 1980; Schwindt and Crill 1980a) or *indirectly*, through the activation of other ionic currents by raised intracellular Ca. Two species of Ca-activated ionic currents have so far been recorded in mammalian central neurones – K-currents (Barrett et al. 1980; Brown and Griffith 1983a; Lancaster and Adams 1984) and Cl-current (Owen et al. 1984) – but others may be anticipated from studies on other tissues (e.g. Colquhoun et al. 1980). It seems clear, therefore, that a knowledge of the physiological and pharmacological properties of Ca-currents in central neurones may provide considerable information about the control of neuronal behaviour. In this paper an attempt is made to assess the current state of knowledge regarding Ca-currents in mammalian brain cells, with particular reference to hippocampal neurones.

I_{Ca} In Hippocampal Neurones

The presence of a voltage-activated Ca-current in hippocampal neurones was first inferred from the observation that, in TTX-solution, all-or-nothing slow spikes could still be evoked by intracellular current which were inhibited by Mn (Schwartzkroin and Slawsky 1977). In addition to single Ca-spikes, neurones in the CA_3-region show grouped spikes superimposed on a slow depolarizing "envelope" ("burst-firing": Kandel and Spencer 1961). This burst-firing is also blocked by Mn, suggesting that the depolarizing envelope also depends on an inward Ca-current (Wong and Prince 1978). A similar burst-firing pattern has been recorded in the dendrites of both CA_3 neurones and their follower CA_1 neurones (Wong et al. 1979). CA_1 neurones do not normally show burst-firing, but can be induced to do so if outward currents are inhibited by (e.g.) tetraethylammonium (Schwartzkroin and Prince 1980) or acetylcholine (Benardo and Prince 1981), and respond to synaptic activation by burst-firing if recurrent inhibition is inhibited (Wong and Prince 1979). Thus, Ca-currents appear to be responsible for two potentials in hippocampal neurones – individual Ca-spikes and slow depolarizations – both of importance to the characteristic "behaviour" of the neurones.

Persistent Ca-Current

Johnston et al. (1980) first recorded an inward Ca-current in voltage-clamped hippocampal CA_3-neurones in vitro using intracellular Cs to suppress outward currents. This appeared as a slow (50–100 msec) inward current at membrane potentials positive to -45 mV. The current was resistant to TTX, intensified by Ba and blocked by Co. Brown and Griffith (1983 b) confirmed that such a current could be recorded from both CA_1 and CA_3 neurones when outward currents were reduced with TEA. Under these conditions both CA_1 and CA_3 neurones generated TTX-resistant action potentials; application of voltage-clamp revealed a region of net inward current at membrane potentials positive to -40 mV which was again augmented by Ba and reduced by omitting Ca or by adding 200 μM Cd or 100 μM verapamil.

The most interesting feature of this inward Ca-current is its prolonged duration. Currents remained net inward after 0.5 s depolarization, and evidence was presented to suggest that the current does not completely inactivate over very much longer periods, but remains to contribute a steady inward component to the total membrane current at potentials down to at least -50 mV (Brown and Griffith 1983 b). Both Johnston et al. (1980) and Brown and Griffith (1983 b) suggested that this slow inward current might be responsible for the depolarizing envelope underlying the burst discharge. Since the slow inward current did not show clear inactivation over the time-scale of the burst-duration (< 0.1 s), it was further suggested that termination of the burst depended on the generation of a Ca-activated outward K-current: a slowly-developing Ca-dependent and TEA-sensitive outward current has been recorded in these neurones (Brown and Griffith 1983 a).

One objection to this hypothesis for the generation of the burst-envelope was that, although the slow inward current induced a region of diminished or negative slope to the current-voltage curve, in the absence of TEA it was rarely, and at most transiently, *net* inward (see, for example, Fig. 1 of Brown and Griffith (1983 a). Recent studies suggest that this may be a function of temperature, since a true net inward current can be detected in cells bathed in normal Ca-solution without added TEA on warming to 35 °C (Brown et al. 1984).

Transient Ca-Currents

Because of clamp-limitations, the kinetics of the slow inward current described by Johnston et al. (1980) and Brown and Griffith (1983 b) could not be pursued into depolarized ranges where strong Ca-spiking occured, so it was unclear whether this slow inward current accelerated sufficiently to generate the Ca-spike, or whether this involved another Ca-current. Traub (1982) has successfully modelled both burst and spike using a single set of kinetic parameters, by incorporating partial inactivation. On the other hand, Brown and Griffith (1983 b) argued in favour of a second spike-current on the grounds that spiking could be inactivated by a depolarizing prepulse which did not reduce the slow inward current (see also Eckert and Lux 1976 for a comparable case in molluscan neurones). Recent recordings in Cs-filled tissue-cultured hippocampal cells have revealed an early, transient component to the slow inward current activated at fairly positive potentials (< −35 mV; Gahwiler and Brown 1985), though again compromised by space-clamp limitations. Likewise, Constanti and Brown (see Brown et al. 1984) have recorded a high-thresold (< −40 mV) inactivating component of inward current in Cs-filled olfactory cortex neurones, of sufficiently rapid kinetics to form the basis for a high-threshold Ca-spike.

Halliwell (1983) has reported a rather different form of transient current in Cs-filled hippocampal neurones, which is activated at a 10–20 mV *lower* threshold than the slow inward current when primed by a short (1 sec) hyperpolarizing prepulse to −70 mV or beyond (Fig. 1).

This current is resistant to TTX but depressed in a Ca-free solution or by 200 μM Cd, so is either a Ca-current or an inward current triggered by Ca-entry. This type of current appears to behave rather like the low-threshold Ca-conductances described by Llinas and Yarom (1981 a) in inferior olivary neurones and by Deschennes et al. (1982) in thalamic neurones, in generating a rebound depolarization (with superimposed Na-spike in the absence of TTX) after a hyperpolarizing current injection: it may therefore provide the initial trigger for the hippocampal burst potential.

The characterization of these hippocampal Ca-currents is, at present, very incomplete – partly because of the limited performance of the single-microelectrode

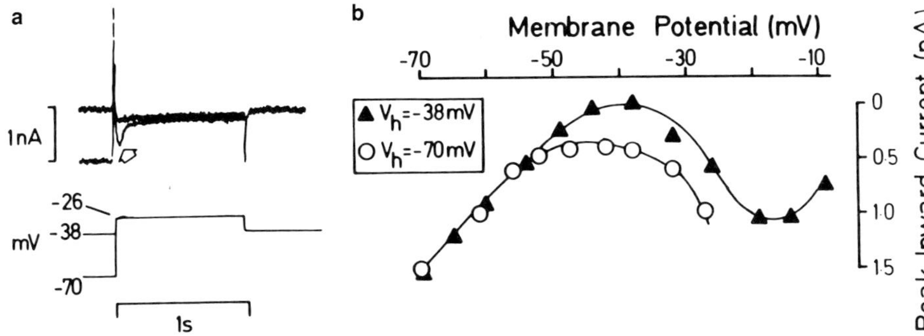

Fig. 1 a, b. Two TTX-insensitive inward currents in a Cs-loadad hippocampal neurone. **a** shows supperimposed membrane currents (*upper record*) induced by depolarizing voltage steps (*lower records*) to −26 mV from prepotentials of −70 mV and −38 mV. The step from −38 mV elicited a sustained inward current lasting for the 1 s step duration (see Brown and Griffith 1983b). The step from −70 mV elicited an initial transient current (*arrowed*) superimposed on the sustained current. The graphs in **b** show peak inward current plotted against command potential for 1 s voltage steps from −70 mV (○) and −38 mV (▲). (Guinea-pig CA_1 neurone impaled with a 3 M CsCl-filled microelectrode and bathed in Krebs' solution containing, *inter alia*, 0.5 µM TTX and 3 mM CsCl, to suppress I_Q. See Halliwell and Adams 1982, and Halliwell 1983 for technical details

voltage clamp technique used in these experiments (exacerbated by the need to use high resistance microelectrodes to minimize cell damage), and partly because of uncertainties regarding the adequacy of the space clamp. Although hippocampal neurones appear reasonably compact electronically (Brown et al. 1980; Turner and Schwartzkroin 1981), the fact that the Ca-current is strongly developed in the dendrites (Wong et al. 1979) places more stringent demands on the space-clamp than can probably be met in practice. Because of possible potential inhomogeneity, measured values of voltage-threshold at the soma may be appreciably in error, particularly for the faster currents. Nevertheless, the impression gained from these experiments of at least two species of Ca-current – one sustained and one of lower somatic threshold which more rapidly inactivates – accords with current information gained from more precise recording techniques in cultured dorsal root ganglion cells (Carbonne and Lux 1984; Nowycky et al. 1984).

Other Membrane Currents in Hippocampal Neurones

The role of hippocampal Ca-currents cannot be assessed in isolation from other membrane currents. Currents so far recorded under voltage-clamp, or known to be present on other criteria include the following (see Table 1):

(1) A fast, Na-current responsible for TTX-sensitive spikes has been recorded in cultured cells (Segal and Barker 1984).

(2) A rather slow K-current resembling a delayed-rectifier current has also been recorded, which appears not to be activated by the Ca-current(s) (Segal and Barker 1984).

Table 1. Hippocampal currents recorded under voltage-clamp

Current	Symbol	Blocked by	Reference
Na-current	I_{Na}	TTX	Segal and Barker (1984)
Persistent Ca-current	$I_{Ca(1)}$	Cd, Mn	Johnston et al. (1980), Brown and Griffith (1983)
Transient, low threshold Ca-current	$I_{Ca(2)}$	Cd	Halliwell (1983)
Sustained delayed rectifier K-current	I_K	TEA	Segal and Barker (1984)
Transient K-current	I_A	4-AP	Gustafsson et al. (1982), Segal and Brown (1984)
Slow, sustained subthreshold K-current	I_M	Acetylcholine Ba	Halliwell and Adams (1982)
Fast, V-sensitive Ca-activated K-current	I_c	TEA	Brown and Griffith (1983)
Slow, V-insensitive Ca-activated K-current	I_{AHP}	Acetylcholine Noradrenaline	Lancaster and Adams (1984)
Inward rectifier current activated by hyper-polarization	I_Q	Cs (external)	Halliwell and Adams (1982)

(3) A very rapidly-activating (<5 ms) transient K-current (Gustafsson et al. 1982; Segal and Barker 1984) resembles the molluscan A-current, I_A (cf. Neher 1971; Connor and Stevens 1971). This current is both activated and then inactivated at membrane potentials positive to -60 mV, so does not contribute a major steady component of membrane current; inactivation can be progressively removed by hyperpolarizing prepules negative to -60 mV, to an extent depending on both the magnitude and duration of the hyperpolarizing prepulse. I_A is blocked by 4-aminopyridine at 10–100 µM (Gustafsson et al. 1982) and also by a snake venom, dendrotoxin at 0.3 µM (Dolly et al. 1984). It is resistant to TEA. I_A exerts a very distinctive effect on the voltage trajectory following the injection of depolarizing current at membrane potentials negative to -60 mV, delaying the first spike.

(4) A slow sustained K-current, I_M, activates positive to -70 mV (i.e. below the threshold for the Na-spike) (Halliwell and Adams 1982). This current is analogous to that previously described in sympathetic neurones (Brown and Adams 1980; Constanti and Brown 1981). It persists after inhibiting I_{Ca} with Cd, so appears not to be primed by Ca-entry. It is characteristically inhibited by muscarinic (atropine-sensitive) acetylcholine-receptor agonists, and also by Ba (Adams et al. 1981; Halliwell and Adams 1982). Inhibition by Ba persists in Cd-solution, so is probably exerted externally (Gahwiler and Brown, unpublished observations). I_M is relatively insensitive to 4-AP and TEA. I_M plays a role in spike adaptation (Madison and Nicoll 1984). Also, since inhibition of I_M by acetylcholine leads to membrane depolarization and "burst-firing" (Dodd et al. 1980; Benardo and Prince 1981; Gahwiler and Dreifuss 1982), I_M appears to exert a considerable stabilizing effect on these cells.

(5) A large Ca-activated K-current I_c (Brown and Griffith 1983 a) is activated above the threshold for I_{Ca} (at about -30 mV), rapidly abbreviating the inward current during a depolarizing command. On repolarization to rest potential I_c is deactivated with a time-constant of <100 ms at room temperature. I_c is readily blocked by TEA at 1–5 mM but not by 4-AP or acetylcholine. Since TEA greatly prolongs Ca-spikes and induces or accelerates burst-firing, I_c probably plays a major role in the termination of both the Ca-spike and the burst-envelope.

(6) A second, smaller but more sustained Ca-dependent K-current, I_{AHP} has recently been described (Lancaster and Adams 1984). Unlike I_c, I_{AHP} persists for hundreds of msec at hyperpolarized potential and appears to be responsible for the long after-hyperpolarization following an action potential and for the late phase of the post-burst hyperpolarization. It probably also assists in slow spike adaptation (Madison and Nicoll, 1984). I_{AHP} is relatively insensitive to TEA, but is blocked by Cd (which inhibits the primary Ca-current) and is exquisitely sensitive to muscarinic agonists (Cole and Nicoll 1984; Lancaster and Adams 1984). It also appears to be inhibited by some other putative neurotransmitters such as noradrenaline (Madison and Nicoll 1982; Haas and Konnerth 1983) and histamine (Haas and Konnerth 1983).

(7) A slow inward rectifier current I_Q is activated by hyperpolarization beyond -70 mV (Halliwell and Adams 1982; see also Segal and Barker 1984). This current accounts for one form of "anomalous rectification" in hippocampal neurones, in which electrotonic potentials generated by hyperpolarizing current injections show a secondary depolarizing sag, giving an apparent fall in membrane resistance (Purpura et al. 1968).

The magnitude and significance of these different currents appears to vary with cell types and with experimental conditions. For example, no Ca or Ca-activated currents were detected in dissociated hippocampal cultures (Segal and Barker 1984) but are strongly developed in organotypic culture (Gahwiler and Brown, unpublished; cf. Gahwiler 1981).

Some indication of how the interplay of some to these currents might affect neuronal behaviour is provided by the control of *endogenous burst-firing* behaviour. The usually postulated mechanism of endogenous burst-firing is that of a time-sequential interplay of inward Ca and outward Ca-activated K-currents (Schwartzkroin 1980; Hotson and Prince 1981; Traub 1982; Wong et al. 1984; Johnston and Brown 1984). It is envisaged that inward Ca-current(s) generate a slow depolarization, which initially triggers a few Na-spikes. As these inactivate, slow, high-threshold Ca-spikes appear. The event is then terminated by the activation of Ca-dependent K-currents by the Ca-entry. The immediately-terminating current is probably the large, voltage-dependent outward current I_c, but the subsequent hyperpolarization may be maintained (and interburst interval determined) by the slower Ca-activated current I_{AHP}. Burst-potentiality is very susceptible to a change in the balance between inward and outward currents, including other "background" currents not directly involved in the burst-process itself. Thus, burst-firing in otherwise quiescent neurones can be induced by reducing the amplitude of the repolarizing Ca-activated K-currents with TEA (Schwartzkroin and Prince 1981) or Cs-injections (Hablitz and Johnston 1981); by increasing the inward current amplitude with Ba (Hotson and Prince 1981; Hablitz and

Johnston 1981) (Ba also reduces outward currents); by acetylcholine, which reduces the amplitude of the "background" outward current I_M and the slow Ca-activated hyperpolarizing current, I_{AHP} (see above); or simply by raising external K^+ which reduces the driving force for all outward currents (Ogata et al. 1976; Prince 1978).

The endogenous burst-firing potentiality of hippocampal pyramidal cells – particularly of the "pacemaker" cells in area CA_3 – plays an important part in the spread of epileptiform seizure activity within the hippocampus and may be analogous to seizure-generating mechanisms in human brain (Prince 1983; Wong et al. 1984). For this reason, if for no other, some knowledge of the pharmacological properties of hippocampal Ca-currents might be useful.

Pharmacology of Hippocampal Ca-Currents

1. Divalent Cations. The slow inward Ca-current in hippocampal neurones resembles those recorded in peripheral neurones and heart in their sensitivity to divalent cations. Thus, Johnston et al. (1980) showed that I_{Ca} in guinea-pig CA_3 neurones was blocked by Co applied as a 10 mM "drop" via a coarse micropipette. Brown and Griffith (1983 b) further showed that the same current was almost eliminated by adding 200 µM Cd to the bath perfusion fluid. Recent tests on rat CA_3 cells in organotypic slice-cultures indicate that the sensitivity of this current to Cd under perfusion conditions allowing rapid diffusion (cf. Gahwiler 1981) may be quite close to that of the cardiac slow I_{Ca} (Lee and Tsien 1983), in that substantial block occurred at Cd concentrations down to 10 µM (Gahwiler and Brown, unpublished data). Conversely, the hippocampal I_{Ca} is strongly potentiated by Ba (Johnston et al. 1980; Brown and Griffith 1983 b). This seems unlikely to be due to added depression of residual outward current, since potentiation is seen in the presence of both intracellular Cs and extracellular TEA; nor can it necessarily be ascribed to loss of Ca-induced I_{Ca}-inactivation (cf. Tillotson 1979). As in other cells (Hagiwara and Byerly 1981) it seems likely that Ba is a more efficient charge carrier than Ca. Thus, although present information is admittedly limited, it does not suggest any unique property of the slow inward Ca-current in hippocampal neurones in respect of ionic affinities. Halliwell (1983) reports that the *transient* current is also sensitive to Cd at 200 µM, though a precise comparison of the sensitivities of the transient and sustained currents to Cd at similar activation voltages has not yet been completed.

2. Organic Ca-Antagonists. Brown and Griffith (1983 b) reported that 100 µM verapamil strongly reduced the slow inward current in guinea-pig hippocampal neurones. Although this is similar to the concentrations required to block Ca-uptake into brain synaptosomes, or Ca-currents in invertebrate neurones, this does not argue for any particular sensitivity of hippocampal Ca-channels to organic Ca-antagonists since such concentration can also affect Na-channels (see Miller and Freedman 1984, for review). More recently, however, Brown et al. (1984) have obtained evidence that the slow Ca-current in hippocampal neurones approaches that of cardiac cells in its sensitivity to dihydropyridine compounds.

Thus, *nimodipine* produced substantial (50%) block of the slow inward current at 1 μM and 80% block at 2 μM (see Fig. 2a). B. H. Gahwiler (unpublished observations) has also observed a substantial and reversible depression of I_{Ca} in hippocampal neurones in culture by nifedipine at concentrations of 0.1 to 1 μM. Conversely, the "Ca-agonist", *Bay K 8644*, was capable of augmenting the slow Ca-current at 5 μM, although rather erratically (Fig. 2b). These effects on macroscopic Ca-currents in hippocampal cells appear broadly comparable to those analysed in more detail in cultured chick dorsal root ganglia cells (Fox, Nowycky and Tsien 1984; see also P. Hess et al., this volume). Thus far, we have not detected any gross difference in the sensitivities of the persistent and transient components of the hippocampal Ca-currents to the dihydropyridines.

Dihydropyridine-sensitive Ca-channels also appear to be present in the *terminals* of hippocampal neurones, since nimodipine (2 μM) rapidly and reversibly depresses transmission from the Schaffer collateral axons of CA_3 neurones onto CA_1 neurones (Fig. 3). This is probably due to an effect of nimodipine on Ca-dependent release processes since conduction in the Schaffer collaterals themselves was unimpaired.

In one sense, the sensitivity of these neurones to the dihydropyridine compounds might not be that unexpected, since brain tissue, including the hippocampus (Cortes et. al. 1983) contains an abundance of dihydropyridine binding sites (e.g. Glossmann et al. 1982, Bellemann et al. 1983; Curtis and Catterall 1983). There remains the question of the 1,000-fold difference in affinities measured by radioligand binding and Ca-current inhibition: interestingly, this difference seems not to occur in clonal cell lines (Toll 1982; Freedman et al. 1984) when Ca-current inhibition is assessed by K-stimulated ^{45}Ca-uptake.

3. Neurotransmitters. Several neurotransmitters or putative neurotransmitters have been reported to reduce Ca-dependent potentials in hippocampal neurones. These include noradrenaline (via β-receptors) (Madison and Nicoll 1982; Haas and Konnerth 1983), acetylcholine (Cole and Nicoll 1984), histamine (Haas and Konnerth 1983), CRF (Aldenhoff et al. 1983) and adenosine (Proctor and Dunwiddie 1983). We have tested the effects of several of these agents (noradrenaline, acetylcholine and adenosine) on the slow Ca-currents in voltage-clamped, Cs-filled hippocampal neurones but have not observed a consistent depression of I_{Ca} under these conditions (Halliwell and Scholfield 1984a, b; Brown and Griffith, unpublished; Brown and Gahwiler, unpublished). We therefore suppose – in agreement with Madison and Nicoll (1982), Haas and Konnerth (1983) and Cole and Nicoll (1984) – that the depression of such Ca-dependent phenomena as spike after-hyperpolarization produced by these compounds occurs at a step beyond the priming Ca-entry.

In this respect, hippocampal neurones appear to differ from certain peripheral neurones such as sympathetic and sensory ganglion cells where noradrenaline and adenosine have been observed to affect the Ca-current itself (e.g. Dunlap and Fischbach 1981; Galvan and Adams 1982; Henon and McAfee 1984). Some observations on peripheral neurones also suggest that another substance which might inhibit Ca-currents is GABA, acting via the bicuculline-insensitive $GABA_B$-receptor (Dunlap 1981; Cherubini and North 1984; but see Schlichter et

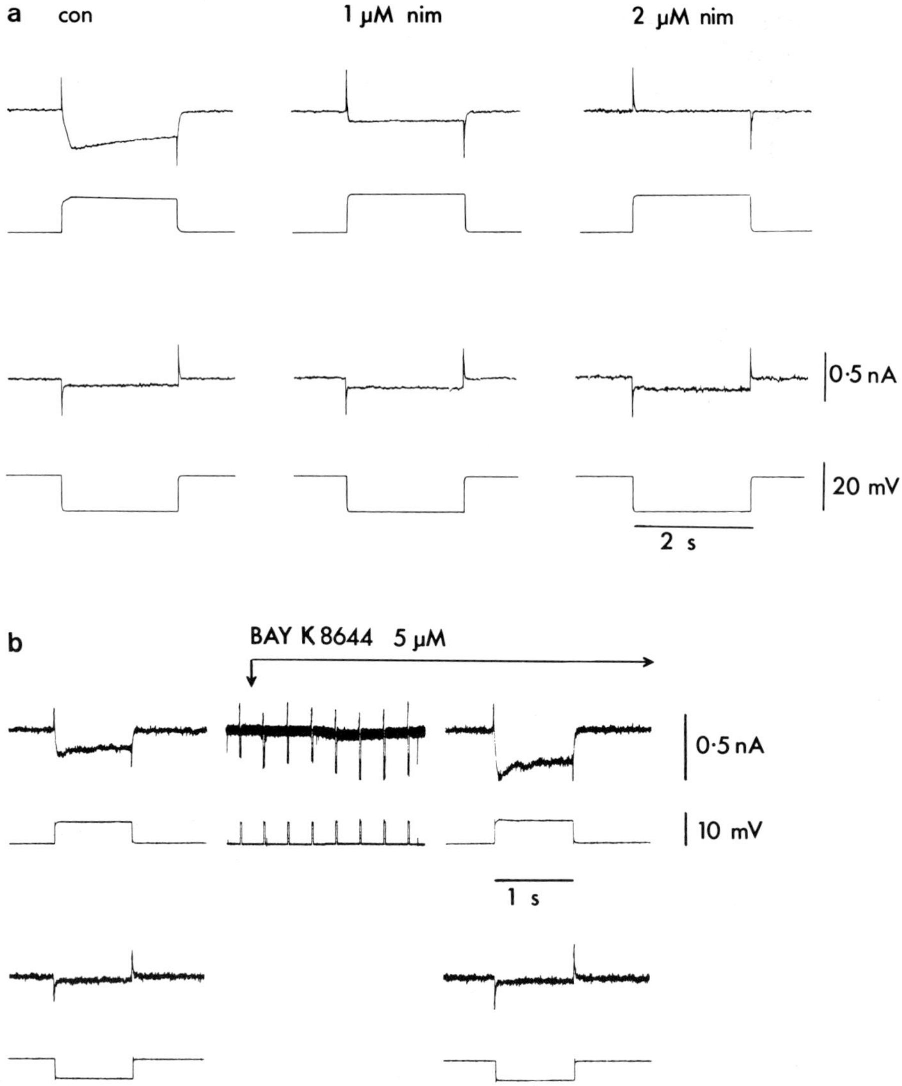

Fig. 2. Effects of **a** nimodipine (*nim*) and **b** bay K 8644 on inward currents recorded from two different Cs-loaded guinea-pig hippocampal Ca_1-neurones. Records show current responses to depolarizing (*upper pair*) and hyperpolarizing (*lower pair*) voltage commands from a holding potential of −42 mV. *Upper records*, current; *lower records*, voltage. Adapted with permission of Macmillan Press from Brown et al. (1984 q.v. for technical details)

al. 1984 for a contrary view). We have tested GABA and its $GABA_B$-selective analogue, baclofen, on I_{Ca} in hippocampal neurones, and find no evidence for a direct effect on I_{Ca}; instead – and in agreement with Newberry and Nicoll (1984) – we find these compounds generate a Ca-independent outward K-current (Gahwiler and Brown 1984).

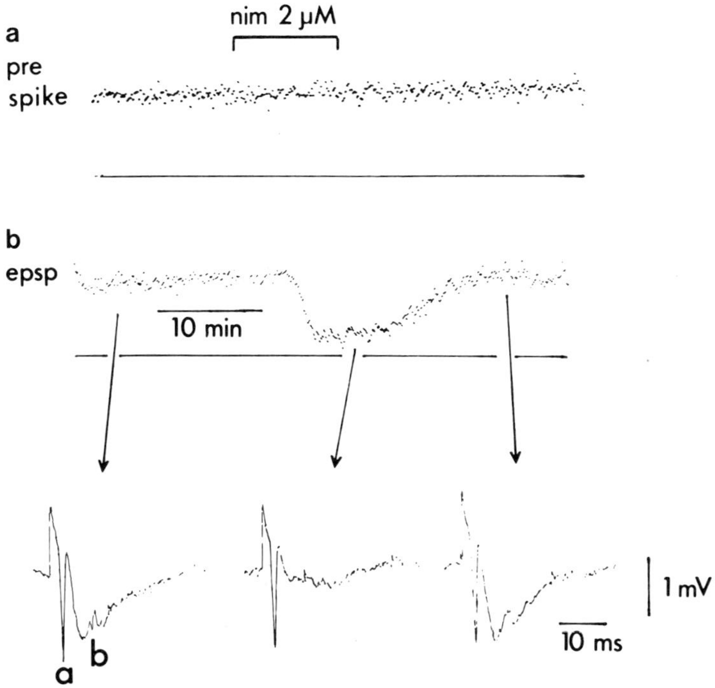

Fig. 3a, b. Effect of nimodipine (*nim*) on transmission from CA_1 and to CA_3 regions in the isolated rat hippocampus preparation. Lower records show extracellular field potentials recorded from the Ca_1 region with a glass microelectrode following single shocks to the Schaffer collaterals. **a** and **b** are the presynaptic volley and postsynaptic excitatory potential respectively. The peak amplitude of these two potentials are plotted on a continuous time-base in the upper records: continuous lines are baselines. Note that nimodipine (2 μM) strongly and reversibly depressed the postsynaptic potential without affecting the presynaptic spike

Conclusions

Even though Ca-currents in hippocampal neurones have been studied to a greater extent than those in any other central neurones, information is still rudimentary when compared with that now available for (e.g.) cardiac cells (see Reuter 1983) or even peripheral mammalian neurones (Kostyuk et al. 1981; Nowycky et al. 1984; Fox et al. 1984). Appropriate voltage-clamp experiments on intact hippocampal neurones, even in slice preparations, are not simple either in execution or interpretation, so progress is likely to remain slow unless new experimental approaches become feasible. Possibilities would include the application of patch-clamp or whole-cell clamp to dispersed or tissue-cultured neurones (e.g. Bormann et al. 1983; Numann and Wong 1984) or incorporation of hippocampal cell membrane vesicles into lipid membranes (Nelson et al. 1984). Nevertheless, it is always necessary to keep in mind the function which these currents play in the behaviour of the intact cell, for which experiments on single cells in organized systems will continue to be necessary.

Acknowledgment. Supported by a grant from the Medical Research Council. We thank Mrs. Jenny Hollington for processing this manuscript.

References

Adams PR, Brown DA, Halliwell JV (1981) Cholinergic regulation of M-current in guinea-pig hippocampal neurones. J Physiol Lond 317:29–30P

Aldenhoff JB, Gruol DL, Rivier J, Vale W, Siggins GR (1983) Corticotrophin releasing factor decreases postburst hyperpolarizations and excites hippocampal neurons. Science NY 221:875–877

Barrett JF, Barrett JN, Crill WE (1980) Voltage-sensitive outward currents in cat motoneurones. J Physiol Lond 304:251–276

Bellemann P, Schade A, Towart R (1983) Dihydropyridine receptor in rat brain labelled with ^3H nimodipine Proc Natl Acad Sci USA 80:2356–2360

Benardo LS, Masukawa LM, Prince DA (1982) Electrophysiology of isolated hippocampal pyramidal dendrites. J Neurosci 2:1614–1622

Benardo LS, Prince DA (1981) Acetylcholine induced modulation of hippocampal pyramidal neurons. Brain Res 211:227–234

Bormann J, Sakmann B, Seifert W (1983) Isolation of GABA-activated single-channel Cl^- currents in the soma membrane of rat hippocampal neurones. J Physiol, Lond, 341:9–10P

Brown DA, Adams PR (1980) Muscarinic suppression of a noval voltage-sensitive K-current in voltage-clamped hippocampal cell somata. Nature, Lond, 183:673–676

Brown DA, Griffith WH (1983 a) Calcium-activated outward current in voltage-clamped hippocampal neurones of the guinea-pig. J Physiol, Lond, 337:287–301

Brown DA, Griffith WH (1983) Persistent slow inward current in voltage-clamped hippocampal neurones of the guinea-pig. J Physiol, Lond, 337:303–320

Brown DA, Constanti A, Docherty RJ, Galvan M, Gahwiler B, Halliwell JV (1984) Pharmacology of calcium currents in mammalian central neurons. Proc 9th Int. Pharmacol Congress (in press)

Brown TH, Fricke RA, Perkel DH (1980) Passive electrical constants in three classes of hippocampal neurons. J Neurophysiol 46:812–827

Carbonne E, Lux HD (1984) A low voltage-activated, fully inactivating Ca-channel in vertebrate sensory neurones. Nature, Lond, 310:501–502

Cherubini E, North RA (1984). Actions of γ-aminobutyric acid on neurones of guinea-pig myenteric plexus. Br J Pharmac 82:93–100

Cole AE, Nicoll RA (1984) The pharmacology of cholinergic excitatory responses in hippocampal pyramidal cells. Brain Res 305:283–290

Colquhoun D, Neher E, Reuter H , Stevens CF (1981) Inward current channels activated by intracellular Ca in cultured cardiac cells. Nature, Lond, 294:752–754

Connor JA, Stevens CF (1971) Voltage-clamp studies of a transient outward membrane current in gastropod neural somata. J Physiol Lond 213:21–30

Constanti A, Brown DA (1981) M-currents in voltage-clamped mammalian sympathetic neurones. Neurosci Lett 24:289–294

Cortes R, Supavilai P, Karobath M, Palacois JM (1983) The effect of lesions in the rat hippocampus suggest the association of calcium channel blocker binding sites with specific neuronal population. Neurosci Lett 42:249–254

Curtis BM, Catterall WA (1983) Solubilization of the calcium antagonist receptor from rat brain. J Biol Chem 258:7280–7283

Desarmenien M, Feltz P, Occhipinti G, Santangelo F, Schlichter R (1984) Coexistence of $GABA_A$ and $GABA_B$ receptors on A and C primary afferents. Br J Pharmac 81:327–334

Deschenes M, Roy JP, Steriade M (1982) Thalamic bursting mechanism: an inward slow current revealed by a membrane hyperpolarization. Brain Res 239:289–293

Dodd J, Dingeldine R, Kelly JS (1980) The excitatory action of acetylcholine on hippocampal neurones of the guinea-pig and rat maintained in vitro. Brain Res 207:109–127

Dolly J, Halliwell JV, Black JD, Williams RS, Pelchen-Matthews A, Breeze AL, Mehraban F, Othman IB, Black AR (1984) Botulinum neurotoxin and dendrotoxin as probes for studies on transmitter release. J Physiol Paris (in press)

Dunlap K (1981) Two types of γ-aminobutyric acid receptor on embryonic sensory neurones. Br J Pharmac 74:579–585

Dunlap K, Fischbach GD (1981) Neurotransmitters decrease the calcium conductance activated by depolarization of embryonic chick sensory neurones. J Physiol, Lond 317:519–535

Eckert R, Lux HD (1976) A voltage-sensitive persistent calcium conductance in neuronal somata of *Helix*. J Physiol, Lond 254:129–152

Fox AP, Nowycky MC, Tsien RW (1984) Single Ca channel in dorsal root ganglion cells are shifted between modes of gating by the calcium agonist Bay K 8644. Neurosci Abstr 10:526

Freedman SB, Dawson G, Villereal ML, Miller RJ (1984) Identification and characterization of voltage-sensitive calcium channels in neuronal clonal lines. J Neurosci 4:1453–1467

Gahwiler B (1981) Organotypic monolayer cultures of nervous tissue. J Neurosci Meth 4:329–342

Gahwiler B, Brown DA (1985) $GABA_B$-receptor activated K^+-current in voltage-clamped CA_3 pyramidal cells in hippocampal cultures. Proc Natl Acad Sci USA 82:1558–1562

Gahwiler BH, Dreifuss JJ (1982) Multiple actions of acetylcholine on hippocampal pyramidal cells in organotypic explant cultures. Neuroscience 7:1243–1256

Galvan M, Adams PR (1982) Control of calcium-current in rat sympathetic neurons by norepinephrine. Brain Res 244:135–144

Glossman H, Ferry DR, Lubbecke F, Mewes R, Hofmann F (1982) Calcium channels: direct identification with radioligand binding studies. Trends in Pharmacol Sci 3:431–437

Gustafsson B, Galvan M, Grafc P, Wigstrom H (1982) A transient outward current in a mammalian central neurone blocked by 4-aminopyridine. Nature, Lond 299:252–254

Haas HL, Konnerth A (1983) Histamine and noradrenaline decrease calcium-activated potassium conductance in hippocampal pyramidal cells. Nature, Lond 302:432–434

Hablitz JJ, Johnston D (1981) Endogenous nature of spontaneous bursting in hippocampal pyramidal neurons. J Cell Molec Neurobiol 1:325–334

Hagiwara S, Byerly L (1981) Calcium channel. Ann Rev Neurosci 4:69–125

Halliwell JV (1983) Caesium-loading reveals two distinct Ca-currents in voltage-clamped guinea-pig hippocampal neurones *in vitro*. J Physiol, Lond 341:10–11P

Halliwell JV, Adams PR (1982) Voltage-clamp analysis of muscarinic excitation in hippocampal neurons. Brain Res 250:71–92

Halliwell JV, Scholfield CN (1984a) Adenosine-resistant Ca-currents in mammalian central nervous system. J Physiol, Lond 349:52P

Halliwell JV, Scholfield CN (1984b) Somatically-recorded Ca-currents in guinea-pig hippocampal and olfactory cortex neurones are resistant to adenosine action. Neurosci Lett 50:13–18

Henon BK, McAfee DA (1983) Modulation of calcium currents by adenosine receptors on mammalian sympathetic neurones. In: Berne RM, Rall TW, Rabio R (eds) Regulatory function of adenosine. Martinus Nijhoff, The Hague, pp 455–466

Hotson JR, Prince DA (1981) Penicillin- and barium-induced epileptiform bursting in hippocampal neurons: actions on Ca^{2+} and K^+-potentials. Ann Neurol 10:11–17

JohnstonD (1981) Passive cable properties of hippocampal CA_3 pyramidal neurons. Cell Mol Neurobiol 1:100–110

Johnston D, Brown TH (1984) Mechanisms of neuronal burst generation. In: Schwartzkroin PA, Wheal HV (eds) Electrophysiology of epilepsy. Academic Press, London, pp 278–301

Johnston D, Hablitz JJ, Wilson WA (1980) Voltage-clamp discloses slow inward current in hippocampal burst-firing neurones. Nature, Lond 286:391–393

Kandel ER, Spencer WA (1961) Electrophysiology of hippocampal neurons. II. After-potentials and repetitive firing. J Neurophysiol 24:243–259

Kostyuk PG (1981) Calcium-channels in the neuronal membrane. Biochem Biophys Acta 650:128–150

Lancaster B, Adams PR (1984) Single electrode voltage clamp of the slow AHP current in rat hippocampal pyramidal cells. Neurosci Abstr (in press)

Lee KS, Tsien RW (1983) Mechanism of calcium channel blockade by verapamil, D 600, diltiazem and nitrendipine in single dialysed heart cells. Nature, Lond 302:790–794

Llinas R, Sugimori M (1980) Electrophysiological properties of in vitro Purkinje cell dendrites in mammalian cerebellar slices. J Physiol, Lond 305:197–213

Llinas R, Walton K (1980) Voltage-dependent calcium conductances in neurons. In: Cotman CW, Poste G, Nicolson GL (eds) The cell surface and neuronal function. Elsevier, North Holland, pp 87–118

Llinas R, Yarom Y (1981) Electrophysiology of mammalian inferior olivary neurones in vitro. Different types of voltage-dependent ionic conductances. J Physiol, Lond 315:549–567

Madison DV, Nicoll RA (1982) Noradrenaline blocks accommodation of pyramidal cell discharge in the hippocampus. Nature, Lond 299:636–638

Madison DV, Nicoll RA (1984) Control of the repetitive discharge of CA_1 pyramidal neurones in vitro. J Physiol Lond 354:318–331

Miller RJ, Freedman SB (1984) Are dihydropyridine binding sites voltage-sensitive calcium channels? Life Sci 34:1205–1221

Neher E (1971) The fast transient current components during voltage clamp on snail neurons. J Gen Physiol 58:36–53

Nelson MT, French RJ, Krueger BK (1984) Voltage-dependent calcium channels from brain incorporated into planar lipid bilayers. Nature, Lond 308:77–80

Newberry NR, Nicoll RA (1984) Direct hyperpolarizing action of baclofen on hippocampal pyramidal cells. Nature, Lond 308:450–452

Nowycky M, Fox AP, Tsien RW (1984) Two components of calcium channel currents in chick dorsal root ganglion cells. Biophys J, 45:36 a

Numann R, Wong RKS (1984) Voltage-clamp study on GABA response desensitziation in single pyramidal cells dissociated from the hippocampus of adult guinea-pigs. Neurosci, Lett 47:289–294

Ogata N, Hori N, Katsuda N (1976) The correlation between extracellular potassium concentration and hippocampal epileptic activity in vitro. Brain Res 110:371–375

Owen DG, Segal M, Barker JL (1984) A Ca-dependent Cl^- -conductance is present in cultured mouse spinal neurones. Nature, Lond 311:567–570

Prince DA (1978) Neurophysiology of epilepsy. Ann Rev Neurosci 1:395–415

Prince DA (1983) Mechanisms of epileptogenesis in brain-slice model systems. In: Ward AA Jr, Penny JK, Purpura D (eds) Epilepsy. Raven Press, New York, pp 29–52

Proctor WR, Dunwiddie TV (1983) Adenosine inhibits calcium spikes in hippocampal pyramidal neurons in vitro. Neurosci. Lett 35:197–201

Purpura DP, Prelevic S, Santini M (1968) Hyperpolarizing increase in membrane conductance in hippocampal neurons. Brain Res 7:310–312

Reuter H (1983) Calcium channel modulation by neurotransmitters, enzymes and drugs. Nature, Lond 301:569–574

Schlichter R, Demeneix BA, Desarmenien M, Desaulles E, Loeffler JP, Feltz P (1984) Properties of the GABA receptors located on spinal primary afferent neurones and hypophyseal neuroendocrine cells of the rat. Neurosci Lett 47:257–263

Schwartzkroin PA (1980) Ionic and synaptic determinants of burst generation. In: Lockard JS, Ward Jr AA (eds) Epilepsy: A window to brain mechanisms. Raven press, New York, pp 83–95

Schwartzkroin PA, Prince DA (1980) Effect of TEA on hippocampal neurons Brain Res 185:169–181

Schwartzkroin PA, Slawsky M (1977) Probable calcium spikes in hippocampal neurones. Brain Res 135:157–161

Schwindt PC, Crill W (1980 a) Role of a persistent inward current in motoneuron bursting during spinal seizures. J Neurophysiol 43:1296–1318

Schwindt PC, Crill W (1980 b) Properties of a persistent inward current in normal and TEA-injected motoneurons. J Neurophysiol 43:1700–1724

Segal M, Barker JL (1984) Rat hippocampal neurones in culture: potassium current. J Neurophysiol 51:1409–1433

Tillotson D (1979) Inactivation of Ca conductance dependent on entry of Ca ions in molluscan neurons. Proc Nat Acad Sci USA, 76:1497–1500

Toll L (1982) High-affinity binding and inhibition of calcium transport in a clonal cell line. J Biol Chem 257:13189–13192

Traub RD (1982) Simulation of intrinsic bursting in CA_3 hippocampal neurons. Neuroscience 7:1233–1242

Turner DA, Schwartzkroin PA (1980) Steady-state electrotonic analysis of intracellularly stained hippocampal neurons. J Neurophysiol 44:184–199

Wong RKS, Prince DA (1978) Participation of calcium spikes sharing intrinsic burst firing in hippocampal neurons. Brain Res 159:385–390

Wong RKS, Prince DA (1979) Dendritic mechanisms underlying penicillin-induced epileptiform activity. Science, NY 204:1228–1230

Wong RKS, Prince DA, Basbaum AI (1979) Intradendritic recordings from hippocampal neurons. Proc Natl Acad Sci 76:986–990

Wong RKS, Traub RD, Miles R (1984) Epileptogenic mechanisms as revealed by studies of the hippocampal slice. In: Schwartzkroin PA, HV Wheal (eds) Electrophysiology of epilepsy. Academic Press, London, pp 254–275

Discussion

(pp. 74–87)

Kass: The possible existances of different kinds of calcium channels in this preparation is very interesting. You didn't mention whether in your experiments for a prepulse-dependence of the fast component tetrodotoxin was present.

Brown: Yes, tetrodotoxin was present in all the clamp records.

Kass: Have you tested the relative sensitivity of those components to any of the organic blockers?

Brown: Yes, but we have only checked them in a qualitative sense. The difficulty with voltage-clamp experiments in brain slices is to get quantitative data. All I can say at the moment is that the transient current is reduced by nimodipine at about 2 μM/l. The problem with the transient current is that we are not actually activating it near the same opening probability as that for the slow Ca-current, because we cannot clamp it adequately. We have to test it just suprathreshold whereas we can clamp the slow Ca current pretty near the peak.

Session II: Molecular Interactions

Chairman: D. J. Triggle

Bayer-Symposium IX
Cardiovascular Effects of Dihydropyridine-Type
Calcium Antagonists and Agonists, 90–103

Chemistry of Dihydropyridines [1 – 4]

H. MEYER, E. WEHINGER, F. BOSSERT, H. BÖSHAGEN, G. FRANCKOWIAK,
S. GOLDMANN, W. SEIDEL and J. STOLTEFUSS

A. Syntheses

Arthur Hantzsch, who can really by called the first heterocyclic chemist, studied the reaction of aldehydes with β-dicarbonyl compounds and ammonia as part of his "Habilitation" work at the University of Leipzig, where he was a young assistant lecturer in the Chemistry Institute. The results of this work were first published by Hantzsch in the year 1882 [5].

Hantzsch synthesis

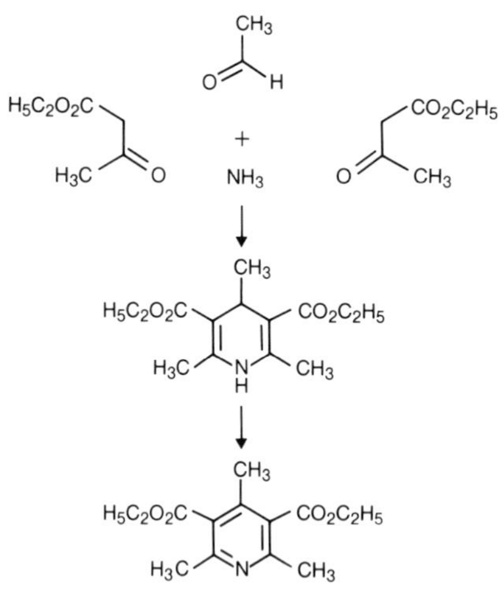

From the reaction of acetaldehyde, ethyl acetoacetate and ammonia he obtained a crystalline intermediate which he was able to convert by oxidation into diethyl 2,4,6-trimethyl-pyridine-3,5-dicarboxylate. The structure of this final product was then confirmed by degradation reactions. By logical deduction he allocated a dihydropyridine constitution to the intermediate obtained in the primary reaction. Later, he, and other workers, showed that this reaction is widely variable with respect to the aldehyde, β-dicarbonyl and amine components. This reaction provided the first access to numerous pyridine derivatives to be independent to coal tar, the sole source of nitrogen heterocycles up to that time.

Variants of Hantzsch synthesis

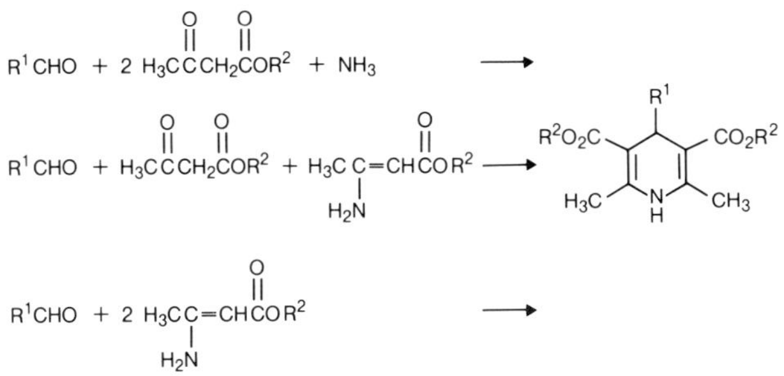

Apart from Hantzsch's one-pot synthesis – the reaction of an aldehyde with two molar equivalents of acetoacetate and ammonia, preferably in alcohol – there are two variations which also lead to the identical 1,4-dihydropyridine derivative. The aldehyde can either be condensed with one mole of β-ketoester and one mole of β-aminocrotonate [6] or it can be condensed directly with two moles of β-aminocrotonate [7].

Synthesis of DHPs with different ester groups

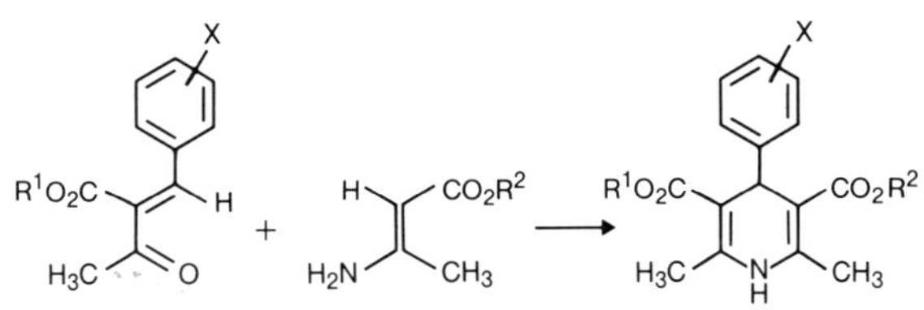

With respect to the chemistry the Hantzsch pyridine synthesis is a cyclising Michael addition. The primary Knoevenagel condensation of the aldehyde with the β-dicarbonyl compound giving the aralkylidene-acetoacetate is followed by a Michael addition of the aminocrotonate, formed from the second acetoacetate molecule and ammonia, to this highly reactive substrate. The final step is a condensation reaction, closing the ring and giving the 1,4-dihydropyridine. This chemistry provides the entry into 1,4-dihydropyridines with non-identical ester groups if one utilises the so-called two component variation [8]. In this case the aralkylidene-acetoacetate obtained by Knoevenagel condensation is isolated, and the cyclising Michael addition of an aminocrotonate having a different ester function is carried out in a second, separate reaction step. This variation multiplies considerably the number of 1,4-dihydropyridinedicarboxylates that can be synthesised.

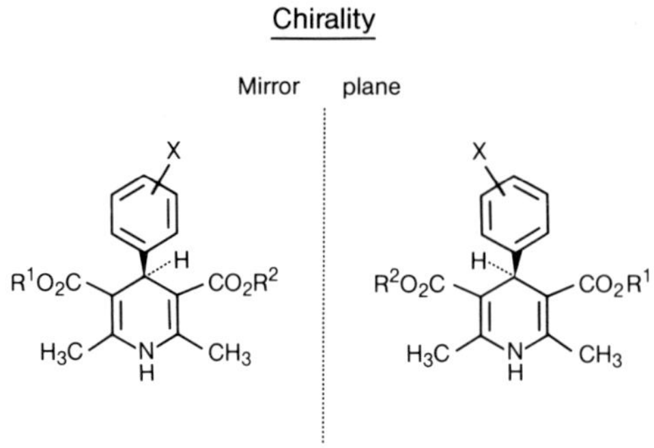

Furthermore, in contrast to the symmetrically substituted products obtained by the classical Hantzsch synthesis, 1,4-dihydropyridines with non-identical substituents in the 3- and 5-positions are chiral, that is, they exist in two enantiomeric forms which bear an object/mirror-image relationship to each other.

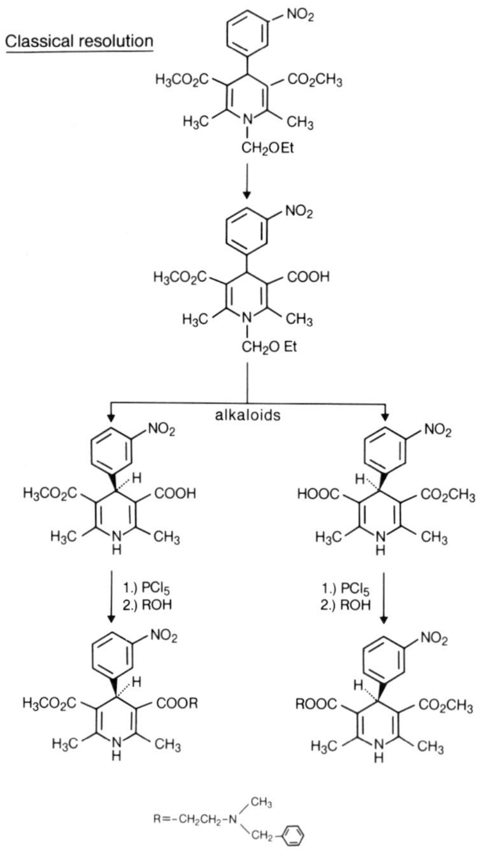

The classical route to obtaining enantiomerically pure dihydropyridine-diesters was chosen by a Japanese research group [9]. The key step in this route is the separation of a 1,4-dihydropyridine-monocarboxylic acid using an optically active alkaloid base. The re-esterification of the enantiomeric monocarboxylic acids so obtained then leads to the target molecules. However, it is first necessary to protect the nitrogen with an alkoxyalkyl group, and to deblock later.

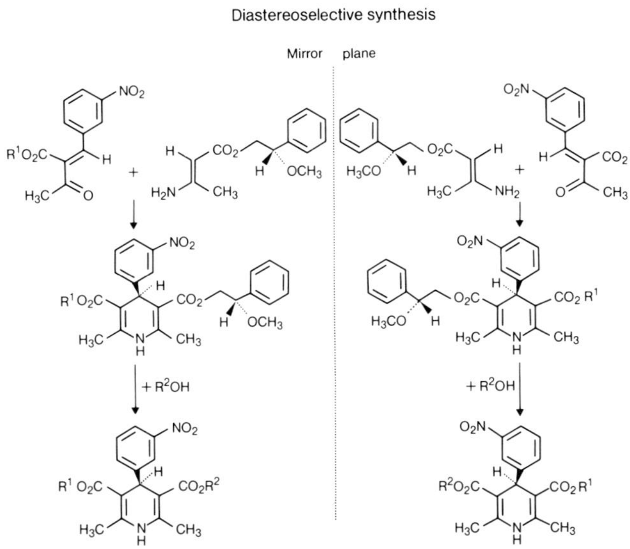

An alternative route, which also permits conclusions concerning the absolute configuration at the C-4 of the dihydropyridine, was discovered in the form of a diastereoselective cyclising Michael addition [10]. 2-Methoxy-2-phenylethanol, an alcohol readily available in enantiomerically pure form, functions as inductor of the diastereoselectivity; it is converted into the enantiomeric aminocrotonate by standard reactions. Cyclising Michael addition of this aminocrotonate to the prochiral centre of the aralkylidene-acetoacetate leads diastereoselectively to two enantiomeric 1,4-dihydropyridine intermediates whose X-ray crystal structure analysis permits conclusions concerning the configuration at C-4. Due to the inductive effect of the methoxy group it is then possible to transesterify the chiral ester function selectively with other alcohols, in the presence of a simple alkyl ester function, to give the enantiomeric 1,4-dihydropyridines with achiral ester groups.

B. Reactions of 1,4-Dihydropyridines

The best-known reaction of 1,4-dihydropyridines is of course the second step in the Hantzsch pyridine synthesis, namely their oxidation to the corresponding pyridine derivatives, which can be carried out with a wide variety of oxidants such as chromium(VI)oxide, nitric acid, tetrachlorobenzoquinone etc. [3]. More difficult is the reduction of 1,4-dihydropyridines to 1,2,3,4-tetrahydropyridines, which requires drastic conditions due to the resonance stabilisation of the 3,5-acceptor-substituted 1,4-dihydropyridine. The cathodic reduction of 1,4-dihydro-

Oxidation and reduction

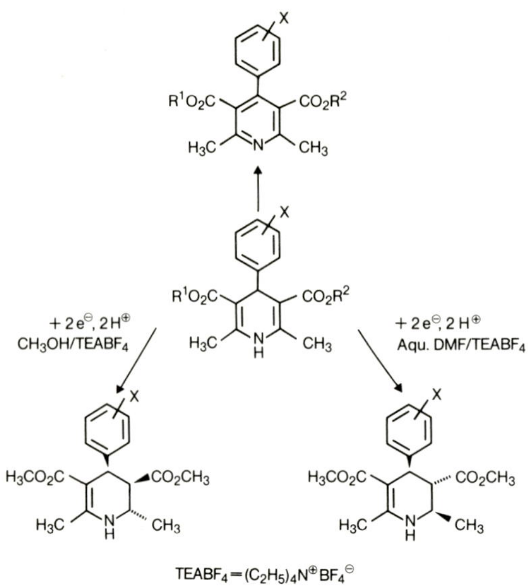

pyridines using tetraethylammonium fluoroborate as supporting electrolyte in various solvents has been found to be particularly facile [11]. This reduction is the equivalent of a trans addition of hydrogen across the 2,3-double bond of the 1,4-dihydropyridine. The two possible stereoisomers can be obtained selectively by a suitable choice of solvent: reduction in methanol provides the "trans-cis" tetrahydropyridine whereas the "trans-trans" stereoisomer is obtained selectively in aqueous dimethyl formamide.

Hydrolysis of one ester group

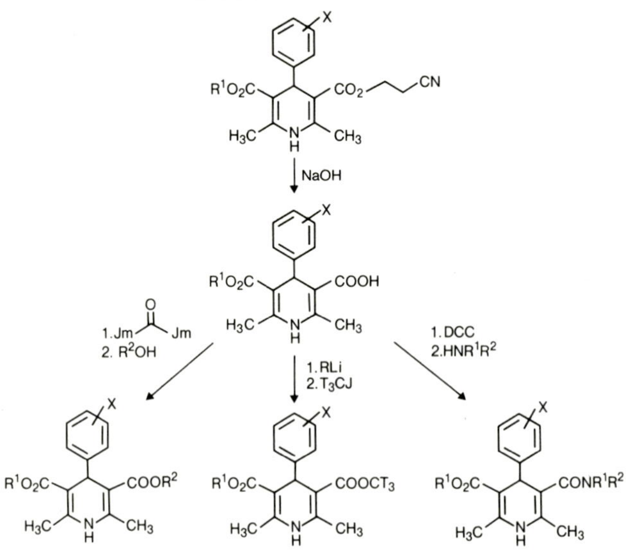

Another important reaction of 1,4-dihydropyridines is the saponification of an ester group to the monocarboxylic acid, which, as a key intermediate, opens up access to numerous carboxylic acid derivatives. The hydrolysis of an ester group after prior protection of the nitrogen atom has already been mentioned. It has been shown that 1,4-dihydropyridine-dicarboxylates can also be hydrolysed without prior protection when the ester groups bear an inductive substituent. The 2-cyanoethyl ester group has been found to be particularly valuable [12]. This can be hydrolysed by alkali under very mild conditions. The monocarboxylic acids thus obtained can then be re-esterified, providing for example the possibility for isotopic labelling, or converted into amides.

C. Introduction of Substituents

The low basicity of the 1,4-dihydropyridine nitrogen, surprising at first glance, is easily explained by resonance with the carbonyl groups in the 3,5-positions. This electronic interaction manifests itself not only in the ^{13}C NMR and IR spectroscopic data of the 1,4-dihydropyridines, but also in their low tendency to undergo alkylation and acylation reactions under classical conditions. It is first necessary to deprotonate with sodium hydride in an inert solvent. The resulting anion can then be alkylated regioselectively at nitrogen [13]. 1-Alkyl-dihydropyridines are also accessible by Hantzsch synthesis, acetoacetate being added to aralkylidene-acetoacetate in pyridine in the presence of an alkylamine hydrohalide [14].

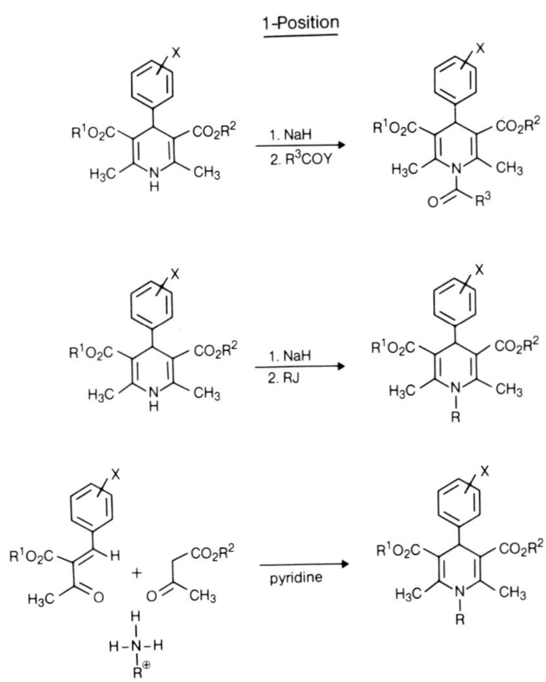

2-Position

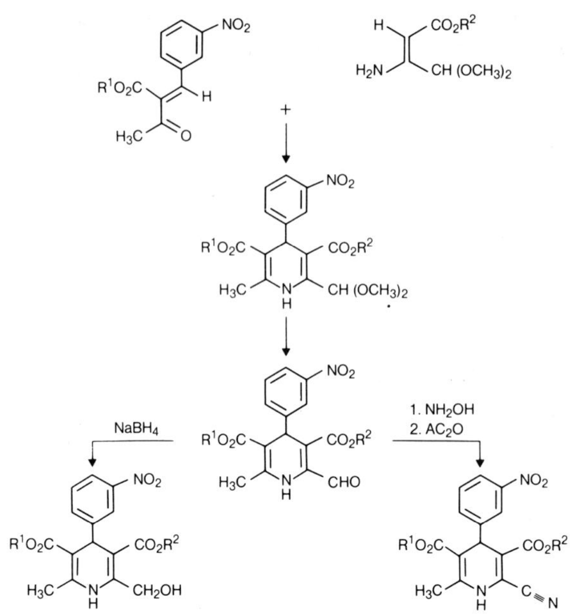

The Hantzsch synthesis and its variations permit a wide spectrum of the substituent in the 2 position as long as an alkyl or aryl substituent is desired. The introduction of functionalised carbon or hetero substituents is, however, also possible by varying the enaminocarbonyl component in the two component reaction. The use of an aminocrotonate bearing a terminal acetal substituent leads to a 2-dialkoxymethyl-substituted 1,4-dihydropyridine which provides the dihydropyridine 2-aldehyde upon acid hydrolysis. This aldehyde undergoes classical carbonyl reactions such as the reduction to alcohol or conversion to nitrile after prior oximation [15].

2-Position

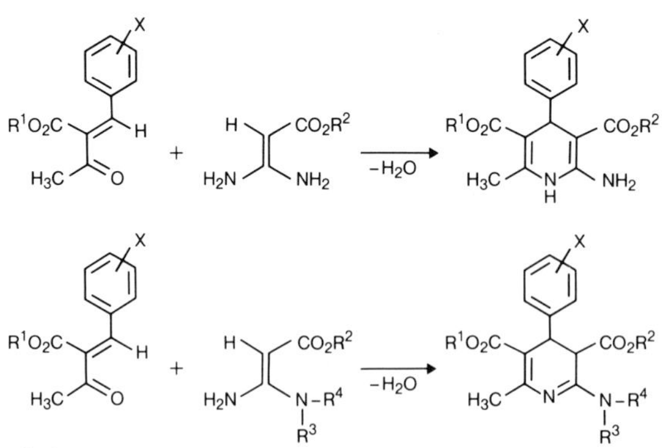

R^3, R^4 = alkyl
$R^3 + R^4$ = alkylen

The formal replacement of the methyl group in an aminocrotonate by an amino group leads to the ene-diamino form of an amidinoacetic ester. The presumption that an amidinoacetic ester should be an excellent Michael addend because of the additional donor function of the second amino group was confirmed by its behaviour in the two-component dihydropyridine synthesis [16]. The 2-amino-1,4-dihydropyridines thus obtained can be subsequently derivatised in many new ways. If one of the amino groups in the amidinoacetic ester is substituted by two alkyl groups, the two-component synthesis surprisingly no longer yields 1,4-dihydropyridines but rather 2-dialkylamino-3,4-dihydropyridine-3,5-dicarboxylates. This deviation from the rule is explicable from steric considerations, but also by the fact that the dialkylamino-dihydropyridines, in contrast to the amino derivatives, cannot form hydrogen bridge bonds.

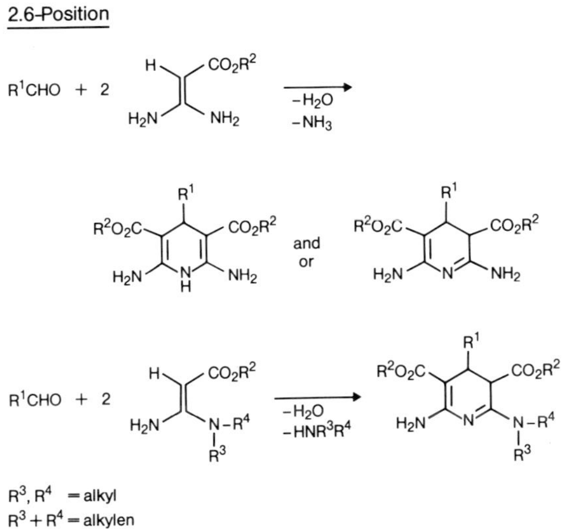

One of the variations of the Hantzsch synthesis mentioned at the beginning was the condensation of an aldehyde with two molar equivalents of aminocrotonate. The use of amidinoacetic esters in this variation leads analogously to 2,6-diamino-substituted dihydropyridines where, depending on the further substitution of the heterocycle, 1,4- or 3,4-dihydropyridines, or mixtures of the two are isolated [17]. In contrast, the reaction of an amidinoacetic ester having a dialkylamino group with an aldehyde leads selectively to 6-amino-2-dialkylamino-3,4-dihydropyridine derivatives with the elimination of water and dialkylamine.

As was demonstrated in the synthesis of 3,5-dicarboxylates with non-identical ester functions, the two-component synthesis also enables the introduction of a substituent in the 3-position by simple means. This possibility embraces a wide variety of other acceptor substituents such as acyl, cyano, alkyl or aryl sulphonyl, NO_2, dialkoxyphosphoryl etc. The acceptor substituent can either be incorporated into the Michael substrate (Knoevenagel condensation product) or, alternatively, into the Michael addend (acceptor-substituted enamine). An example of this is the synthesis of the 3-nitro-1,4-dihydropyridine-5-carboxylate BAY k 8644

3-Position

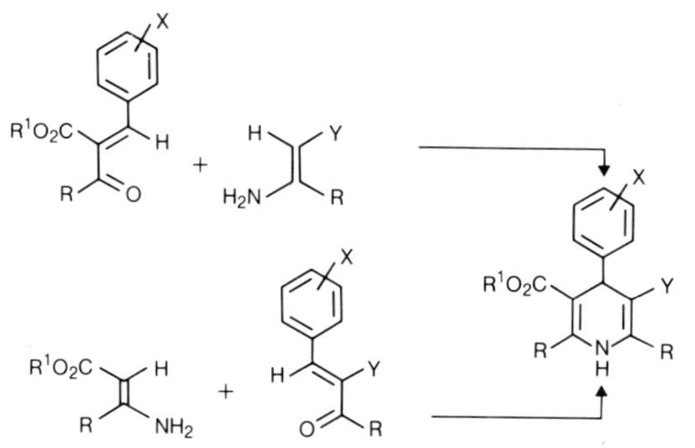

Y = CO_2R^2, COR, CN, SO_2R, NO_2, PO $(OR)_2$

For example:

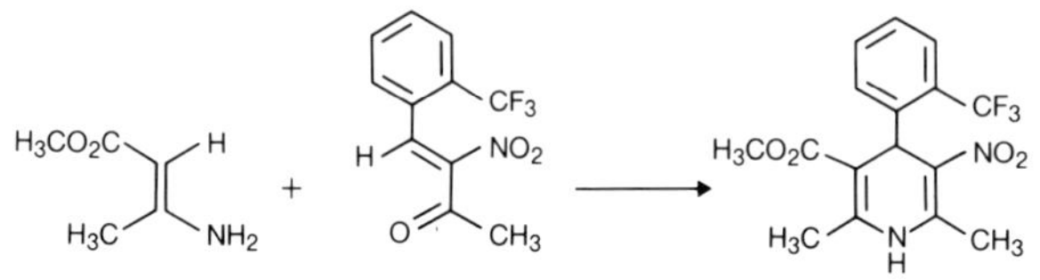

by cyclising Michael addition of methyl aminocrotonate to the nitrosubstituted enone available from Knoevenagel condensation of 2-trifluoromethylbenzaldehyde and nitroacetone [18].

4-Position

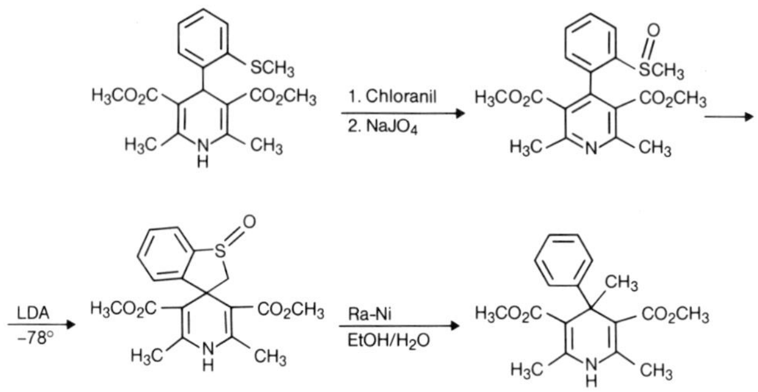

Apart from the substitution at the nitrogen atom mentioned before, the 1,4-dihydropyridines available by the Hantzsch synthesis also provide the possibility of a second substitution in the 4-position, i.e. the replacement of the hydrogen atom introduced from the formyl group of the aldehyde. Because the Hantzsch synthesis fails with ketones (for simultaneous introduction of ester functions in the 3,5-positions), the synthesis of such 4,4-disubstituted dihydropyridines is only possible by a roundabout route [19]. The starting materials are 4-(2-alkylthiophenyl)-substituted 1,4-dihydropyridines. Two selective oxidation steps with tetrachlorobenzoquinone and sodium periodate lead to the alkylsulphinyl-substituted pyridine derivative. Deprotonation of this intermediate by lithium diisopropylamide provides a carbanion which reacts by an intramolecular 1,4-addition reaction to give a spirodihydropyridine. Desulphurisation of this product using Raney nickel in aqueous ethanol leads to the desired 4,4-disubstituted molecule.

D. Annellations

1.2-Annellation

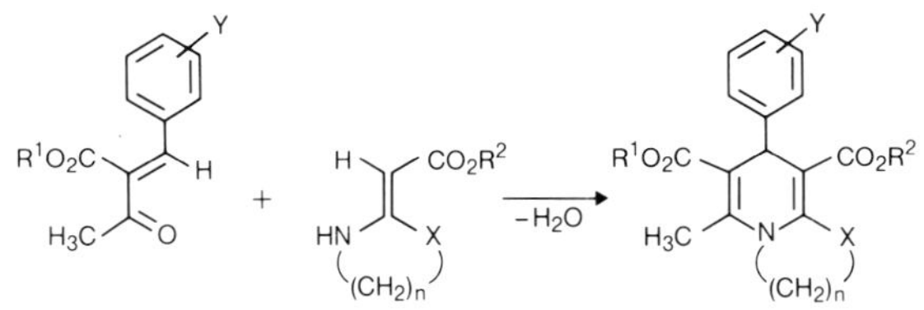

$X=CH_2$, O, S, NH

Use of acceptor-substituted enamines in which the nitrogen atom is incorporated into a ring to the α-position leads to 1,4-dihydropyridines with a 1,2-annellation in the two component synthesis. Heteroatoms (O, S, NH) flanking the double-bond can also be introduced [20].

2.3-Annellation

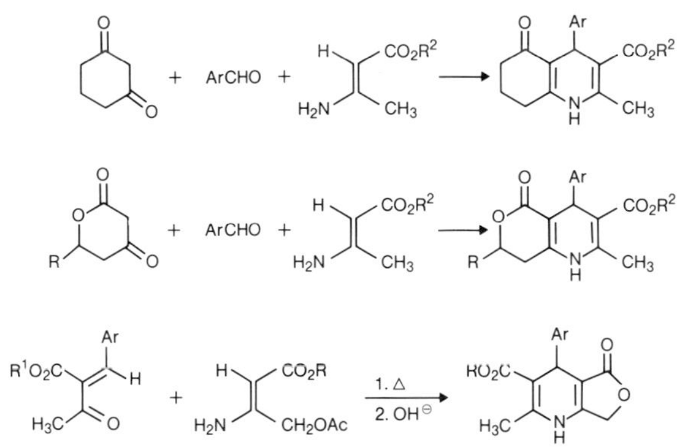

2,3-Annellated dihydropyridines are accessible by a three component variation. The condensation of an aldehyde with a cyclic β-dicarbonyl compound, especially a cyclic β-diketone or β-ketolactone, and an aminocrotonate leads selectively to a 2,3-annellated dihydropyridine [21]. The annellating using a γ-lactone, however, requires a two component reaction. The cyclising Michael addition of a terminally acetoxy-substituted aminocrotonate to an aralkylidene-acetoacetate yields a 2-acetoxymethyl-substituted dihydropyridine intermediate that can be cyclised by alkali treatment, without isolation, to give the five-membered lactone [22].

1.2.3-Bisannellation

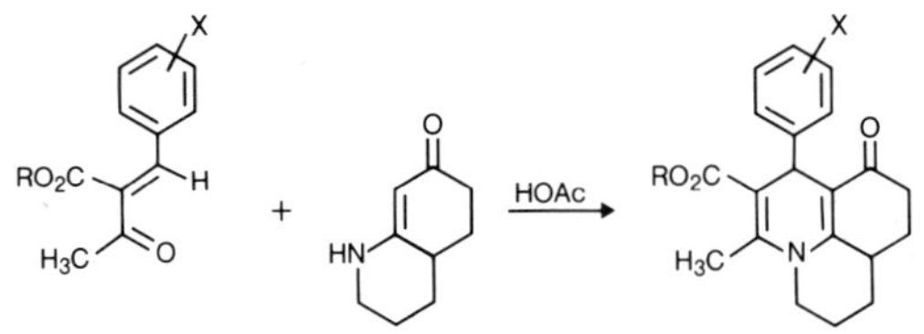

A 1,2,3-bisannellation of the dihydropyridine core is possible with the use of a special enamino-carbonyl compound. The partially hydrogenated quinolone described by Grob, in which the enamino-carbonyl entity is integrated into both rings, can be condensed with an aralkylidene-acetoacetate to a tricyclic dihydropyridine with a bridgehead nitrogen [20].

3.2'-Lactonisation

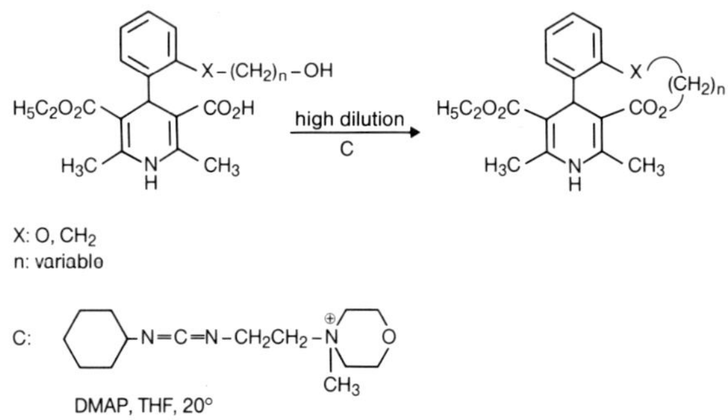

The linking of the dihydropyridine core to an aromatic ring in the 4-position is possible by means of a lactone bridge from the 3-position to the ortho-position of the aromatic ring. The starting materials for the synthesis of such compounds are 1,4-dihydropyridine-monocarboxylic acids, available in several steps, which bear an ortho-alkyl or ortho alkoxy substituent in the aromatic ring that is terminally functionalised by a hydroxy group. Lactonisation of such intermediates can be achieved under high dilution conditions using standard reagents, preferably carbodiimides. The number of atoms in the lactone ring can be varied within wide limits [23].

E. Variations of the Heterocycle

The 2-aza analogues of the Hantzsch-type 1,4-dihydropyridines, the 1,4-dihydropyridazine-dicarboxylates, are also accessible via a cyclising Michael addition [24]. The starting materials are the trusty aralkylidene-acetoacetates from the dihydropyridine synthesis. The base-catalysed addition of nitroacetic ester provides a Michael adduct which can be converted to the nitronate with sodium methoxide. Low-temperature ozonolysis of this nitronate in methanol yields a tetracar-

1.4-Dihydropyridazine

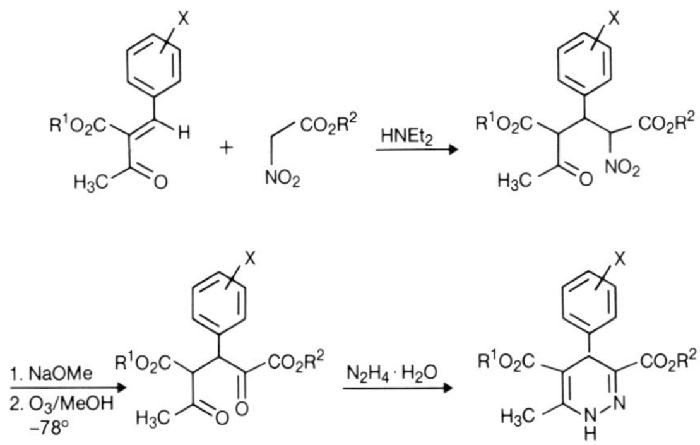

bonyl compound which can be condensed with hydrazine hydrate to give a 1,4-dihydropyridazine-3,5-dicarboxylate. The fact that the 1,4-dihydropyridazines are formed selectively in this cyclisation is further evidence for the stabilisation of the 1,4-dihydroazine system by resonance of the 1-nitrogen atom with the acceptor substituents in the 3,5-positions.

2-Amino-4H-pyrane

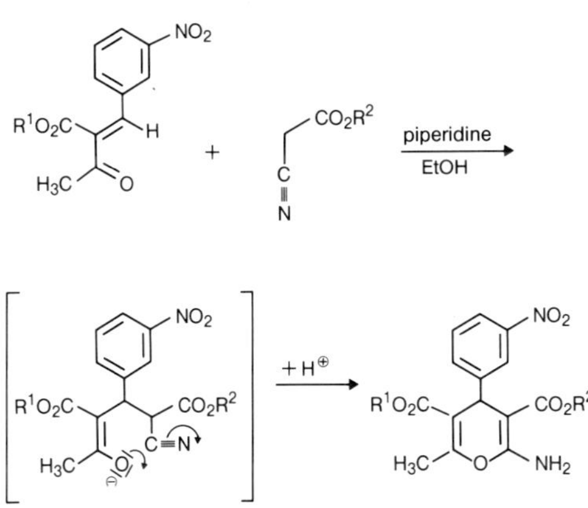

The 2-amino-6-alkyl-4H-pyran-3,5-dicarboxylates are an interesting bioisosteric variation of the Hantzsch dihydropyridines. As was the case with the 1,4-dihydropyridazine synthesis, the chemistry is again related to that of the Hantzsch pyridine synthesis. The primary addition of a cyanoacetate to a 3-nitrobenzylidene-acetoacetate under base catalysis yields a nonisolable Michael adduct whose enolate anion carries out a nucleophilic attack at the nitrile carbon [25]. In this case a tautomerisation to the "1,4-dihydro" system of the 4-H-pyrans is again observed due to resonance stabilisation. In contrast to the other heterocyclic syntheses discussed so far this synthesis is characterised by a double addition without a condensation step.

F. Active 1,4-Dihydropyridine Structures

The parent compound of the 1,4-dihydropyridine calcium antagonists, the achiral Nifedipine [26], has been modified in numerous analogue structures. The development products Darodipine [27] and the N-alkylated Flordipine [28] represent

Calcium antagonists

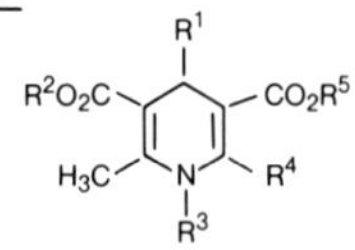

	R^1	R^2	R^3	R^4	R^5
Nifedipine	2-NO_2-C_6H_4	CH_3	H	CH_3	CH_3
Nicardipine	3-NO_2-C_6H_4	CH_3	H	CH_3	CH_2-$CH_2N(Bz)(CH_3)$
Nitrendipine	3-NO_2-C_6H_4	CH_3	H	CH_3	C_2H_5
Nimodipine	3-NO_2-C_6H_4	$CH(CH_3)_2$	H	CH_3	$CH_2CH_2OCH_3$
Nisoldipine	2-NO_2-C_6H_4	CH_3	H	CH_3	$CH_2CH(CH_3)_2$
Felodipine	2.3-Cl_2-C_6H_3	CH_3	H	CH_3	C_2H_5
FR 7534	3-NO_2-C_6H_4	C_2H_5	H	CH_2OH	C_2H_5
Nilvadipine	3-NO_2-C_6H_4	$CH(CH_3)_2$	H	CN	CH_3
Darodipine	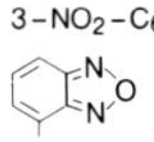	C_2H_5	H	CH_3	C_2H_5
PN 200-110	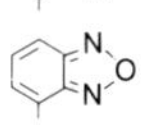	$CH(CH_3)_2$	H	CH_3	CH_3
Flordipine	2-CF_3-C_6H_4	C_2H_5	CH_2CH_2-N O	CH_3	C_2H_5
PO 219	3-NO_2-C_6H_4	CH_3	H	CH_3	CH_2-CH_2-N N-Ph

achiral symmetrically substituted 1,4-dihydropyridines. The majority of the Nifedipine analogues are, however, chiral due to non-identical ester groups, as in the development products Nitrendipine [29], Nimodipine [29], Nisoldipine [30], Nicardipine [31], PN 200–110 [32] and PO 219 [33], or due to non-identical 2,6-substituents, as in FR 7534 [34] and Nilvadipine [15].

Calcium agonists

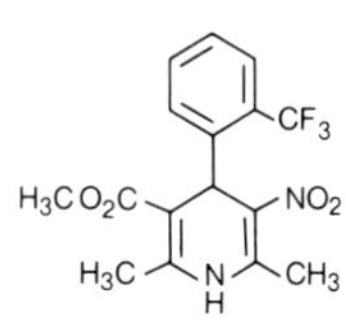

BAY K 8644

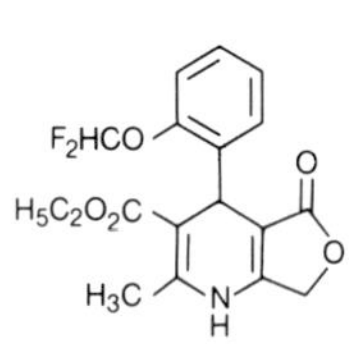

CGP 28 392

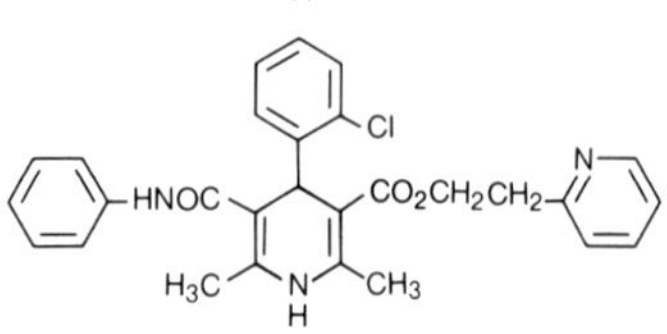

YC 170

The structures of the 1,4-dihydropyridine calcium agonists worked on recently are characterised mainly by a 3-nitro substitution, as in BAY k 8644 [18], or by a lactone annellation, as in the case of the agonist CGP 28–392 [35]. Weak agonistic properties have also been reported for the 3-carboxanilide YC-170.

In conclusion it can be said that the intensive chemical research on 1,4-dihydropyridines – initiated by their excellent calcium modulating properties – has produced many variations that should permit qualitative and quantitative deductions about structure and activity.

References

1. Eisner U, Kuthan J (1972) Chem Rev 72:1
2. Bossert F, Meyer H, Wehinger E (1981) Angew Chem 93:755
3. Kuthan J, Kurfürst A (1982) Ind Eng Chem Prod Res Dev 21:191
4. Stout DM, Meyers AI (1982) Chem Rev 82:223
5. Hantzsch A, (1882) Justus Liebigs Ann Chem 215:1
6. Fox HH, Lewis JI, Wenner W (1951) J Org Chem 16:1259
7. Cook AH, Heilbron IM, Steger L (1943) J Chem Soc 413
8. Meyer H, Bossert F, Wehinger E, Stoepel K, Vater W (1981) Arzneim-Forsch/Drug Res 31:407
9. Shibanuma T, Iwanami M, Okuda K, Takenaka T, Murakami M (1980) Chem Pharm Bull 28:2809
10. Ger Offen 2935451 (Bayer; Prior 1.9.1979)
11. Wehinger E (1984) 5th International Conference on Organic Synthesis, Freiburg i Br, 27.8.–30.8.1984, Abstracts, p 122
12. Ger Offen 2921429 (Bayer; Prior 26.5.1979)
13. Paleček J, Kuthan J (1976) Synthesis 550
14. Ger Offen 2210672 (Bayer; Prior 6.3.1972)
15. U.S. 4338322 (Fujisawa; GB Prior 2.7.1975)
16. Meyer H, Bossert F, Horstmann H (1977) Liebigs Ann Chem 1895
17. Meyer H, Bossert F, Horstmann H (1978) Liebigs Ann Chem 1476
18. Franckowiak G, Schramm M, Thomas G, Towart R (1984) 188th ACS National Meeting, Philadelphia, 26.8.–31.8.1984, Abstr MEDI 8
19. Goldmann S (1981) Angew Chem 93, 798
20. Meyer H, Bossert F, Horstmann H (1977) Liebigs Ann Chem 1888
21. Meyer H, unpublished results
22. Meyer H, Wehinger E, Bossert F, Scherling D (1983) Arzneim-Forsch/Drug Res 33:106
23. Seidel W, Meyer H, Born L, Kazda S, Dompert W (1984) 187th ACS National Meeting, St. Louis, 8.4.–13.4.1984, Abstr MEDI 14
24. Franckowiak G, Meyer H (1981) 8th International Congress of Heterocyclic Chemistry, Graz (Austria), 23.8.–28.8.1981, Abstract Book p 335
25. Ger Offen 2235406 (Bayer; Prior 19.7.1972)
26. Ger 1670827 (Bayer; Prior 20.3.1967)
27. Eur Pat Appl 150 (Sandoz; CH Prior 20.6.1977)
28. Ger Offen 3109794 (USV Pharmaceutical; US Prior 11.4.1980)
29. Ger 2117571 (Bayer; Prior 10.4.1971)
30. Ger 2549568 (Bayer; Prior 5.11.1975)
31. Ger Offen 2407115 (Yamanouchi; JP Prior 20.2.1973)
32. Ger Offen 2949491 (Sandoz; CH Prior 18.12.1978)
33. Eur Pat Appl 97821 (Pierrel; IT 3.6.82)
34. Ger Offen 2629892 (Fujisawa; GB Prior 2.7.1975)
35. Eur Pat Appl 111455 (Ciba-Geigy; CH Prior 10.12.1982)

Bayer-Symposium IX
Cardiovascular Effects of Dihydropyridine-Type
Calcium Antagonists and Agonists, 104–110

Structure-Function Relationships of 1,4-Dihydropyridines: Ligand and Receptor Perspectives

C. M. Su, F. B. Yousif, D. J. Triggle, and R. A. Janis

The synthetic methodology previously outlined (Meyer, this volume) for the 1,4-dihydropyridines has made available numerous analogs with which to generate structure-activity data and attempt to solve a number of important questions concerning the actions of this class of drugs. Amongst the questions to be answered are the following:

1. Are there specific 1,4-dihydropyridine sites?
2. How many classes of such sites exist?
3. What are the structural demands at these sites?
4. How may activator and antagonist ligands be differentiated?
   a) Structure
   b) Mechanism
5. What is the relationship of binding sites to the Ca^{2+} channel and channel permeation processes?
6. What relationship does this site(s) have to the actions of other structural categories of Ca^{2+} channel ligands?
7. What is the basis for any tissue selectivity of the 1,4-dihydropyridines?
8. Are there endogenous ligands for the Ca^{2+} channel?

A number of structure-activity analyses derived from in vivo and in vitro pharmacologic and radioligand binding experiments (inter alia, Loev et al. 1974; Rosenberger and Triggle 1978; Mannhold et al. 1982; Janis and Triggle 1983; Bolger et al. 1983) indicate that the basic structural requirements for the expression of antagonist activity are as shown in Fig. 1. The general conformational requirements are, as deduced from the analysis of solid state structures (Triggle et al. 1980; Fossheim et al. 1982) and the synthesis of 1,4-dihydropyridines with restricted conformational mobility (Seidel et al. 1984), represented schematically in Fig. 2.

The availability of 1,4-dihydropyridines which possess Ca^{2+} channel activating properties but which are of close structural similarity to the ligands with antagonist structures (Fig. 3; Schramm et al. 1983) raises important questions concerning the sites and mechanisms of action of the 1,4-dihydropyridines. From very limited structural studies it is clear that these activators share the same gen-

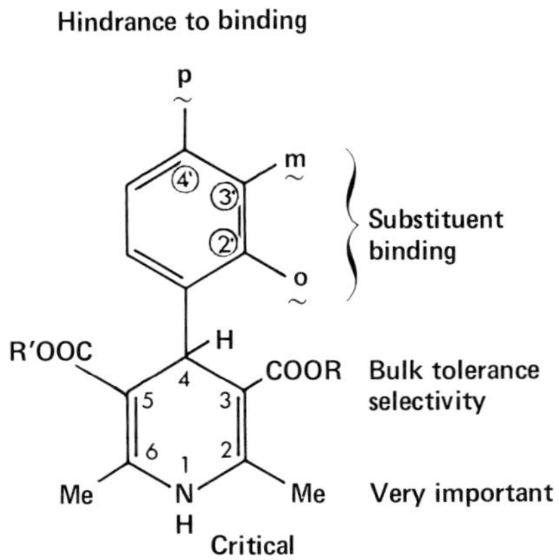

Nifedipine: R = R' = Me; 2' = NO_2
Nimodipine: R = $CHMe_2$; R' = $MeOCH_2CH_2$; 3' = NO_2
Niludipine: R = R' = $C_3H_7OCH_2CH_2$; 3' = NO_2

Fig. 1. Schematic representation of structural requirements for expression of antagonist activity in 1,4-dihydropyridines

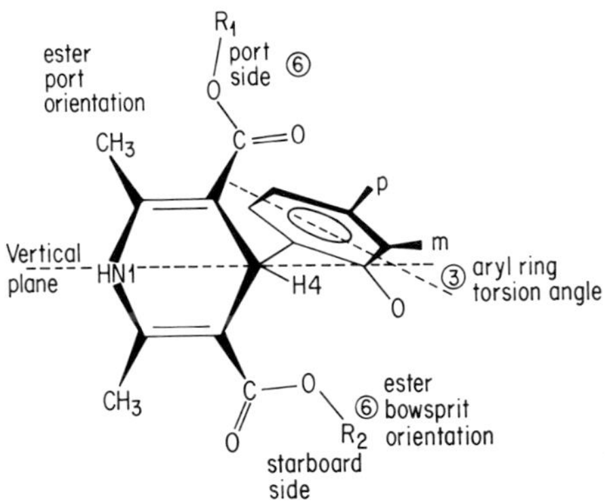

Fig. 2. Solid state conformation of 2,6-dimethyl-3,5-dicarboxylic ester-4-phenyl-1,4-dihydropyridines as revealed from solid state structural studies

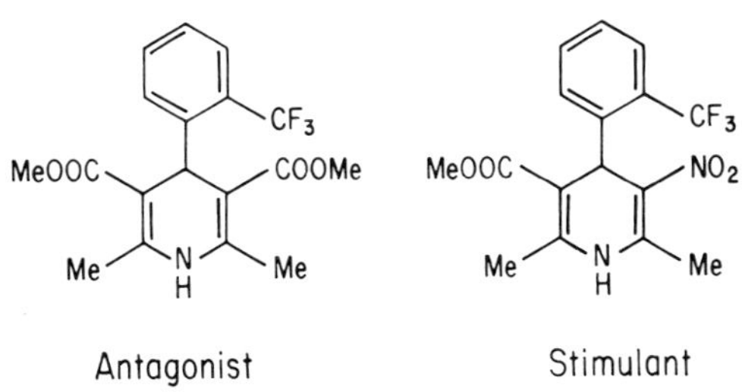

Fig. 3. Structural formulae of 1,4-dihydropyridines with antagonist or activator properties

eral conformational requirements demonstrated by the antagonists (Langs and Triggle 1984); however, it is clear from radioligand binding studies that their interactions with the binding sites are very different, antagonist and activator binding being entropically and enthalpically controlled respectively (R. A. Janis, D. Rampe and D. J. Triggle, unpub. observations).

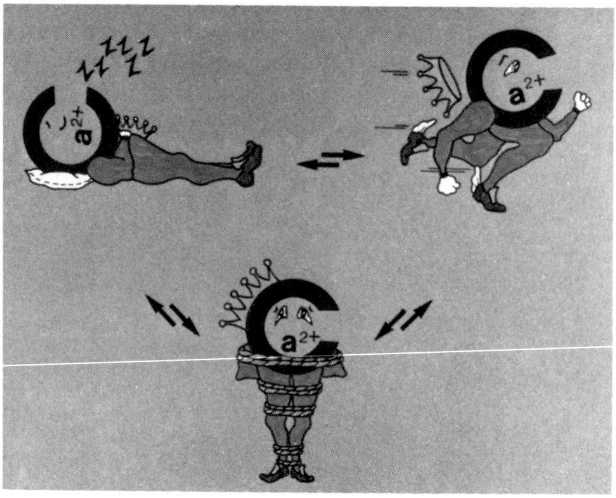

Fig. 4. Representation of Ca^{2+} channels existing in several states (or families of states) and intended to correspond approximately to the resting, activated and inactivated states

The studies just summarized represent one perspective, that from the receptor, but one which is routinely adopted in the analysis of structure-activity relationships. Such structural demands for activity may, however, not be uniformly expressed at the different functional states of the Ca^{2+} channel (Fig. 4). Thus an additional perspective, that from the ligand, must be considered. Electrophysiologic data bearing on this point are presented elsewhere in this volume (Tsien et al., Kass et al.). Other functional and radioligand binding studies also lead to the conclusion that the affinities of 1,4-dihydropyridines for Ca^{2+} channel binding sites are dependent on the channel state.

The data of Fig. 5 represent several different functional and binding correlations in smooth and cardiac muscle. There exists an excellent, virtually 1:1 correlation (Fig. 5 A), for a series of 1,4-dihydropyridines as antagonists of [3H]nitrendipine binding and the tonic (slow, sustained) component of the response to a K^+ depolarizing stimulus in intestinal smooth muscle. An analysis of cardiac binding and response, shown in Figure 5 B, shows a high affinity binding and low affinity correlation. The remaining correlations demonstrate an essentially 1:1 correlation between [^{3}H]nitrendipine binding in cardiac and smooth muscle (Fig. 5 C) and the functional correlation in the same tissues (Fig. 5 D). Despite the expression of low and high affinity activities it is important to note that the same rank order sequences of activity are observed. This suggests that these affinities may reflect different states of the same receptor rather than different receptors. Similar conclusions may be reached for other systems, including both vascular and nonvascular smooth muscles. In a number of smooth muscles showing a high dependence on $[Ca^{2+}_{ext}]$, the Ca^{2+} channel antagonists inhibit both the phasic (fast) and tonic (slow) components of response, the tonic response being more sensitive than the phasic component (Bolger et al. 1983; Yousif et al. 1985). However, the same rank order expressions of Ca^{2+} channel antagonist activity are seen (Yousif et al. 1985; F. B. Yousif and D. J. Triggle, unpub. observations), suggesting a fundamentally similar expression of activity rather than the operation of discrete structure-activity sequences. Additionally, when functional data for cardiac and smooth muscle

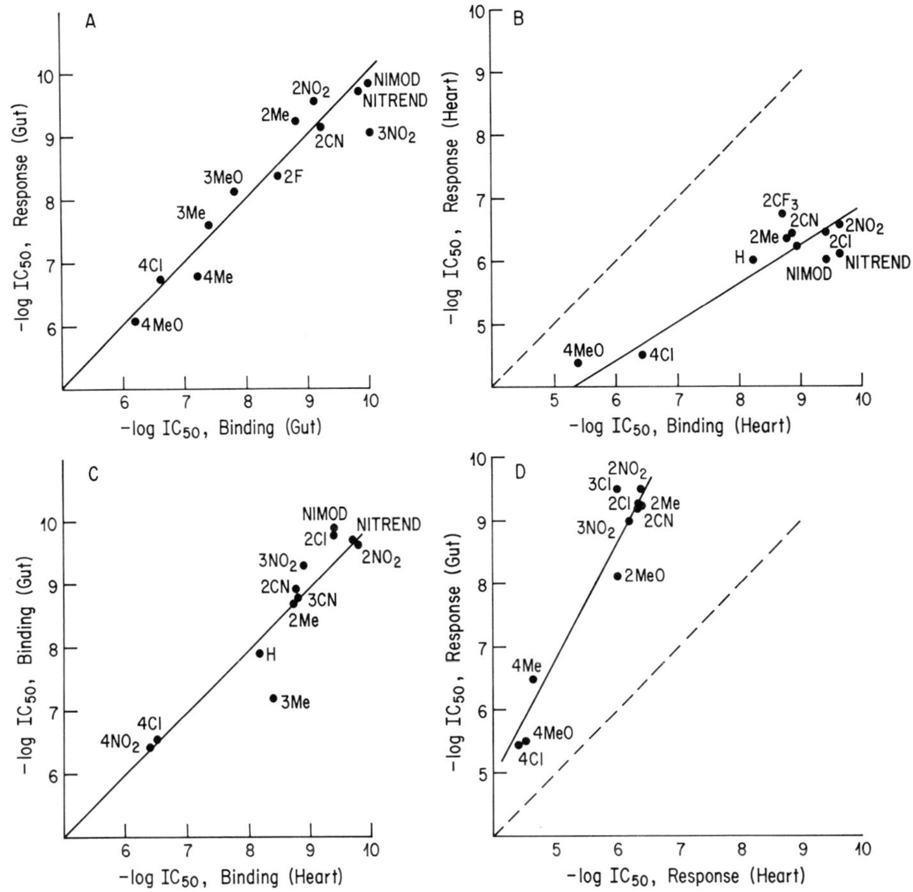

Fig. 5 A–D. Correlations between binding and pharmacological activities for a series of 1,4-dihydropyridines in smooth and cardiac muscle. **A** Abilities to inhibit specific [^{3}H]nitrendipine binding in guinea pig ileal longitudinal muscle membranes and to inhibit the tonic component of K^+-induced tension response in the same smooth muscle. **B** Abilities to inhibit specific [^{3}H]nitrendipine binding to rabbit cardiac membranes and to inhibit tension responses in driven cat papillary muscles. **C** Abilities to inhibit specific [^{3}H]nitrendipine binding to rabbit cardiac membranes and to guinea pig ileal longitudinal smooth muscle membranes. **D** Abilities to inhibit K^+-induced responses in guinea pig ileal smooth muscle and tension responses in the driven cat papillary muscle. Data from Bolger et al. (1983), Mannhold et al. (1982) and Janis et al. (1984). The *symbols* refer to the position of the substituent in the 4-phenyl ring of 2,6-dimethyl-3,5-dicarbomethoxy-4-phenyl-1,4-dihydropyridine, $X = 2-NO_2$ = nifedipine; *Nimod* = nimodipine; *Nitr* = nitrendipine

contractility are compared a virtually 1:1 correlation is obtained when data for the phasic component of response rather than for the tonic component of response are employed (compare Fig. 6 A, B).

One interpretation of such data is that they represent interaction of the antagonists with different functional states of the Ca^{2+} channel. The differential sensitivity of the phasic and tonic components of K^+ depolarization may reflect in-

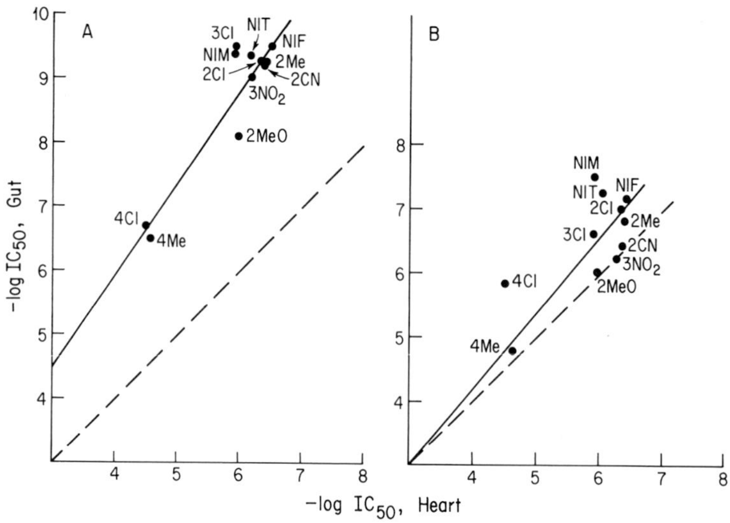

Fig. 6 A, B. Comparison of abilities of a series of 1,4-dihydropyridines (as in Fig. 5) to inhibit K^+ depolarization induced responses in guinea pig ileal longitudinal smooth muscle and driven cat papillary muscles. **A** Tonic (slow) component of the K^+ induced response in smooth muscle. **B** Phasic (fast) component of the K^+ induced response in smooth muscle. Data from Bolger et al. (1983) and Mannhold et al. (1982)

teraction of the antagonist initially with the resting state (phasic) and subsequently with an activated or inactivated state (tonic component, typically measured 10–20 min after depolarization). From electrophysiologic data (Sanguinetti and Kass 1984; Kass et al., this volume; Bean et al. 1984), this later interaction likely represents an inactivated state which also describes the high affinity interactions of [^{3}H]1,4-dihydropyridines with (depolarized) membrane fragments from smooth and cardiac muscle. The low affinity cardiac pharmacology data may also represent interaction with primarily a resting state of the Ca^{2+} channel since the stimulus frequency rate was probably too low to inactivate channels.

The affinities of 1,4-dihydropyridines for the Ca^{2+} channel can also be quantitated from their properties as competitive antagonists of responses to the Ca^{2+} channel activator Bay k 8644. Such data (Table 1) suggests an intermediate affinity state, clearly of lower affinity than that observed for the apparently competitive inhibition of responses to Ca^{2+} in K^+ depolarizing media. If Bay k 8644 acts to stabilize an open state of the Ca^{2+} channel (Hess et al. 1984; Tsien et al., this

Table 1. pA_2 values for nifedipine antagonism of responses in rat tail artery. Data from Su et al. (1984)

System	pA_2	Slope
Bay k 8644	8.27 ± 0.09	1.01
Ca^{2+}/K^+ 25 mM	9.35 ± 0.10	1.14
Ca^{2+}/K^+ 80 mM	9.65 ± 0.13	0.98

Table 2. Antagonism by nifedipine of Bay k 8644 responses in rat tail artery. Data from Su et al. (1984)

Activator	pA_2	Slope
Bay k 8644 – K^+	8.27 ± 0.19	1.01
Bay k 8644 – PE	8.20 ± 0.15	1.04
Bay k 8644 – BHT – 920	8.04 ± 0.08	0.94

volume; Kokubun and Reuter 1984) then this intermediate affinity state may represent interaction with an open or activated channel state.

Such considerations, although clearly speculative, may be of value for interpretation of the basis of tissue selectivity. The selectivity offered by the 1,4-dihydropyridines, and Ca^{2+} channel antagonists in general, may in principle arise from a variety of causes:

1. Pharmacokinetic factors
2. Relative extent of mobilization of Ca^{2+} sources
3. Physiologic reflex mechanisms
4. Differences in Ca^{2+} channels
   - structure
   - kinetics
5. State dependent block
6. Agonist-antagonist ratio (ligand efficacy)
7. Pathological state of the tissue

Thus the extent to which a particular ligand exhibits state-dependent affinities and the extent to which the channels in a particular tissue may exist in the resting, activated or inactivated states, could be powerful determinants of tissue selectivity. The ratio of these states may be controlled by specific receptor activation processes. Thus, in vascular smooth muscle in vivo and in vitro vasoconstriction can be initiated by both α_1- and α_2-adrenoceptor agonists. These can substitute for the modest levels of K^+ needed in some vascular tissues to permit Bay k 8644 actions (Schramm et al. 1983; Su et al. 1984). However, the identical pA_2 values for nifedipine against Bay k 8644 action regardless of promotion by K^+ or by the α_1- and α_2-adrenoceptor selective agonists phenylephrine and BHT 920 respectively (Table 2) indicate that the same Ca^{2+} channel state is probably produced. Nonetheless, BHT 920 is a superior promoter of Bay k 8644 action than is phenylephrine. This may indicate a preferential association of α_2-adrenoceptors with the Ca^{2+} channels. It is possible that similar preferential associations of channels with other categories of receptors also exist.

Acknowledgements. This work was supported in part by grants from The National Institutes of Health (HL 16003).

References

Bean B (1984) Nitrendipine block of cardiac calcium channels: high affinity binding to the inactivated state. Proc Nat Acad Sci USA

Bolger GT, Gengo P, Klockowski R, Luchowski E, Siegel H, Janis RA, Triggle AM, Triggle DJ (1983) Characterization of binding of the Ca^{2+}-channel antagonist [^{3}H]nitrendipine, to guinea pig ileal smooth muscle. J Pharmacol Exptl Therap 225:291–310

Fossheim R, Svarteng K, Mostad A, Rømming C, Shefter E, Triggle DJ (1982) Crystal structures and pharmacological activity of calcium channel antagonists. J Med Chem 25:126–131

Hess P, Lansman JB, Tsien RW (1984) Different modes of Ca channel gating behaviour favored by dihydropyridine Ca agonists and antagonists. Nature

Janis RA, Sarmiento JG, Maurer SC, Bolger GT, Triggle DJ (1984) Characteristics of the binding of [^{3}H]nitrendipine to rabbit ventricular membranes: modification by other Ca^{++} channel antagonists and by the Ca^{2+} channel agonist BAY K 8644. J Pharmacol Exptl Therap 231:8–15

Janis RA, Triggle DJ (1983) New development in Ca^{2+} channel antagonists. J Med Chem 26:775–785

Kokubun S, Reuter H (1984) Dihydropyridine derivatives prolong the open state of Ca^{2-} channels in cultured cardiac cells. Proc Nat Acad Sci USA 81:4824–4827

Langs DA, Triggle DJ (1984) Chemical structure and pharmacologic activities of Ca^{2+} channel antagonists. In: Proc 9th International Congress of Pharmacology, London, 1984

Loev B, Goodman KM, Snader KM, Tedeschi R, Macko E (1974) "Hantzsch-type" dihydropyridine hypotensive agents. J Med Chem 17:956–965

Mannhold R, Rodenkirchen R, Bayer R (1982) Qualitative and quantitative structure-activity relationships of specific Ca antagonists. Prog Pharmacol 5:25–52

Rosenberger LB, Triggle DJ (1978) Calcium, calcium translocation and specific calcium antagonists. In: Weiss GB (ed) Calcium and drug action. Plenum Press, New York, pp 3–31

Sanguinetti MC, Kass RS (1984) Voltage-dependent block of calcium channel current in calf cardiac Purkinje fiber by dihydropyridine calcium channel antagonists. Circ Res 55:336–348

Schramm M, Thomas G, Towart R, Franckowiak G (1983) Novel dihydropyridines with positive inotropic action through activation of Ca^{2+} channels. Nature 303:535–538

Seidel W, Meyer H, Born L, Kazda S, Dompert W (1984) Rigid calcium antagonists of the nifedipine type: geometrical requirements for the dihydropyridine receptor. Abs 14 Div Med Chem American Chemical Society, 187th National Meeting, St. Louis, MO, April 8–13

Su CM, Swamy VC, Triggle DJ (1984) Calcium channel activation in vascular smooth muscle by BAY K 8644. Can J Physiol Pharmacol 62:1401–1410

Yousif FB, Bolger GT, Ruzycky A, Triggle DJ (1985) Ca^{2+} channel antagonist actions in smooth muscle: Pharmacologic and radioligand binding studies. Can J Physiol Pharmacol 63:453–462

Triggle AM, Shefter E, Triggle DJ (1980) Crystal structures of calcium channel antagonists. J Med Chem 23:1442–1445

Discussion

(pp. 104–110)

Schwartz: In terms of what we heard today, it is clear that the "state" of the channel is extremely important with respect to correlating pharmacology with binding. So the "grinders and binders" need to be aware that what preparation we use may not really reflect what is desirable: An excellent membrane preparation not only with the appropriate sidedness, but one that has a measurable functioning calcium channel. That has not been yet done.

Van Breemen: You are referring to the initial phasic and tonic components of the contraction, due to high K^+, and suggesting that they may be different of channels states, but we have found that the initial component may be related to the release of surface-bound calcium which increases the flux perhaps through the same channel about 4-fold. If you have an increased rate of calcium entry then apparently you also diminish the effect of the intercellular buffering system, the SR. When the calcium enters faster, it also becomes more effective. And that would all explain why those contractions are less senstitive to the calcium antagonist, too.

Triggle: It was not my intention to provide, from the sorts of studies that we do, an over-interpretation of data from cellular systems that have inherent limitations for the provision of quantitative data. However, when we examine the rapid initial component, we have a system which has been preequilibrated with a calcium channel antagonist. The system is then activated and one interpretation of the lower sensitivity of this component with the same rank order correlation as the high sensitivity components, is that is reflects the interaction of the calcium channel antagonist with one state of the calcium channel (resting?) prior to its being turned on. The slower, sustained component which you and I measure typically some 15 or 20 minutes later represents the reequilibration to a state of the channel in which the preparation is being either significantly or even fully depolarized. This presumably represents interactions of a Ca^{2+}-channel blocker with another (inactivated?) state of the Ca^{2+}-channel.

Fleckenstein: Have you included into your consideration the effects of other calcium antagonists, like verapamil or diltiazem? We have found that diltiazem is also effective in suppressing the effects of the BAYER Calcium agonist. Have you seen differences between nifedipine, verapamil and diltiazem in antagonizing this calcium agonist?

Triggle: The effects of the Ca^{2+}channel antagonists on BAY K 8644 responses was originally described by Schramm et al. (1983). The 1,4-dihydropyridines are competitive inhibitors of BAY K 8644 whereas diltiazem, verapamil, D 600 etc. are non-competitive antagonists. Therefore, we deliberately chose to attempt to quantitate possible channel differences by BAY K 8644/nifedipine competition because it is difficult to quantitate affinity with non-competitive antagonists. So we preferred to quantitate using the competitive PA2 values that we got.

Bayer-Symposium IX
Cardiovascular Effects of Dihydropyridine-Type
Calcium Antagonists and Agonists, 113–139

Calcium Channels: Introduction into Their Molecular Pharmacology

H. GLOSSMANN, D. R. FERRY, A. GOLL, J. STRIESSNIG, and G. ZERNIG

1. Introduction

Calcium has a central role in cellular physiology. It mediates contraction of cardiac, smooth and skeletal muscle, neurotransmitter and hormone release, egg fertilization, acts as an intracellular signal regulating key enzymes in metabolism, controls cell differentiation and growth and plays a role in the immune response. Voltage- or receptor operated calcium specific channels in plasmamembranes are important regulators of calcium entry into cells. Despite sophisticated electrophysiological methods, the structural features and the molecular pharmacology of the calcium channel remained completely unexplored until 1981. In this year our group reported that the radiolabelled 1,4-dihydropyridine ^{3}H-nitrendipine binds to stereoselective drug receptor sites in cardiac membranes [1]. Since that time rapid progress has been made with respect to the biochemical characterisation of the calcium channel. These findings have advanced our understanding of the action of drugs which alter the channel function and have led to new concepts and hypotheses. The german physiologist Fleckenstein [2] not only paved the way for a new useful pharmacodynamic concept (with important therapeutic consequences) but also discovered and classified the tools which were essential to extend calcium channel research to the molecular level. As the calcium antagonist binding sites are evolutionary preserved and occur in plants, electric eel membranes, non electrically excitable tissues (as are human red blood cells), calcium channel drug research will grow in the next few years and extend from agriculture to neurochemistry.

In the following we will report on the biochemical analysis of Ca^{2+}-channels and the concepts which were derived from these studies. The strategy we have employed is to use radiolabelled ligands which block (or activate) Ca^{2+}-channels selectively with ED_{50} values in the picomolar, nanomolar or submicromolar range. Tritiated d-*cis*-diltiazem and (±) verapamil can be used to label calcium channels. Their K_D values are in the 20–40 nM range. The 1,4-dihydropyridines and the (−) enantiomer of the potent phenylalkylamine desmethoxyverapamil offer the following advantages: The affinity and selectivity for their channel drug receptor sites can be very high [e.g. for (+) PN 200–100 the K_0 can be $\leqq 50$ pM] and their interaction with other membrane components is often neglegible. This makes the choice of tissue preparation and purity of the respective membrane fraction less critical. However, as will shown below, there are low affinity sites for Ca^{2+} antagonists not linked to Ca^{2+} channels. ^{3}H-d-cis-diltiazem is very useful to discriminate 1,4-dihydropyridines which activate or block the Ca^{2+} channel. In the following we describe the experimental procedures including the autoradiographic techniques to visualize 1,4-dihydropyridine and phenylalkylamine binding sites linked to Ca^{2+} channels in brain. Results on photoaffinity labelling of the calcium channel with ^{3}H-azidopine and evidences for the oligomeric structure of the channel are given. A chapter on low affinity binding sites for Ca^{2+} antagonists is included, to emphasize that strict criteria have to be met before a binding site for Ca^{2+} channel drugs can be identified as a domain of the Ca^{2+} channel.

2. Reagents and Chemicals

The following buffers were employed. Buffer A: Buffer for homogenization of tissues: Fresh hypotonic, ice-cold 20 mM $NaHCO_3$, containing 0.1 mM phenylmethylsulfonylfluride (PMSF) is prepared. PMSF is kept as a 40 mM stock solution in absolute ethanol and stored at – 20 °C. Buffer B: Buffer for washing of tissues pellets and for incubation: ice-cold 50 mM TRIS HCl, 0.1 mM PMSF, (pH 7.4 measured at 37 °C). Buffer C: Buffer for solubilization: 500 mM NaCl, 50 mM TRIS HCl, 0.1 mM PMSF with 10 mM 3-(3-cholamidopropyl)-dimethylammonio 1-propanesulfonate (CHAPS), (pH 7.4 measured at 37 °C). Buffer D: Buffer for filtration and precipitation (Filtrationmedium): 10% (w/v) polyethyleneglycol 6,000 in 10 mM $MgCl_2$, 20 mM TRIS HCl, pH 7.4. A trace of sodium azide (0.01% w/v) is added. Buffer E: Divalent cation free buffer B: 500 ml 50 mM TRIS HCl (pH 7.4 at 37 °C) is pumped through 8 ml of Chelex-100 ion exchange resin (Biorad) in the sodium form in a plastic column at a flow rate of 1.0 ml/min^{-1} at 4 °C. The divalent cation-depleted buffer is collected and stored in a plastic container. PMSF is added as above. Buffer F: Buffer for autoradiographic localization studies: Isoosmotic (0.170 M) TRIS-HCl (pH 7.6 to 7.7 at 23 °C). Buffer G: Buffer for washing of labelled tissue sections: Buffer F, supplemented with 0.25 mg/ml bovine serum albumin (essentially fatty acid free, obtained from Sigma). Buffer H: Buffer for preparing red blood cell ghosts and for labelling experiments of low affinity Ca binding sites: 11.4 mM TRIS HCl, supplemented with 0.1 mM PMSF (pH 7.4).

Radiochemicals

Racemic ^{3}H nimodipine (140–160 Ci/mmol), the optical enantiomers of the unlabelled compound [(−) nimodipine and (+) nimodipine], (−) and (+) Bay e 6927, (−) and (+) nitrendipine, (−) Bay M 5579, (+) Bay K 8644 and (−) ^{3}H Bay K 8644 (75 Ci/mmol) were from Bayer AG (Wuppertal, FRG). (+) PN 200–110, (−) PN 200–110, (±) PN 200–110 and the optically pure enantiomers of the 1,4 dihydropyridine 202–791 (isopropyl 4-(2,1,3 benzoxadiazol-4-yl)-1,4-dihydro-2-6-dimethyl-5-nitro-3-pyridine carboxylate) were from Sandoz AG (Basel, Switzerland), (+) and (−) nicardipine from Syntex Ltd. (Glasgow, Scotland), (−) ^{3}H desmethoxyverapamil (85 Ci/mmol), the enantiomers of desmethoxyverapamil, D-600 and verapamil from Knoll AG (Ludwigshafen, FRG) and CGP 28392 from Ciba-Geigy AG (Basel, Switzerland); ^{3}H nitrendipine (78 Ci/mmol), d-cis ^{3}H diltiazem (72.3 Ci/mmol) and ^{3}H verapamil (83,9 Ci/mmol) were from NEN (Dreieich, FRG), (+) ^{3}H PN 200–110 (60 Ci/mmol) were from Amersham (Braunschweig, FRG); (±) ^{3}H azidopine (54 Ci/mmol) and (±) ^{125}I iodipine (2,000 Ci/mmol) were prepared as described (3,4). Radioligands are stored in ethanol at 100 °C/ml for up to 3 months at −25 °C, and remain stable. In the presence of a large receptor excess the bindability fraction of the chiral ^{3}H-1,4-dihydropyridines is (and stays for 3 months) in the range of 40–50% and for the pure (+) enantiomer of PN 200–110 85%. The coelution or comigration of the radioligand with the unlabelled compound is tested by HPLC or TLC. All 1,4-dihydropyridines are handled in the absence of UV light. Sodium lighting or dimmed, diffuse daylight is also suitable. D-*cis* (0-methyl-^{3}H)-Diltiazem (85–145 Ci/mmol), ^{125}I-Iodipine, (−) ^{3}H-desmethoxyverapamil and ^{3}H-azidopine are also available from Amersham. ^{125}I-Iodipine and ^{3}H-azidopine can be used for up to five weeks after synthesis when stored in ethanol at −25 °C.

Other Chemicals

Nitrophenyl 1,4-dihydropyridine derivatives (not mentioned above) are obtained from Bayer AG, Wuppertal, FRG, Benzothiazepines (l- and d-cis-diltiazem) are from Gödecke AG. Freiburg, FRG Tiapamil [N-(3,4-dimethoxyphenethyl)-2-(3,4-deimethoyphenyl)-N-methyl-m-dithiane-2 propylamine-1,1,3,3-tetraoxide] is from Hoffmann La Roche, Basel, Switzerland. (+) and (−) Prenylamine are from Hoechst AG, Frankfurt, FRG. Dipyridamole was from Thomae (Biberach, FRG), hexobendine from Chemie Linz AG (Linz, Austria) and dilazep from Degussa (Frankfurt, FRG). Nitrobenzylthioinosine [S-(p-nitrobenzyl)-6-thioinosine], the corresponding guanosine analogue nitrobenzylthioguanosine [S-(p-nitrobenzyl)-6-thioguanosine], nucleosides and nucleotides, trypsin (L-1-tosylamide-2-phenylethylchloromethyl ketone-treated) and trypsin inhibitor (from lima bean) were from Sigma (Munich, FRG).

3. Methods

Preparation of Membrane Fragments

Cardiac Muscle and Smooth Muscle Organs. Organs (cleaned from connective tissue and fat) are finely minced with scissors and homogenized in ice-cold buffer A with a wet weight to volume ratio of 1:3 by an ultraturrax for 2 × 15 s at 3/4 maximal speed and then have buffer A added to give a wet weight to volume ratio of

1:7. The diluted homogenate is subjected to a 15 min 1,500 × g centrifugation. The supernatants are centrifuged at 45,000 × g for 15 min, the pellets are resuspended in buffer B and washed twice as above.

Brain. Whole brain (minus medulla and cerebellum) is homogenized at a wet weight to volume ratio as above and then subjected to a 45,000 × g (15 min) centrifugation. Pellets are washed twice in buffer B as above.

Skeletal Muscle. 15 g of guinea-pig hind limb skeletal muscles are finely minced in buffer A and homogenized at a wet weight to volume ratio of 1:5 with an ultraturrax as above using 2–3 × 20 s bursts of 3/4 maximal speed. Disrupted muscle is filtered through two layers of cheese cloth and then centrifuged as described for cardiac muscle. This membrane fraction is referred to as the partially purified skeletal muscle transverse tubule membrane. For preparation of t-tubules the 45,000 × g pellet is taken up in 0.25 M sucrose in buffer B (45 ml for 15 g original wet weight tissue) and is homogenized with seven complete strokes of a Dounce homogenizer (tight pestle). 7 ml fractions are overlayed on a discontinous sucrose gradient [8 ml of 40%, 35%, 30%, 7 ml 25% (w/w) sucrose in buffer B]. Gradients are spun in a Beckman SW 27 rotor for 150 min at 2°–4 °C at 113,000 × g (25,000 rpm). The material collecting at the 25% (w/w) sucrose layer/overlay interface is removed with a syringe, diluted 20-fold in buffer B and centrifuged for 120 min at 45,000 × g. The membranes were kept in 2 ml aliquots in polypropylene vials and could be stored in liquid nitrogen for up to 3 months.

Hippocampus. The hippocampal formation is dissected out of the guineapig brain on ice. After gentle homogenisation (10 complete strokes) in a Dounce homogenizer (Blaessig Glass Company, Rochester N.Y.), equipped with the tight pestle, in ice-cold buffer A at a wet-weight to volume ratio of 1:10, the homogenate is spun at 45,000 × g (15 min) at 2 °C.

The resulting pellet is resuspended in ice-cold buffer B by 4 strokes of the homogenizer and the centrifugation repeated twice as before. The final pellet is flash frozen in liquid nitrogen and was stored for up 4 weeks without loss of binding.

Red Blood Cell Ghosts. They were prepared from human erythrocytes according to Dodge et al. [5].

Solubilization of Calcium Channels

For solubilization the skeletal muscle partially purified transverse tubule membrane (6 mg of protein) is suspended in 5 ml ice-cold buffer B and 2.5 ml of 2 M NaCl are added. 2.5 ml of 40 mM CHAPS in buffer B are dropped into the gently shaken mixture which is kept on ice for 30 minutes and then centrifuged for 45,000 × g for 60 min at 4 °C. The supernatant is filtered through a disposable 0.2 μm nitrocellulose filter with a syringe. At the above protein to detergent ratio, CHAPS solubilizes 90% of the protein and 20–40% of the 1,4-dihydropyridine and ^{3}H-desmethoxyverapamil binding sites (present in the starting membranes) are recovered.

Basic Ligand Binding Assay for High Affinity Receptors on Ca^{2+} Channels

In this laboratory filtration manifolds (12–48 places), strong vacuum pumps and polystyrol incubation tubed are used. The manifold is loaded with prewetted Whatman GF/C filters. Immediately before filtration the vacuum pump is turned on, 1 ml of buffer E is poured on each filter and filters are dried by vacuum prior to filtration of the diluted contents of the assay. For separation of bound and free ligand 3.5 ml of buffer D was added to the contents of the assay tubes and poured through the filters. Two washes, each with 3.5 ml of the buffer, followed. Dried filters (at 45 °C) were then counted for retained radioactivity after adding a suitable liquid scintillation cocktail, or directly in a gamma counter (^{125}I-iodipine). For low affinity binding sites (e. g. on human red blood cell ghosts) the blank definition was 3 μM (+) nimodipine, for Ca^{2+} channel linked receptors, see [6].

Assay with Solubilized Calcium Channels

The incubation is as above but the assay is performed in the presence of 0.2 mg/ml fat free bovine serum albumin. After incubation, assay tubes were transferred into melting ice and 0.1 ml of an ice-cold mixture of bovine serum albumin/rabbit gamma globulin (5 mg of each per ml) as carrier protein, in buffer B was added followed by 3.5 ml of filtration medium (and precipitation) buffer D. After 5–10 min bound and free ligand were separated as above. This method can be used successfully to precipitate prelabelled and not prelabelled solubilized channels.

Autoradiographic Procedures

Unfixed tissues are used. Brains are frozen at −20 °C and are mounted onto microtome chucks using mounting media. They are cut with a microtome cryostate into 8 μm thick sections. Sections are thaw-mounted onto gelatine-coated microscope slides. The slides can be stored for up to 7 days at −20 °C before deterioration of binding activity is observed. Radioactivity bound to tissue sections was measured by wiping off the wet tissues, with a glass fiber filter paper, from the slide. The binding of labelled 1,4-dihydropyridines to e. g. guinea-pig brain sections is reversible, saturable, of high affinity (dissociation constants are in the nanomolar range) and with the appropriate pharmacology. Labelled 1,4-dihydropyridines are bound to tissue sections in buffer F at 23 °C for 60 min, (−) ^{3}H-desmethoxyverapamil at 2 °C for 60 min. Loosely bound radioactivity is then washed away by the following procedure. A short dip in buffer F is followed by a 30 minute "wash" in ice-cold buffer G, followed by a 15–30 second dip in ice-cold distilled water to remove salt and thereby facilitate drying with a stream of cooled (< 10 °C) air. This takes 30–60 s. Failure to include albumin in the wash buffer results in unacceptable high blank values. Even in brain sections including the heavily specifically labelled hippocampal formation the signal to noise ratio is at best very unfavourable. In rat brain sections the high affinity binding is almost unmeasureably low, relative to blank binding without the use of albumin in the wash buffer. The inclusion of albumin in the wash buffer has no effect on the K_D or B_{max} of ^{3}H-nimodipine or ^{3}H-PN 200–110 in guinea-pig brain sections. In mapping experiments the following concentrations are used; 0.1 nM ^{3}H-nimodipine, 0.1 nM ^{3}H-PN 200–110, 0.01 nM ^{125}I-iodipine, 1 nM (−) ^{3}H-desmethoxyverapamil. Blanks were generated with sections consecutive to those used for "total binding" by adding 2 μM nimodipine or other blank definitions (see above) to the incubation media. Before being exposed to radioligands, blanks are preincubated with unlabelled ligands for 10–15 minutes. Dried, labelled tissue sections are mounted on a square of adhesive plastic foil placed on an X-ray cassette and a ^{3}H-Ultrafilm (LKB, Stockholm, Sweden) is placed against them. The cassettes are stored, at room temperature, for the exposure period. Exposure time ranges from 3 to 8 weeks for the ^{3}H-ligand-labelled tissues or 1–2 days for ^{125}I-iodipine. Films are developed in D-19 for 5 min at 20 °C, rinsed in water and fixed 5 min at 20 °C in Ektaflo Fixer (1:4 with water). After 20 min of rinsing in running water the films are dried in air. Sections can be re-exposed or counted for radioactivity.

Photoaffinity Labelling

Guinea-pig skeletal muscle membranes (protein: 1–2 mg/ml) in buffer B are incubated with 2.5 nM of ^{3}H-azidopine (total binding) or with 2.5 nM ^{3}H-azidopine in the presence of 100 nM of the (+) enantiomer of PN 200–110 (blank binding) or other drugs in a volume of 4 ml. After 60 min incubation at 25 °C the assay mixture is centrifuged at 35,000 × g for 10 min at 2 °C. The first supernatant is discarded and the pellets are resuspended in 4 ml of ice-cold buffer B, supplemented with 0.25 mg/ml bovine serum albumin (fat free; Sigma, Munich). The centrifugation is repeated, the supernatant is discarded and the pellets are resuspended in 4 ml of ice-cold buffer B. The suspensions are irradiated with a Philips TL 40 W/OB black-light lamp in a 8 cm diameter Petri dish at a distance of 10 cm for 3 min on ice. The irradiated suspensions are spun down as above and the pellets were resuspended in 50 μl of buffer B. 0.02 ml of a protease inhibitor mix containing 0.14 mg/ml leupeptin, 0.7 mM benzamidine, 0.7 mM PMSF, 2.8 mM EDTA, 0.02 mg/ml Trasylol and 0.14 mg/ml Pepstatin A was added to the pellet. After 20 min 0.2 ml of boiling stop solution was added. This solution was composed of 2.5 ml of 20% SDS, 0.5 ml of 2-mercaptoethanol (reducing condition) or 1 mg/ml N-ethylmaleimide (nonreducing conditions), 1.0 ml glycerol, 1.0 ml of 0.625 M TRIS HCl, 0.1 mM PMSF (pH 7.5) with 1.8 g of urea. After 10 min at 25 °C the solubilized membranes were applied to a 4–12% polyacrylamide gel.

Following electrophoresis slab gels were either cut and counted for radioactivity after 3 days of solubilization in Lipoloma/Liposolve liquid scintillation cocktail or fixed for 30 min, and then impregnated with Amersham Amplify for 30 min before being dried and exposed to Kodak XO-mat films for 20–40 days at −70 °C. Molecular weights of bands identified in fluorograms were calculated by linear interpolation.

For two-dimensional gel-electrophoresis, column gels of the first dimension were of 0.4 cm internal diameter and were 8 cm long; 8% polyacrylamide were employed with a 1 cm stacking gel. After the column gel has been run it was fused and covered with a 4–12% slab gel by 2 cm of 2% agar which contained either 0.55 ml of βmercaptoethanol and 7.5 mg of dithiothreitol per 5 ml (second dimension reduced) or 1 mg/ml N-ethylmaleimide (second dimension non-reduced) then left to stand for 1 hour at room temperature before running the second dimension. The second dimension gels were calibrated by 1 cm position of column gels which contained ^{14}C-marker proteins and were applied to the second dimension along with the photolabelled first dimension gel.

4. Results and Interpretation

The Three Drug Receptor Sites of the Ca^{2+}-Channel

1,4-Dihydropyridines, developed mainly by chemists and pharmacologists of the Bayer company in Germany have been essential in the initial biochemical characterization of calcium channels (6). ^{3}H-Nitrendipine, ^{3}H-nimodipine and ^{3}H-nifedipine as well as ^{3}H-PN 200–110 (a potent benzoxadiazol 1,4-dihydropyridine from the Sandoz AG in Switzerland) bind to high affinity, stereospecific receptor sites in brain, heart, ileum and skeletal plasma membranes. Nitrendipine, PN 200–110, nimodipine, Bay K 8644, iodipine and azidopine are chiral whereas nifedipine is not. The racemic nature of some of the ligands has to be taken into account for the data calculation. E. g. the bindability of ^{3}H-(±)PN 200–110, ^{125}I-iodipine, ^{3}H-azidopine and ^{3}H-nimodipine is $\approx 50\%$ whereas that of (+) ^{3}H-PN 200-110 is $\geqq 85\%$.

Figure 1 shows the radiolabelled 1,4-dihydropridines which can be used to characterize, what we term "receptor site 1" or the 1,4-dihydropyridine selective site of the channel, namely the chiral 1,4-dihydropridines nitrendipine, nimodipine, PN 200–110, Bay K 8644, the first iodinated 1,4-dihydropyridine, ^{125}I-iodipine, the arylazide photoaffinity ligand azidopine and the nonchiral nifedipine. One may wonder why so many ligands are necessary to characterize this particular domain of the calcium channel. However, without them we would not have been able to understand the concept of agonists, antagonists and dualists for the channel, predict the tissue selectivity of a given 1,4-dihydropyridine by in vitro receptor and gain insight the structure of the channel as well as into the mechanism by which the drugs act.

Figure 2 shows the drugs which are employed to characterize the drug receptor site "2" or the verapamil-selective site: Racemic ^{3}H-verapamil and the optically pure (−) ^{3}H-desmethoxyverapamil. This latter drug is 25 times more potent than verapamil in both, functional studies and with respect to receptor affinity [7, 8]. The only drug so far employed to characterize the third receptor site, the diltiazem selective site, is ^{3}H-d-*cis*-diltiazem [9]. The three distinct domains (with given selectivities for the chemically heterogeneous calcium channel blockers and activators) are linked one to another through bidirectional allosteric coupling processes (Fig. 3). The three drug receptor sites are arranged in our model [10] in

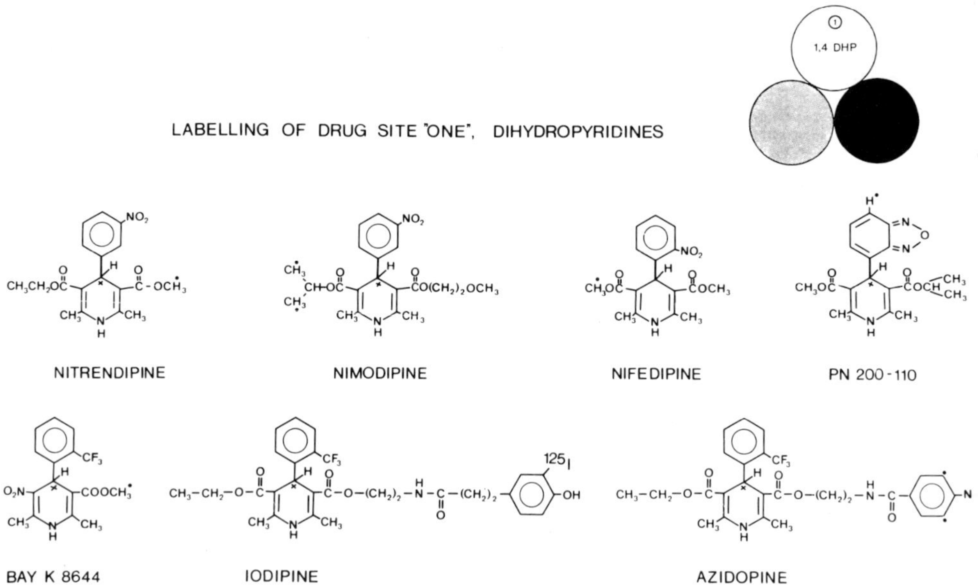

Fig. 1. Ligands for receptor site "1"

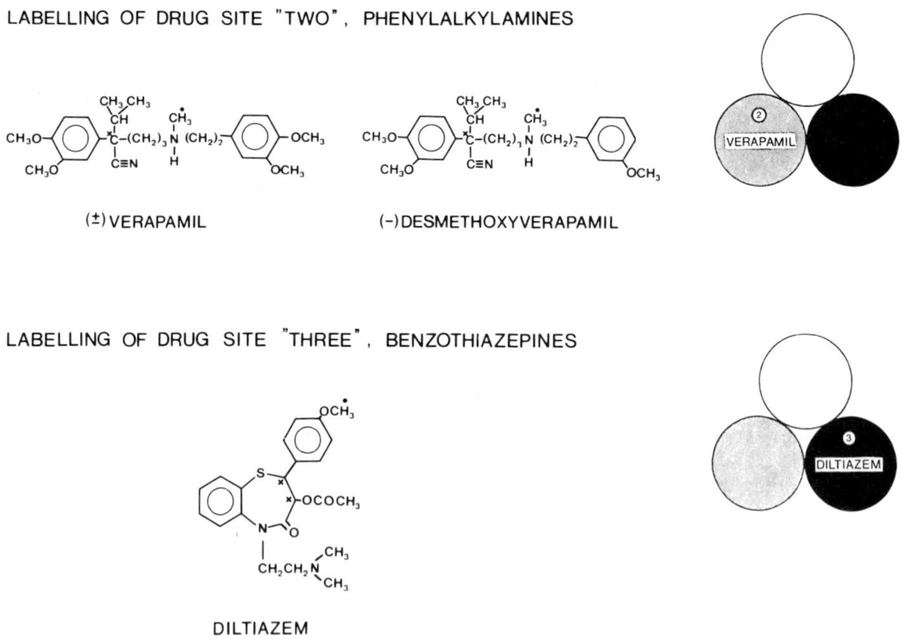

Fig. 2. Ligands for receptor site "2" and "3"

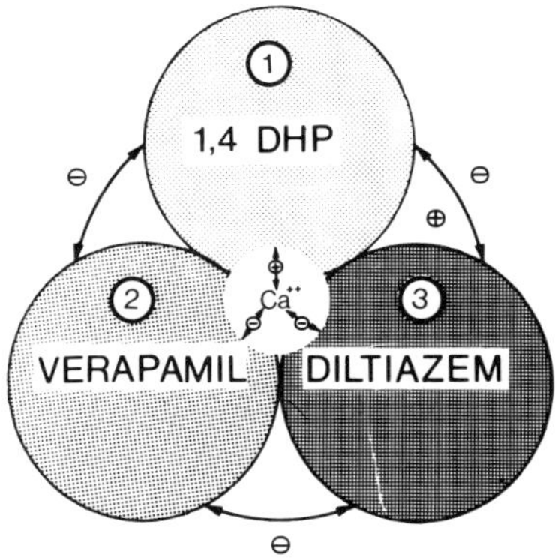

Fig. 3. Interaction of receptor sites "1", "2", and "3" with Ca^{2+} binding sites (see [10])

a circular manner and they are connected by bidirectional arrows. These arrows symbolize allosteric interactions and the effects of a drug binding to a receptor site on the adjacent one is indicated by plus and minus sign. Each of the three drug receptor sites can exist in low or high affinity states and the equilibrium between these states is determined by the intrinsic activity of a given drug. Although electro-physiologists question that a Ca^{2+} channel can exist open or closed in a broken cell preparation, the high and low affinity states which we observe in vitro can be conveniently envisaged as being equivalent to the nonconducting or conducting states of the channel in the intact membrane. In the center of the model are the divalent cation binding sites. These divalent cation binding sites are the key to understand calcium channel function and how drugs can stabilize the open or closed state of the channel. The model also explains the interaction of drugs at the receptor level and predicts, in analogy to the GABA-benzodiazepine-chloride ionophore complex, that for each site (perhaps there are even more than three), agonists, inverse agonists and antagonists exist. The most intriguing prediction [15] is, that the optical antipodes of chiral drugs may stabilize different conformations (e.g. open vs closed).

The Divalent Cation Binding Sites of the Channel

In vitro binding studies from our group have led to the identification of two classes of cation binding sites. The first class has micromolar dissocation constants for Ca^{2+} and high selectivity for divalent cations since it will not accept sodium or potassium. This class of sites is coupled to the 1,4-dihydropyridine receptor. Any drug which will increase the fraction of receptor site "one" having high affinity, will increase the fraction of channels holding the divalent cation very tightly. Conversely, drugs which will increase the fraction of receptor sites "one" having low affinity will convert channels into ones holding the divalent cations less tightly. ^{3}H-Dihydropyridine binding to brain membranes is strictly dependent upon Me^{2+}. Using EDTA washed membranes and Chelex 100 treated buffers, Ca^{2+} can be shown to have an ED_{50} of $\approx 2\ \mu M$ to facilitate high affinity ^{3}H-1,4-dihydropyridine binding (Fig. 4). Monovalent cations are, in contrast, in-

a

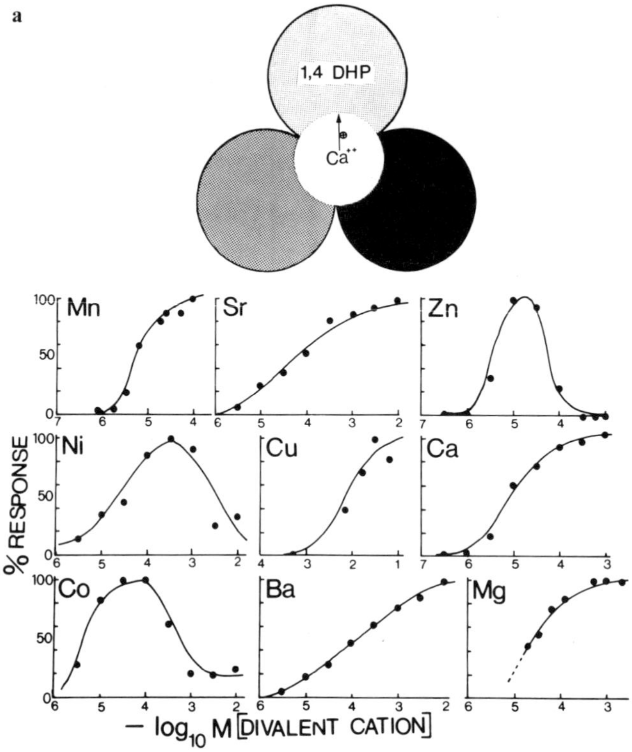

Fig. 4. a Refilling of Ca^{2+} channels (guinea-pig brain isochannel) with divalent cations. Channels were depleted (see [6]) for divalent cations as described and 1,4-dihydropyridine binding (^{3}H-nimodipine) recovered as a function of Me^{2+}. **b** Refilling of the brain isochannel in the presence (*closed symbols*) or absence (*open symbols*) of 10 μM d-*cis* diltiazem. Note that the apparent affinity for ions, which pass, is increased

effective and La^{3+} inhibits Ca^{2+}-dependent, high affinity ^{3}H-1,4-dihydropyridine binding. In other tissues, e.g. heart and skeletal muscle, the binding is less sensitive (or even insensitive) to chelators. However, if the skeletal muscle channel solubilized, a constraint is removed and 1,4-dihydropyridine binding is as sensitive to chelators as seen in partially purified brain membranes (6,11). Fig. 5 shows the different states of the receptor site 1 induced by chelators, calcium, agonists or antagonists. The low affinity, low selectivity cation binding sites have close to millimolar dissociation constants for divalent cations. Binding of, for example ^{3}H-verapamil, ^{3}H-desmethoxyverapamil or ^{3}H-d-*cis*-diltiazem, is inhibited by divalent cations with millimolar K_D values (Fig. 6). This class of sites will also accept sodium or potassium (Table 1).

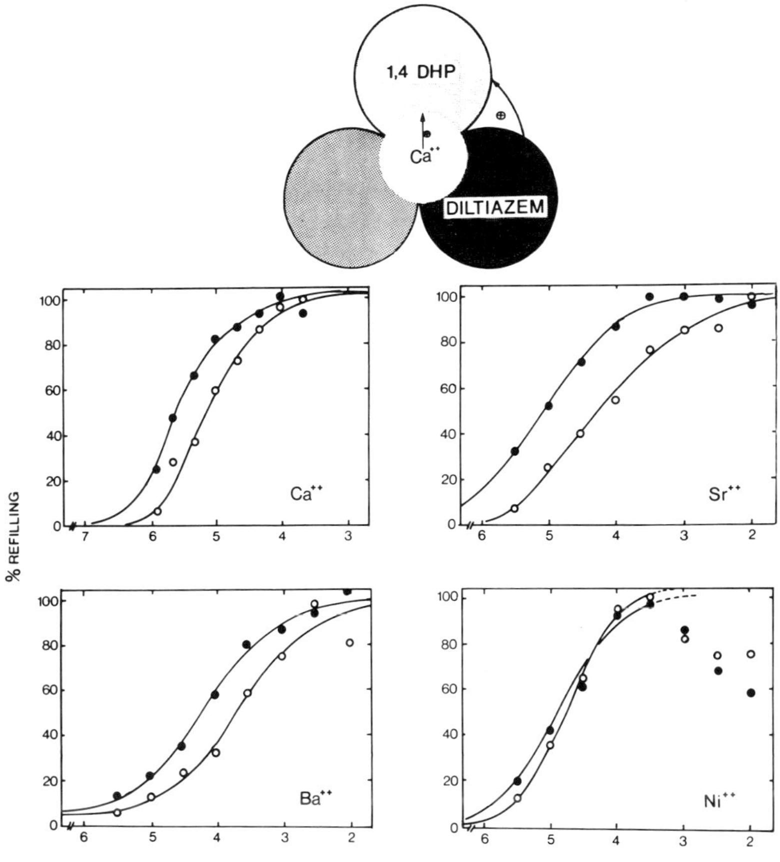

Fig. 4 b.

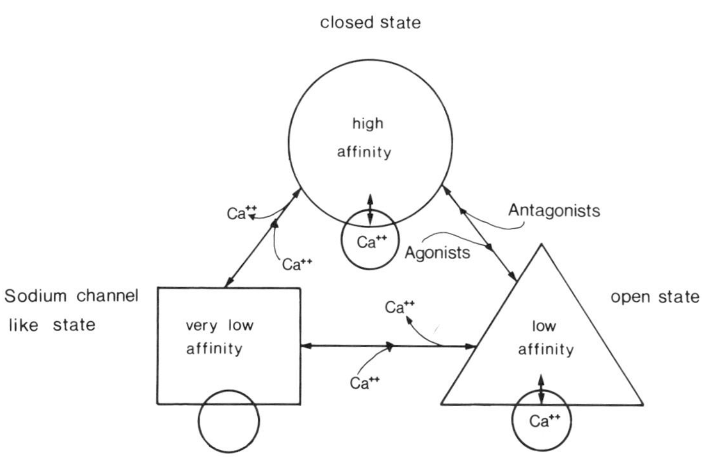

Fig. 5. Three different states of receptor site "1" induced by agonists, antagonists or by removal of Ca^{2+}

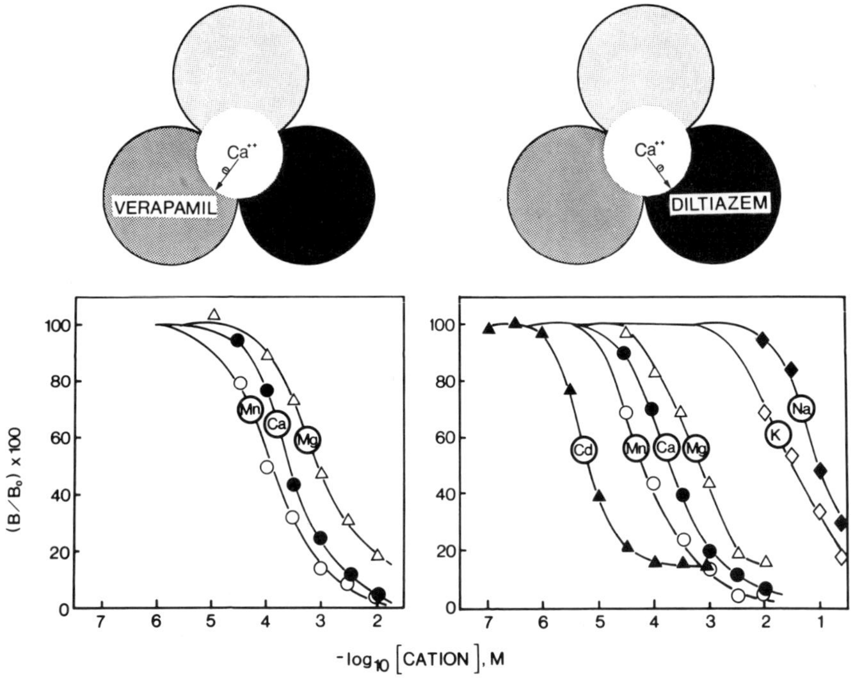

Fig. 6. Interaction of cations with receptor sites "2" and "3". The skeletal muscle isochannel (partially purified transverse tubule membranes) was probed with ^{3}H-verapamil (*left*) or ^{3}H-d-*cis* diltiazem (*right*). B_O is the specific binding (at equilibrium) in the absence. B in the presence of ions (all as chloride salts)

Table 1. Properties of calcium channel metal ion binding sites. For further details see [6] and Fig. 4a, b

	High affinity sites	Low affinity sites
Dissociation constants Me^{2+}	μM range	mM range
Specificity for Me^{2+}	Yes	No
Coupled to	1,4-DHP site	Verapamil, diltiazem sites
Coupling	Positive	Negative

The Concept of Isochannels

Figure 7 shows the saturation analysis of drug receptor site "1", labelled with ^{3}H-nimodipine at 37 °C in the absence (open circles) and presence of d-*cis*-diltiazem (filled circles) in different membranes. In brain, diltiazem increases the affinity, in skeletal muscle dramatically the fraction of sites stabilized in high affinity, whereas in heart there is only a modest increase in B_{max}. These differential effects of diltiazem are tissue but not species specific and were the first evidence that calcium channels are heterogeneous [12].

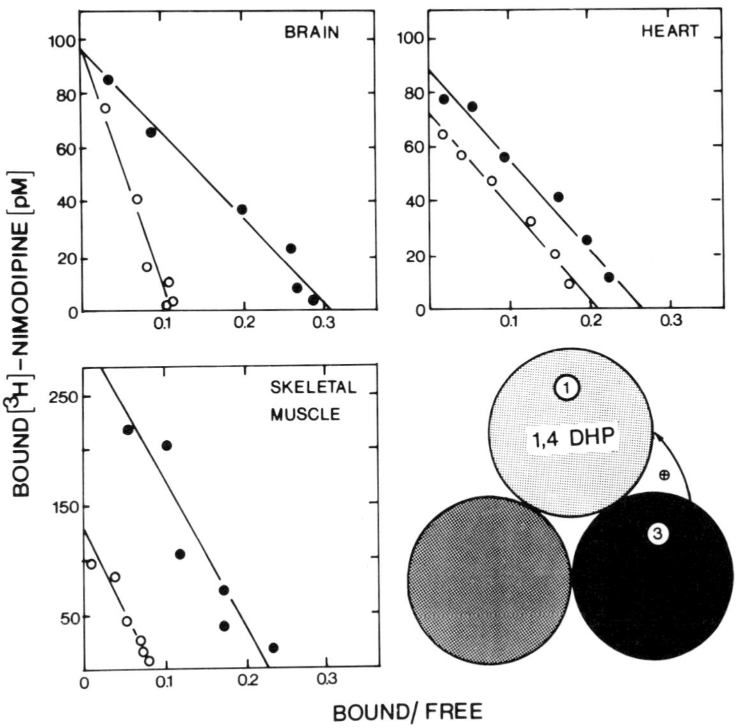

Fig. 7. Saturation analysis for receptor site "1" for the three subtypes (isochannels) brain, heart and skeletal muscle (transverse tubule membranes) in the absence (*open circles*) or presence (*closed circles*) of an allosteric regulator (d-*cis* diltiazem, binding to receptor site "3") at 37 °C

Table 2. The concept of calcium isochannels. Adapted from [13]

Property	Isochannel		
	Brain	Heart	Skeletal muscle
Target size Mr ^{3}H-nimodipine	180,000	180,000	180,000
Target size Mr reduction by diltiazem (~60,000)	+	+	+
pH profile	Biphasic	n. d.	Monophasic
^{3}H-nimodipine dissociation constant	0.6 nM	0.25 nM	2 nM
AQA-39 regulation	−	+	+++
EDTA sensitivity	+++	++	(+)
Heparin sensitivity	−	+	+++
SH-groups (essential)	+	+	+++

In Table 2 we summarize our findings which argue for subtypes of channels, which we call "isochannels". These isochannels have the same molecular weight (as calculated from target size analysis experiments with high enery electrons) and display the same reduction of the size of receptor site "1", when d-*cis*-diltiazem occupies drug receptor site "3", that is by 60,000 mass units. Differences reside in the pH profile for 1,4-dihydropyridine binding, the dissociation constant for a given 1,4-dihydropyridine in a given tissue, sensitivity to subtype-selective drugs, such as AQA-39, sensitivity of 1,4-dihydropyridine binding to chelators, to heparin and sulfhydryl reagents [13].

Reciprocal Allosteric Regulation

Reciprocal allosteric regulation between the three different drug receptor sites. ^{3}H-d-*cis*-diltiazem and (−) ^{3}H-desmethoxyverapamil have been most helpful to advance this concept. Figure 8 shows the stabilisation of channels in high affinity for drug receptor site "3", labelled by ^{3}H-d-*cis*-diltiazem in skeletal muscle transverse tubule membranes as a function of 1,4-dihydropyridine structure and concentration. Clearly, individual 1,4-dihydropyridines differ in their capacity to stabilize. Agonists such as Bay K 8644 and CGP 28392 have much less conversion power than the antagonists, (−) Bay e 6927 or (−) nimodipine. If one quantitates the capacity for stabilization of site "3" in high affinity by different 1,4-di-

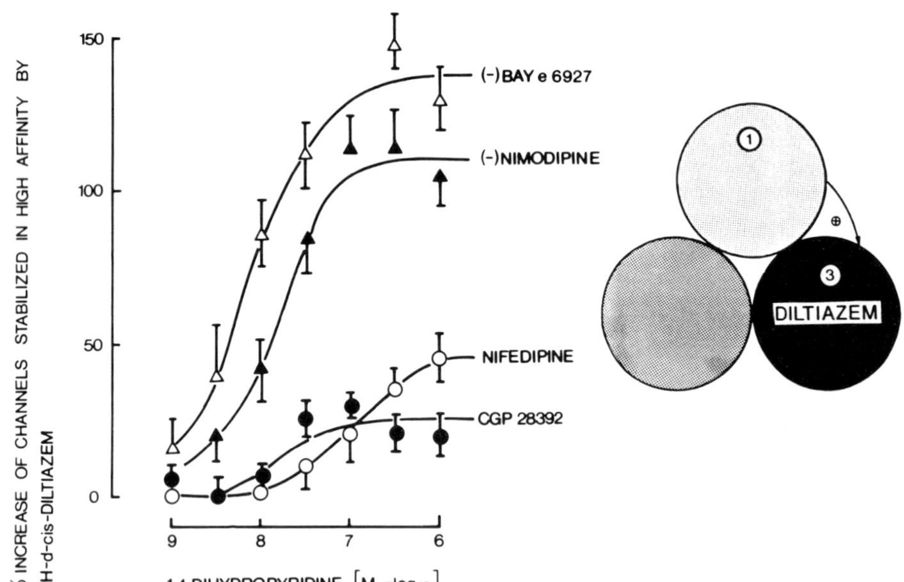

Fig. 8. Stabilization of skeletal muscle transverse tubulus calcium channels in high affinity for ^{3}H-d-*cis* diltiazem (at 30 °C) by different 1,4-dihydropyridines. Note that EC_{50} and maximal effect differentiate the individual 1,4 dihydropyridines

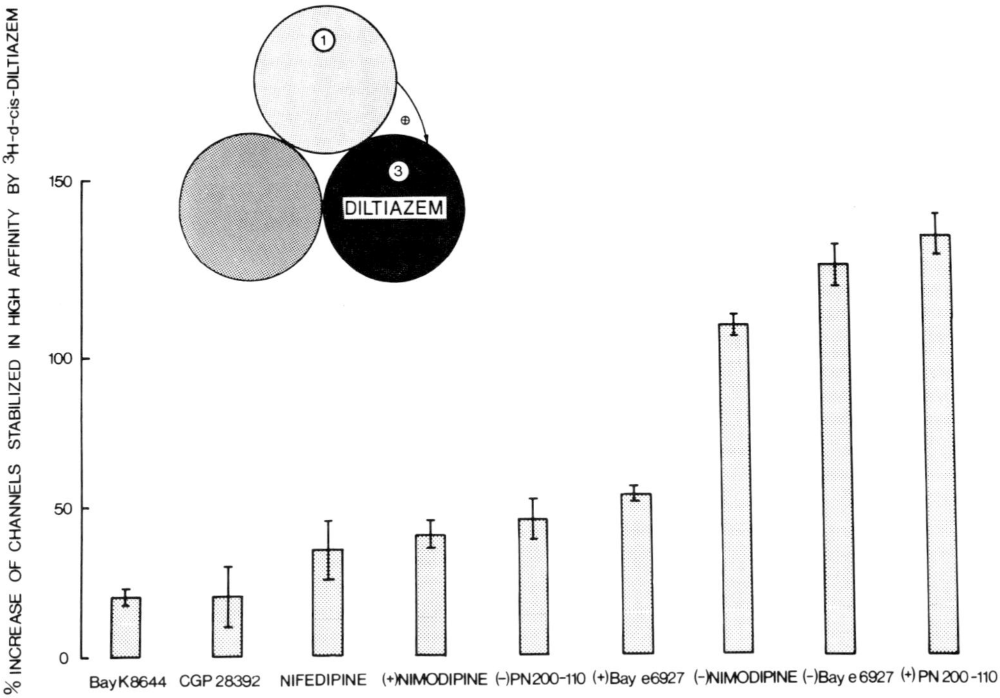

Fig. 9. Computer optimized maximal effects for conversion of receptor site "3" into the high affinity state by drugs acting on receptor site "1" are plotted. Data were generated as in Fig. 8. Means from 3–5 experiments

hydropyridines, acting via receptor site "1" a continuum is found for these drugs, with the agonists to the left and the antagonists to the right. This is shown in Fig. 9

The Concept of Intrinsic Activity

A more direct way to quantitiate the intrinsic activity of a radiolabelled 1,4-dihydropyridine to stabilize either the low or high affinity states of its receptor site is, to measure the fraction of channels labelled with high affinity. In the graph shown in Fig. 10 we have plotted the fraction of channels stabilized in high affinity for two isochannels. One immediately sees that the agonist ^{3}H-Bay k 8644 stabilizes only a small percentage of both isochannels in high for drug receptor site "1". ^{125}I-iodipine, however, is a fully antagonistic 1,4 dihydropyridine for the heart isochannel but similar in behaviour as ^{3}H-Bay K 8644 for the skeletal muscle isochannel. As above, using ^{3}H d-*cis*-diltiazem as label for drug receptor site "3", a continuum is seen by directly labelling drug receptor site "1", ranging from agonists to antagonists. The fraction of channels stabilized in high affinity at site "1" by each 1,4-dihydropyridine is a tissue and drug specific constant and is the

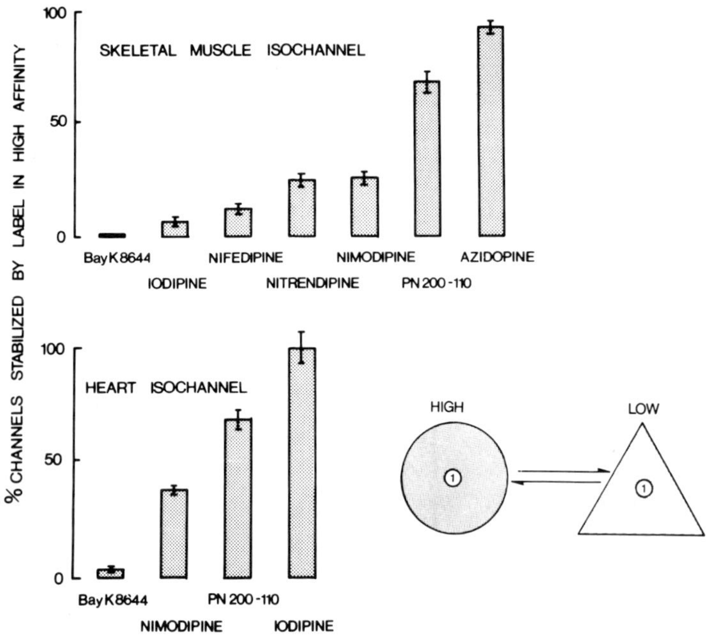

Fig. 10. Saturation analysis of Ca^{2+} channels with radiolabelled 1,4-dihydropyridines. The B_{max} values from 3–10 experiments are plotted for the two isochannels. Note, that ^{125}I iodipine labels more sites in the heart than any other 1,4 dihydropyridine whereas azidopine stabilizes more channels in high affinity in the skeletal muscle than any other 1,4-dihydropyridine. The low-affinity state of the channel is not detected in direct binding experiments with labelled 1,4-dihydropyridines (fast off-kinetics) but easily recognized in competition experiments. Thus, unlabelled Bay K 8644 has a biphasic displacement curve (at 37 °C) for (+) ^3H PN 200 110. The equilibrium distribution of the receptor site "1" in high and low affinity states stabilized by the ligands is symbolized at the *right*

basis for the tissue-selectivity of the different 1,4-dihydropyridines. The heart isochannel selectivity of iodipine was confirmed in pharmacological studies with the unlabelled compound (not shown).

The Concept of the Reciprocal Allosteric Regulation is Valid Not Only for Skeletal Muscle Isochannel but also in Brain Tissue

The evidence is strong that the concept of reciprocal allosteric regulation of the three receptor sites is valid for the skeletal muscle isochannel. This has been demonstrated by labelling each of the three distinct drug receptor sites individually. Does this model also apply to other isochannels? The hippocampal formation is one of the brain region with the highest density of neuronally localized calcium channels. In membranes prepared from hippocampus, the allosteric coupling between receptor sites "2", labelled by (−) ^3H-desmethoxyverapamil and the drug receptor site "3" can be easily demonstrated. We could show that d-*cis*-diltiazem

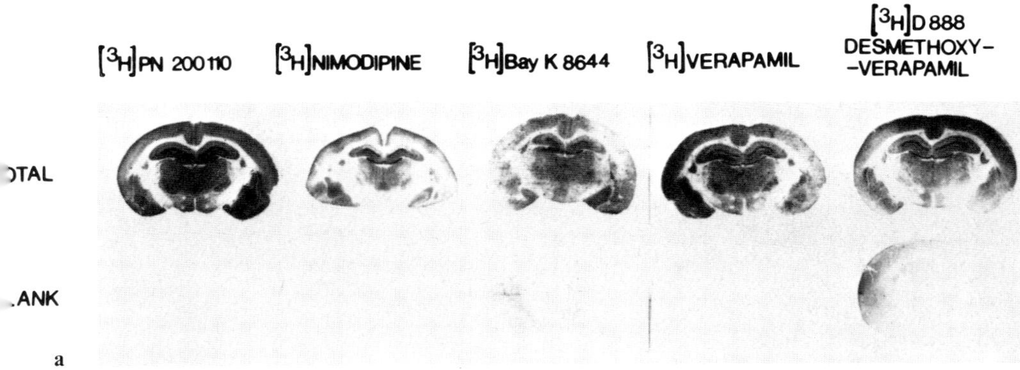

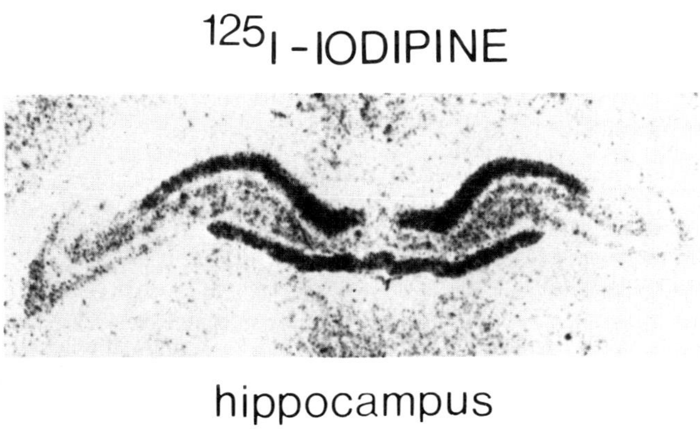

Fig. 11. a Autoradiographic distribution of 1,4-dihydropyridine and phenylalkylamine binding sites in thaw-mounted coronal sections of the guinea-pig brain. Note the identical distribution in the hippocampus formation. Autoradiographic grains indicate the presence of bound ligand. **b** Same as in **a** but the label is ^{125}I-iodipine (photographically enlarged)

is not a simple, competitive ligand for the drug receptor site "2" because it causes only a limited increase in the dissociation constant of the ^{3}H-desmethoxyverapamil label [7]. In the same membranes one can also demonstrate the allosteric link between the receptor site "1" and the receptor site "2". Thus, the concept of reciprocal allosteric regulation is valid for two of the isochannels. This was not unexpected as the autoradiographic distribution study with the different ligands shows a similar labelling pattern for the different ligands (Fig. 11).

Calcium Channels are Oligomeric Structures

The first evidence that the calcium channels are oligomeric structures came from our radiation inactivation experiments using high energy electrons to determine the size of the channel in situ, labelled at the different drug receptor sites. The size

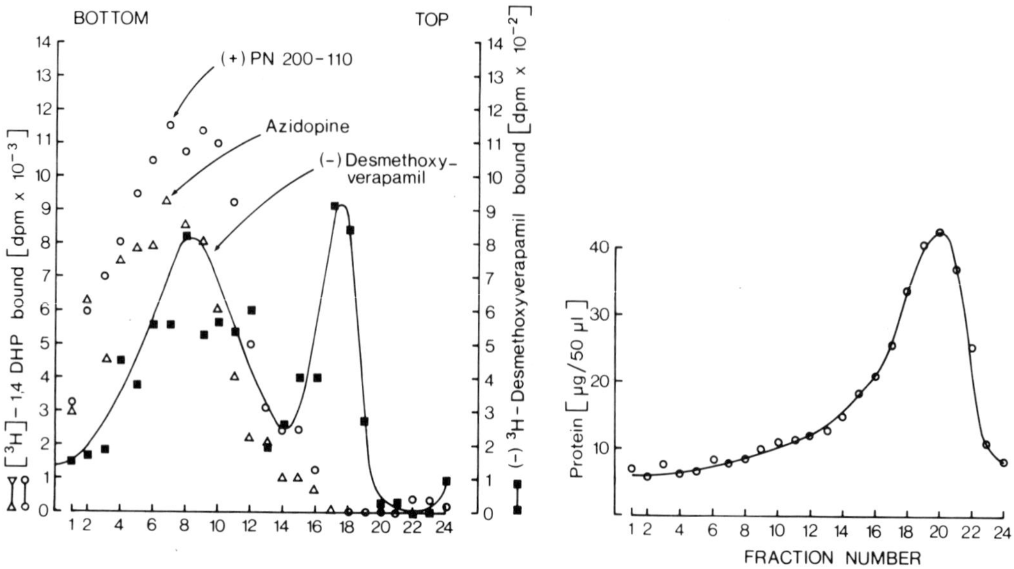

Fig. 12. Sucrose gradient centrifugation of solubilized skeletal muscle transverse tubule channels (see [6]). Note, that the ligands ^{3}H azidopine and ^{3}H PN 200–110 label a peak which comigrates with the receptor site "2" label (Fraction 8). In this peak allosteric (reciprocal) regulation is preserved: d-*cis* diltiazem (via receptor site "3") stimulates 1,4-dihydropyridine binding (receptor site "1"), verapamil and desmethoxyverapamil (via receptor site "2") inhibit allostericly receptor site "1", however ^{3}H-desmethoxyverapamil binding (receptor site "2") is regulated by receptor site "1" ligands in a fashion which discriminates agonists (Bay K 8644, CGP 28392) from antagonists (e. g. (+) PN 200–110). The former inhibit, the latter stimulate. d-*cis* Diltiazem (via receptor site "3") inhibits stereospecifically. The receptor site "2" ligand peak at fraction 17 is not regulated by ligands acting on site "1" or "3". It is yet not known whether this fraction is a component of the channel or originates from other, perhaps intracellular components which contaminate the transverse tubules membranes. However, the sites in this peak are stereospecific. From [19]

of the 1,4-dihydropyridine selective domain, as labelled by nimodipine, is 178,000. If the channel drug receptor site "3" is occupied by d-*cis*-diltiazem, the size of the 1,4-dihydropyridine receptor decrease by $\approx$60,000 mass units. If, however, the more antagonistic 1,4-dihydropyridine PN 200–110, labels the drug receptor site "1", we measure a molecular size, which is smaller than that with nimodipine, namely by 40,000 mass units. But, as for nimodipine, d-*cis*-diltiazem still induces the reduction of size by 60,000 mass units [14]. The sizes of the drug receptor sites "2" and "3" differ from the sizes measured for the 1,4-dihydropyridine receptor. Receptor site "2" has an Mr 110,000, whereas drug receptor site "3" has 130,000. This suggests that the channel may be composed of subunits and that channel drugs not only alter channel function but simultaneously change the architecture of the ionic pore. When the skeletal muscle isochannel is solubilized we observe a partial separation of receptor sites "2" from the receptor sites "1" upon sucrose gradient centrifugation (Fig. 12).

Photoaffinity Labelling of the Ca^{2+} Channel

Photoaffinity labelling has become a key approach to explore the structure of active sites of enzymes or receptors for hormones, neurotransmitters and toxins. The advantages of photoaffinity labelling with e. g. arylazides over simple affinity labelling are well known. The principle advantage is the stability in aqueous solutions in the absence of ultraviolet light, therefore the reversible binding characteristics can be examined. In addition, it is often possible to wash out much of the non-receptor bound ligand prior to ultra-violet light exposure in order to minimize non-receptor covalent incorporation. ^{3}H-Azidopine is highly suitable as a photoaffinity ligand of the calcium channel. First, it has high affinity ($K_D \approx$ 350 pM). Second, the 1,4-dihydropyridines exhibit a spectrum ranging from "agonists", which activate the calcium channel (causing e. g. positive inotropic effects or releasing neurotransmitters) to "antagonists" which block the ionic pore. Radiolabelled agonistic 1,4-dihydropyridines stabilize in high affinity only a fraction of the sites recognized e. g. by the potent antagonist (+) ^{3}H-PN 200–110 (see above). Other labelled 1,4-dihydropyridines are intermediate in their behavior. ^{3}H-Azidopine lies to the "antagonistic" side of this spectrum and stabilizes at least as many transverse-tubule calcium channels in high affinity as does the benzoxadiazol 1,4-dihydropyridine (+) ^{3}H-PN 200–110. This is the third valuable property of our photoaffinity probe. Fourth, the extremely slow dissociation of ^{3}H-azidopine at 4 C allows the use of the cold-trap method, i. e. washing out non-receptor bound label at low temperatures. Reducing agents such as dithiothreitol can activate calcium channels and thiol-selective alkylating agents have the opposite effect. Apparently both, free thiol groups and disulfide bridges, are part of the channel structure and are relevant for function [15]. Previously we have shown that the binding of the phenylalkylamine calcium antagonist (±) ^{3}H-verapamil [14] and of ^{3}H-nimodipine to skeletal muscle transverse tubule calcium channels [13] is sensitive to sulfhydril group alkylation. The reversible interaction of the photoaffinity ligand ^{3}H-azidopine is also sensitive to p-chloromercuriphenylsulfonic acid, N-ethylmaleimide and, to a lesser degree, iodoacetamide (not shown). Dithiothreitol also inhibits ^{3}H-azidopine binding, indicating the presence of not easily cleavable but essential disulfide bonds for the channel to bind drugs of the 1,4-dihydropyridine class.

Because of the presence of both, essential free sulfhydril groups and disulfide bridges, we first examined the photolabelled calcium channel with SDS-PAGE under non-reducing but alkylating conditions. We consistently observed the specific labelling of three bands with Mr's 240 kDa, 158 kDa and 99 kDa, which we term the A, B and C components, respectively. The stereoselective protection by the enantiomers of the benzoxadiazol 1,4-dihydropyridine PN 200–110, and the partial but stereoselective protection by the enantiomers of the negative allosteric regulator verapamil and the protection by La^{3+} (but not Ca^{2+}) is compelling evidence for the pharmacological specificity of these bands. In some of our experiments two specific bands with Mr's 55 kDa/52 kDa (termed components D1 and D2) were also observed.

When alkylated photolabelled membranes were separated under nonreducing conditions in the first dimension and reduced in the second dimension, the B, C,

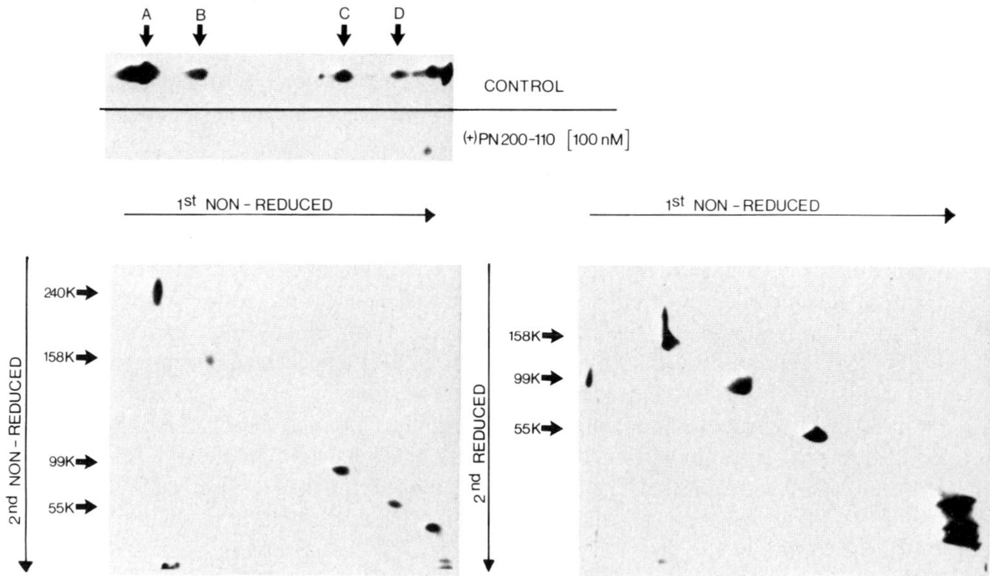

Fig. 13. Photolabelling of guinea-pig skeletal muscle transverse tubulus channels with ^{3}H-azidopine, SDS-Page and fluorograms. *Upper:* first dimension non-reduced but alkylated. 4 components (*A, B, C, D*) are specifically labelled (control). The gel with 0.1 μM (+) PN 200–110 (blank) shows complete (stereospecific, not shown) protection. *Lower panels: Left* (second dimension non-reduced): the A, B, C, D components run at the diagonal. Sometimes the D component resolve in D1, D2 (not shown). Right (Second dimension reduced): The B, C and D components run on the diagonal. However, A runs now identical to C. From [20]

and D components run close to or on the diagonal, indicating that B, C and D are subunits not linked by interchain disulfide bonds. For the A component only one labelled spot with Mr$\approx$99 kDa, was found. This spot was equal in Mr to the C subunit (Fig. 13). It is highly unlikely that A is disulfide bridged trimer of three C subunits. Instead, we favour the idea that A consists of the B subunit, disulfide-bonded to C and is, in contrast to B and C not photolabelled. Radiation inactivation experiments with partially purified transverse-tubule membranes prior to photoaffinity labelling show that the larger A component is much more radiation-sensitive than the B or C components (not shown). This indicates that A, B and C decay as independent targets and must be present as such in the membrane. The finding that more than one component of the channel is photolabelled is not unusual as photoaffinity ligands are known to incorporate into more than one subunit of oligomeric enzymes and hormone- or neurotransmitter receptors. It is, of course, possible that the A, B, and C components may not actually carry the 1,4-dihydropyridine recognition sites. Perhaps these may reside on smaller polypeptides, e.g. the D components. Previous radiation inactivation studies from our group came to the conclusion that the 1,4-dihydropyridine binding component has a Mr of <75 kDa [14]. This appears to be supported by experiments using ^{3}H-nitrendipine as a photolabel for cardiac membranes where a 30 kDa peptide was identified [16]. However, concentrations of ^{3}H-nitrendipine were employed

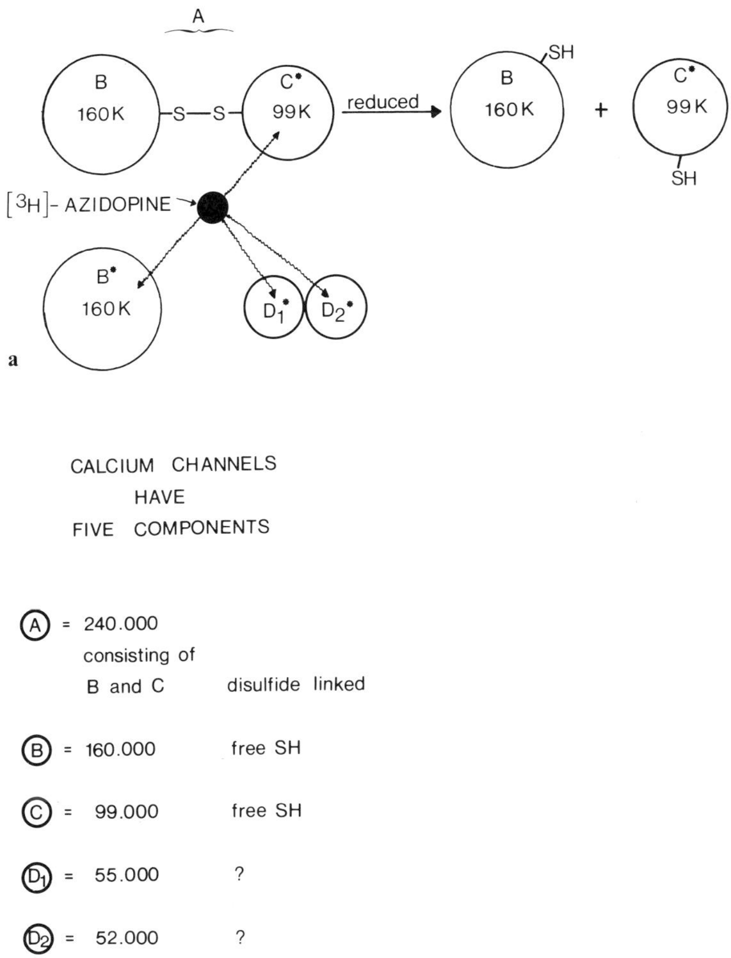

a

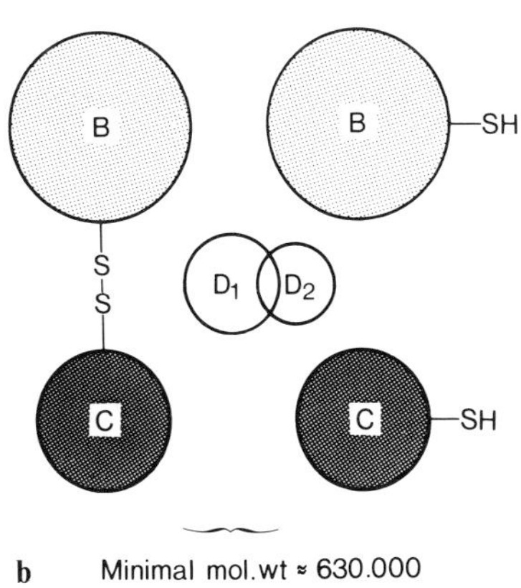

b

Fig. 14a, b. Interpretation of the photoaffinity labelling experiments. Labelled subunits are indicated by the *asterik*. The disulfide-linked B component is assumed not to be labelled by the nitrene forming radical of azidopine whereas free B is labelled. D1, D2 may actually represent the 1,4-dihydropyridine binding subunits. The model assumes that free sulfhydril groups are essential for function and that opening or closing of channels could be accompanied with disulfide bridge formation and breakage under conditions (150 mM NaCl) where mainly a low affinity site, unrelated to Ca^{2+} channels, is labelled. Low affinity 1,4 dihydropyridine sites have now been shown to reside on the nucleoside transporter, a 45 to 60 kDa peptide (see below). As Campbell et al. (16) also found that 50 μM nifedipine suppresses labelling only by 50% (although nifedipine blocks reversible ^{3}H-nitrendipine binding with a K_D of ≈1 nM) this casts doubts on the conclusion that a component of the calcium channel was identified by this procedure. Horne et al. [17] have presented data on an isothiocyanate-substituted 1,4-dihydropyridine in heart membranes where 50 μM nicardipine blocked irreversible binding by only 50% into a band of Mr ≅ 42 kDa. Affinity labelling is an approach which is very unlikely to succeed with unpurified receptor sources. Unless it is demonstrated that ^{3}H-nitrendipine photolabelling or affinity labelling with the isothiocyanate ligand is blocked stereoselectively by low concentrations of the 1,4-dihydropyridine enantiomers it cannot be accepted that Campbell et al. [16] or Horne et al. [17] recognized calcium channel subunits. It is interesting that in rabbit skeletal muscle we also find, as in the guinea-pig, specifically photolabelled bands of 240 kDa and 99 kDa (not shown). In conclusion, the arylazide 1,4-dihydropyridine, ^{3}H-azidopine, can photoincorporate into three (possibly five) distinct components of the calcium channel. The highest Mr component, A, maybe a disulfide-bridged heterodimer of B and C. The 140 kDa mass units loss which is observed when A is reduced in the second dimension could indicate a disulfide linkage of labelled C to an unlabelled B subunit. Perhaps B, because it is disulfide linked to C, is not within the reach of the nitrene forming moiety of ^{3}H-azidopine. C and B, which are not linked by disulfide bridges, are, on the other hand, accessible to the label. Although this is a hypothesis, which will require peptide mapping for final proof, it provides an extremely attractive working model (see Fig. 14) which combines evidence for the role of essential sulfhydril groups and disulfide bonds in calcium channel function with structural data.

Properties of Low Affinity Ca^{2+}-Antagonist Binding Sites

Figure 15 shows the ability of different radiolabelled Ca^{2+} channel ligands to interact in a saturable manner with human red blood cell membranes. From all labels (belonging to different chemical classes) the 1,4 dihydropyridine, ^{3}H-nimodipine, as was reported in 1982 [18], gave a favourable signal (see Table 3) and was therefore selected for all further studies. Most notable was that (+) ^{3}H PN 200–110, an optically pure enantiomer, which always has higher affinity for Ca^{2+} channels in membranes from excitable tissues (brain, heart and skeletal muscle) compared to racemic nimodipine [6], failed to label saturable sites in ghosts. This finding and the observation that ^{125}I-iodipine, a ligand which has the highest specific activity of all Ca^{2+} channel ligands, had a similar low labelling efficiency prompted further studies on the stereospecificity of the Ca^{2+} antagonist binding sites in the ghost. Saturable binding of ^{3}H nimodipine was linear with respect to the concentration of ghost protein. The sites are an intrinsic component of the red cell surface. Evidence for a proteinaceous nature of the binding site was obtained by experiments with trypsin digestion. The sulfhydryl group alkylating

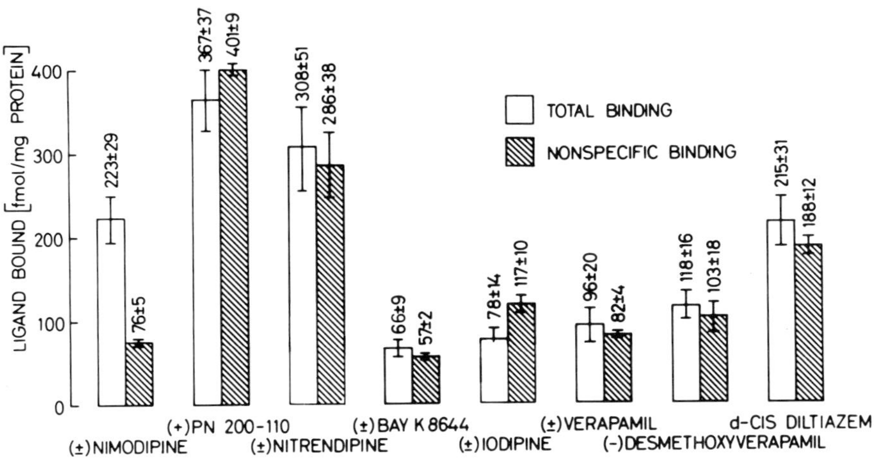

Fig. 15. Ability of different radiolabelled Ca^{2+} channel probes to label saturable sites in human red blood cell membranes. Radioligands (2–8 nM) were incubated with 0.040–0.045 mg of ghost protein for 60 min at 25 °C in the absence or presence of excess unlabelled ligand. To determine nonsaturable binding the following concentrations of unlabelled ligands were used: 1 μM (−) nimodipine, 1 μM (+) PN 200–110, 10 μM (−) Bay K 8644, 10 μM (−) nitrendipine, 1 μM (−) desmethoxyverapamil, 10 μM (−) verapamil and 10 μM d-*cis* diltiazem, for the respective radioligands, 10 μM (±) nimodipine in the case of ^{3}H azidopine and ^{125}I iodipine, respectively. Results are means from triplicates ± S.D.

Table 3. Tissue distribution of ^{3}H-nimodipine binding. The data for the table were obtained in 1981 and (without skeletal muscle and electric eel membranes) published in [18]. Electrophorus electricus membranes were a kind gift from Dr. Grünhagen (Homburg, Saar). The human red blood cell ghost binding site has now been shown to reside on the nucleoside carrier and not on Ca^{2+} channels

Tissue	Specific bound (fmol/mg of protein)
Duodenum	124
Uterus	152
Heart	371
Lung	106
Kidney	31
Liver	48
Cerebral cortex	153
Cerebellum	119
Medulla/pons	42
Striatum	90
Hypothalamus	82
Hippocampus	200
Thalamus/midbrain	68
Olfactory tubercle	163
Adrenal	212
Fat cell membranes (Hamster)	0
Platelet membrane (human)	0
Erythrocyte ghosts (human)	26
Electrophorus electricus	1,680
Skeletal muscle	1,770

reagents N-ethylmaleimide and p-chloromercuriphenylsulfonic acid inhibited saturable binding of ^{3}H nimodipine. The binding sites were heat stable and withstood lyophilization. In contrast, the high affinity binding of ^{3}H nimodipine to 1,4 dihydropyridine-selective sites on skeletal muscle transverse tubule membranes is inactivated by $\gg 90\%$ after lyophilization (not shown). At 25 °C the dissociation constant of the human red blood cell ghost for ^{3}H-nimodipine [calculated for the bindable (+) enantiomer] was 51.7 ± 6.3 nM (mean ± S.E.M from 9 experiments) and the B_{max} 9650 ± 4470 fmoles per mg of protein. The apparent Hill slope was close to unity. Association kinetics at 2 °C was a second-order reaction, whereas the dissociation kinetics was a first-order process. Computer fitting of the association data gave a $K_{+1} = 9.15 \pm 0.47 \times 10^5$ $nM^{-1}min^{-1}$ and a $K_{-1} = 1.58 \pm 0.14$ min^{-1}. The K_{-1} was confirmed by dissociation experiments with unlabelled nimodipine ($K_{-1} = 2.23$ min^{-1}).

It was surprising that the tritiated optically pure (+) enantiomer of PN-200 110 failed to label the red blood cell ghost binding site. In membranes from excitable tissues this ligand has, as a rule, always higher affinity than nimodipine or labels more sites at 37 °C or 25 °C than ^{3}H-nimodipine e.g. in skeletal muscle (see above and [6]). This indicated, among other possibilities, that the stereoselectivity of the ghost binding site was different (in fact opposite) to that observed for the calcium channel linked receptors. The first tool to prove or disprove this hypothesis were displacement studies with the enantiomers of nimodipine. Indeed, the (+) enantiomer of nimodipine was 14 times more potent than the (−) enantiomer ($p < 0.01$). As expected the IC_{50} value for racemic nimodipine was twice that of the more potent (+) enantiomer. When the racemic ligand ^{3}H nimodipine was depleted for the (−) enantiomer with an excess of skeletal muscle Ca^{2+} channel receptor sites, the residual ligand (enriched for the (+) enantiomer) displayed a higher bindability for the ghost receptor than the native, racemic ligand. To further explore the apparently opposite stereospecificity, the optical enantiomers of Bay e 6927 and of PN 200–110 were used. As for nimodipine the stereoselectivity was found to be reversed for the benzoxadiazol 1,4-dihydropyridine PN 200–110 and for Bay e 6927 (Table 4). The question arised if the ghost Ca^{2+} antagonist site, labelled by ^{3}H nimodipine, was able to interact with other Ca^{2+}-channel regulators from chemically totally different classes. We have found that the optical enantiomers of verapamil, D-600 and desmethoxyverapamil were able to allostericly regulate ^{3}H nimodipine binding. The (−) enantiomers of verapamil and desmethoxyverapamil stimulated, whereas the respective optical antipodes were inhibitory. Interestingly, both enantiomers of methoxyverapamil inhibited nimodipine binding. In steady state saturation experiments it was found that (−) methoxyverapamil decreased the affinity of ^{3}H nimodipine, whereas (−) verapamil decreased the K_D and increased B_{max} to a limited extend. La^{3+}, an inorganic Ca^{2+} channel blocker, is inhibitory in membranes from excitable tissues for e.g. the 1,4 dihydropyridine-selective site and the d-*cis* diltiazem-selective site. The ghost Ca^{2+} antagonist binding site interaction with ^{3}H nimodipine was affected in an opposite manner. The stimulating effect of La^{3+} on ^{3}H-nimodipine binding ($EC_{50} = 1$ nM) was mainly caused by increasing B_{max}. In order to exclude that the effects of La^{3+} were of a nonspecific nature a variety of monovalent and divalent cations were investigated. Divalent

Table 4. Pharmacological profile of the human red blood cell ghost Ca^{2+}-antagonist binding sites in comparison to the Ca^{2+} channel binding site in excitable tissues

Compound	Red blood cell ghost		Electrically excitable tissues
	IC_{50} or EC_{50} (nM)	Maximal inhibition or stimulation	IC_{50} or EC_{50} (nM)
(+) Nimodipine	67 ± 10	100	17.6
(−) Nimodipine	940 ± 450	100	3.24
(±) Nimodipine	123 ± 19	100	6.68
(−) PN 200–110	820 ± 230	100	198
(+) PN 200–110	> 6,000	100	2
(−) Nitrendipine	810 ± 240	100	0.24
(+) Nitrendipine	545 ± 228	100	31.8
(−) Nicardipine	n. e. (10 μM)	–	42
(+) Nicardipine	167 ± 71	100	7
(−) Bay e 6927	1,000 ± 460	100	3
(+) Bay e 6927	370 ± 50	100	420
Nifedipine	16,400 ± 5,300	100	8.2
(±) Bay M 5579	> 10,000	100	1,860
(±) VO 2605	201 ± 84	100	320
(±) Bay K 8644	25,000 ± 12,000	100	37
(±) CGP 28392	11,371 ± 5,800	100	1,250
(−) Verapamil	17,000 ± 11,000	231	98
(+) Verapamil	2,300 ± 580	61	54
(−) Methoxyverapamil	3,180 ± 820	80	21
(+) Methoxyverapamil	10,800 ± 9,800	37	190
(−) Desmethoxyverapamil	7,100 ± 2,500	198	n. d.
(+) Desmethoxyverapamil	3,100 ± 940	75	n. d.
(±) D-619	> 10,000	–	n. d.
Tiapamil	> 10,000	100	292
d-cis Diltiazem	n. e. (100 μM)	–	960
l-cis Diltiazem	n. e. (100 μm)	–	3,000
Trifluoperazine	n. e. (10 μM)	–	2,500, 4,100
Pimozid	447 ± 144	100	13, 100
W7	> 10,000	–	
Cinnarizine	n. e. (10 μM)	–	29.0
Flunarizine	n. e. (10 μM)	–	12.6

cations (Ca^{2+}, Mg^{2+}) were ineffective, except Cd^{2+} (exhibiting very high affinity for the Me binding sites of the Ca^{2+}-channel in excitable tissues) which was inhibitory. Monovalent cations were ineffective. D- and l-*cis*-diltiazem, flunarizine, the calmodulin antagonist W7, the benzodiazepine diazepam or the hydrophobic β-adrenoceptor blocker propranolol were without effect. It was observed that nucleotides (ATP, GTP) at high concentrations caused only a very small inhibition of ^{3}H nimodipine binding in the human red blood cell ghost in contrast to e.g. brain membranes [18]. Most interestingly, however, nucleosides were inhibitory. Inosine and adenosine were the most potent in this series. Inosine was a competitive inhibitor in steady state saturation experiments. In order to explore the possibility that the ^{3}H nimodipine labelled site was a component of the nucleoside carrier we tested a series of nucleoside transport inhibitors and found that they were extremely potent with respect to inhibition of ^{3}H-nimodipine binding. Nitrobenzylthioinosine and nitrobenzylthioquanosine were the most effective compounds, dilazep, hexobendine and dipyridamole were of lesser potency. The nature of inhibition was evaluated for nitrobenzylthioinosine and was of a noncompetitive nature. Erythrocytes from most ($\geqslant$95%) sheep are known to be almost completely impermeable to inosine. These "nucleoside-impermeable" sheep erythrocytes were tested for adenosine uptake and specific ^{3}H-nimodipine binding. The absence of any high affinity adenosine transport was found to be accompanied by a lack of specific ^{3}H-nimodipine binding to ghosts prepared from these erythrocytes. When the human red blood cell ghost nucleoside transporter was covalently photoinactivated with nitrobenzylthioinosine, ^{3}H-nimodipine binding was irreversibly lost. The loss was strictly dependent upon ultraviolet irradiation and required the presence of the nucleoside transport inhibitor.

We have also investigated the influence of several Ca^{2+} channel drugs on the high-affinity saturable nucleoside transporter in human red blood cells and compared it to well-known adenosine uptake inhibitors such as nitrobenzylthioinosine or dipyridamole. Our analysis indicates that (+) nimodipine is a competitive inhibitor (with respect to adenosine) whereas nitrobenzylthioinosine acts non-competitively. The relationship between the inhibition or stimulation of ^{3}H-nimodipine binding and the adenosine-uptake inhibition in red blood cells by the same drug was investigated for 18 compounds. The relationship closely approached 1:1 equivalence (slope = 0.95, r = 0.82), the IC_{50} of uptake inhibition being on average 1.7 times higher than that of binding inhibition or EC_{50} for stimulation. Our labelling experiments with ^{3}H nimodipine make it likely that the high capacity, low affinity sites for 1,4-dihydropyridines are linked to the nucleoside carrier not only in the red blood cell but in other tissues as well.

These results have important consequences. Affinity and photoaffinity labelling experiments of putative Ca^{2+} channel components will require the demonstration that incorporation of the ligand is stereoselectively inhibited with a Ca^{2+}-channel typical pharmacological profile. Otherwise incorporation into unrelated membrane structures (such as the nucleoside carrier) cannot be excluded. Our results may help to understand the pharmacological effects (unrelated to Ca^{2+} channel blockade) of racemic 1,4 dihydropyridines and have important implications for drug development. (+) Nimodipine is preferentially a nucleoside transport inhibitor whereas (−) nimodipine preferentially blocks the Ca^{2+} channel. Finally it is surprising that two different plasma membrane structures, the voltage-dependent Ca^{2+}-channel and the nucleoside carrier share binding sites for phenylalkylamines and 1,4 dihydropyridines but differ with respect to the benzothiazepine d-*cis* diltiazem. Perhaps, the carrier and the channel are structurally related [21].

Acknowledgements. The authors wish to thank their collegues at the pharmaceutical companies, especially Drs. Hoffmeister, Meyer and Wehinger (Bayer AG); Dr. Traber (Tropon AG), Drs. Karobath, Palacios, Tobler, Hauser and Lindenmann (Sandoz Ltd), Drs. Bahrmann and Satzinger (Goedecke AG), Drs. Unger, Lietz, Hollmann and Traut (Knoll AG), Drs. Sombroek, Schmitges, Häusler (Merck AG), Dr. Nitz (Casella AG), Dr. Schölkens (Hoechst AG), C. Auriga, C. Gadow, A. Goll, B. Habermann, M. Rombusch, I. Seidel, T. Linn, A. Rücker and W.

Nürnberger shared our enthusiasm in the laboratory. We like to pay tribute to Prof. A. Fleckenstein, the scientific father of the concept of calcium antagonism. Our work is supported by Deutsche Forschungsgemeinschaft, Bonn-Bad Godesberg, Legerlotz-Foundation, Fonds der chemischen Industrie and by Österreichische Nationalbank.

References

1. Bellemann P, Ferry D, Lübbecke F, Glossmann H (1981) Drug Res 31:2064–2067
2. Fleckenstein A (1983) Calcium antagonism in the heart and smooth muscle. Experimental facts and therapeutic prospects. Wiley, New York
3. Ferry DR, Glossmann H (1984) Naunyn-Schmiedeberg's Arch Pharmacol 325:186–189
4. Ferry DR, Rombusch M, Goll A, Glossmann H (1984) FEBS Lett. 169:112–118
5. Dodge JT, Mitchell C, Hanahan DJ (1963) Arch Biochem Biophys 100:119–130
6. Glossmann H, Ferry DR (1985) Methods in Enzymology 109:513–550
7. Ferry DR, Goll A, Gadow C, Glossmann H (1984) Naunyn-Schmiedeberg's Arch Pharmacol 327:183–187
8. Goll A, Ferry DR, Striessnig J, Schober M, Glossmann H (1984) FEBS Lett 176:371–377
9. Glossmann H, Linn T, Rombusch M, Ferry DR (1983) FEBS Lett 160:226–232
10. Glossmann H, Ferry DR, Goll A (1984) In: Proc IUPHAR 9th Internat Congress Pharmacol 2:329–336
11. Glossmann H, Ferry DR (1983) Naunyn-Schmiedeberg's Arch Pharmacol 323:279–291
12. Ferry DR, Glossmann H (1983) Brit J Pharmacol 78:81 P
13. Glossmann H, Ferry DR, Goll A, Rombusch M (1984) J Cardiovasc Pharmacol 6:S608–S621
14. Goll A, Ferry DR, Glossmann H (1983) FEBS Lett 157:63–69
15. Goll A, Ferry DR, Glossmann H (1984) Eur J Biochem 141:177–186
16. Campbell KP, Lipshutz GM, Denney GH (1984) J Biol Chem 259:5384–5387
17. Horne P, Triggle DJ, Venter JC (1984) Biochem Biophys Res Comm 121:890–898
18. Glossmann H, Ferry DR, Lübbecke F, Mewes R, Hofmann F (1982) Trends Pharmacol Sci 3:431–437
19. Glossmann H, Ferry DR, Goll A, Striessnig J, Schober M (1985) J Cardiovasc Pharmacol 7:S20–S30
20. Ferry DR, Kämpf K, Goll A, Glossmann H (1985) EMBO J 4:1933–1940
21. Striessnig J, Zernig G, Glossmann H (1985) Eur J Pharmacol 150:67–77

Bayer-Symposium IX
Cardiovascular Effects of Dihydropyridine-Type
Calcium Antagonists and Agonists, 140–155

The Dihydropyridine Receptors *

R. A. JANIS, P. BELLEMANN, J. G. SARMIENTO, and D. J. TRIGGLE

A. Introduction

The purpose of this chapter is to review some of the recent studies on the characterization of 1,4-dihydropyridine receptors (DHPRs). In this respect the chapter will complement the contributions of Glossmann, Nayler and Schwartz (this volume) and the previously published reviews of 1,4-dihydropyridine (DHP) binding studies (Meyer et al. 1983; Janis and Triggle 1984; Triggle and Janis 1984).

The most important recent developments in the field of DHPRs include electrophysiological studies which demonstrate the voltage dependency of the action of Ca^{2+} channel antagonists and provide, therefore, an explanation for some of the discrepancies between the binding activity and the pharmacological effects of these drugs. There is a considerable amount of new information on the development of DHPRs in various organs of different species, although the ontogeny of DHPRs is not yet fully correlated with the pharmacological effects of Ca^{2+} channel antagonists or agonists in whole animals or in isolated organs. The development of DHPRs in clonal cell lines were correlated with some aspects of their morphological differentiation and with some pharmacological effects, i. e. an effect on Ca^{2+} uptake.

Of considerable pharmacological and potentially clinical importance were the recent findings that the density of DHPRs and the affinity for ligands can be modulated by hormones, drugs, tissue innervation and even disease states. Nucleotides, enzymes and some environmental factors were also shown to affect the affinity of DHPRs for their ligands or the interaction of drug-receptor complexes with Ca^{2+} channels. The in vivo activity of drugs affecting Ca^{2+} channels is, therefore, likely to be also modified by the same factors. The nature, size and structure of DHPRs and their subunits received considerable attention during the past year but still remain a subject of controversy.

* Research from the University of Connecticut and the State University of New York at Buffalo was supported, in part, by Grants HL 07420, HL 16003, HL 21812 and HL 32588

This chapter updates the reader on the above mentioned aspects of the physiology and pharmacology of DHPR. The discovery (Schramm et al. 1983) and use of the Ca^{2+} channel activator, BAY K 8644 [1,4-dihydro-2,6-dimethyl-3-nitro-4-(2-trifluoromethylphenyl)-5-pyridine-carboxylic acid methyl ester] has been of equal importance to that of the Ca^{2+} channel antagonists in characterizing DHPRs (Gross et al., this volume; Hess et al. 1984; Kokubun and Reuter 1984; Thomas et al. 1985).

B. Multiple Affinities and Apparent DHPR Densities Are Dictated by Multiple States and Gating Modes of the Ca^{2+} Channel

A major point of discussion in this area has been the apparent discrepancy between the dissociation constants of binding of DHPs to isolated membranes and the concentrations of these drugs needed for half-maxi mal inhibition of cardiac muscle contraction or Ca^{2+} current. This inconsistency, along with certain others, such as the lack of stereoselective binding of gallopamil (Holck et al. 1983), resulted in the suggestion that the high affinity binding sites may be unrelated to a physiological Ca^{2+} channel (i.e. see Bristow et al. 1984). However, the demonstration that the effect of these drugs is extremely voltage-dependent (see Kass et al., this volume; Bean 1984; Sanguinetti and Kass 1984) appears to explain this lack of agreement. Considerable evidence supports the view that DHP binding in smooth and cardiac muscle is to Ca^{2+} channels in the inactivated state and, therefore, the information from binding and from electrophysiological studies may be related to each other (Kass et al., this volume; Janis et al. 1984b). There are, however, many complexities that must be considered.

Any description of the DHPRs is complicated by the following:

(a) There are multiple types of Ca^{2+} channels (e.g. Bean 1985; Cota and Stefani 1985; Nowycky et al. 1985a; Tsunoo and Narahashi 1985) and only some of these are sensitive to DHPs, (e.g. Brown et al., this volume, and references therein; Cohen and McCarthy 1985; Gould et al. 1985; Miller 1985; Nilius et al. 1985; Turner and Goldin 1985). As discussed below, there is also evidence for multiple types of DHPRs, so that information from one type of DHPR-Ca^{2+} channel complex is not necessarily applicable to another type. It is not yet known whether a given type of DHPR is invariably associated with a single type of Ca^{2+} channel.

(b) The Ca^{2+} channel exists in multiple states which are determined by voltage, drugs and both reversible and covalent endogenous modifiers, such as Ca^{2+}, GTP, and protein phosphorylation.

(c) Response is determined by simultaneous voltage-dependent binding of drug to the Ca^{2+} channel in multiple states (Kass et al., this volume), and in multiple modes of gating (Hess et al., this volume).

(d) The intrinsic activity of activators may be much greater than that of inhibitors of the Ca^{2+} channel because activators produce a dramatic increase in the duration of channel opening in smooth, cardiac and skeletal muscle and neurons

(Caffrey et al. 1985; Hess et al., this volume; Kokubun and Reuter 1984; Coronado and Affolter 1985; Nowycky et al. 1985b). In addition, in cardiac cells, activators promote Ca^{2+} influx at a time in the cardiac cycle when contraction will be most effectively increased (Thomas et al. 1985). Therefore, a small amount of activator binding (e.g. BAY K 8644) may have far more effect on contraction than the specific binding of a larger amount of Ca^{2+} channel antagonist.

Many predictions about the expected results from ligand binding experiments can be made from the published electrophysiological data. The results indicate that the DHPR will have *no* unique affinity to intact cells because the affinity will change with membrane potential. It could also be predicted that, in isolated membranes, which are in the depolarized state, the binding affinity to the inactivated channels would be 0.25–0.36 nM for nitrendipine at 37 °C, which is, in fact, the same as that obtained from binding studies (Bellemann et al. 1981; Janis and Triggle 1984). It could be further expected that in spontaneously beating cells the affinity of binding will change with each contraction cycle, and therefore, measurement of affinity represents the average state of the channel in the contraction cycle.

The voltage dependence of binding also predicts that the apparent DHPR density, as measured by the filtration assay, will vary with membrane potential. The low affinity binding of nitrendipine and nisoldipine ($K_d = 0.7–1.3$ μM) associated with resting channels at −80 mV (Bean 1984; Sanguinetti and Kass 1984b) may not be detected with the filtration assay because "pseudo-resting state" Ca^{2+} channels can not exist in isolated membranes. With an appropriate amount of depolarization, these low affinity sites will be converted to the high affinity sites ($K_d = 0.2–0.3$ nM) associated with inactivated Ca^{2+} channels. This would be detectable in the filtration assay as an apparent increase in the number of high affinity binding sites if conversion of low affinity sites to high affinity sites occurs. An increase in site density for [^{3}H]nitrendipine binding to depolarized cardiac myocytes has been reported (Green et al. 1985). Ligand binding studies have also predicted the presence of a very low affinity state of the DHP receptor, which in isolated membranes, is in equilibrium with the high affinity binding site (Weiland and Oswald 1985; Shrikhande et al. 1985). It remains to be determined whether one of the low affinity states detected or predicted by electrophysiological studies corresponds to those detected using ligand binding, and represents a "frozen" resting or open state of the channel. The low affinity site for DHP antagonists reported in both intact cells (Marsh et al. 1983; Green et al. 1985) and isolated membranes (Bellemann et al. 1981; Kennesey et al. 1984; Kunze et al. 1985; McBride et al. 1984; Rogart et al. 1984), may have too large a density in some cells to be associated 1:1 with Ca^{2+} channels (Schilling et al. 1985).

Another prediction from the results of Bean (1984) is that Ca^{2+} will not compete with DHPs for their receptor. Ligand binding studies have also supported this view (Janis and Triggle 1984). Ca^{2+} does not decrease the binding of DHP to isolated membranes, but is required for binding to occur (Gould et al. 1982; Bolger et al. 1983; Luchowski et al. 1984; Bellemann 1984a, and references in Glossmann et al., this volume).

The qualitative change in the activity of BAY K 8644, from activator to antagonist (Sanguinetti and Kass 1985), is consistent with the idea that DHPs exert both effects by acting at a common binding site; this has been supported by ligand binding studies (Bellemann 1984b, 1985; Janis et al. 1984a, b). However, Hof et al. (1985) have demonstrated that one enantiomer of the 202–791 (isopropyl 4-(2,1,3-benzoxadiazol-4-yl)-1,4-dihydro-2,6-dimethyl-5-nitro-3-pyridine carboxylate) exhibits all of the Ca^{2+} channel activator activity and the other exhibits all of the antagonistic activity. These results may indicate that different states of the Ca^{2+} channel may exhibit opposite stereoselectivities.

C. Ontogeny and Differentiation of Clonal Cell Lines

1. Ontogeny

The density of DHPRs per unit protein is generally low at the early fetal stage and then it increases at various rates, depending on the tissue and species, to maximal developmental levels by birth, or in the case of the chick heart, by 6–9 days post-natal. The density of receptors increases from 50 fmoles at 17 days post-coitum to 175 fmoles per milligram of protein at 7 to 60 days post-natal in rat heart homogenates (Kazazoglou et al. 1983). Marangos et al. (1984) found that [^{3}H]nitrendipine binding increased in chick heart membranes by about 50% from day 3 to day 7–14; thereafter no further increase was seen up to day 20. In another study, binding site density of chick heart was found to increase from 40 fmol/mg protein at 3 days of development in ovo to 100 fmol/mg protein at day 14; after a 4 day lag, the receptor density again increased rapidly to 210 fmol/mg protein at 4 to 8 days post-natal (Renaud et al. 1984).

The early DHP binding sites, like the tetrodotoxin and the muscarinic receptors present at this early stage of development, are apparently not pharmacologically functional: nitrendipine (0.1 μM) did not affect either the slow action potential nor the contraction of 3-day-old aggregates. These results contrast with the complete inhibition by 50 nM nitrendipine of both of these parameters in 11-day-old heart cells (Renaud et al. 1984). The membrane potential of the 3-day-old cells were −50 mV, and that of the 11-day-old cells, −60 mV, suggesting that the insensitivity was not due to the younger cells being less depolarized. It remains to be determined whether the apparently silent DHP binding sites in the early embryonic cardiac cells are analogous to those in some neuronal cells.

The rate of appearance of DHP binding sites varies between tissues. For example, rat cerebellum shows a slow increase in sites from about 6 days post-coitum to 30 days post-natal, whereas sites in brain appear to plateau at least 12 days sooner. Rat heart, in contrast to chick heart, exhibits a very rapid increase in binding sites between birth and day 5, at which time adult levels appear to be reached. Both rat cardiac and skeletal muscle exhibit very high rates of appearance of sites just after birth, approximately 30 fmol/mg protein/day, whereas for cerebellum, the rate is less than 1/30 of this value (Kazazoglou et al. 1983). The number of DHPRs in chick heart on the third gestational day is already relatively high, whereas that in chick brain is almost undetectable until day 6, after which an increase is seen (Marangos et al. 1984).

2. Differentiation of Clonal Cell Lines

The synthesis of DHPR increases dramatically in neuronal clonal Nbr10-A cells that have been treated with PGE_1 and other agents that cause morphological differentiation by increasing cyclic AMP levels (Nirenberg et al. 1983). This increase is associated with a similar increase in the apparent number of Ca^{2+} channels. Differentiation of NG108-15, NCB-20 and N4TG1 cells with 10 μM PGE_1 and 50 μM 3-isobutylmethylxanthine for 4 days produced an increase in depolarization-induced uptake of $^{45}Ca^{2+}$ which was sensitive to 1 nM nitrendipine, suggesting that there was an associated increase in the number of Ca^{2+} channels (Freedman et al. 1984). Other agents that increase cyclic AMP, such as dimethyl sulfoxide, forskolin, and cholera toxin (with isobutylmethylxanthine present) also increased K^+-sensitive Ca^{2+} uptake. It is not known whether cyclic AMP is also a physiological signal for Ca^{2+} channel synthesis in normal mammalian cells in situ. Some cell lines, such as human neuroblastoma MC9C, do not appear to contain-voltage-sensitive Ca^{2+} channels that stay open long enough for measuring $^{45}Ca^{2+}$ uptake, irrespective of the growth conditions (Freedman et al. 1984).

In all of the above studies, in which binding to isolated membranes was studied at 25 °C, only a high affinity site was noted, and there was no change in this affinity during development. In contrast, both high and low affinity [^{3}H]nitrendipine binding was seen in intact developing fetal mouse spinal cord neurons studies at 37 °C (Litzinger and Brenneman 1984). The K_d values changed from 0.3 and 22 nM on day 3 in culture to 1.1 and 50 nM on day 21, for the high and low affinity sites, respectively. Another change that was noted in these neurons was a loss of sensitivity of nitrendipine binding to tetrodotoxin from day 5 to day 27 in culture (Litzinger and Brenneman 1984).

D. Effect of Hormonal State, Denervation, Drug Treatment, and Hypertension

1. Hormonal State

A study of the affinity and density of the DHPRs did not reveal any marked differences between the myometrium of pregnant and non-pregnant rats (Huszar et al. 1983). Similarly, there were no differences in the binding of DHP to adenohypophysis homogenates from female rats in proestrus and estrus; however, differences were seen in the ability of verapamil to inhibit DHP binding (Moscona-Amir and Sokolovsky 1984).

2. Denervation

The effect of denervation of chick and rat lower leg skeletal muscles on DHPR, tetrodotoxin (TTX) binding sites, and ouabain binding sites were compared (Schmid et al. 1984). DHPR density was found to approximately double at 10–12 days after denervation, whereas the apparent density of both Na^+ channels and

Na^+,K^+-ATPase molecules decreased by 40–60%. The changes in DHPR density tended to reverse over the following 20 days, but the changes in TTX and ouabain binding sites were maintained. Further evidence for an increase in DHPR in skeletal muscle following neural section is seen in results obtained with denervated rat gastrocnemius muscle: binding site density increased from 6 to 12 pmol/mg without a change in the affinity of binding (E. Luchowski, A. Rutledge, and D.J. Triggle, unpublished).

The effect of reserpine, which depletes norepinephrine levels without loss of adrenergic nerve endings, was studied on chick cardiac DHPR by Renaud et al. (1984). Reserpine increased both DHP binding sites (35%) and muscarinic binding sites (48%), but reduced TTX binding sites by 30%. The new densities of channels and receptors remained stable for at least a week. Reserpine treatment was without effect on the binding affinity of ligands for DHP, muscarinic and TTX binding sites.

3. Effect of Drug Treatment

Changes in the density of DHP binding sites in morphine-tolerant mice have also been reported (Ramkumar and El-Fakahany 1984). Three days after morphine pellet implantation, synaptosomal membranes from treated rats had B_{max} values of 174 fmol/mg whereas those of control mice had only 109 fmol/mg protein. It had been previously reported that chronic morphine or levorphanol treatment increased vesicular Ca^{2+} uptake and that acute morphine treatment caused Ca^{2+} depletion of the synaptic vesicles in various brain regions (see Ross and Cardenas 1977). Taken together, the above results support the hypothesis that opiate receptor occupation can regulate the number of neuronal Ca^{2+} channels and that this change in number may be relevant to the development of physical dependence.

4. Effect of Hypertension

Ishii et al. (1983) reported that there was a greater number of nitrendipine binding sites (107 fmol/mg vs 68 fmol/mg) in membranes from the brain of hypertensive (SHR) compared with normotensive (WKY) rats; no change in DHPRs in the heart was noted. Similarly, no change in the DHPR of the cardiac membranes from 9-week-old SHR was found in most studies (Chatelain et al. 1984).

E. Kinetics and Thermodynamics of Binding

1. Kinetics of Binding

Initial reports of the kinetics of DHP binding were usually consistent with single association processes (Triggle and Janis 1984). Recent evidence, however, using generally higher free concentrations of [^{3}H]DHPs, indicate that the rate of binding of both [^{3}H]nitrendipine to brain membranes (Weiland and Oswald 1985) and [^{3}H]BAY K 8644 to cardiac membranes (Shrikhande et al. 1985) is not consistent with a simple association process. There appears to be two interconvertible forms of the DHPR, one of which exhibits a much higher affinity than the other. The rate of isomerization of the low to high affinity site, rather than the free ligand concentration, dominates the rate of formation of the high affinity complex. It is not known if the low affinity binding site reflects the existence of DHPRs which are analogous to those occurring in Ca^{2+} channels in the resting state.

2. Thermodynamics of Binding

The affinity of Ca^{2+} channel antagonists is relatively independent of temperature. The equilibrium dissociation constant at 37 °C is usually only 2 to 4 times greater than that at 15 °C to 25 °C (Triggle and Janis 1984). In contrast, the K_d values for the high affinity binding of BAY K 8644 and CGP 28392 increase at least 10-fold over this temperature range. The binding of the activators, but not the antagonists was associated with an unfavorable change in entropy (Shrikhande et al. 1985). The results are consistent with the hypothesis that these activators produce a conformational change in the Ca^{2+} channel complex such that long openings are favored.

F. Cellular and Subcellular Localization

Ligand binding studies agree with electrophysiological studies in detecting high affinity sites for DHPs in most excitable cells that contain Ca^{2+} channels (Janis and Scriabine 1983; Triggle and Janis 1984). Autoradiographic studies of [^{3}H]nitrendipine binding to brain indicate that only certain synaptic areas contain a high density of DHPRs (Cortes et al. 1983; Quirion 1983; Gould et al. 1985). The light microscopic techniques used in these studies did not allow specific localization to dentrites, nerve endings or neuronal cell bodies. Snyder and Reynolds (1985) suggest that the pronounced regional variation in DHP binding in brain suggests that these receptors normally interact with some neurotransmitters or neuromodulators.

Ligand binding studies also agree with electrophysiological data demonstrating the presence of Ca^{2+} channels in smooth and cardiac muscle sarcolemma (Grover et al. 1984; Sarmiento et al. 1984b), skeletal muscle transverse tubules (Fosset et al. 1983; Brandt et al. 1985; Chin and Beeler 1985) and neuronal plasma membranes (Marangos et al. 1982; Janis and Scriabine 1983; Triggle and Janis 1984). Sarcoplasmic reticulum and mitochondrial membranes from heart contain few DHP binding sites (Sarmiento et al. 1984; Brandt et al. 1985a). In agreement with these results, calmodulin inhibitable Ca^{2+} release from skeletal muscle sarcoplasmic reticulum was found to be insensitive to nitrendipine (Meissner and Darling 1985). It has been demonstrated that skeletal muscle contraction is sensitive to Ca^{2+} channel antagonists when that contraction is directly dependent on extracellular Ca^{2+} (Frank 1984).

G. Modification of 1,4-Dihydropyridine Binding by Non-Dihydropyridines

Many aspects of the allosteric regulation of DHPRs have been recently reviewed (Janis and Triggle 1984). Initial studies by Roeske, Yamamura and co-workers (see Boles et al. 1984 for references) demonstrated that verapamil was a negative heterotropic regulator of the DHPR. In contrast, diltiazem was found to be a positive heterotropic regulator of the DHPR (Bolger et al. 1983; Murphy et al. 1983; Janis et al. 1984b; see also chapters in this volume by Glossmann and by Schwartz et al.).

Murphy and co-workers (1983) had proposed that many of the non-DHP Ca^{2+} channel antagonists, including verapamil and diltiazem, act at a common allosteric site to modify the DHPR. However, the results of Bolger et al. (1984) and Glossmann et al. (1984) have suggested that there are at least two types of allosteric sites for organic ligands that regulate the DHPR, one for diltiazem-type drugs, and one for verapamil-type drugs. Recent studies have shown that some neuroleptics and antidiarrheal drugs affect Ca^{2+} channels and the DHPRs (Snyder and Reynolds 1985).

The reversal of the inhibitory effects of DHP-type Ca^{2+} channel antagonists by Ca^{2+} in contractile and electrophysiological studies is due to neither a direct nor an allosteric type of competition with Ca^{2+}, but rather a surface charge effect (Bean 1984). The recent studies of Bean (1984) and Kass et al. (this volume) indicate that the antagonistic effect of Ca^{2+} is due to hyperpolarizing shift in the relationship between Ca^{2+} channel availability and membrane potential.

The requirement for a divalent cation at the DHPR for DHP binding to occur has been well established (Gould et al. 1984, Bellemann 1984a; Glossmann et al. 1984; Janis et al. 1984b). The data indicate that the divalent cation must have similar charge density to that of Ca^{2+} for restoration of binding to EDTA treated membranes. In contrast, binding to calmodulin requires an ionic radius similar to Ca^{2+} (see Luchowski et al. 1984). Glossmann et al. (1984) have proposed that the DHPR contains two to four interacting divalent cation sites.

H. Effect of GTP, Enzymes, pH, and Sulfydryl Reagents

1. Guanyl Nucleotides

Galizzi et al. (1984b) reported that the apparent density of verapamil binding sites in transverse tubular membranes of skeletal muscle is decreased by GTP, ATP and Gpp(NP)p (5′-guanyl-imidodiphosphate). This decrease appeared to be due to a conversion of high to low affinity binding sites. In these t-tubular membranes GTP at 0.13 mM did not inhibit [^{3}H]nitrendipine binding.

In contrast to the above results, the binding affinity of [^{3}H]nitrendipine to guinea pig heart and brain membranes was decreased by guanyl nucleotides. Gpp(NH)p (0.2 mM) decreased the affinity of [^{3}H]nitrendipine binding to guinea pig synaptosomal membranes from 162 pM to 82 pM (A. Rutledge and D.J. Triggle, unpublished); no change in binding site density was found with

Gpp(NH)p treatment. Although the change in affinity was observed in only one-half of the experiments, it was always in the direction of a decrease. Glossmann et al. (1982) have reported that the inhibitory effect of ATP and GTP (10 mM) on [^{3}H]nimodipine binding to guinea pig brain membranes was overcome by 10 mM Mg^{2+}. However, the above studies were carried out with a large excess of divalent cation (1.2 mM Ca^{2+} and 1.3 mM Mg^{2+}) relative to guanyl nucleotide (0.2 mM). Although guanyl nucleotides usually decrease the affinity of agonist binding in a large number of adenylate cyclase linked systems, they have also been reported to prevent antagonist (spiroperidol) binding (Andron and Kohagen 1984).

2. Effect of Degrading Enzymes

Trypsin, α-chymotrypsin, phospholipase A_2, and phospholipase C either reduced or eliminated specific binding in smooth and cardiac muscle membranes (Bolger et al. 1983; Janis et al. 1984 b). In addition to these enzymes, β-galactosidase and β-glucosidase, but not phospholipase D, neuraminidase, adenosine deaminase or phosphodiesterase, were reported to decrease [^{3}H]nimodipine binding to brain membranes (Glossmann et al. 1982). The DHPR in skeletal muscle t-tubular membranes was degraded by trypsin, pronase and papain, and, at a lower rate, by chymotrypsin and leucine aminopeptidase (Fosset et al. 1983). These results and those of others (Borsotto et al. 1984; Curtis and Catterall 1984) indicate that the DHPR is a glycoprotein with a phospholipid requirement for binding.

3. Protein Phosphorylation

No effect of cyclic AMP dependent protein kinases on the binding of nitrendipine was observed under conditions that produced phosphorylation (Bowling et al. 1984). Similarly, neither cyclic AMP- nor cyclic GMP-dependent protein kinases were found to change nitrendipine binding to purified canine cardiac sarcolemma (J. G. Sarmiento, unpublished studies). In contrast, nitrendipine, but not BAY K 8644, was found to stimulate the calcium-dependent phosphorylation of a 42,000 dalton protein in canine cardiac membranes (Horne et al. 1984). Cyclic AMP-dependent protein kinase has been found to stimulate the phosphorylation of the 50,000 dalton subunit of the putative skeletal muscle Ca^{2+} channel (B. M. Curtis and W. A. Catterall, Proc. Natl. Acad. Sci., to be published).

4. Effect of pH

[^{3}H]Nitrendipine binding to t-tubular membranes from skeletal muscle increased with an increase in pH from 4 to 6.5 and then remained constant (Fosset et al. 1984). The DHPR, like the Ca^{2+} channel in barnacle muscle, appears to contain an external ionizable group with a pK_a of 5.3 which must be in the basic form for binding.

The pH dependence of nitrendipine binding to ileal, brain, and cardiac membranes was found to be maximal over the 6.5 to 8 range; a marked decrease in binding was found at pH values above 8.5 (Bolger et al. 1983; Glossmann et al. 1984; Janis et al. 1984b). In contrast, skeletal muscle membranes exhibit increased binding with increased pH up to 9.5. This is one of nine differences between the binding of [^{3}H]nimodipine to brain and skeletal muscle membranes listed by Glossmann et al. (1984).

5. Effect of Heat

Heating membranes from excitable cells at or above 50–65 °C for 5–10 min produced a marked decrease in high affinity specific binding of DHPs (Bolger et al. 1983; Glossmann et al. 1982; Bellemann et al. 1983; Janis et al. 1984b). Of further interest is the lower binding site density observed in some preparations at 37 °C relative to lower temperatures (Gould et al. 1982; Janis et al. 1984b) but not others (Boles et al. 1984). In cardiac membranes this decrease in binding is reversed by 1–10 μM diltiazem (Janis et al. 1984b).

6. Effect of Sulfhydryl Reagents

Initial reports stated that neither reducing nor alkylating agents changed nimodipine binding to the DHPR, but subsequent studies have indicated that the DHPRs in membranes from rat brain were sensitive to sulfhydryl reagents (Marangos et al. 1982). The sensitivity of the receptor in brain and heart to these reagents was subsequently reported to be lower than that of skeletal muscle (Glossmann et al. 1984). Curtis and Catterall (1984) found that treatment of digitonin-solubilized skeletal muscle DHPR with the strong reducing agent, dithiothreitol, resulted in a change in the apparent molecular weight of the largest subunit from 160,000 to 130,000. The affinity of the DHPR in transverse tubules from skeletal muscle is also decreased by treatment with dithiothreitol, further demonstrating the sensitivity of the DHPR to the oxidation of a critical cysteine residue (Brandt et al. 1985b).

I. Estimates of Macromolecular and Subunit Sizes

Radiation inactivation analysis of membranes from ileal smooth muscle, cardiac muscle and brain membranes have yielded molecular weight values of 278,000; 180,000 and 100,000, respectively (Venter et al. 1983; Venter and Triggle, unpublished). These results support other lines of evidence that indicate that there are chemical differences in the DHPR of these three types of tissue. In contrast, Norman et al. (1983) have found a similar value of 210,000 for both skeletal muscle and brain membranes. Glossmann et al. (1984) reported that the apparent target size is the same for skeletal and cardiac muscle, and brain, and that it varies from 75,000 to 178,000 depending on the ligand and preincubation conditions used (see also Glossmann et al., this volume).

Estimates of the macromolecular complex size have also been obtained from the apparent subunit composition of the solubilized receptor from skeletal muscle. Curtis and Catterall (1984) obtained a molecular weight of 213,000 from subunits of 130,000; 50,000 and 33,000, whereas Borsotto et al. (1984) reported a molecular weight of 205,000 from subunit sizes on sodium dodecyl sulfate gels of 142,000; 33,000 and 32,000. The apparent molecular weights of the DHP binding subunit (or a neighboring subunit) range from 32,000 to 145,000 (Borsotto et al. 1984; Glossmann et al. 1984). Labeling with both tritiated and iodinated photoaffinity ligands and with an isothiocyanate affinity label (Venter et al. 1983) have yielded subunits with values from 32,000 to 50,000 (e.g. Campbell et al. 1984; Sarmiento et al. 1985). Both nitrendipine and isoproterenol were found to stimulate the phosphorylation of a 42,000 dalton peptide in canine cardiac membranes, and this component was found to co-migrate with that protein labeled by treatment of the DHP isothiocyanate derivative (Horne et al. 1984), whereas Curtis and Catterall observed cyclic AMP-dependent phosphorylation at the 50,000 dalton protein. Comparative studies of several ligands and tissues in the same laboratory will be necessary before it will be possible to establish that differences exist in the molecular weight of the DHP recognition site in various tissues.

The characterization of DHPRs purified by DHP-specific antibodies (Campbell et al. 1985) may resolve some of the controversy in this field. The DHPR-linked binding site for non-DHP Ca^{2+} channel antagonists remains coupled to the DHPR after solubilization (Curtis and Catterall 1983; Borsotto et al. 1984b). However, differences in the affinity of the d-*cis*-diltiazem site and, independently, the (+)verapamil site, were found in different fractions of solubilized DHPR (Borsotto et al. 1984b).

The ratio of DHP binding sites to verapamil, and diltiazem sites in skeletal muscle membranes has been reported to be 2:4:1 (Glossmann et al. 1984) and 1:1 for DHPR and verapamil sites by Gallizzi et al. (1984a). Garcia et al. (1984) have found that the 4-fold excess of verapamil sites over DHP sites in *crude* canine heart membranes, was lost on purification, to yield an equal density of DHP, verapamil and diltiazem binding sites, in agreement with the results (Gallizzi et al. 1984a).

J. Summary

Both electrophysiological and ligand binding studies indicate that the DHPR is closely associated with Ca^{2+} channel in smooth and cardiac muscle, and that inhibition of the Ca^{2+} current by DHPs is not a steric block of the channel. The excellent correlation in a series of DHPs between the affinity for the [^{3}H]DHP binding site and for the inhibition of smooth muscle contraction is key evidence in relating the high affinity [^{3}H]DHP binding site with Ca^{2+} channels. Differences in absolute potencies for binding and contractility in cardiac muscle are consistent with electrophysiological studies indicating the voltage dependence of binding. The change in potency of antagonists with membrane potential also indicates that the DHPR is linked to the Ca^{2+} channel. Voltage-dependence of binding dictates that there will be no unique affinity of this receptor for a given

DHP. Differences between the DHPs and non-DHPs in use-dependence support the idea that there are fundamental differences in the sites or mechanisms of action of these types of drugs, a view demonstrated independently by ligand binding studies. That receptor affinity is dependent on the state of the Ca^{2+} channel is consistent with the hypothesis that the DHP binding causes conformational changes in the channel structure to produce alterations in channel activity. The DHPR also appears to be part of the Ca^{2+} channel of skeletal muscle, nerve and endocrine cells. The ontogenesis of the DHP binding sites appear to precede that of active Ca^{2+} channels in some tissues.

The extent to which chemical differences in the DHP binding site exist and can account for tissue selectivity of DHPs remains to be determined. The available evidence is consistent with the view that tissue selectivity at the receptor level is due to both conformational and chemical differences in the DHPR/Ca^{2+} channel complex.

References

Andorn AC, Kohagen KR (1984) Guanyl nucleotides decrease antagonist binding at high affinity dopamine receptors. Eur J Pharmacol 103:127–131

Bean BP (1984) Nitrendipine block of cardiac calcium channels: High-affinity binding to the inactivated state. Proc Natl Acad Sci USA 81:6388–6392

Bean BP (1985) Two kinds of calcium channels in atrial cells from dog and frog hearts. Biophys J 497a

Bellemann P (1984a) Observations on receptor sites for dihydropyridines. In: Reid E, Cook GMW, Moore DJ (eds) Investigation of membrane-located receptors. Plenum, New York, pp 513–518

Bellemann P (1984b) Binding properties of a novel calcium channel activating dihydropyridine in monolayer cultures of beating myocytes. FEBS Lett 167:88–92

Bellemann P (1984c) Interaction of the calcium channel activating [^{3}H]BAY K 8644 and inhibiting [^{3}H]verapamil with specific receptor sites on cultured beating myocardial cells. J Recept Res 4:571–585

Bellemann P, Ferry D, Lübbecke F, Glossmann H (1981) [^{3}H]Nitrendipine, a potent calcium antagonist, binds with high affinity to cardiac membranes. Arzneim Forsch 31:2064–2067

Bellemann P, Schade A, Towart R (1983) Dihydropyridine receptor in rat brain labeled with [^{3}H]nimodipine. Proc Natl Acad Sci USA 80:2356–2360

Boles RG, Yamamura HI, Schoemaker H, Roeske WR (1984) Temperature-dependent modulation of [^{3}H]nitrendipine binding by the calcium channel antagonists verapamil and diltiazem in rat brain synaptosomes. J Pharmacol Exp Ther 225:291–309

Bolger GT, Gengo P, Klockowski R, Luchowski E, Siegel H, Janis RA, Triggle AM, Triggle DJ (1983) Characterization of binding of the Ca^{2+} channel antagonist, nitrendipine, to guinea pig ileal smooth muscle. J Pharmacol Exp Ther 225:291–309

Borsotto M, Barhanin J, Norman RI, Lazdunski M (1984a) Purification of the dihydropyridine receptor of the voltage-dependent Ca^{2+} channel from skeletal muscle transverse tubules using (+) [^{3}H]PN 200–110. Biochem Biophys Res Commun 122:1357–1366

Borsotto M, Norman RI, Fosset M, Lazdunski M (1984b) Solubilization of the nitrendipine receptor from skeletal muscle transverse tubule membranes: Interactions with specific inhibitors of the voltage-dependent Ca^{2+} channel. Eur J Biochem 142:449–455

Bowling N, Conrey BG, Kauffman RF, Hayes JS (1984) Phosphorylation of dog heart sarcolemmal vesicles does not alter nitrendipine binding properties. Fed Proc 43:549 (abstract)

Brandt NR, Kawamoto RM, Caswell AH (1985a) Dihydropyridine binding sites on transverse tubules isolated from triads of rabbit skeletal muscle. J Receptor Res 5:155–170

Brandt NR, Kawamoto RM, Caswell AH (1985b) Effects of mercaptans upon dihydropyridine binding sites on transverse tubules isolated from triads of rabbit skeletal muscle. Biochem Biophys Res Commun 127:205–212

Bristow MR, Ginsburg R, Laser JA, McAuley BJ, Minobe W (1984) Tissue response selectivity of calcium antagonists is not due to heterogeneity of [^{3}H]nitrendipine binding sites. Br J Pharmac 82:309–320

Caffrey JM, Josephson IR, Brown AM (1985) Calcium channels in smooth muscle: dihydropyridine action. Biophys J 47:265a

Campbell KP, Lipshutz GM, Denny GH (1984) Direct photoaffinity labeling of the high affinity nitrendipine-binding site in subcellular membrane fractions isolated from canine myocardium. J Biol Chem 259:1–4

Campbell KP, Strom M, Sharp A (1985) Development of an affinity column for the purification of the dihydropyridine receptor. Biophys J 47:514a

Chatelain P, Demol D, Roba J (1984) Comparison of [^{3}H]nitrendipine binding to heart membranes of normotensive and spontaneously hypertensive rats. J Cardiovasc Pharmacol 6:220–223

Chin H, Beeler T (1985) Nitrendipine binding to transverse tubule and plasma membrane vesicles purified from rat skeletal muscle. Biophys J 47:265a

Cohen CJ, McCarthy RT (1985) Differential effects of dihydropyridines on two populations of Ca channels in anterior pituitary cells. Biophys J 47:513a

Coronado R, Affolter H (1985) Kinetics of dihydropyridine-sensitive single calcium channels from purified muscle transverse tubules. Biophys J 47:434a

Cortes R, Supavila P, Karobath M, Palacios JM (1983) The effect of lesions in the rat hippocampus suggest the association of calcium channel binding sites with a specific neuronal population. Neurosci Lett 42:249–254

Cota G, Stefani E (1985) Fast and slow Ca channels in twitch muscle fibers of the frog. Biophys J 47:65a

Curtis BM, Catterall WA (1984) Purification of the calcium antagonist receptor of the voltage-sensitive calcium channel from skeletal muscle transverse tubules. Biochem 23:2113–2118

Fairhurst AS, Thayer SA, Colker JE, Beatty DA (1983) A calcium antagonist drug binding site in skeletal muscle sarcoplasmic reticulum: evidence for a calcium channel. Life Sci 32:1331–1339

Ferry DR, Goll A, Gadow C, Glossmann H (1984) (−)-[^{3}H]-Desmethoxyverapamil labeling of putative calcium channels in brain: autoradiographic distribution and allosteric coupling to 1,4-dihydropyridine and diltiazem binding sites. Naunyn-Schmiedeberg's Arch. Pharmacol 327:183–187

Frank GB (1984) Blockade of Ca channels inhibits K^+ contractures but not twitches in skeletal muscle. Can J Physiol Pharmacol 62:374–378

Freedman SB, Dawson G, Villercal ML, Miller RJ (1984) Identification and characterization of voltage-sensitive calcium channels in neuronal clonal cell lines. J Neurosci 4:1453–1467

Fosset M, Jaimovich E, Delmont E, Lazdunski M (1983) [^{3}H]Nitrendipine receptors in skeletal muscle. J Biol Chem 258:6086–6092

Galizzi J-P, Fosset M, Lazdunski M (1984a) [^{3}H]Verapamil binding sites in skeletal muscle transverse tubule membranes. Biochem Biophys Res Commun 118:239–245

Galizzi J-P, Fosset M, Lazdunski M (1984b) Properties of receptors for the Ca^{2+} channel blocker verapamil in transverse-tubule membranes of skeletal muscle: Stereospecificity, effect of Ca^{2+} and other inorganic cations, evidence for two categories of sites and effect of nucleoside triphosphates. Eur J Biochem 1–5

Garcia ML, Trumble MJ, Reuben JP, Kaczorowski J (1984) Characterization of verapamil binding sites in cardiac membrane vesicles. J Biol Chem 259:15013–15016

Glossmann H, Ferry DR, Lübbecke F, Mewes R, Hofmann F (1982) Calcium channels: Direct identification with radioligand binding studies. Trends Pharmacol Sci 3:431–437

Glossmann H, Ferry DR, Goll A, Rombusch M (1984) Molecular pharmacology of the calcium channel: evidence for subtypes, multiple drug receptor sites, channel subunits and the development of a radioiodinated 1,4-dihydropyridine calcium channel label, ^{125}I-iodipine. J Cardiovasc Pharmacol 6:S608–S621

Goll A, Ferry DR, Glossmann H (1983) Target size analysis of skeletal muscle Ca^{2+} channels. Positive allosteric heterotropic regulation by d-*cis*-diltiazem is associated with apparent channel oligomer dissociation. FEBS Lett 157:63–69

Gould RJ, Murphy KMM, Snyder SH (1984) Tissue heterogeneity of calcium channel antagonist binding sites labeled by [^{3}H]nitrendipine. Molec Pharmacol 25:235–241

Gould RJ, Murphy KMM, Snyder SH (1985) Autoradiographic localization of calcium channel antagonist receptors in rat brain with [^{3}H]nitrendipine. Brain Res 330:217–224

Green FJ, Farmer BB, Wiseman GL, Jose MJL, Watanabe AM (1985) Effect of membrane depolarization on binding of [^{3}H]nitrendipine to rat cardiac myocytes. Circ Res 56:576–585

Grover AK, Kwan CY, Luchowski E, Daniel EE, Triggle DJ (1984) Subcellular distribution of [^{3}H]nitrendipine binding in smooth muscle. J Biol Chem 259:2223–2226

Hess P, Lansman JB, Tsien RW (1984) Different modes of calcium channel gating favored by Ca agonists and antagonists. Nature 311:538–544

Hof RP, Rüegg UT, Hof A, Vogel A (1985) Stereoselectivity at the calcium channel: opposite action of the enantiomers of a 1,4-dihydropyridine. J Cardiovasc Pharmacol 7:689–693

Holck M, Thorens S, Haeusler G (1983) Does [^{3}H]nifedipine label the calcium channel in rabbit myocardium? J Receptor Res 3:191–198

Horne P, Triggle DJ, Venter JC (1984) Nitrendipine and isoproterenol induce phosphorylation of a 42,000 Dalton protein that comigrates with the affinity labeled calcium channel regulatory subunit. Biochem Biophys Res Common 121:890–898

Huszar G, Janis RA, Sakamoto H, Scriabine A (1983) A calcium entry blocker and the control of labor. Proc of Soc for Gynecologic Investigation, Abstr 448

Ishii K, Kano T, Kurobe Y, Ando J (1983) Binding of [^{3}H]nitrendipine to heart and brain membranes from normotensive and spontaneously hypertensive rats. Eur J Pharmac 88:277–278

Janis RA, Rampe D, Sarmiento JG, Triggle DJ (1984a) Specific binding of a Ca^{2+} channel agonist to membranes from cardiac muscle and brain. Biochem Biophys Res Common 121:317–323

Janis RA, Sarmiento JG, Maurer SC, Bolger GT, Triggle DJ (1984b) Characteristics of the binding of [^{3}H]nitrendipine to rabbit ventricular membranes. Modification by other Ca^{2+} channel antagonists and by the Ca^{2+} channel agonist, BAY K 8644. J Pharmacol Exp Ther 231:8–15

Janis RA, Scriabine A (1983) Sites of action of Ca^{2+} channel inhibitors. Biochem Pharmacol 32:3499–3507

Janis RA, Triggle DJ (1984) 1,4-Dihydropyridine Ca^{2+} channel antagonists and agonists. A comparison of binding characteristics with pharmacology. Drug Dev Res 4:257–274

Kazazoglou T, Schmid A, Renaud J-F, Lazdunski M (1983) Ontogenic appearance of Ca^{2+} channels characterized as binding sites for nitrendipine during development of nervous, skeletal and cardiac muscle systems in the rat. FEBS Lett 164:75–79

Kenessey A, Cantor EH, Spector S (1984) Low affinity dihydropyridine binding site in rat heart membranes. Fed Proc 43:1548 (abstract)

Kirley TL, Schwartz A (1984) Solubilization and affinity labeling of a dihydropyridine binding site from skeletal muscle: Effects of temperature and diltiazem on [^{3}H]dihydropyridine binding to transverse tubules. Biochem Biophys Res Commun 123:41–49

Kokubun S, Reuter H (1984) Dihydropyridine derivatives prolong the open state of Ca channels in cultured cardiac cells. Proc Natl Acad Sci USA 81:4824–4827

Kunze DL, Hawkes MJ, Hamilton SL, Brown AM (1985) Binding and pharmacological studies of nitrendipine on PC12 cells. Biophys J 47:264a

Litzinger MJ, Brenneman DE (1984) TTX displacement of [^{3}H]nitrendipine binding in developing spinal cord neurons. Biochem Biophys Res Commun 124:979–987

Luchowski EM, Yousif F, Triggle DJ, Maurer SC, Sarmiento JG, Janis RA (1984) The effects of metal cations and calmodulin antagonists on [^{3}H]nitrendipine binding in smooth and cardiac muscle. J Pharmacol Exp Ther 230:607–613

Marangos PJ, Patel J, Miller C, Martino AM (1982) Specific calcium antagonist binding sites in brain. Life Sci 31:1575–1585

Marangos PJ, Sperelakis N, Patel J (1984) Ontogeny of calcium antagonist binding sites in chick brain and heart. J Neurochem 42:1338–1342

Marsh JD, Loh E, Lachance D, Barry WH, Smith TW (1983) Relationship of binding of a calcium channel blocker to inhibition of contraction on intact cultured embryonic chick ventricular cells. Circ Res 53:539–543

Matsubayashi H, Kito S, Itoga E, Mizuno K, Miyoshi R (1984) Ontogenic development of the specific [^{3}H]nitrendipine binding sites in the rat brain. Adv Exp Med Biol 175:193–204

McBride W, Mukherjee A, Haghani Z, Wheeler-Clark E, Brady J, Gandler T, Bush L, Buja ML, Willerson JT (1984) Nitrendipine: effects on vascular responses and myocardial binding. Am J Physiol 247:H775–H783

Meissner G, Darling E (1985) Kinetics of rapid Ca^{2+} release by sarcoplasmic reticulum. Biophys J 47:285a

Meyer S, Kazda S, Bellemann P (1983) Calcium antagonists – New opportunities. Annu Repts Med Chem 18:79–88

Miller RJ (1985) How many types of calcium channels exist in neurons? Trends in Neurosci 8:45–47

Moscona-Amir E, Sokolovsky M (1984) Interactions between Ca^{2+} antagonist binding sites in rat adenohypophysis: dependence on estrous cycle. Life Sci 35:1043–1050

Murphy KMM, Gould RJ, Largent BL, Snyder SH (1983) A unitary mechanism of calcium antagonist drug action. Proc Natl Acad Sci USA 80:860–864

Nilius B, Hess P, Lansman JB, Tsien RW (1985) A novel type of calcium channel in ventricular heart cells. Nature 316:443–446

Nirenberg M, Wilson S, Higashida H, Rotte A, Krueger K, Busis N, Ray R, Kenimer JG, Alder M (1983) Modulation of synapse formation by cyclic adenosine monophosphate. Science 222:794–799

Norman RI, Borsotto M, Fosset M, Lazdunski M (1983) Determination of the molecular size of the nitrendipine-sensitive Ca^{2+} channel by radiation inactivation. Biochem Biophys Res Commun 111:878–883

Nowycky MC, Fox AP, Tsien RW (1985a) Three types of calcium channels in chick dorsal root ganglion cells. Biophys J 67a

Nowycky MC, Fox AP, Tsien RW (1985b) Novel mode of neuronal calcium channel gating and its promotion by the dihydropyridine calcium agonist BAY K 8644. Proc Natl Acad Sci USA 82:2178–2182

Quirion R (1983) Autoradiographic localization of a calcium channel antagonist, [^{3}]nitrendipine binding site in rat brain. Neurosci Lett 36:267–271

Rampe D, Janis RA, Triggle DJ (1984) BAY K 8644, A 1,4-dihydropyridine Ca^{2+} channel activator: Dissociation of binding and functional effects in brain synaptosomes. J Neurochem 43:1688–1692

Ramkumar V, El-Fakahany EE (1984) Increase in [^{3}H]nitrendipine binding sites in the brain in morphine-tolerant mice. Eur J Pharmacol 102(2):371–372

Renaud J-F, Kazazoglow T, Schmid A, Romey G, Lazdunski M (1984) Differentiation of receptor sites for [^{3}H]nitrendipine in chick hearts and physiological relation to the slow Ca^{2+} channel and to excitation-contraction coupling. Eur J Biochem 139:673–681

Rogart RB, Bruyn, Kops A De, Janis RA, Dzau VJ (1984) Nimodipine binding to two calcium channel subtypes in rat heart. IUPHR 9 Int Congr Pharmacology, London, Abstr 409

Ross DH, Cardenas HL (1977) Effects of levorphanol on Ca^{2+} binding to synaptic membranes in vitro. Life Sci 20:1455–1462

Sanguinetti MC, Kass RS (1984) Voltage-dependent block of calcium channel current in the calf cardiac Purkinje fiber by dihydropyridine derivatives. Circ Res 55:336–348

Sanguinetti MC, Kass RS (1985) Voltage selects activity of the Ca channel modulator BAY K 8644. Biophys J 47:513a

Sarmiento JG, Janis RA, Katz AM, Triggle DJ (1984a) Comparison of high affinity binding of calcium channel blocking drugs to vascular smooth muscle and cardiac sarcolemmal membranes. Biochem Pharmacol 33:3119–3123

Sarmiento JG, Janis RA, Jenkins D, Triggle DJ (1984b) Characteristics of [^{3}H]nitrendipine binding to vascular smooth muscle membranes. In: Scriabine A, Vanov S, Deck K (eds) Nitrendipine. Urban & Schwarzenberg, Baltimore, pp 153–160

Sarmiento JG, Epstein PM, Smilowitz H, Chester DW, Wehinger E, Janis RA (1985) Photoaffinity labeling of the 1,4-dihydropyridine Ca^{2+} channel binding site in cardiac, skeletal and smooth muscle membranes. Fed Proc 44:1640 (abstract)

Schilling WP, Hamilton SL, Yatini A, Brush K, Brown AM (1985) High and low affinity nitrendipine binding in membrane preparations from guinea pig ventricle. Biophys J 47:264 a

Schmid A, Kazazoglou T, Renaud J-F, Lazdunski M (1984) Comparative changes of levels of nitrendipine Ca^{2+} channels, of tetrodotoxin-sensitive Na^+ channels and of ouabain-sensitive $(Na^+ + K^+)$-ATPase following denervation of rat and chick skeletal muscle. FEBS Lett 172:114–118

Schramm M, Thomas G, Towart R, Franckowiak G (1983) Novel dihydropyridines with positive inotropic action through activation of Ca^{2+} channel. Nature 303:535–537

Shrikhande AV, Sarmiento JG, Janis RA, Rutledge E, Triggle DJ (1985) Characteristics of binding of BAY K 8644 to high and low affinity sites on cardiac membranes. Biophys J 47:265 a

Snyder SH, Reynolds IJ (1985) Calcium antagonist drugs. Receptor interactions clarify therapeutic effects. N Eng J Medicine (to be published)

Su CM, Swamy VC, Triggle DJ (1984) Calcium channel activation in vascular smooth muscle of BAY K 8644. Can J Physiol Pharmacol 62:1401–1410

Thayer SA, Stein L, Fairhurst AS (1984) Endogenous modulator of calcium channels. IUPHAR 9th Int Congress of Pharmacol, Abs 892 p

Thomas G, Groß R, Schramm M (1984) Calcium channel modulation: ability to inhibit or promote calcium influx resides in the same dihydropyridine molecule. J Cardiovasc Pharmacol 6:1170–1176

Thomas G, Chung M, Cohen CJ (1985) A dihydropyridine (BAY K 8644) that enhances calcium currents in myocardial cells. A new type of positive inotropic agent. J Cardiovasc Pharmacol 56:87–96

Triggle DJ, Janis RA (1984) Ca^{2+} channel antagonists. New perspectives from the radioligand binding assay. In: Back N, Spector S (eds) Modern methods in pharmacology, vol 2. Alan R Liss, New York, pp 1–28

Tsunoo MY, Narahashi T (1985) Differential block of two types of calcium channels in neuroblastoma cells. Biophys J 47:433 a

Turner TJ, Goldin SM (1985) Identification and pharmacological characterization of calcium channels in rat brain synaptosomes. J Neurochem 5:841–849

Venter JC, Fraser JC, Schaber JS, Jung CY, Bolger G, Triggle DJ (1983) Molecular properties of the slow inward calcium channel. J Biol Chem 258:9344–9348

Weiland GA, Oswald RE (1985) The mechanism of binding of dihydropyridine calcium channel blockers to rat brain membranes. J Biol Chem 260:8456–8464

Bayer-Symposium IX
Cardiovascular Effects of Dihydropyridine-Type
Calcium Antagonists and Agonists, 156–184

A Proposed Pharmacological Role for Dihydropyridine Binding Sites in Heart and Coronary Smooth Muscle

P. L. VAGHY, G. P. DUBÉ, I. L. GRUPP, G. GRUPP, J. S. WILLIAMS, Y. H. BAIK, and A. SCHWARTZ

Introduction

The recent discovery of the dihydropyridine derivatives Bay k 8644 [55, 56, 62] YC-170 [61] and CGP 28392 [14, 68] together with the well-known nifedipine-like drugs have provided an avenue for a classification of dihydropyridines (DHPs) into two separate groups (Table 1). The members of the first group are termed "Ca^{2+} antagonists" or "Ca^{2+} channel inhibitors." These drugs inhibit voltage-dependent Ca^{2+} influx both in smooth and cardiac muscle. This results in vasodilation in the former and negative inotropy in the latter [38, 58]. The second group of compounds activate Ca^{2+} channels, producing vasoconstriction and positive inotropy, i.e., effects which are opposite to those produced by the "Ca^{2+} antagonists" [55, 56, 61–63, 68]. These drugs have been termed "Ca^{2+} agonists" or "Ca^{2+} channel activators" [35, 55, 56, 65].

We have studied the pharmacological effects of DHPs of both groups on isolated heart and coronary smooth muscle preparations with the goal of correlating these effects with putative DHP binding sites identified by employing radioligand binding techniques in canine cardiac sarcolemmal membranes. Our data show

Table 1. Classification of dihydropyridines

I. "Ca^{2+} Antagonists"	II. "Ca^{2+} Agonists"
Nifedipine	Bay k 8644
Nitrendipine	CGP 28392
Nimodipine	YC-170
Nisoldipine	
Nicardipine	
Niludipine	
Felodipine	
PN 200–110	

that the DHPs we have studied possess biphasic contraction-relaxation effects which suggest the intriguing possibility of interaction with more than one DHP binding site.

Experimental Procedures

Materials

Nitrendipine, nimodipine, nifedipine and Bay k 8644 were supplied by Miles Pharmaceuticals, courtesy of Dr. Alexander Scriabine. Diltiazem was supplied by Marion Laboratories, courtesy of Dr. Ronald K. Browne. Isosorbide dinitrate was a gift from Ives Laboratories, courtesy of Drs. Robert Piwonka and Alfred Ling. Histamine was purchased from Sigma Chemical Co., St. Louis, MO. [^{3}H]Nitrendipine (specific activity 70–79.5 Ci/mmol) was purchased from New England Nuclear, Boston, MA.

Methods

Pharmacological Experiments. Inverted Rings from porcine coronary arteries were mounted on stainless steel hooks in muscle baths containing physiological salt solution (PSS) of the following composition (mM/l): 126.9 NaCl, 4.7 KCl, 1.6 $CaCl_2$, 1.17 $MgSO_4$, 1.18 KH_2PO_4, 18 $NaHCO_3$ and 5.5 glucose. The solution was aerated with 95% O_2/5% CO_2, and maintained at pH 7.35, 37 °C. Changes in tension were measured by an isometric force transducer (Model FT.03, Grass Instrument Co.) connected to a Grass polygraph.

Myocardial contractile force in atrial and ventricular strips, trabeculae, and isolated hearts was measured using methods described elsewhere [23]. Generally, the experiments were run at 37 °C in Krebs-Henseleit solutions containing 1.3 to 2 mM Ca^{2+} and 5.9 mM K^+, pH 7.4. When required, the tissues were stimulated through needle electrodes with Grass S8 stimulators, voltage 20% above threshold [41].

Bay k 8644, nimodipine and isosorbide dinitrate stock solutions were prepared in absolute ethanol, propylene glycol or dimethyl sulfoxide. Diltiazem and histamine were dissolved in water. Control experiments were carried out with the appropriate solvent.

Radioligand Binding Experiments. Canine cardiac sarcolemma was isolated by the method of Van Alstyne et al. [71]. Protein was determined by the Lowry procedure [39] using bovine serum albumin as standard.

Cardiac sarcolemmal membranes (23–50 μg protein) were incubated in a total volume of 1 ml of 50 mM Tris-HCl buffer, pH 7.4, containing 150 mM NaCl and 1 mM $CaCl_2$ with varying concentrations of [^{3}H]nitrendipine. The specific activity of [^{3}H]nitrendipine used for studying high affinity binding sites ranged from 70–79.5 Ci/mmol. For measurement of low affinity binding, the specific activity of [^{3}H]nitrendipine was reduced to 8 or 1 Ci/mmol by diluting it with nonlabeled nitrendipine. After 50 minutes of incubation, the bound [^{3}H]nitrendipine was separated by a filtration method and the radioactivity was measured with a Beckman LS 8100 liquid scintillation counter as described previously [69, 70]. The filter paper binding was measured by carrying out the experiments in the absence of the sarcolemmal membranes. Specific [^{3}H]nitrendipine binding was linear with protein concentrations ranging from 5 to 100 μg/ml both at low and high [^{3}H]nitrendipine concentrations. All experiments involving light sensitive drugs were carried out under a sodium lamp.

Data Analysis. Dose-response data obtained in studies with coronary arteries were analysed using the iterative, nonlinear, least squares computer program (ALLFIT) of DeLean et al. [6] converted to Apple Pascal by Dr. C. L. Johnson of this Department. Statistical differences were determined for multiple comparisons using the Student-Neumann-Kuels (SNK) multiple range test [54]. Comparisons of only two data sets were made using the T-test for grouped or paired data, according to the experimental protocol used. P values <0.05 were considered to indicate statistical significance.

ED_{50}, i.e., the drug concentration that produced a 50% increase in contractility, and IC_{50}, i.e., the drug concentration that produced a 50% decrease in contractility of heart muscle preparations were determined graphically in each experiment. Care was taken to reach a steady-state with each drug concentration. Because of the varying negative inotropic effects of Bay k 8644, the IC_{50} was determined from the contractile force decrease from maximal inotropy to control. Values are means ± SEM.

The radioligand binding data were analyzed using a nonlinear least squares Ligand program [42, 43] converted to Applesoft by M. H. Teicher, MED-50 ligand program (Biomedical Computing Technology Information Center).

Results

Effects of Dihydropyridines on Isolated Porcine Coronary Arteries

Bay k 8644 produced a biphasic, contraction-relaxation response in isolated coronary arteries (Fig. 1). The ED_{50}, i.e., the concentration of Bay k 8644 that produced a 50% increase in developed tension, was 11 nM. Maximal tension development occurred at 350 nM when Bay k 8644 was given in a cumulative manner, and at 100 nM when Bay k 8644 was given as a single concentration. Concentrations of Bay k 8644 higher than these produced a dose-dependent *relaxation* of the coronary arteries, with an IC_{50} of 6 μM. The relaxation effect of Bay k 8644 could be washed out rapidly ($t^1/_2 = 4$ min), but the contractile response could not.

Since Bay k 8644-induced contraction was well maintained for several hours, this model proved to be excellent for testing the effects of several vascular smooth muscle relaxants. The effects of isosorbide dinitrate (ISDN), diltiazem and nimodipine (NIMO) on coronary arteries contracted by 100 nM Bay k 8644 or on contractions of equal magnitude induced by 35 mM KCl were studied. All the drugs studied relaxed both the KCl- and the Bay k 8644-induced contractions in a dose-dependent manner (Fig. 2). The KCl-induced contraction was most sensitive to

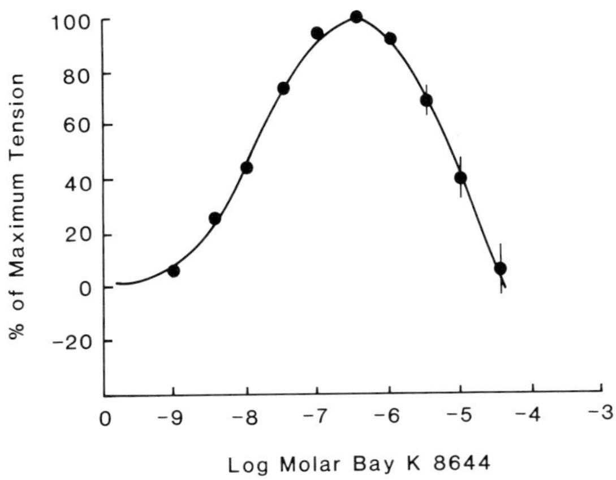

Fig. 1. Dose-response curve for the effect of Bay k 8644 in porcine coronary artery rings. Bay k 8644 was added to the muscle bath in a cumulative fashion waiting until equilibrium tension was obtained before delivering the next dose. The highest Bay k 8644 concentration employed was 35 μM due to a limitation of solubility above 40 μM. Each point represents the mean response ± S.E.M. of 16 to 27 coronary rings from 8 to 14 animals. Taken from [11]

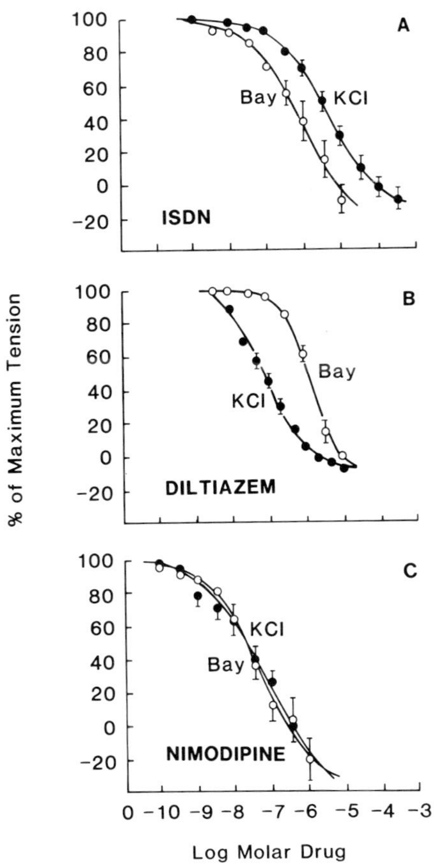

Fig. 2 A–C. Dose-response curves for isosorbide dinitrate (ISDN)-, diltiazem- and nimodipine-induced relaxation of high potassium and Bay k 8644 induced contractions. Porcine coronary artery rings were contracted by either 35 mM KCl or 100 nM Bay k 8644 which yielded equal developed tensions. **A** ISDN, **B** diltiazem, or **C** nimodipine was then added to the muscle bath in a cumulative fashion. Each point represents the mean response ± S.E.M. of 4 to 15 rings from 4 to 15 animals. Taken from [11]

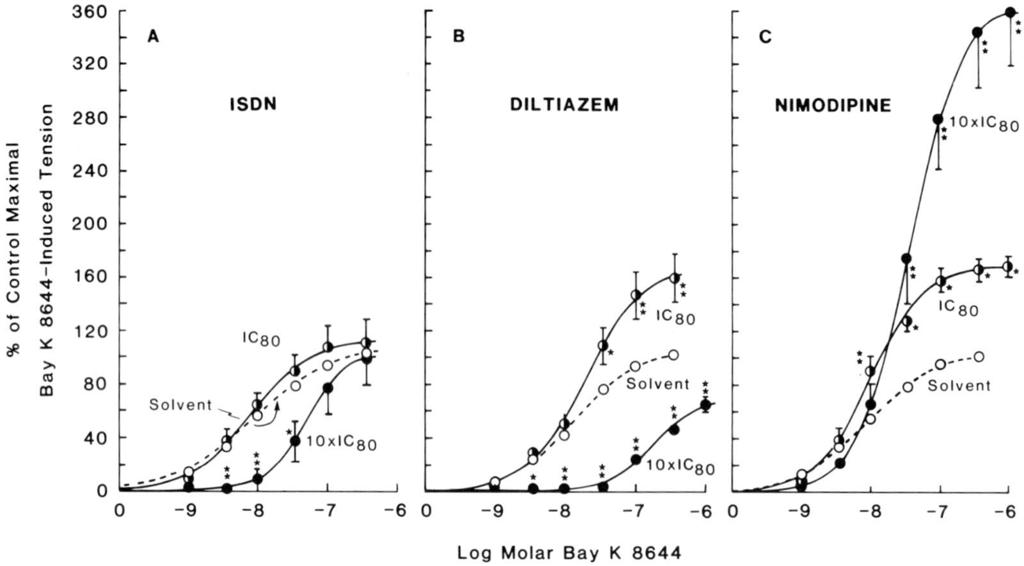

Fig. 3 A–C. Effect of ISDN, diltiazem, and nimodipine pretreatment on the Bay k 8644 dose-response curve. Two equipotent doses of each of three vasodilators were selected from the dose-response curves for relaxation of Bay k 8644 contractions shown in Fig. 2. In panels **A, B,** and **C**, coronary artery test rings were pretreated with concentrations of ISDN (2.4 μM, 25 min), diltiazem (3.57 μM, 30 min), or nimodipine (0.089 μM, 90 min), respectively, which relaxed a 100 nM Bay k 8644-induced contraction 80% (IC_{80}) or with concentrations of ISDN (24.0 μM), diltiazem (35.7 μM), or nimodipine (0.89 μM) which were 10-fold higher than the IC_{80} ($10 \times IC_{80}$). For each vasodilator, paired control rings, in a separate muscle bath, were pretreated with the appropriate corresponding volume of solvent. Following the pretreatment period, the resting tensions, which were reduced by the vasodilators, were mechanically restored to the original 5 gram baseline tension. Solvent had no effect on the resting tension of control tissues. Bay k 8644 was then delivered to both the test and control muscle baths in a cumulative fashion, waiting until equilibrium tension had been obtained before delivering the next dose. The highest Bay k 8644 concentration point shown for each curve was the maximally effective contractile concentration for that group of tissues; the next dose of Bay k 8644 produced relaxation. Each point represents the mean response ± S.E.M. of 4 to 12 rings from 4 to 12 animals. Significant difference from control is indicated by * ($p<0.05$) or ** ($p<0.01$). Taken from [11]

NIMO (IC_{50}=25 nM) followed by diltiazem (IC_{50}=0.1 μM) and ISDN (IC_{50}=4.2 μM). Similarly, NIMO was the most potent (IC_{50}=20 nM) on the Bay k 8644-induced contraction. In this model, however, ISDN was found to be more effective (IC_{50}=0.5 μM) than diltiazem (IC_{50}=1.6 μM). The different orders of effectiveness in producing vasodilation suggest that KCl and Bay k 8644 activate the potential-operated channels (POCs) by different mechanisms in coronary arteries and/or that Bay k 8644 activates receptor-operated channels in addition to POCs.

In subsequent experiments, the effects of pretreatment of the coronary artery rings with these vasodilators on Bay k 8644-induced contraction were studied. The coronary rings were pretreated with equipotent concentrations of ISDN, dil-

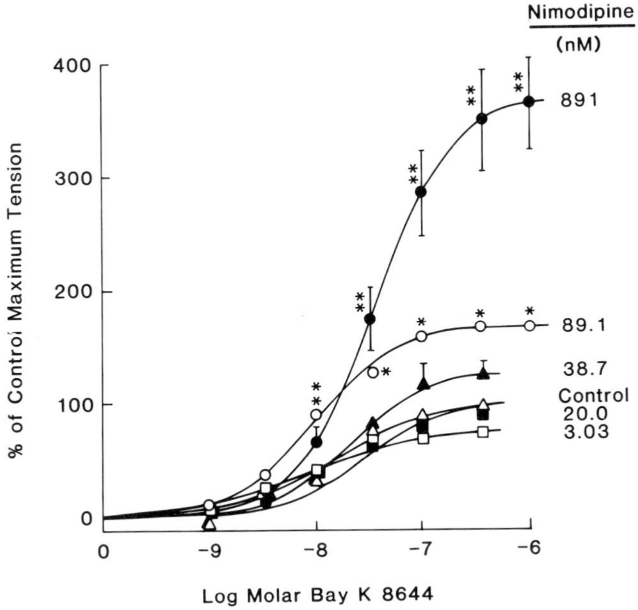

Fig. 4. Effect of pretreatment with different concentrations of nimodipine on the Bay k 8644 cumulative dose-response curve. Coronary artery test rings were pretreated for 90 min with concentrations of nimodipine, selected from Fig. 2, for relaxation of a maximal Bay k 8644 contraction. The nimodipine concentrations used and the extent to which they relaxed the maximal Bay k 8644 contraction of Fig. 2 were: 3.03 nM = IC_{20}; 20.0 nM = IC_{50}; 37.8 nM = IC_{63}; 89.1 nM = IC_{80}; and 891 nM = $10 \times IC_{80}$; solvent = control. Following the pretreatment period, resting tensions, which were reduced by nimodipine, were mechanically restored to the original 5 gram baseline tension. Solvent had no effect on the resting tension of control tissues. Bay k 8644 was then delivered to both test and control tissues in a cumulative fashion. The highest Bay k 8644 concentration point shown for each curve was the maximally effective contractile concentration for that group of tissues; the next dose of Bay k 8644 produced relaxation. Each point represents the mean response ± S.E.M. of 4 to 28 rings from 4 to 28 animals. Significant difference from control is indicated by * ($P<0.05$) or ** ($P<0.01$). Taken from [11]

tiazem or NIMO followed by the cumulative addition of Bay k 8644. The concentration of the inhibitors that produced an 80% inhibition of a preexisting Bay k 8644-induced contraction (IC_{80}) and a concentration 10 times higher than this ($10 \times IC$ 80) were selected for these studies, since lower concentrations had little or no effect when used in the pretreatment experiments. While the IC_{80} concentration of ISDN had no significant effect, IC_{80} concentrations of diltiazem and NIMO surprisingly *stimulated* the Bay k 8644-induced contraction (Fig. 3). When $10 \times IC_{80}$ concentrations were used for pretreatment, ISDN and diltiazem inhibited Bay k 8644-induced contraction but NIMO caused an even further stimulation of contraction.

The effect of pretreatment with five different concentrations of NIMO on Bay k 8644-induced contraction is illustrated in Fig. 4. Low concentrations of NIMO had no significant effect or showed a tendency to inhibit maximal and

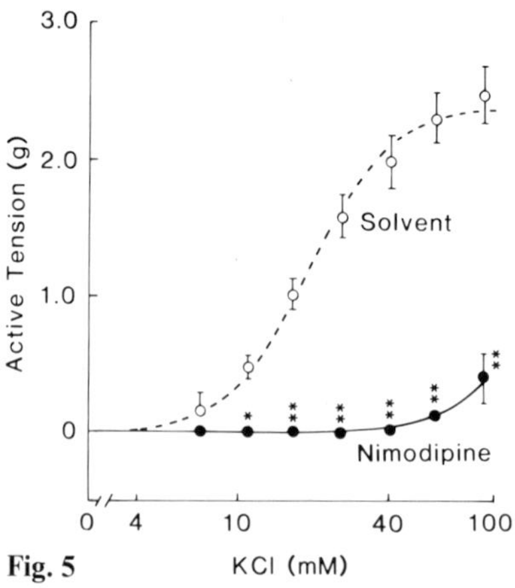

Fig. 5

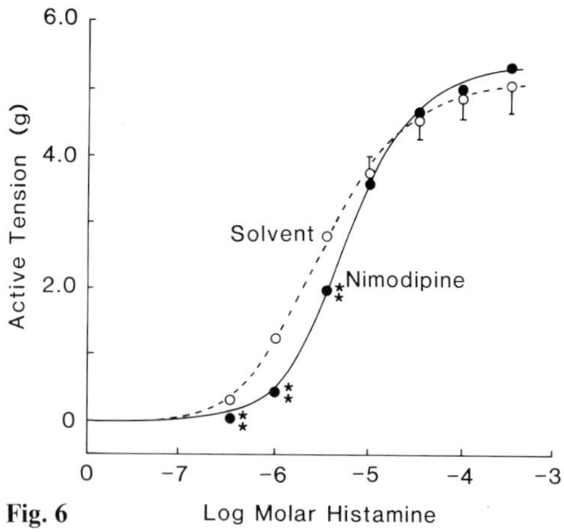

Fig. 6

Fig. 5. Effect of nimodipine pretreatment on the KCl dose-response curve. Coronary artery test rings were pretreated with a concentration of nimodipine (891 nM, 90 min), selected from Fig. 2, which was ten-fold higher than the concentration required to relax a maximal Bay k 8644 contraction by 80%. Paired control rings in a separate muscle bath were pretreated with the corresponding volume of solvent. Following the pretreatment period, the resting tensions of test rings, which had been reduced by nimodipine, were mechanically restored to the original 5 gram baseline. Solvent had no effect on the resting tension of control tissues. KCl was then delivered to both test and control tissues in a cumulative fashion. Each point represents the mean response ± S.E.M. of 4 rings from 4 hearts. Significant difference from control is indicated by * ($p<0.05$) or ** ($p<0.01$). Taken from [11]

Fig. 6. Effect of nimodipine pretreatment on the histamine dose-response curve. Coronary artery test and control rings were pretreated with nimodipine (891 nM) or solvent as described for Fig. 4. Following the pretreatment period, the resting tensions of test rings, which had been reduced by nimodipine, were mechanically restored to the original 5 gram baseline tension. Solvent had no effect of the resting tension of control tissues. Histamine was then delivered to both test and control tissues in a cumulative fashion. Each point represents the mean response ± S.E.M. of 4 rings. Significant difference from control is indicated by ** ($P<0.01$). Taken from [11]

near maximal Bay k 8644-induced contraction in a noncompetitive manner. As the NIMO concentrations were increased above IC_{50}, however, the Bay k 8644-induced contraction was stimulated in a dose-dependent manner as was shown above (Fig. 3).

In an attempt to analyse the mechanism of stimulation of Bay k 8644-induced contraction by NIMO, the effect of NIMO pretreatment on KCl- and histamine-induced contraction was also investigated. Pretreatment with the $10 \times IC_{80}$ concentration of NIMO (891 nM), which stimulated the Bay k 8644-induced contraction, inhibited the KCl-induced contraction (Fig. 5). Pretreatment with the $10 \times IC_{80}$ concentration of NIMO had only a slight inhibitory effect on the histamine dose-response curve (Fig. 6). These results indicate that the NIMO-induced stimulation of Bay k 8644-induced contraction is specific for DHP receptor-mediated contractions.

The data presented here, specifically the biphasic, contraction-relaxation response of coronary arteries to Bay k 8644 and the paradoxical stimulation of

Bay k 8644 contraction by NIMO pretreatment demonstrate the complexities involved in the action of DHP "Ca^{2+} agonists" and "antagonists" in coronary smooth muscle. Our data suggest that the assumption of a single binding site for both DHP "Ca^{2+} agonists" and "antagonists" and their competitive interaction is too simple and does not sufficiently explain the pharmacological effects of these compounds in porcine coronary artery.

Effects of Dihydropyridines on the Heart

Bay k 8644 produced concentration-dependent positive inotropy followed by negative inotropic effects in atrial and ventricular strips from rat, guinea pig, and dog, in isolated, perfused rat hearts, and in isolated dog Purkinje strands (Table 2, Fig. 7). It is of considerable interest that a "traditional Ca^{2+} antagonist," NIMO, produced a consistent small but significant positive inotropy followed by the usual negative inotropic effect (Fig. 7). This phenomenon has been reported with respect to DHPs, verapamil and diltiazem in isolated and intact preparations [22, 28, 29, 57, 59, 62, 63].

If the negative inotropic actions of Bay k 8644 were due simply to excessive accumulation of cellular calcium, i.e., "calcium overload," addition of calcium to tissues treated with high concentrations of the drug would be expected to produce further negative inotropic effects and irreversible damage. The opposite was observed, namely, calcium at least partially overcame the negative inotropy (Fig. 8). An analysis of the effects of calcium in the presence and absence of Bay k 8644 revealed a shift to the left of the calcium dose-response curve by 1 μM Bay k 8644 (Fig. 9, left panel). Calcium was also able to partially restore the contractility decreased by 10 μM Bay k 8644 in a concentration-dependent manner (Fig. 9, right panel). These data suggest that Bay k 8644 acts as a "Ca^{2+} agonist" at low concentrations and as a "Ca^{2+} antagonist" at high concentrations.

Table 2. Positive and negative inotropic effects of Bay k 8644. Adopted from [57]

	Positive inotropic effect. Control to maximum		Negative inotropic effect. Maximum to control
	N	ED_{50} (nM)	IC_{50} (μM)
Rat Langendorff	7	35 ± 15	6.8 ± 2.1
Atria	5	74 ± 45	12.4 ± 3.1
Ventricles	13	91.6 ± 21.7	9.9 ± 1.34
Guinea pig atria	6	104 ± 28	4 ± 1.7
Ventricles	6	120 ± 34	6.6 ± 1.6
Dog atria	8	30.5 ± 9.7	3.71 ± 1.48
Ventricles	8	29.5 ± 8.0	4.65 ± 2.31
Purkinje	2	67.5	7.5
Pig coronary artery rings	16	11.4 ± 1.0	5.7 ± 1.0

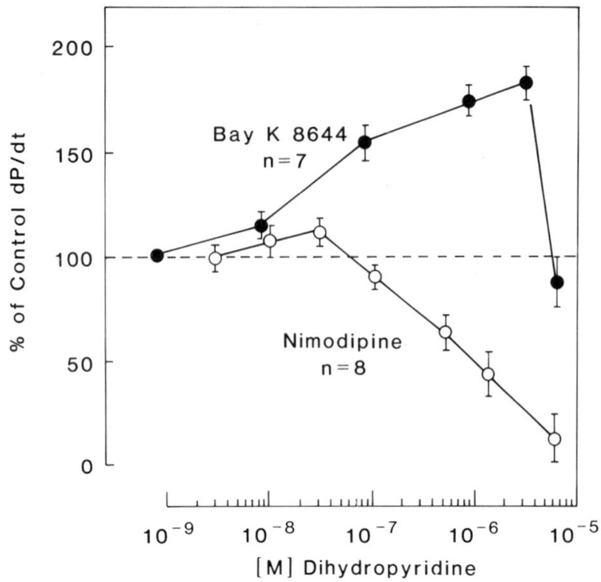

Fig. 7. Concentration-dependent effect of Bay k 8644 (*closed circles*) and nimodipine (*open circles*) on contractility (dP/dt) of isolated, retrogradely perfused rat heart preparations. The drugs were added in a cumulative manner. Each point represents the mean response ± S.E.M. of 7 or 8 experiments. Taken from [57]

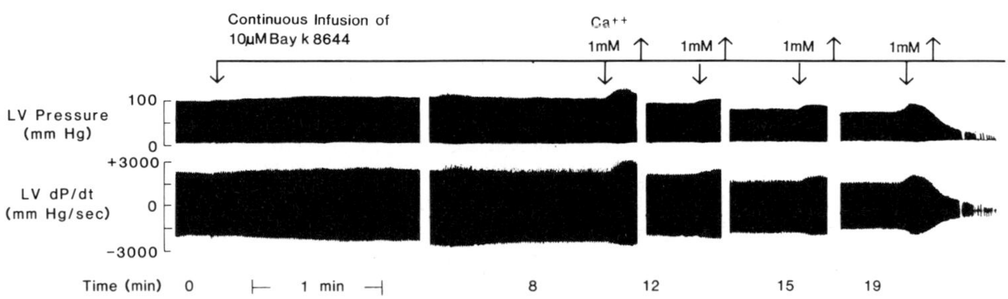

Fig. 8. Reversal by Ca^{2+} of the Bay k 8644-induced negative inotropic effect in an isolated, retrogradely perfused rat heart preparation. A continuous infusion of 10 μM Bay k 8644 produced a transient increase in contractility followed by a time-dependent decreased in contractility. Short term (20 s) infusions of 1 mM $CaCl_2$ (Ca^{2+}) were applied where indicated by *arrows*. Taken from [57]

Fig. 10. Effects of washout on the contractility of isolated, retrogradely perfused rat heart preparations after Bay k 8644 treatment. The abscissa indicates the time and the ordinate represents the percentage change in contractility (dP/dt). The results of two different sets of experiments are shown. The first one is indicated by closed circles and the second is indicated by open circles. The first part (i.e., from zero to 60 min) of the two sets of experiments are identical. In both cases, Bay k 8644 was delivered at the indicated time in a cumulative manner. Addition of the last Bay k 8644 concentration (8 μM) at 40 min produced only a transient increase in contractility which was followed by a rapid decrease (40–50 minutes). From this time point, (i.e. 50 minutes), the hearts were perfused with a Bay k 8644-free Krebs-Henseleit solution. Initiation of Bay k 8644

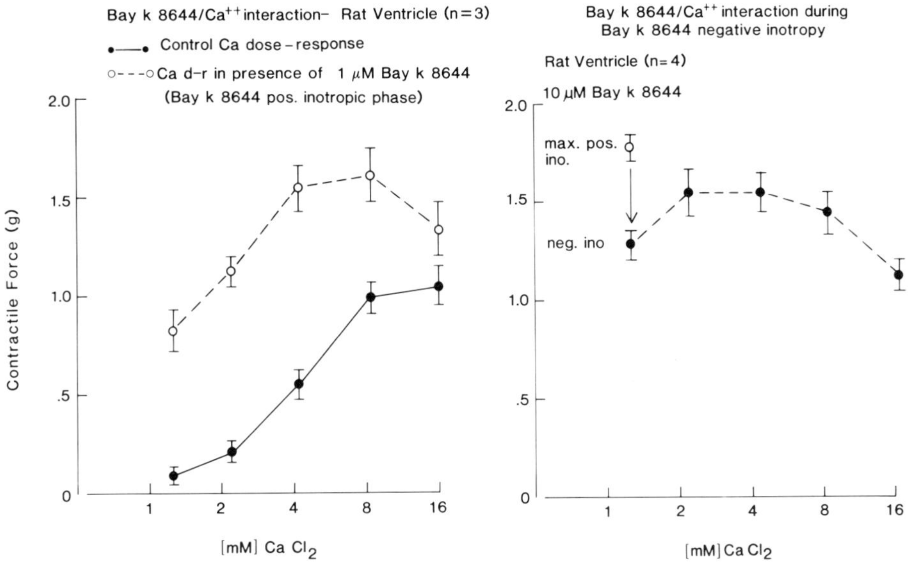

Fig. 9. Effect of Ca^{2+} on the Bay k 8644-induced positive and negative inotropic effects in isolated rat ventricular strips. *Left panel:* Calcium dose-response curves in the absence (*closed circles*) and in the presence of 1 μM Bay k 8644 (*open circles*). *Right panel:* Rat ventricular strips were treated with 10 μM Bay k 8644 in the presence of 1.3 mM $CaCl_2$. Bay k 8644 induced first an increase in contractile force (*open circle*) followed by a decrease (*arrow*). During the negative inotropic phase, calcium dose-response curves were constructed (*closed circles*). Taken from [57]

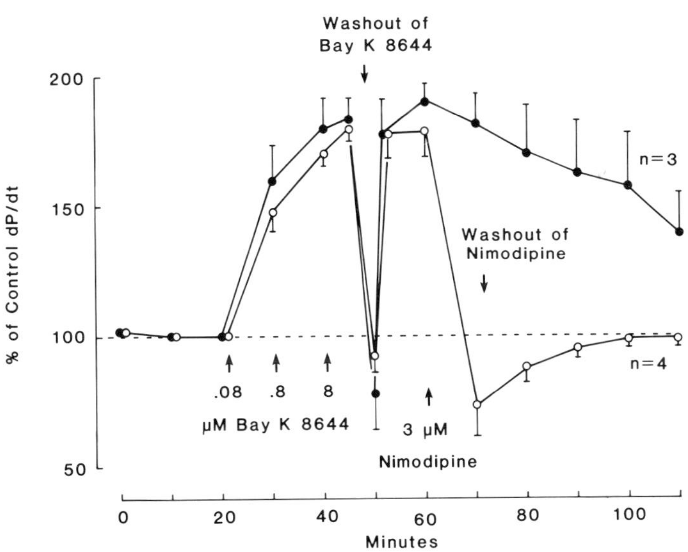

washout is indicated by an arrow. In the first set of experiments (*closed circles*), no other additions were made. In the second set of experiments (*open circles*), infusion with 3 μM nimodipine was started at 60 minutes as indicated by the arrow. The nimodipine infusion was stopped at 70 minutes and then the hearts were perfused with a drug free Krebs-Hanseleit solution (washout of nimodipine)

The positive and negative inotropic effects of Bay k 8644 respond at different rates to washout of the drug (Fig. 10). The negative inotropic effect of Bay k 8644 was washed out rapidly but its positive inotropic effect was not. When NIMO was added during the washout period, it rapidly abolished the Bay k 8644-induced positive inotropy and actually produced a negative inotropy. The latter effect was washed out as indicated, i. e., contractility was returned to control. NIMO therefore apparently "chased" Bay k 8644 from the "receptor."

High and Low Affinity Binding Sites in Isolated Canine Cardiac Sarcolemma

Parallel to the pharmacological studies, radioligand binding experiments were carried out to identify binding sites that may be involved in the pharmacological effects. Competition binding experiments were employed in which the [^{3}H]nitrendipine (NTD) concentration was kept constant at different levels and the non-labeled NTD concentration was varied. The shape of the competition binding curves was dependent on the [^{3}H]NTD concentration (Fig. 11). At 0.3 nM [^{3}H]NTD, a monophasic inhibition curve was obtained. Analyzing these data with a nonlinear least squares Ligand program, a one binding site model fitted the data significantly better than a two-site model. This indicates that under these conditions, only one set of high affinity NTD binding sites with a K_D of 0.3 nM and a B_{max} of 1.8 pmol/mg protein can be demonstrated. When the [^{3}H]NTD concentration was kept constant at 7 nM or 25 nM, biphasic competition binding

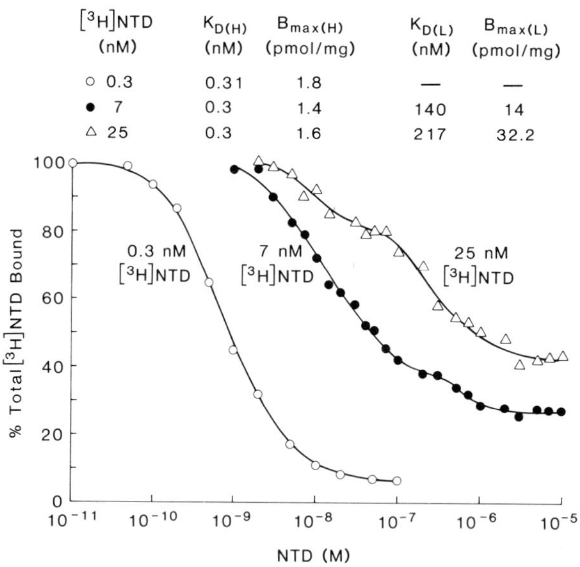

Fig. 11. Inhibition binding studies for the identification of high (*H*) and low (*L*) affinity nitrendipine (*NTD*) binding sites. Canine cardiac sarcolemma (25 μg protein) was incubated with 0.3, 7 or 25 nM [^{3}H]NTD in the absence or presence of varying concentrations of nonlabeled NTD. The percentage inhibition of total [^{3}H]NTD binding by nonlabeled NTD is demonstrated. Taken from [57]

curves were obtained, suggesting either cooperativity in binding or the presence of more than one set of binding sites (Fig. 11). When biphasic competition binding curves were analyzed with the Ligand program, the K_D for the high affinity site was kept constant at 0.3 nM. In these cases, the data were fitted better by a two binding site model. The K_D of 0.3 nM and B_{max} of 1.4–1.6 pmol/mg protein obtained for the first site were the same as those values generally considered as characteristics of the high affinity binding site in cardiac membrane preparations [2, 8–10, 12, 13, 19, 44, 52, 53, 58, 66, 67].

We would like to stress that two plateau phases were observed in the competition binding curve when a high, i.e., 25 nM [^{3}H]NTD concentration was used as labeled ligand (Fig. 11). The first plateau was seen at 0.05–0.1 μM nonlabeled NTD. This is the range of NTD concentrations which has frequently been used for measurement of nonspecific binding of NTD in conditions where only the high affinity binding sites were investigated [3, 52, 69]. The second plateau phase was observed at around 10 μM nonlabeled NTD. We assume that this second plateau phase is the one corresponding to the true nonspecific binding of NTD. If this assumption is correct, then the use of 10–15 μM nonlabeled NTD may be appropriate for measurement of nonspecific binding in conditions where the putative low affinity binding site is also investigated. We tested this assumption by carrying out saturation binding experiments. Figure 12 illustrates saturation binding isotherms obtained under conditions where the [^{3}H]NTD concentration was varied between 0.8 and 23 nM and the nonspecific binding was measured in the presence of 15 μM nonlabeled NTD. The inset which shows the specific bind-

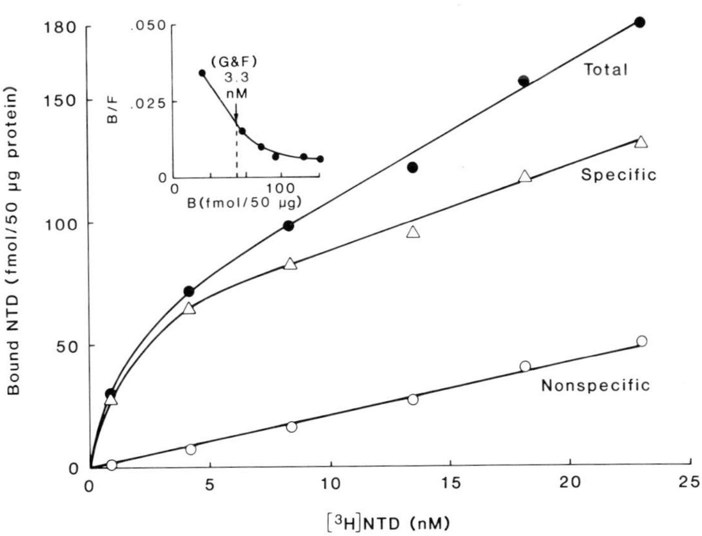

Fig. 12. Saturation binding studies for the identification of high and low affinity nitrendipine (*NTD*) binding sites. Cardiac sarcolemma (50 μg protein) was incubated with [^{3}H]NTD concentrations ranging from 0.8 to 23 nM both in the absence (total binding) and in the presence of 15 μM nonlabeled NTD (nonspecific binding). The *inset* shows the specific binding data in Scatchard format. The *arrow* indicates the value which corresponds to the specific binding obtained at 3.3 nM [^{3}H]NTD. *G* and *F* refers to Glossmann and Ferry [19]

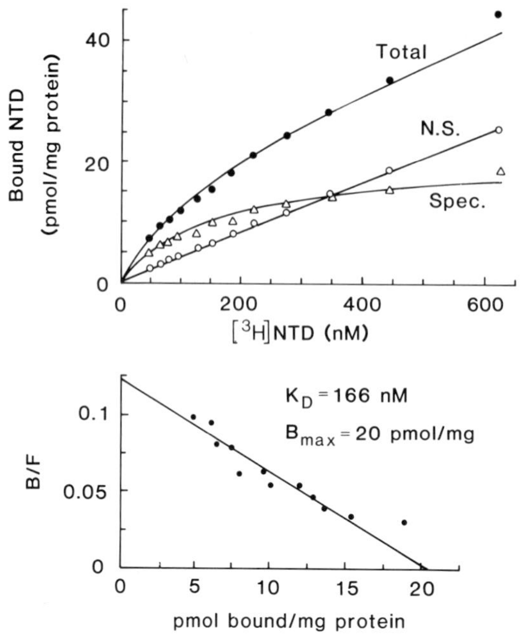

Fig. 13. Measurement of nitrendipine (*NTD*) binding to the low affinity binding sites by the saturation binding method. Cardiac sarcolemma (50 μg protein) was incubated with [^{3}H]NTD concentrations ranging from 50 to 625 nM both in the absence (total binding) and in the presence of 15 μM nonlabeled NTD (nonspecific binding). The *upper part* of the figure demonstrates saturation binding isotherms. The *lower part* of the figure shows specific binding data in Scatchard format. For these experiments the specific activity of [^{3}H]NTD was decreased from 79 Ci/mmol to 1.126 Ci/mmol by diluting it which nonlabeled NTD

ing data in Scatchard format, reveals a curvilinear shape. This suggests that under these conditions, either cooperativity in NTD binding occurs or NTD binds to more than one set of binding sites. Also shown in Figure 12 is that both high and low affinity binding sites may have been occupied by the labeled ligand when 3.3 nM [^{3}H]NTD is used. This will be of significance in a subsequent section of this paper.

The upper part of Fig. 13 shows saturation binding isotherms obtained using [^{3}H]NTD concentrations ranging from 50 to 625 nM. Nonspecific binding was measured in the presence of 15 μM unlabeled NTD. In spite of the fact that nonspecific binding was more than 50% of the total binding at [^{3}H]NTD concentrations higher than 400 nM, saturable, reversible and low affinity specific NTD binding was clearly demonstrated. In the lower part of Fig. 13 the specific binding data are shown in Scatchard format. Under these conditions a K_D of 166 nM and a B_{max} of 20 pmol/mg protein were obtained. These values are very similar to those obtained from competition binding experiments for the low affinity NTD binding site.

To characterize the NTD binding sites in isolated cardiac sarcolemmal preparations, their heat sensitivity was investigated. In a previous study, Bolger et al. [3] found that high affinity NTD binding to guinea pig ileal smooth muscle was destroyed by heating. Glossmann and Ferry [19] reported that the high affinity NIMO binding site in guinea pig cardiac membranes was also destroyed by heating, but they found a *stimulation* of NTD binding to guinea pig heart membrane fractions when they tested the effect of heat treatment both at low and at high ionic strength. They used 3.3 nM [^{3}H]NTD for these studies and measured nonspecific binding in the presence of 10 μM nonlabeled NTD. They showed that in-

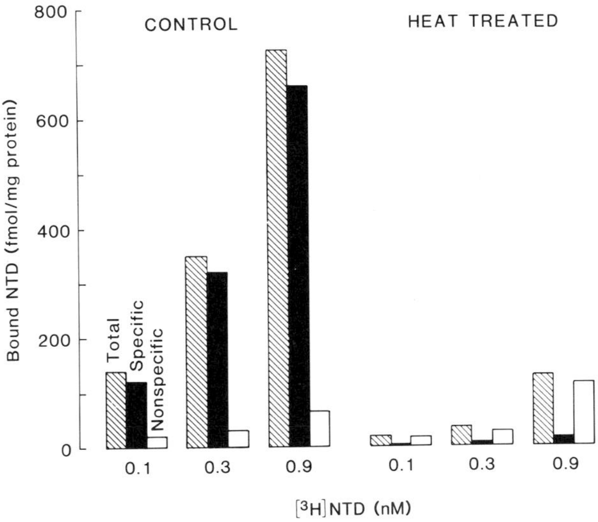

Fig. 14. Effect of heat treatment of sarcolemma on high affinity nitrendipine (*NTD*) binding. A cardiac sarcolemmal preparation was divided into two portions. One was kept on ice, and the other was incubated for 10 minutes at 90 °C and subsequently placed on ice. After this treatment, saturation binding experiments were carried out with both control and heat treated sarcolemmal preparations. The [^{3}H]NTD concentrations were varied between 0.1 and 0.9 nM and 0.1 μM nonlabeled NTD was used to measure nonspecific binding

cubation of heart membranes at 56 °C resulted in a time-dependent *stimulation* of NTD binding. The heat stimulation was much higher at high ionic strength than at low ionic strength.

We reexamined the effect of heating on NTD binding to cardiac sarcolemmal preparations in high ionic strength medium. In the first set of experiments, the [^{3}H]NTD concentration were varied between 0.1 and 0.9 nM, and 0.1 μM nonlabeled NTD was used to measure nonspecific binding. These conditions are appropriate for measurement of high affinity NTD binding. Our data show that specific NTD binding was destroyed by heat treatment (Fig. 14).

Figure 15 demonstrates the effect of heating on low affinity NTD binding. In these experiments, the [^{3}H]NTD concentration was varied between 50 and 400 nM and the nonspecific binding was measured in the presence of 15 μM nonlabeled NTD. The data indicate that heat treatment stimulated the total, nonspecific and specific low affinity NTD binding. There was only a small increase in K_D, but the B_{max} was increased five fold. These data are in agreement with the observations of Glossmann and Ferry [19], although our data strongly suggest that the reason that they found a stimulation of NTD binding to cardiac membranes was that they used 3.3 nM [^{3}H]NTD to measure binding, i.e., a concentration which resulted in the occupation of not only the high, but a portion of the low affinity sites as well. It was previously demonstrated (Fig. 12 inset) that at this concentration the specific binding falls on the curvilinear portion of the Scatchard plot. We assume that in their case, heat treatment destroyed the high affinity NTD binding sites and substantially stimulated the low affinity NTD binding re-

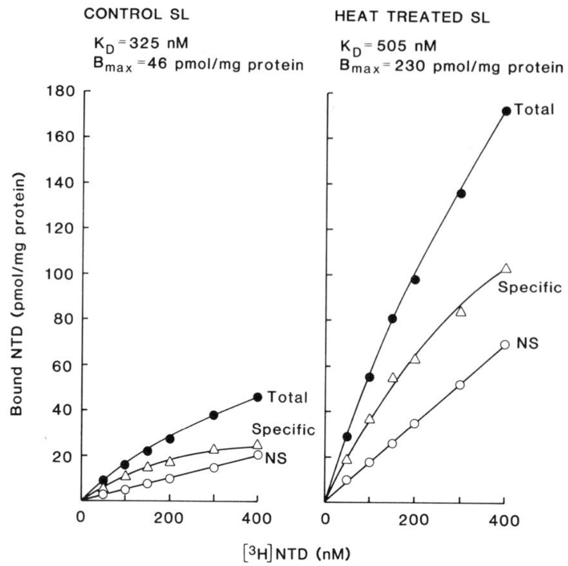

Fig. 15. Effect of heat treatment of sarcolemma on low affinity nitrendipine (*NTD*) binding. The heat treatment was carried out as described for Fig. 14. For saturation binding, the [^{3}H]NTD concentrations were varied between 50 and 400 nM and 15 μM nonlabeled NTD was used to measure nonspecific binding. For these experiments [^{3}H]NTD with a specific activity of 1.126 Ci/mmol was used

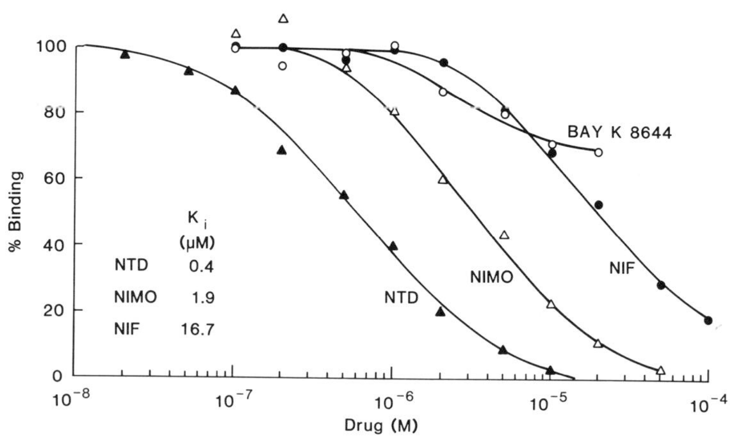

Fig. 16. Effects of nitrendipine (*NTD*), nimodipine (*NIMO*), nifedipine (*NIF*) and Bay k 8644 on low affinity NTD binding. For these experiments heat treated sarcolemmal preparations and 100 nM [^{3}H]NTD with a specific activity of 1.126 Ci/mmol were used. The nonspecific binding was measured in the presence of 15 μM nonlabeled NTD. The horizontal axis indicates the concentration of nonlabeled drugs and the vertical axis indicates the percentage specific NTD binding

sulting in a net stimulation of the binding. Thus, the data suggest the interesting possibility that the heat sensitive high affinity binding sites may act as regulators of the heat resistant low affinity sites. Alternatively, an endogenous regulator independent of the high affinity sites may exist in cardiac tissue which, like the high affinity binding sites, is destroyed by heating.

Specific low affinity NTD binding to heat treated sarcolemmal preparations can be selectively measured by competition binding methods (Fig. 16). For these experiments, 100 nM [^{3}H]NTD with a specific activity of 1.126 Ci/mmol was used as labeled ligand, and the nonspecific binding was measured in the presence of 15 μM nonlabeled NTD. It is apparent that under these conditions a monophasic displacement curve was obtained with nonlabeled NTD with a K_D of 0.4 μM (Fig. 16). It is also shown that NIMO and nifedipine (NIF), two DHP "Ca^{2+} antagonists," inhibited low affinity NTD binding apparently in a competitive manner. However, Bay k 8644 which is structurally very similar to NIF, produced only a partial inhibition of low affinity NTD binding in concentrations ranging from 1 to 20 μM.

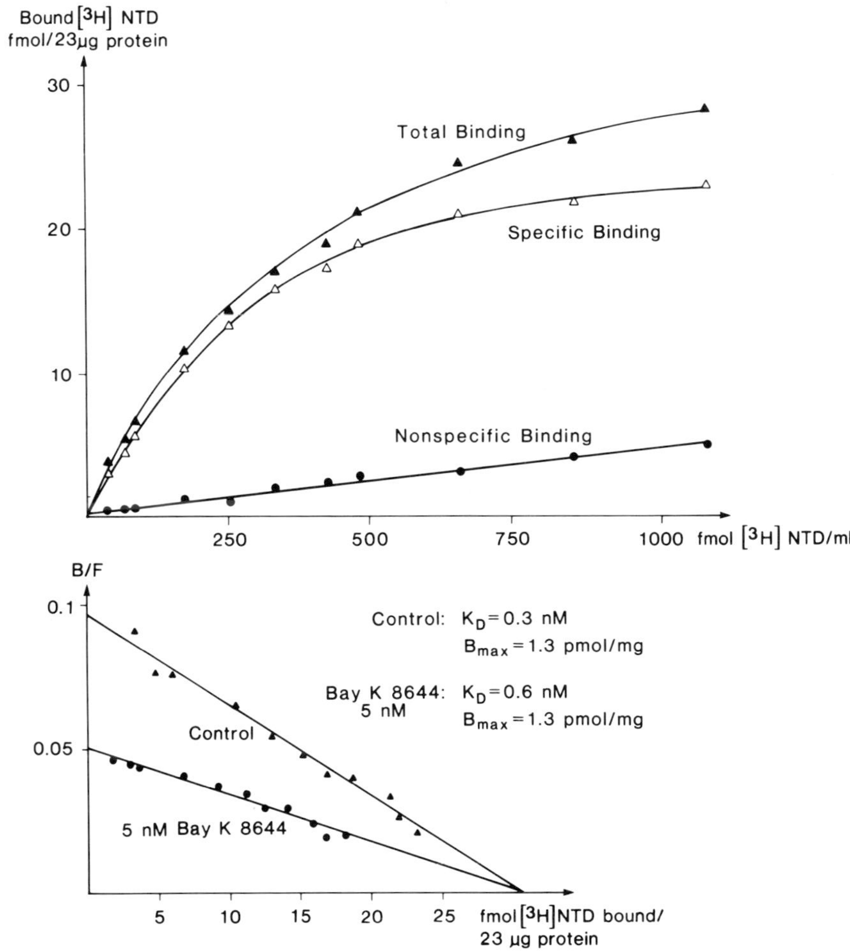

Fig. 17. Effect of Bay k 8644 on high affinity nitrendipine (*NTD*) binding. The upper part of the figure demonstrates saturation binding isotherms in the absence of Bay k 8644. The [^{3}H]NTD concentration (specific activity 70 Ci/mmol) was varied between 0.05 and 1.1 nM and 0.1 μM nonlabeled NTD was used to measure nonspecific binding. The lower part of the figure demonstrates the specific binding data in the absence (control) and in the presence of 5 nM Bay k 8644 in Scatchard format. Adopted from [69]

It is well known from previous studies that DHP "Ca^{2+} antagonists" competitively inhibit [^{3}H]NTD binding to the high affinity binding site [3, 13, 53, 66]. In subsequent experiments we studied the effect of Bay k 8644, a "Ca^{2+} agonist," on high affinity NTD binding both in saturation and competition binding experiments in canine cardiac sarcolemma. Figure 17 demonstrates saturation binding experiments carried out by varying the [^{3}H]NTD concentration between 0.05 and 1.1 nM. The nonspecific binding was measured in the presence of 0.1 μM nonlabeled NTD. The upper part of the figure shows saturation binding isotherms obtained under control conditions. The lower part of the figure demonstrates the specific binding data in Scatchard format. In control conditions, a K_D of 0.3 nM and a B_{max} of 1.3 pmol/mg protein were obtained. A Hill plot of specific binding data revealed a straight line with a Hill coefficient of 0.99 indicating that under these conditions, NTD interacted with only one set of high affinity binding sites. The presence of 5 nM Bay k 8644 did not influence the B_{max} but resulted in an apparent increase in the K_D, which suggests that Bay k 8644 may be a competitive inhibitor of high affinity NTD binding.

In order to further analyze this possibility, we conducted competition binding experiments. The specific NTD binding data obtained using 0.3 nM [^{3}H]NTD as the labeled ligand are demonstrated in Fig. 18. The nonspecific binding was again measured in the presence of 0.1 μM nonlabeled NTD. It is apparent that both nonlabeled NTD and Bay k 8644 completely inhibited the specific NTD binding to the high affinity site (Fig. 18). Bay k 8644 was, however, about 30 times less effective than NTD. Logit-log plots of specific binding data revealed straight lines with slopes close to 2.3. This, together with the saturation binding data shown above, suggests that NTD and Bay k 8644 bind to and compete for the high affinity DHP binding sites in heart. A similar conclusion was recently reached by Belleman [1] and by Janis et al. [33, 34], who used radiolabeled Bay k 8644.

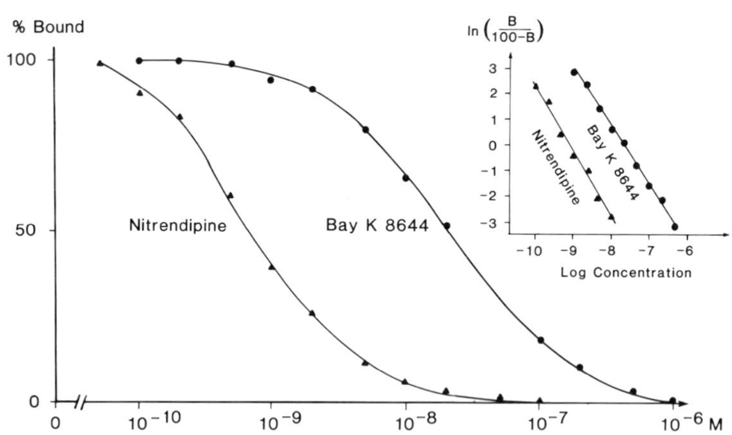

Fig. 18. Inhibition of specific high affinity nitrendipine (*NTD*) binding by nonlabeled NTD and Bay k 8644. In these experiments 0.3 nM [^{3}H]NTD (specific activity 70 Ci/mmol) was used and the concentration of the nonlabeled drugs were varied as indicated on the *abscissa*. The *ordinate* indicates percentage specific binding. The *inset* shows logit-log plots of specific binding data. Taken from [69]

A Comparison of Binding Data with Pharmacological Effects

In order to identify possible receptors for DHP "Ca^{2+} agonists" and "antagonists," we have compared equilibrium dissociation constants (K_D) obtained from radioligand binding experiments with drug concentrations that produced either a 50% increase (ED_{50}) or a 50% decrease (IC_{50}) in contractility measured in isolated canine heart trabecular muscles (Table 3). We have found that NTD produced a small positive inotropic effect in concentrations ranging from 1 to 20 nM. This positive inotropic effect may correspond to the binding of NTD to the high affinity sites, which has a K_D of 0.3 nM.

The partial effect of NTD may be the result of its low intrinsic activity at the high affinity sites. Bay k 8644 produced a 50% increase in contractility at around 30 nM. This concentration is very similar to that producing a 50% occupancy of the high affinity DHP binding sites (Table 3). These data suggest that binding of DHPs to the high affinity sites may correlate with this positive inotropic effect and not to the negative inotropic effect as has been suggested [19, 35, 53, 58, 67].

NTD produced a 50% decrease in contractility at around 600 nM. This concentration is very similar to that resulting in a 50% occupation of the low affinity binding sites, i.e., 140–400 nM. Bay k 8644 produced a partial negative inotropic effect in concentrations ranging from 1 to 20 μM. In the same concentration range, Bay k 8644 partially inhibited the NTD binding to the low affinity sites (Table 3). Therefore, binding of DHPs to the low affinity binding site can be correlated with a negative inotropic effect, which was also recently suggested by Marsh et al. [40] and by us [57, 70].

Table 3. Correlation of inotropic effects with equilibrium dissociation constants (K_D) in canine cardiac sarcolemma

	Nitrendipine	Bay k 8644
ED_{50} (positive inotropy)	Partial effect at 1–20 nM	29.5 nM
K_D(H)	0.3 nM	10.0 nM
IC_{50} (negative inotropy)	600 nM	Partial effect at 1–20 μM
K_D(L)	140–400 nM	Partial effect at 1–20 μM

Discussion

It has been demonstrated that Ca^{2+}-channel modulating drugs can bind to at least three different putative receptors, which are assumed to be part of, or closely related to, the Ca^{2+}-channel [15, 17–20, 32, 35, 46, 53, 58, 66, 67, but see 4, 60]. These sites or receptors, namely, the "DHP, verapamil and diltiazem binding sites," appear to interact with each other in a complex manner [20, 45, 46, 58, 67].

We have presented in this study data obtained by a combined pharmacological and radioligand binding approach. We feel that binding and pharmacology need to be related if a putative receptor is to be given any credence. It was found that DHPs can produce both positive and negative inotropy in isolated heart preparations and contraction and relaxation in isolated pig coronary smooth muscle. As a possible related corollary, we have demonstrated two DHP binding sites in canine cardiac sarcolemma preparations.

In an attempt to explain the complex effects of DHPs, we have suggested that DHP receptor subtypes may exist in both cardiac [57, 69, 70] and coronary smooth muscle [11], perhaps analogous to the well-known α and β adrenergic subtypes of receptors. To reconcile our observations in cardiac and smooth muscle to a single hypothesis, we propose that binding of DHPs to one set of binding sites, which we term *DHP_ε (excitatory)* binding sites, mediates positive inotropy and coronary smooth muscle contraction. On the other hand, negative inotropy and coronary smooth muscle relaxation is mediated by DHP interaction with separate *DHP_ι (inhibitory)* binding sites.

In our previous publications [11, 57, 69, 70], the DHP_ε binding site was termed an "agonist receptor" and the DHP_ι binding site was an "antagonist receptor" in order to refer to the drugs (i.e., "Ca^{2+} agonists" and "Ca^{2+} antagonists," respectively) acting at these receptors. However, the terminology we used before, we feel, may be confusing. According to classical pharmacology, in the case of competitive antagonism, agonists and antagonists bind to the same receptors and compete with each other. It is the intrinsic activity or efficacy of a drug which determines whether it is a full agonist, a partial agonist or an antagonist [36]. Keeping these aspects in mind, we assume that DHPs can be divided into theoretical subgroups which are defined as follows:

1. *Selective DHP_ε agonists* which bind to, and have intrinsic activity at, only DHP_ε binding sites. These compounds are expected to open Ca^{2+} channels and enhance muscle function, i.e., positive inotropy in the heart and contraction in smooth muscle, respectively. Depending on their intrinsic activity, full or partial DHP_ε agonists also exist.
2. *Selective DHP_ε* antagonists which bind only to the DHP_ε binding sites but have no intrinsic activity. These compounds have no effect on muscle contraction, but should competitively inhibit the effect of DHP_ε agonists.
3. *Selective DHP_ι agonists* which bind to, and have intrinsic activity at, only DHP_ι binding sites. These compounds are expected to block Ca^{2+} channels and inhibit muscle function, i.e., negative inotropy in the heart and relaxation in smooth muscle, respectively. Depending on their intrinsic activity, full or partial DHP_ι agonists also exist.
4. *Selective DHP_ι antagonists* which bind only to the DHP_ι binding sites but have no intrinsic activity. These compounds have no effect on muscle contraction, but should competitively inhibit the effect of DHP_ι agonists.

According to our hypothesis, positive inotropy and smooth muscle contraction can be produced either by a DHP_ε agonist or by a DHP_ι antagonist. In the first case, a DHP_ε agonist increases contraction from control and in the second case, a DHP_ι antagonist reverses the relaxation effect of a DHP_ε agonist back to control (Fig. 19). Conversely, negative inotropy and smooth muscle relaxation can be produced either by a DHP_ι agonist or by a DHP_ε antagonist. In the first case, DHP_ι agonists produce a relaxation from control. In the second case, posi-

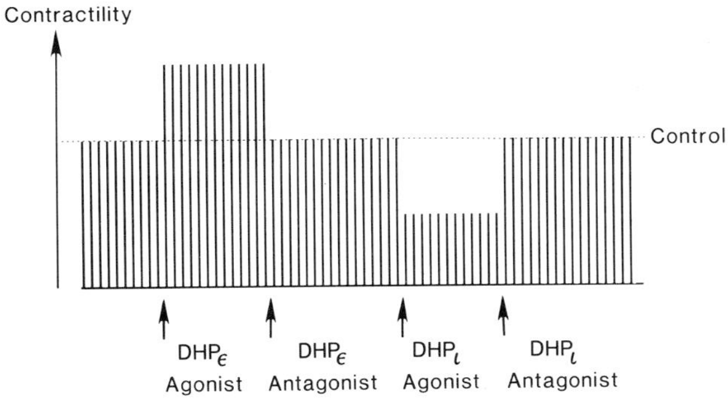

Fig. 19. Theoretical effects of selectively acting dihydropyridines (*DHP*) on contractility of cardiac muscle. A DHP_ε agonist produces only an increase in contractility. The DHP_ε antagonist has no effect on control contractility but competitively inhibits the positive inotropic effect of a DHP_ε agonist. A DHP_ι agonist produces only a decrease in contractility. The DHP_ι antagonist has no effect on control contractility but competitively inhibits the negative inotropic effect of DHP_ι agonist

tive inotropy or smooth muscle contraction produced by a DHP_ε agonist will be abolished by a DHP_ε antagonist and relaxation back to control will be seen (Fig. 19).

This hypothesis is based on the following observations:

1. DHPs bind to high and low affinity binding sites in cardiac membrane preparations (Figs. 11–13 and [2, 19, 33, 37, 48, 57, 70]) and in cultured heart cells [40].
2. Using four different radiolabeled DHPs different B_{max} values were obtained [15] and diltiazem increased the B_{max} for these compounds [3, 8, 9, 15, 33, 58, 72].
3. The DHPs tested so far have a biphasic (positve-negative) inotropic effect in cardiac muscle (Figs. 7–10 and [22, 29, 57, 59, 62, 63, 70]).
4. Concentrations of DHPs producing an *increase* in contractility of cardiac muscle preparations are similar to the concentrations resulting in occupancy of the high affinity binding sites [1, 33, 34, 57, 69, 70].
5. Bay k 8644 produces a biphasic (contraction-relaxation) effect in coronary smooth muscle (Fig. 1 and [11, 62]).
6. NIMO relaxes Bay k 8644-induced contraction of pig coronary arteries (Fig. 2 and [11]), but NIMO *pretreatment* enhances the contractile effect of Bay k 8644 (Figs. 3–4 and [11]).

On the basis of the above observations and criteria, one might speculate that the DHP_ε binding site, as we define it, corresponds to the high affinity DHP binding site, ($K_D = 0.2 - 0.3$ nM), and the DHP_ι binding site corresponds to the low affinity DHP binding site ($K_D = 140 - 400$ nM) present in cardiac tissue. So far, subpopulations of DHP binding sites have not been identified with direct receptor binding techniques in coronary smooth muscle, although high affinity DHP binding has been demonstrated in porcine coronary artery [8]. The assumption that distinct DHP_ε and DHP_ι binding sites exist in coronary smooth muscle as well is therefore, at this time based solely on pharmacological evidence.

The observation that all the tested DHPs have a positive inotropic effect at low concentrations [22, 28, 29, 57, 62, 63, 69, 70] suggests that they can act as DHP_ε agonists. The fact that Bay k 8644 is more effective in this regard than other DHPs tested so far suggests that it simply has a higher intrinsic activity than NIMO, NIF or NTD at the DHP_ε binding site. Using our terminology, NIMO, NIF and NTD are partial DHP_ε agonists. Recent receptor binding data are in agreement with this concept. It has been shown that Bay k 8644, NIMO and NTD bind to, and compete for, the same high affinity DHP binding sites, i.e., DHP_ε binding sites (Figs. 17, 18 and [1, 14, 33, 34, 69]).

Since DHPs can also produce negative inotropy and smooth muscle relaxation even under conditions where the tissues have not been treated with a DHP_ε agonist, this muscle relaxation effect, we suggest, is the result of their *agonist* action at the DHP_ι binding site.

We have demonstrated that in coronary smooth muscle, Bay k 8644 produces a biphasic (contraction-relaxation) effect similar to that seen in cardiac tissue preparations. This suggests that Bay k 8644 may act as a DHP_ε and a DHP_ι agonist in coronary smooth muscle as well. The occurrence of contraction at low concentrations and relaxation at high concentrations suggests that Bay k 8644 interacts with high affinity at DHP_ε binding sites and with low affinity at DHP_ι binding sites. The net response to any given concentration of Bay k 8644 is determined by the fractional occupancy of, and intrinsic activity at, these binding sites [7, 36]. NIMO inhibits the Bay k 8644-induced contraction probably by acting as a DHP_ι agonist. In other words, the DHP_ε agonist effect of Bay k 8644, i.e., the contractile effect, which was dominant when the drug was used alone, was overcome by the combined DHP_ι agonist effects of NIMO and Bay k 8644, resulting in muscle relaxation.

When coronary arteries were pretreated with a relatively high concentration of NIMO and subsequently treated with Bay k 8644, an unmasking of the contractile effect of Bay k 8644 occurred, or stating in another way, its full contractile effect could be realized. We expect that under these conditions, viz., when the maximal DHP_ε agonist effect of Bay k 8644 was demonstrated, other DHPs can be tested for their DHP_ε antagonist effects. DHP_ε antagonists, under these conditions, should result in a parallel shift of the Bay k 8644 dose-response curve to the right indicating competitive antagonism. Actually, even NIMO is able to produce a rightward shift of the Bay k 8644 dose-response curve when very high concentrations are used in the pretreatment experiments with coronary arteries. This implies that NIMO is also acting as a DHP_ε antagonist in coronary smooth muscle. A similar effect, i.e., a rightward shift of the Bay k 8644 dose-response curve by NIF in rabbit aortic strips was demonstrated by Schramm et al. [55, 56]. This indicates that NIF, like NIMO, is acting as a DHP_ε antagonist in smooth muscle. This conclusion is seemingly contradictory to that reached from analyzing the NIMO effect exerted on cardiac muscle, where we suggest that NIMO is a partial DHP_ε *agonist*. To explain this contradiction, we have to remember that there is only a small difference between an antagonist and a very weak partial agonist [36]. The antagonist has no intrinsic activity and a weak partial agonist has a very low intrinsic activity. Therefore, a weak partial agonist, i.e., NIMO, under certain conditions, can antagonize the effects of a DHP_ε agonist, e.g., Bay k 8644.

We suggest that NIF, NIMO and NTD act predominantly as DHP_ι agonists, but they also have partial DHP_ε agonist activity. On the other hand, Bay k 8644 is predominantly a DHP_ε agonist but also has some DHP_ι agonist activity. It remains to be demonstrated whether or not Bay k 8644 acts on the same DHP_ι binding site as NTD, or whether subtypes of DHP_ι binding sites also exist. It is, e. g., possible that two types of DHP_ι exist.

According to this hypothesis, the most effective vasodilators are expected to possess both DHP_ι agonist and DHP_ε antagonist activity. NIMO, NTD and NIF, which have very low intrinsic activity at the DHP_ε binding sites but have a high intrinsic activity at the DHP_ι binding sites, approach these requirements.

A hypothesis very similar to the one presented above has recently been suggested by Thomas et al. [62, 63] based upon pharmacological experiments. Our data confirm these authors' observations and provide additional evidence which support the assumption that DHP receptor subtypes may exist in both cardiac and coronary smooth muscle. However, to prove this hypothesis, further study of DHP receptor subtypes is required. For example, more information is needed to prove that the low affinity DHP binding site demonstrated in cardiac tissue is identical with the putative DHP_ι receptor and does not represent specific nonreceptor binding. Among other points, the stereospecificity of this binding and its relation to the Ca^{2+}-channel remains to be determined. The order of affinity of DHPs for this low affinity site has also to be determined and should be correlated with the order of potency of DHPs in intact tissue. Furthermore, distinct DHP_ε and DHP_ι binding sites have yet to be identified in smooth muscle, particularly coronary tissue.

The hypothesis presented above implies the existence of distinct DHP_ε and DHP_ι receptors both in heart and coronary smooth muscle. However, receptor subtypes can be identified only after the discovery of drugs which selectively act at one of these receptor subtypes [36]. Since we do not have selective DHP_ε or DHP_ι agonists or antagonists, the question of whether or not DHP receptor subtypes exist has yet to be demonstrated. An alternative possibility is that DHPs are multivalent ligands and they bind to only one receptor which has multiple, interacting DHP binding sites. The concept of multisubsite receptors for multivalent ligands has been proposed to explain the effects of drugs, hormones and neurotransmitters [7]. The application of this concept for DHPs may be a fruitful approach in determining their mechanism of action.

If this hypothesis proves to be correct, it may explain the well-known discrepancy existing between high affinity binding and the negative inotropic effect of DHPs in cardiac muscle [8, 38, 52, 53, 58, 65–67]. It may further explain why there is no such discrepancy between binding of Bay k 8644 to the high affinity sites and its positive inotropic effect [1, 33, 34, 57, 69, 70]. This hypothesis also provides a molecular explanation for the recently observed partial agonist effects of DHPs [22, 29, 57, 59, 62, 63]. However, it does not exclude other possibilities. We are still unable to prove a one to one correlation between binding and pharmacological effects. The reason for this may be the voltage dependence of effects [49–51] and/or the presence of endogenous regulator(s) [19, 55, 64], both of which may exist in vivo but not in isolated membrane preparations.

Possible Relationship of Pharmacological and Radioligand Binding Data to Electrophysiological Studies

This Bayer Symposium was unusually successful in that it brought together several scientists all studying the same class of drugs, namely dihydropyridines, from different aspects. Although information is still limited, it is stimulating, intellectually, to formulate concepts and models to explain results. The following is a presentation of our interpretation of the available pharmacological, electrophysiological and radioligand binding data.

The positive inotropic and smooth muscle contraction effects of DHPs may be related to an activation of Ca^{2+} channels, and the negative inotropic and smooth muscle relaxation to inactivation of Ca^{2+} channels. Indeed, electrophysiological data indicate that DHPs can, in fact, either activate or inactivate Ca^{2+} channels [5, 24, 31, 38, 47, 49–51]. The Modulated Receptor Model, which was originally proposed to explain use-, frequency- and voltage-dependent effects of antiarrhythmic drugs on Na^{+} channels [25–27, 30, 31], has recently been applied to Ca^{2+} channels to interpret the use- and voltage-dependent effects of Ca^{2+} channel blocking DHPs [31, 49, 51]. The Modulated Receptor Model assumes that the channel states, when associated with a drug, are nonfunctional [27, 31]. This assumption explains the use- and voltage-dependent *inhibition* of the Ca^{2+} channel by DHPs, but it does not explain the recently demonstrated *activation* of the calcium channel by Bay k 8644 [5, 24, 47] which is also voltage-dependent [50]. Using the available pharmacological and receptor binding data, we propose a model to explain both the activation and the inactivation of the Ca^{2+} channel by DHPs (Figs. 20, 21). This model is based on the following assumptions:

1. The Ca^{2+} channel exists in three different states, namely open (activated) state (0), rested state (R), and inactivated state (I).

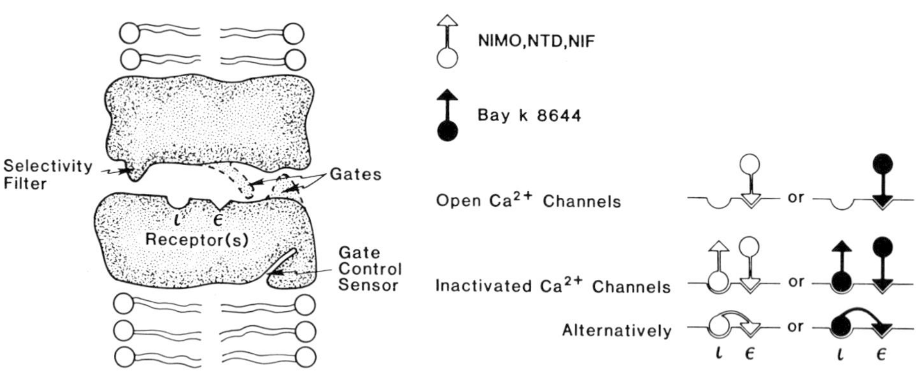

Fig. 20. Possible localization of DHP binding sites, namely DHP_ε (ε) and DHP_ι (ι) in the Ca^{2+} channel. Nimodipine (*NIMO*), nitrendipine (*NTD*), nifedipine (*NIF*) and Bay k 8644 can bind to the DHP_ε binding site with a high affinity and to the DHP_ι binding site with a low affinity. Binding to the DHP_ε binding site may result in an activation of Ca^{2+} channels. Binding to the DHP_ι binding site results in an inactivation of Ca^{2+} channels. Two alternatives are presented: 1. One molecule binds to the DHP_ε and the other binds to the DHP_ι binding site. 2. The same molecule binds to both the DHP_ε and DHP_ι binding sites

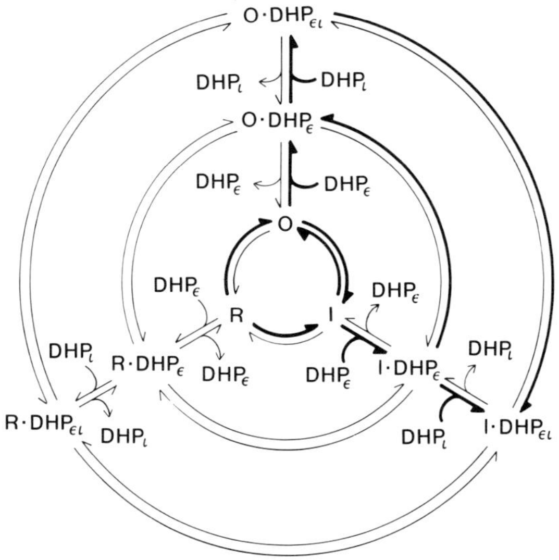

Fig. 21. Interaction of DHP Ca^{2+} channel modulators with the Ca^{2+} channel states, namely activated (open) (*O*), rested (*R*) and inactivated (*I*). The inner circle represents the turnover of channel states in the absence of drug. DHP$_e$ and DHP$_\iota$ stand for the DHP$_\varepsilon$ agonist and DHP$_\iota$ agonist respectively. Heavy arrows indicate the preferred direction of channel state interconversion. Binding of a DHP$_\varepsilon$ agonist stabilizes the O · DHP$_\varepsilon$ complex and accelerates the conversion of other channel states to O · DHP$_\varepsilon$ and keeps the Ca^{2+} channel open and functional. On the other hand, binding of a DHP$_\iota$ agonist stabilizes the I · DHP complex and accelerates the conversion of other channel states to I · DHP$_{\varepsilon\iota}$ and keeps the Ca^{2+} channel in an inactive, nonfunctional form

2. The channel states are *similar* to each other in that they have both high affinity, excitatory (DHP$_\varepsilon$) and low affinity, inhibitory (DHP$_\iota$) binding sites.
3. The channel states are *different* from each other in that their DHP binding sites are not equally available for DHPs. In the rested state, the accessibility of the binding sites for DHPs is less than in open or inactivated states. The accessibility of binding sites may be controlled by activation and inactivation gates [21].
4. DHP Ca^{2+} channel modulators are bivalent drugs and therefore can bind to one (DHP$_\varepsilon$) or two (DHP$_\varepsilon$ plus DHP$_\iota$) binding sites (Figs. 20 and 21).
5. DHPs at low concentrations bind to the high affinity, excitatory binding site (DHP$_\varepsilon$) of the open and inactivated channel states, and O · DHP$_\varepsilon$ and I · DHP$_\varepsilon$ complexes will be formed. The O · DHP$_\varepsilon$ complex is stable, open and functional. The labile I · DHP$_\varepsilon$ complex can rapidly be converted to O · DHP$_\varepsilon$. The net result of these changes is that most of the Ca^{2+} channels are converted to a stable, activated and functional state, i. e., to O · DHP$_\varepsilon$ (Fig. 21).
6. DHPs at high concentrations bind to the low affinity, inhibitory binding site (DHP$_\iota$) of the open and inactivated channel states, and O · DHP$_{\varepsilon\iota}$ and I · DHP$_{\varepsilon\iota}$ complexes will be formed. The I · DHP$_{\varepsilon\iota}$ complex is stable, inactivated and nonfunctional. The labile O · DHP$_{\varepsilon\iota}$ complex can rapidly be converted to

$I \cdot DHP_{\varepsilon\iota}$. The net result of these changes is that most of the Ca^{2+} channels are converted to a stable, inactivated and nonfunctional state, i.e., to $I \cdot DHP_{\varepsilon\iota}$ (Fig. 21).

Both the original Modulated Receptor Theory [26, 27, 31] and its modified version presented here assume that drugs bind to a receptor(s) which is on, or very close to, the transmembrane ionic channel, and that binding of a drug to its receptor(s) is dependent on the channel state. However, in our modified model, we eliminate the assumption that drugs bind with a "low affinity" to the rested channels and with a "high affinity" to the open and inactivated channels. In this respect, our model is consistent with the most recent concept, called the "Guarded Receptor Hypothesis" [21], which maintains that the same binding site(s) are associated with *each channel* state and only the *accessibility* of the binding sites for the drug is different in different channel states [21]. Our model (Figs. 20 and 21) also assumes that drug-associated channels are different from the drug-free channels not only in that they are nonfunctional, but in that they may be *even more functional* than the drug-free channels as illustrated by the Bay k 8644-induced activation [50].

Summary

An hypothesis is presented which predicts that dihydropyridine (DHP) Ca^{2+}-channel modulators act at distinct but interacting binding sites, designated DHP_ε and DHP_ι both in cardiac and coronary smooth muscle. The terms DHP_ε and DHP_ι agonists and antagonists are introduced which refer to the binding sites with which DHPs interact, and define the subgroups. Using this terminology, (1) DHP_ε agonists bind to DHP_ε binding sites, open Ca^{2+} channels, produce positive inotropy in the heart and contraction of coronary smooth muscle. (2) DHP_ε antagonists bind to DHP_ε binding sites but have no intrinsic activity. (3) DHP_ι agonists bind to the DHP_ι binding sites, block Ca^{2+} channels, produce negative inotropy in the heart and relaxation of coronary smooth muscle. (4) DHP_ι antagonists bind to the DHP_ι binding sites but have no intrinsic activity.

Nimodipine, nitrendipine and Bay k 8644 are bivalent drugs which interact with both DHP_ε and DHP_ι binding sites. Nimodipine and nitrendipine are predominantly DHP_ι agonists with a partial DHP_ε agonist activity at least in the heart. The intrinsic activity of these drugs at the DHP_ε binding sites is very low and, therefore, in most cases, they act as DHP_ε antagonists. Conversely, Bay k 8644 can be best described as a DHP_ε agonist. However, at high concentrations, it may also act as a partial DHP_ι agonist.

Acknowledgements. We thank Mr. Gilbert Newman for technical assistance, Ms. Gwen Kraft for the art work, and Mrs. Janet Duritsch and Ms. Janet Simons for typing the manuscript. We should like to extend our special appreciation to Dr. Carl L. Johnson, Dr. Earl T. Wallick and Mr. Richard Wagner for their critical review of the manuscript. This work was supported by a grant from the American Heart Association, Southwestern Ohio Chapter (G. G.) and by National Institutes of Health grant PO1 HL 22619-07 (I–C). We hereby acknowledge that permission has been granted by the American Heart Association, Inc., Academic Press, and Raven Press to reproduce Figs. 1–11, 17 and 18, and Table 2.

References

1. Bellemann P (1984) Binding properties of a novel calcium channel activating dihydropyridine in monolayer cultures of beating myocytes. FEBS LETT 167:88–92
2. Bellemann P, Ferry D, Lubbecke F, Glossman H (1981) [^{3}H]-Nitrendipine, a potent calcium antagonist, binds with high affinity to cardiac membranes. Arzneim. Forsch Drug Res 31:2064–2067
3. Bolger GT, Gengo P, Klockowski R, Luchowski E, Siegel H, Janis RA, Triggle AM, Triggle DJ (1983) Characterization of binding of the Ca^{++} channel antagonist, [^{3}H]-nitrendipine, to guinea-pig ileal smooth muscle. J Pharmacol Exp Ther 225:291–309
4. Bristow MR, Ginsburg R, Laser JA, McAuley BJ, Minobe W (1984) Tissue response selectivity of calcium antagonists is not due to heterogeneity of [^{3}H]-nitrendipine binding sites. Br J Pharmacol 82:309–320
5. Brown AM, Kunze DL, Yatani A (1984) The agonist effect of dihydropyridine on Ca channels. Nature 311:570–572
6. DeLean A, Munson PJ, Rodbard D (1978) Simultaneous analysis of families of sigmoidal curves: Application to bioassay, radioligand assay, and physiological dose-response curves. Am J Physiol 235:E97–E102
7. DeLean A, Munson PJ, Rodbard D (1979) Multi-subsite receptors for multivalent ligands. Application to drugs, hormones, and neurotransmitters. Molec Pharmacol 15:60–70
8. DePover A, Matlib MA, Lee SW, Dube GP, Grupp IL, Grupp G, Schwartz A (1982) Specific binding of [^{3}H]-nitrendipine to membranes from coronary arteries and heart in relation to pharmacological effects. Paradoxical stimulation by diltiazem. Biochem Biophys Res Commun 108:110–117
9. DePover A, Grupp IL, Grupp G, Schwartz A (1983) Diltiazem potentiates the negative inotropic action of nimodipine in heart. Biochem Biophys Res Commun 114:922–929
10. DePover A, Lee SW, Matlib MA, Withmer K, Davis BA, Powell T, Schwartz A (1983) [^{3}H]-Nimodipine specific binding to cardiac myocytes and subcellular fractions. Biochem Biophys Res Commun 113:185–191
11. Dube GP, Baik YH, Schwartz A (1985) Effects of a novel calcium channel agonist dihydropyridine analogue, Bay k 8644, on pig coronary artery: Biphasic mechanical response and paradoxical potentiation of contraction by diltiazem and by nimodipine. J Cardiovasc Pharmacol 7:377–389
12. Ehlert FH, Itoga E, Roeske WR, Yamamura HI (1982) The interaction of [^{3}H]-nitrendipine with receptors for calcium antagonists in the cerebral cortex and heart of rats. Biochem. Biophys Res Commun 104:937–943
13. Ehlert FJ, Roeske WR, Itoga E, Yamamura HI (1982) The binding of [^{3}H]-nitrendipine to receptors for calcium channel antagonists in the heart, cerebral cortex and ileum of rat. Life Sci 30:2191–2202
14. Erne P, Burgisser E, Buhler FR, Dubach B, Kuhnis H, Meier M, Rogg H (1984) Enhancement of calcium influx in human platelets by CGP 28392, a novel dihydropyridine. Biochem Biophys Res Commun 118:842–847
15. Ferry DR, Glossmann H (1982) Evidence for multiple receptor sites within the putative calcium channel. N.S. Arch Pharmacol 321:80–83
16. Ferry DR, Goll A, Glossmann H (1983) Differential labelling of putative skeletal muscle calcium channels by [^{3}H]-nifedipine, [^{3}H]-nitrendipine, [^{3}H]-nimodipine and [^{3}H]-PN 200 110. N.S. Arch Pharmacol 323:276–277
17. Fosset M, Jaimovich E, Delpont E, Lazdunski M (1983) [^{3}H]Nitrendipine labelling of the Ca^{2+} channel in skeletal muscle. Eur J Pharmacol 86:141–142
18. Glossmann H, Ferry DR, Lubbecke F, Mewes R, Hofmann F (1982) Calcium channels: Direct identification with radioligand binding studies. Trends in Pharmacol Sci 3:431–437
19. Glossmann H, Ferry DR (1983) Molecular approach to the calcium channel. Drug Develop Evaluation 9:63–98
20. Glossmann H, Ferry DR, Goll A, Rombusch M (1984) Molecular pharmacology of the calcium channel. J Cardiovasc Pharmacol 6:S608–S621
21. Grant AO, Starmer CF, Strauss HC (1984) Antiarrhythmic drug action. Blockade of the inward sodium current. Circ Res 55:427–439

22. Grupp IL, Dube GP, Baik YH, Lathrop D, Grupp G, Schwartz A (1984) Effects of dihydropyridine Ca^{++} agonist Bay k 8644 on porcine coronary artery, isolated rat hearts and canine Purkinje and trabecular action potentials. Fed Proc 43:937
23. Grupp IL, Grupp G (1984) Isolated heart preparations perfused or superfused with balanced salt solution. In: Schwartz A (ed) Methods in pharmacology, vol 5. Plenum Press, New York, pp 111–128
24. Hess P, Lansman JB, Tsien RW (1984) Different models of Ca channel gating behaviour favoured by dihydropyridine Ca agonists and antagonists. Nature 311:538–544
25. Hille B (1977) Local anesthetics: Hydrophilic and hydrophobic pathways for the drug-receptor reaction. J Gen Physiol 69:497–515
26. Hille B (1978) Local anesthetic action on inactivation of the Na channel in nerve and skeletal muscle: Possible mechanisms for antiarrhythmic agents. In Morad M (ed) Biophysical aspects of cardiac muscle. Academic Press, New York, pp 55–74
27. Hille B (1984) Ionic channels of excitable membranes. Sinauer publishers, MA
28. Himori N, Ono H, Taira N (1975) Dual effects of a new coronary vasodilator, diltiazem on the contractile force of the blood-perfused papillary muscle of the dog. Japan J Pharmacol 25:350–352
29. Himori N, Ono M, Taira N (1976) Simultaneous assessment of effects of coronary vasodilators on the coronary blood flow and the myocardial contractility by using the blood perfused canine papillary muscle. Japan J Pharmacol 26:427–435
30. Hondeghem LM, Katzung BG (1977) Time- and voltage-dependent interactions of antiarrhythmic drugs with cardiac sodium channels. Biochem Biopyhs Acta 472:373–398
31. Hondeghem LM, Katzung BG (1984) Antiarrhythmic agents: The modulated receptor mechanism of sodium and calcium channel-blocking drugs. Ann Rev Pharmacol Toxicol 24:387–423
32. Janis RA, Scriabine A (1983) Sites of action of Ca^{2+} channel inhibitors. Biochem Pharamcol 32:3499–3507
33. Janis RA, Rampe D, Sarmiento JG, Triggle DJ (1984) Specific binding of a calcium channel activator, [^{3}H] Bay k 8644, to membranes from cardiac muscle and brain. Biochem Biophys Res Commun 121:317–323
34. Janis RA, Sarmiento JG, Maurer SC, Bolger GT, Triggle DJ (1984) Characteristics of the binding of [^{3}H]nitrendipine to rabbit ventricular membranes. Modification by other Ca^{++} channel antagonists and by the Ca^{++} channel agonist Bay K 8644. J Pharmacol Exper Ther 231:8–15
35. Janis RA, Triggle DJ (1984) 1,4-dihydropyridine Ca^{2+} channel antagonists and activators: A comparison of binding characteristics with pharmacology. Drug Dev Res 4:257–274
36. Kenakin TP (1984) The classification of drugs and drug receptors in isolated tissues. Pharmacol Rev 35:165–222
37. Kenessey A, Cantor EH, Spector S (1984) Low affinity dihydropyridine binding site in rat heart membranes. Fed Proc 43:550
38. Lee KS, Tsien RW (1983) Mechanism of calcium channel blockade by verapamil, D600, diltiazem and nitrendipine in single dialysed heart cells. Nature 302:790–794
39. Lowry OH, Rosebrough NJ, Farr AL, Randall RJ (1951) Protein measurements with the Folin phenol reagent. J Biol Chem 193:265–275
40. Marsh JD, Loh E, Lachance D, Barry WH, Smith TW (1983) Relationship of binding of a calcium channel blocker to inhibition of contraction in intact cultured embryonic chick ventricular cells. Circ Res 53:539–543
41. Millard RW, Grupp G, Grupp IL, DiSalvo J, DePover A, Schwartz A (1983) Chronotropic, inotropic and vasodilator actions of diltiazem, nifedipine and verapamil. A comparative study of physiological responses and membrane receptor activity. Circ Res 52 (Suppl I): 29–39
42. Munson PJ (1983) LIGAND: A computerized analysis of ligand binding data. Methods in Enzymology 92:543–577
43. Munson PJ, Rodbard D (1980) LIGAND: A versatile computerized approach for characterization of ligand-binding systems. Anal Biochem 107:220–239
44. Murphy KMM, Snyder SH (1982) Calcium antagonist receptor binding sites labeled with [^{3}H]nitrendipine. Eur J Pharmacol 77:201–202

45. Murphy KMM, Gould RJ, Largent BL, Snyder SH (1983) A unitary mechanism of calcium antagonist drug action. Proc Natl Acad Sci 80:860–864
46. Murphy KMM, Gould RJ, Snyder SH (1984) Regulation of [^{3}H]nitrendipine binding: A single allosteric site for verapamil, diltiazem and prenylamine. In: Scriabine A, Vanov S, Deck K (eds) Nitrendipine. Urban & Schwarzenberg, Baltimore, pp 107–131
47. Ochi R, Hino N, Niimi Y (1984) Prolongation of calcium channel open time by the diyhdropyridine derivative Bay K 8644 in cardiac myocytes. Proc Japan Acad 60:153–156
48. Rogart RB, deBruyn Kops A, Janis RA, Dzau VJ (1984) Nimodipine binding to two calcium channel subtypes in rat heart. Proc IUPHAR, London, 409
49. Uehara A, Hume JR (1984) Voltage clamp comparison of the organic calcium channel blockers D-600 and nisoldipine. Proc West Pharmacol Soc 27:343–347
50. Sanguinetti MC, Kass RS (1984) Regulation of cardiac calcium channel current and contractile activity by the dihydropyridine Bay k 8644 is voltage dependent. J Mol Cell Cardiol 16:667–670
51. Sanguinetti MD, Kass RS (1984) Voltage dependent block of calcium channel current in the calf cardiac Purkinje fiber by dihydropyridine calcium channel antagonists. Circ Res 55:336–348
52. Sarmiento JG, Janis RA, Colvin RA, Triggle DJ, Katz AM (1983) Binding of the calcium channel blocker nitrendipine to its receptor in purified sarcolemma from canine cardiac ventricle. J Mol Cell Cardiol 15:135–137
53. Sarmiento JG, Colvin RA, Janis RA, Messineo FC, Katz AM (1984) Biochemical effects of nitrendipine on membranes from skeletal and cardiac muscle. In: Scriabine A, Vanov S, Deck K (eds) Nitrendipine. Urban & Schwarzenberg, Baltimore, pp 53–66
54. Schefler WC (1979) Statistics for the biological sciences. Addison-Wesley, Reading, Massachusetts
55. Schramm M, Thomas G, Towart R, Franckowiak G (1983) Novel dihydropyridines with positive inotropic action through activation of Ca^{2+} channels. Nature 303:535–537
56. Schramm M, Thomas G, Towart R, Franckowiak G (1983) Activation of calcium channels by novel 1,4-dihydropyridines. A new mechanism for positive inotropics or smooth muscle stimulants. Arzneim Forsch/Drug Res 33:1268–1272
57. Schwartz A, Grupp IL, Grupp G, Williams JS, Vaghy PL (1984) Effects of dihydropyridine calcium channel modulators in the heart: Pharmacological and radioligand binding correlations. Biochem Biophys Res Commun 125:387–394
58. Schwartz A, Triggle DJ (1984) Cellular action of calcium channel blocking drugs. Ann Rev Med 35:325–339
59. Strauer BE (1974) Inotropic effects of nifedipine: A new coronary dilating agent. Int J Clin Pharmacol 9:101–107
60. Surprenant A (1983) Effects of calcium antagonists on action potentials and contractions in peripheral and cerebral arterial smooth muscle. Blood Vessels 20:207
61. Takenaka T, Maeno H (1982) A new vasoconstrictor 1,4-dihydropyridine derivative, YC-170. Japan J Pharmacol 32: Supplement 139p
62. Thomas G, Schramm M, Franckowiak G (1983) Dihydropyridines that exert positive inotropic effects in isolated cardiac muscle: Evidence for Ca channel modulation. Pharmacologist 25:206
63. Thomas G, Gross R, Schramm M (1984) Calcium channel modulation: The ability to inhibit or promote calcium influx resides in the same dihydropyridine molecule. J Cardiovasc Pharmacol 6:1170–1176
64. Towart R, Schramm M (1984) Recent advances in the pharmacology of the calcium channel. Trends in Pharmacol Sci 5:111–113
65. Triggle, DJ (1984) Ca^{2+}channel revisited: Problems and promises. Trends in Pharmacol. Sci 5:4–5
66. Triggle DJ, Janis RA (1984) Ca^{2+} channel antagonists: New Perspectives from the radioligand binding assay. In: Back N, Spector S (eds) Modern methods in pharmacology, vol 2. Alan R Liss, New York, pp 1–28
67. Triggle DJ, Janis RA (1984) Nitrendipine: Binding sites and mechanism of action. In: Scriabine A, Vanov S, Deck K (eds) Nitrendipine. Urban & Schwarzenberg, Baltimore, pp 33–52

68. Truog AG, Brunner H, Criscione L, Fallert M, Kuhnis H, Meier M, Rogg H (1984) CGP 28392, a dihydropyridine Ca^{2+} entry stimulator. In: Weiss GB (ed) Calcium in biological systems. Plenum Press, New York, pp 441–449
69. Vaghy PL, Grupp IL, Grupp G, Schwartz A (1984) Effects of Bay k 8644, a dihydropyridine analog, on [^{3}H]nitrendipine binding to canine cardiac sarcolemma and the relationship to a positive inotropic effect. Circ Res 55:549–553
70. Vaghy PL, Grupp IL, Grupp G, Balwierczak JL, Williams JS, Schwartz A (1984) Correlation of nitrendipine and Bay k 8644 binding to isolated canine heart sarcolemma with their pharmacological effects on the canine heart. Eur J Pharmacol 102:373–374
71. Van Alstyne E, Burch RM, Knickelbein RG, Hungerford RT, Gower EJ, Webb JG, Poe SL, Lindenmayer GE (1980) Isolation of sealed vesicles highly enriched with sarcolemma markers from canine ventricle. Biochim Biophys Acta 602:131–143
72. Yamamura HI, Schoemaker H, Boles RG, Roeske WR (1982) Diltiazem enhancement of [^{3}H]nitrendipine binding to calcium channel associated drug receptor sites in rat brain synaptosomes. Biochem Biophys Res Comm 108:640–646

Discussion

(pp. 113–184)

Thomas: I appreciated very much that you pointed out that the negative inotropic effect of Bay K 8644 at high concentrations is not due to calcium overload. We found in isolated perfused hearts with intermediate concentrations (83 nmol/l) of Bay K 8644 a positive inotropic effect and an increase in perfusion pressure indicating coronary constriction. When the concentration of Bay K 8644 was increased to 28 µmol/l Bay K 8644 had a negative inotropic effect and caused a reduction of perfusion pressure indicating coronary dilation. When under these conditions calcium concentration was increased from 1.2 to 2.4 µmol/l left ventricular pressure increased again. After washing out Bay K 8644, the inotropic effect of addition of Ca^{2+} was even more pronounced. Therefore, there was no calcium overload.

Glossmann: I have a few comments.

First: The work of Prof. Schwartz clearly confirms that with nitrendipine in higher ionic strength media you can label a site which may have nothing to do with the channel because it is not of the same stereoselectivity. This we already know. These results question all the so-called photo-affinity labelling experiments so far published in heart membranes with nitrendipine at 10 nanomolar concentration under high ionic-strength conditions. Here peptides are labeled which have nothing to do with the calcium channel, as we believe.

Second: Peter Bellemann and we found in 1981 that nucleotides inhibit binding of nitrendipine to heart membranes. We were able to show this for the brain and we could clearly show that this is a chelator effect, which has nothing to do with an endogenous regulator. I think, others are wrong in the interpretation of the GTP or ATP effect.

Third: One has to look at the temperature dependence of the B_{max} and then we can fully agree that at a certain temperature all the 1,4-dihydropyridines may label the same number of sites. But, if you do it at 37 °C they don't. And this is our side of the story.

Fourth: We have published that the heart, the skeletal muscle and the brain nimodipine-labeled channels have the same size, namely 180,000. This is of course not the whole channel size, but the size of the 1,4-dihydropyridine receptor domain. In our photo-affinity labelling paper we showed one band (under reduced conditions) of 145,000 dalton. This peptide is clearly a component of the channel. And so far nobody else has as good evidence that their irreversibly labeled or so-called photo-affinity labeled bands are components of the channel.

Fleckenstein: Lidoflazine has some calcium antagonistic effects, but it is primarily a sodium-antagonistic component. It is related to lidocaine, but it is certainly not a specific calcium antagonist.

Session III: Myocardial Effects

Chairman: A. Fleckenstein

Bayer-Symposium IX
Cardiovascular Effects of Dihydropyridine-Type
Calcium Antagonists and Agonists, 188–194

The Effects of 1,4-Dihydropyridine Type Ca^{2+}-Channel Antagonists and Agonists on Intracellular [Ca^{2+}) Transients Accompanying Twitch Contraction of Heart Muscle

W. G. Wier and D. T. Yue

Introduction

We have investigated the cellular mechanism(s) of the inotropic effects in mammalian heart muscle of the 1,4-dihydropyridine compounds, nitrendipine and Bay k 8644. Our primary tool in this work has been the Ca^{2+}-sensitive photoprotein, aequorin (see Blinks et al. 1982), which we have used to observe the changes in cytoplasmic free [Ca^{2+}) that accompany the twitch contraction of mammalian ventricular muscle.

Previously, Morgan et al. (1983) used the aequorin technique to show clearly that one mechanism by which the 1,4-dhp compound, nifedipine, (as well as other Ca^{2+}-channel antagonists) decreases inotropic state is to reduce the the availability of Ca^{2+} to the myofilaments. The diminshed availability of Ca^{2+} almost certainly comes about as a result of the actions of these compounds to decrease Ca^{2+} entry through surface membrane Ca^{2+} channels (Kohlhardt et al. 1972). Nevertheless, there is evidence that suggests that certain Ca^{2+} channel antagonists change the sensitivity of the myofilaments to Ca^{2+} as well. Maryuma et al. (1982) reported that verapamil and diltiazem, in high concentrations (up to 1 mM) increased Ca^{2+}-sensitivity of the myofilaments in glycerinated dog heart muscles. In contrast, in physiological experiments on intact cat heart muscle, Morgan and Colleagues (1983) found that verapamil, diltiazem, nifedipine, and perhexilene apparently decreased myofilament Ca^{2+}-sensitivity.

Direct information on the cellular mechanism(s) of the inotropic effects of the recently discovered Ca^{2+}-channel agonists has, until now been lacking. The 1,4-dhp compound, Bay k 8644 (Schramm et al. 1983), has been reported to have both positive inotropic effects and negative inotropic effects (Sanguinetti and Kass 1984), an interesting property that may be related to its partial agonist activity on Ca^{2+}-current (Sanguinetti and Kass 1984; Hess, Lansman, and Tsien, to be published).

The goals in the present study of both nitrendipine and Bay k 8644 were 1) to demonstrate, and quantify, any change in the availability of Ca^{2+} to the myofilaments and 2) to answer the question of whether or not the change in availability of Ca^{2+} accounts *completely* for the inotropic effects.

Methods

We used small (~.5 mm dia.) papillary muscles taken from the right ventricles of the hearts of young (8 to 10 wk.) ferrets. The muscles were bathed in a solution composed of NaCl, 92 mM; KCl, 5 mM; $MgCl_2$, 1 mM; $NaHCO_3$, 20 mM Na_2HPO_4, 1 mM; $NaC_2H_3O_2$, 20 mM; $CaCl_2$, 6 mM; glucose, 10 mM. It was equilibrated with a mixture of 95% O_2 and 5% CO_2 at 30 °C. Aequorin was micro-injected into more than 40 superficially located cells of the muscle. Aequorin luminescence was measured using a photon-counting system which was also capable of signal averaging. At the end of the experiment, the muscle cells were lysed using the detergent, TX-100, as previously described (Allen and Blinks 1978; Wier and Hess 1984), in order to obtain the fractional luminescence, L/L_{max}. The fractional luminescence was converted by a computer into an upper-limit estimate of spatial average $[Ca^{2+}]$ using an aequorin calibration curve (C–E curve) (Allen et al. 1977). See Blinks et al. (1982) for a discussion of the limitations on the quantitative interpretation of such signals.

Nitrendipine and Bay k 8644 were kept for brief periods as 1 mM stock solutions in polyethylene glycol in opaque containers at 4 °C. Drug-containing experimental solutions were prepared immediately before use by appropriate dilution of the stock solutions. Experiments were performed in a darkened laboratory.

Results

The $[Ca^{2+}]$ transient in ferret ventricular tissue is largely due to Ca^{2+} released from the sarcoplasmic reticulum, according to the results of Wier, Yue, and Marban (to be published). Thus, we do not expect to be able to observe directly the effects of 1,4-dhp compounds on the portion of the $[Ca^{2+}]$ transient that arises directly from Ca^{2+} entering via surface membrane Ca^{2+}-channels.

We performed two basic types of experiments. The first, performed for both nitrendipine and Bay k 8644, was the conventional cumulative dose-response curve. The second was one in which we compared the $[Ca^{2+}]$-tension relations in the presence and absence of nitrendipine, in order to examine directly the possibility that nitrendipine changes the sensitivity of the myofilaments to Ca^{2+}.

Nitrendipine

Figure 1 contains original records from a nitrendipine dose-response experiment. The left column of records contains the original recordings of the force of the isometric contraction (upper trace), the aequorin luminescence (middle trace), and the calculated upper-limit spatial average $[Ca^{2+}]$ transient (lower trace). The right

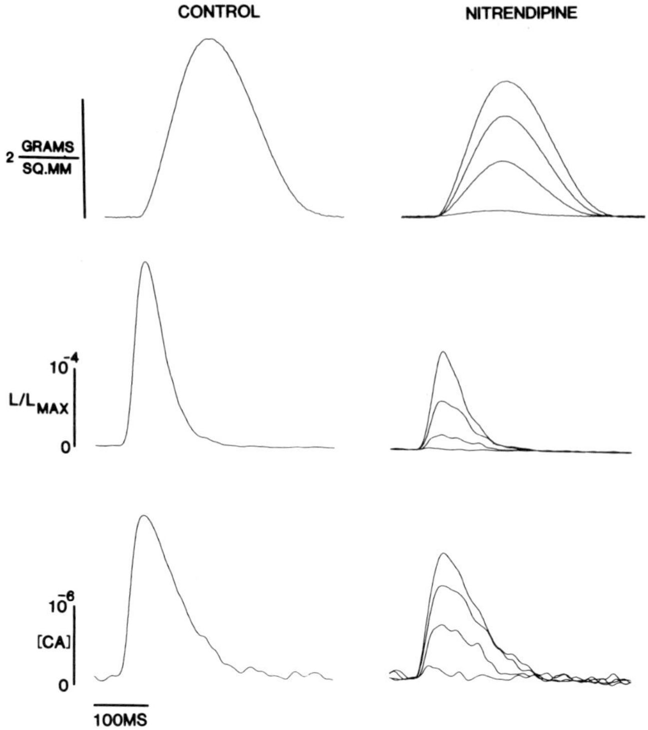

Fig. 1. The effects of nitrendipine on force of the isometric contraction (*upper traces*), aequorin luminescence, (*middle traces*), and calculated upper-limit spatial-average [Ca^{2+}] transient (*lowest traces*). Cumulative dose-response curve; all concentrations of drug applied for 30 minutes. Increasing concentrations of nitrendipine (4 nM, 44 nM, 444 nM, 4.4 μM) successively reduced the force of contraction and the intracellular [Ca^{2+}] transient

column contains the superimposed recordings of contraction, aequorin luminescence and [Ca^{2+}]-transient at 4 different concentrations of nitrendipine (4 nM, 44 nM, 444 nM, 4.44 μM). Each successively higher concentration of nitrendipine was applied for 30 minutes before the records were obtained. The most prominent effect of the drug was to reduce, in a dose-dependent manner, the peak amplitudes of the isometric contraction, aequorin luminescence, and [Ca^{2+}) transient.

Figure 2 A illustrates a plot of the data from this experiment. Peak aequorin luminescence, (filled diamonds), peak tension (open squares), and peak [Ca^{2+}) (crosses) were each plotted as a fraction of their control values at each concentration of nitrendipine. The dose-response curves for the [Ca^{2+}] transient and tension are nearly superimposable on each other, while that for aequorin luminescence is quite different; it lays considerably to the left. Thus, there was an approximately linear relationship between peak [Ca^{2+}] transient and tension, in the presence of the drug, as shown more clearly in Fig. 2 B.

Fig. 3 illustrates the mean results from 3 experiments of this type. It shows mean data for the effects of nitrendipine on contraction (A) and on the [Ca^{2+}]

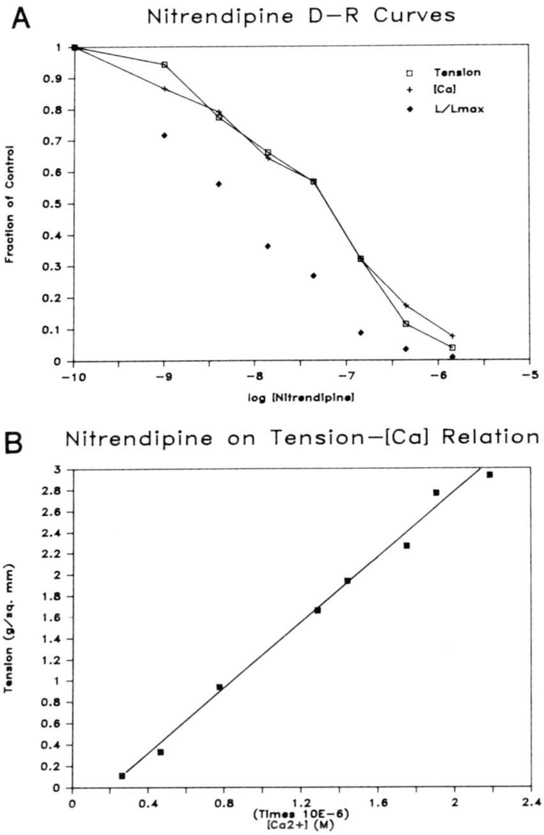

Fig. 2. A Nitrendipine dose-response curve. Complete data from experiment illustrated in Fig. 1. Tension (*open squares*), [Ca^{2+}], (+); L/L_{max}, (*filled diamonds*). **B** The relationship between [Ca^{2+}] and tension obtained in the presence of nitrendipine

transient (B). The smooth curves are plots of the best-fitting Hill equation. For contraction, the Hill coefficient was 1.01 and the IC_{50} was 63 nM (arrow). For [Ca^{2+}] transient, the Hill coefficient was .72 and the IC_{50} was 76 nM (arrow). Thus the IC_{50} values for contraction and [Ca^{2+}] transient are essentially identical.

The experiments shown so far would suggest strongly that the negative intropic effect of nitrendipine is due almost completely to the reduction in availability of intracellular Ca^{2+}. As noted above, however, other effects have been reported for Ca^{2+}-channel antagonists, including nifedipine. Specifically, nifedipine, diltizem, verapamil and perhexilene were all reported to reduce the sensitivity of the myofilaments to Ca^{2+} in addition to reducing the availability of Ca^{2+} (Morgan et al. 1983). The basic observation was this: after twitch tension and aequorin luminescence had been reduced by a Ca^{2+} channel antagonist, the twitch could be completely restored to control by raising extra-cellular [Ca^{2+}], but the fully restored twitch was accompanied by a larger-than-control [Ca^{2+}] transient. Although the present dose-response data argue against such a phenomenon we reinvestigated this issue in more detail. We compared [Ca^{2+}]-tension relations (obtained by varying extracellular [Ca^{2+}]) in the presence and absence of

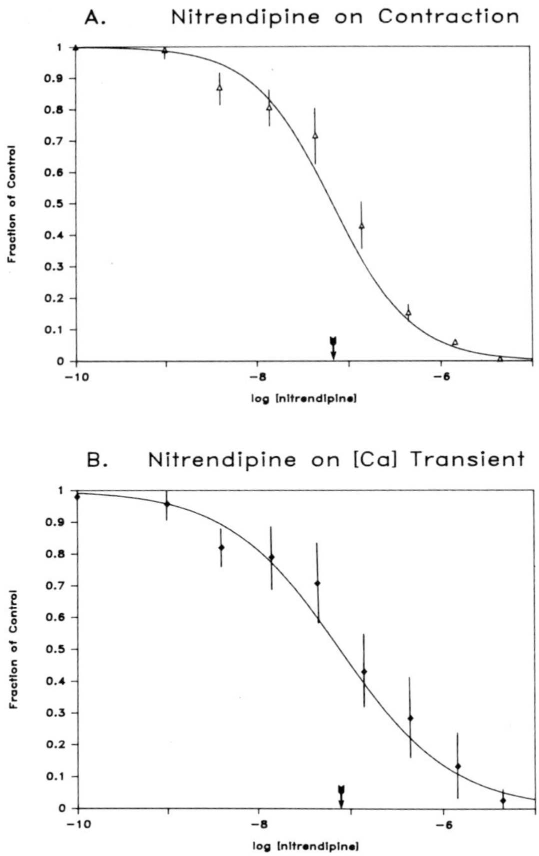

Fig. 3 A, B. Nitrendipine dose-response curves. Mean data (± SEM) from three preparations. Smooth curves are best fitting Hill equation obtained by linear regression. See text for Hill coefficients and IC_{50}s

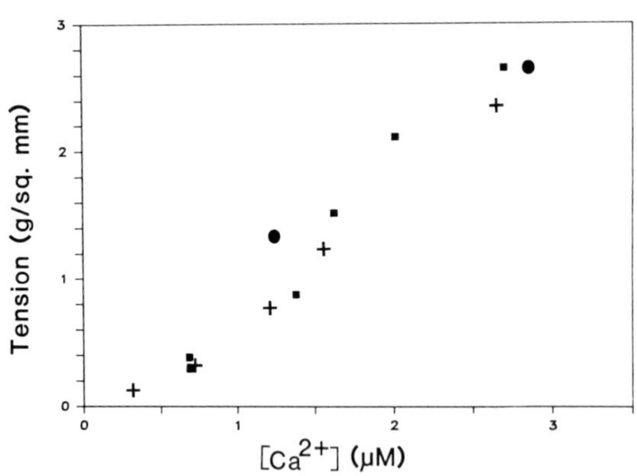

Fig. 4. $[Ca^{2+}]$-tension relations in the presence and absence of nitrendipine. +, $[Ca^{2+}]$-tension relation obtained by varying extracellular $[Ca^{2+}]$ in the absence of nitrendipine; + and (●), $[Ca^{2+}]$-tension relations obtained by vary extracellular $[Ca^{2+}]$ in the presence of 200 nM nitrendipine and 1 uM nitrendipine, respectively

the drug. Figure 4 illustrates such an experiment. The filled squares show the points obtained by varying extracellular $[Ca^{2+}]$ in the absence of the drug. Then 200 nM nitrendipine was added and a $[Ca^{2+}]$-tension relationship was obtained (crosses). The drug concentration was further increased to 1 uM and extracellular $[Ca^{2+}]$ was again elevated (filled circles). The results are clear; at a given intracellular $[Ca^{2+}]$, peak twitch tension is not significantly less in the presence of nitrendipine. In no case (n=4) did the $[Ca^{2+}]$-tension data in the presence of the drug lay below the $[Ca^{2+}]$-tension relation obtained by varying extracellular $[Ca^{2+}]$. Thus the present experiments do not indicate the desensitization of the kind previously reported. In the present experiments, a change of drug concentration is equivalent to a change in extracellular $[Ca^{2+}]$.

Bay k 8644

We have begun experimentation with the 1,4-dhp Ca^{2+}-channel agonist, Bay k 8644. Figure 5 shows the data obtained with this compound, in an experiment exactly analogous to those for nitrendipine. Clearly, the positive inotropic effect of this compound is accompanied by an increase in the $[Ca^{2+}]$ transient. It was

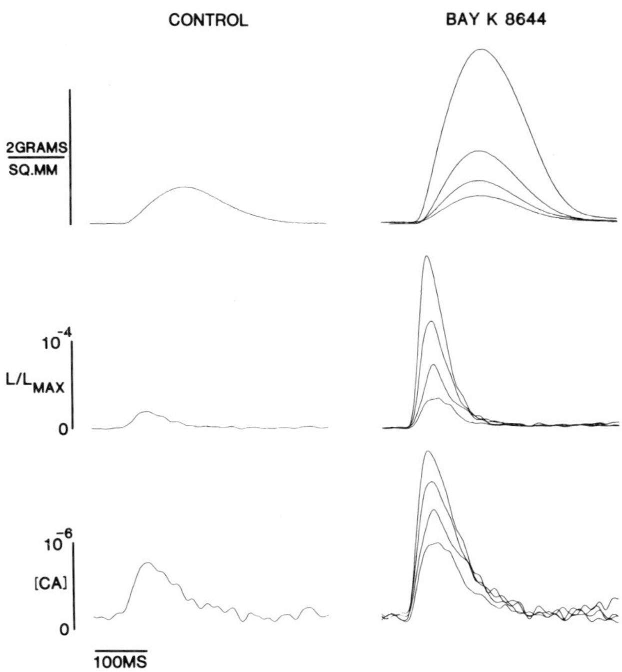

Fig. 5. The effects of Bay k 8644 on force of the isometric contraction (*upper traces*), aequorin luminescence, (*middle traces*), and calculated upper-limit spatial-average $[Ca^{2+}]$ transient (*lowest traces*). Cumulative dose-response curve; all concentrations of drug applied for 30 minutes. Increasing concentrations of Bay k 8644 (1 nM, 4 nM, 44 nM, 144 nM) successively increased the force of contraction and the intracellular $[Ca^{2+}]$ transient. Extracellular $[Ca^{2+}]$ was .25 mM

necessary in these experiments to start with a low extracellular $[Ca^{2+}]$ (.25 mM) in order to avoid Ca^{2+}-overload of the preparation as the concentration of Bay k 8644 was increased.

Discussion

These experiments indicate clearly several points. First, the negative and positive inotropic effects of the 1,4-dhp compounds, nitrendipine and Bay k 8644 are clearly associated with changes in the availability to the myofilaments of intracellular free Ca^{2+}. In ferret ventricular muscle, the drugs thus produce their inotropic effects, indirectly, by changing the amount of calcium released from the sarcoplasmic reticulum. This change almost certainly results from changes in the amount of Ca^{2+} entering through Ca^{2+} channels. For nitrendipine, the IC_{50} is the same for calculated $[Ca^{2+}]$ transient and peak twitch force, strongly suggesting that the reduction of the $[Ca^{2+}]$ transient is of primary importance in the inotropic effect. In ferret muscle, we find no evidence for a desensitization of the myofilaments to Ca^{2+} by nitrendipine.

Acknowledgements. We wish to thank the Miles Institute for Preclinical Pharmacology for providing us with the 1,4-dhp compounds, and for their generous financial support of this project. This work was done during the tenure of an Established Investigatorship (W.G.W) of the American Heart Association and with funds contributed in part by Maryland Affiliate, American Heart Association.

References

Allen DG, Blinks JR (1978) Calcium transients in aequorin-injected frog cardiac muscle. Nature (Lond) 273:509–513

Allen DG, Blinks JR, Prendergast FG (1977) Aequorin luminescence: Relation of light emission to calcium concentration – A clacium-independent component. Science 196:996–998

Blinks JR, Wier WG, Hess PO, Prendergast FG (1982) Measurement of Ca^{2+} concentrations in living cells. Prog Biophys Molec Biol 40:1–114

Hess PO, Lansman JB, Tsien RW (1984) Different modes of Ca channel gating behaviour favoured by dihydropyridine Ca agonists and antagonists. Nature 311:538–544

Kohlhardt M, Bauer B, Krause H, Fleckenstein A (1972) Differentiation of the transmembrane Na and Ca channel in mammalian cardiac fibers by the use of specific inhibitors. Pflugers Arch 335:309–322

Maruyama Y, Okayama H, Ishide N, Takishima T (1982) Effects of Ca antagonist on the contractile force in glycerinated dog heart muscles. Pflugers Arch 395:49–54

Morgan JR, Wier WG, Hess PO, Blinks JR (1983) Influence of Ca^{2+}-channel blocking agents on calcium transients and tension development in isolated mammalian heart muscle. Circ Res 52, Suppl 1:47–52

Sanguinetti MC, Kass RS (1984) Regulation of cardiac calcium channel current and contractile activity by the dihydropyridine Bay k 8644 is voltage-dependent. J Mol Cell Cardiol 16:667–670

Schramm M, Thomas G, Towart R, Franckowiak G (1983) Novel dihydropyridines with positive inotropic action through activation of Ca^{2+} channels. Nature (Lond) 303:535–537

Wier WG, Hess P (1984) Excitation-contraction coupling in cardiac Purkinje fibers: effects of cardiotonic steroids on the intracellular $[Ca^{2+}]$ transient, membrane potential and contraction. J Gen Physiol 83:395–416

Wier WG, Yue DT, Marban E (1984) Effects of ryanodine on intracellular Ca^{2+} transients in canine cardiac Purkinje fibers and ferret ventricular muscle. Fed Proc (to be published)

Discussion

(pp. 188–194)

From the audience: How long did you put on nitrendipine? Presumably there is a time course of the reduction in the amount of intracellular calcium by the diminished entering of Ca^{2+} each excitation. Can you see an immediate effect on force before you see an effect on the calcium transient?

Wier: The experiments were made in a very stereotyped manner and we waited exactly 30 minutes with each drug concentration and measured at the end of that time. The reduction in force was slow during that period at each drug concentration.

Fleckenstein: You reported that there was a dissociation between relatively fast recovery of the light signal and slower restoration of the contractive force. Are you sure that you recorded the light signal from the same fibres in which you measured contractility? We see a similar phenomenon when we insert microelectrodes: the superficial fibres show rapid recovery of the calcium dependent upstroke, but the tension is recorded from the whole papillary muscle. That might be the reason for the phase lag between recovery of the light signal and of contractile force.

Wier: That discrepancy was in the earlier work where we used cat papillary muscles which were considerably larger in diameter than the very small ferret ventricular muscles which we use in this study. This discrepancy disappeared, so that it may very well be related to the phenomenon you mentioned. To make it clear: These experiments do not support any change in sensitivity of the myofilaments to calcium.

From the audience: Did you say that there is an intracellular site for nitrendipine? Is the action connected to a calcium-induced calcium release from the sarcoplasmic reticulum?

Wier: No, I showed in the beginning that the calcium transient in this tissue is due almost entirely to calcium released from the SR. The inotropic effects of these agents are due to changes in the amount of calcium released from the SR. These are a result of changes in the amount of calcium entering and filling the SR.

Nayler: Why do you think that the cardiac cell in your experiments under normal conditions does not have the capacity either to store that calcium in a subcellular compartment or to expel the cytosolic Ca^{2+} from the cell? If ATP levels are normal, why does not the cell extrude the calcium? Any damaged cardiac tissue normally becomes calcium-overloaded if calcium entry is uncontrolled.

Wier: If the extracellular calcium is too high or if you apply very high concentration of ordiac glycosides, any cardiac tissue that that has a sarcoplasmic reticulum will become calcium-overloaded.

Nayler: If you do that by altering sodium-calcium exchange, the cardiac cells are ble to handle that calcium. Why does the cell not handle the excess calcium that enters in response to slow channel stimulation?

Wier: I do not have the data to answer this question; what we observed was that there is an elevation of aequorin luminescence.

Fleckenstein: But if there is an increase of calcium by a factor of four, due to Bay k 8644 we have already a damage of mitochondria and the whole contractile system.

Wier: I do not think it is necessary to invoke damage to explain this. All the data of Fibiato show that the SR can take and release calcium in every intact tissue. Since I could abolish these calcium overload-calcium fluctuations by ryanodine, they are probably SR-dependent.

Fleckenstein: Ryanadine may have effects at high concentrations on Ca^{2+}-exit by influencing $Na^{+} \cdot Ca^{2+}$-exchange.

Wier: I do not have data on that. I do not know that it is ever been shown to influence calcium entry under any circumstances in any concentration. We used five μmol/l.

Thomas: Did you see after-contractions under high calcium and high Bay k 8644 as with cardiac glycosides? We never saw it with high concentrations of Bay k 8644.

Wier: In the first experiments we used normal extracellular calcium and we saw oscillations in calcium. Therefore we reduced the extracellular calcium, so that we raise the drug concentration.

Fleckenstein: If in our experiments extracellular calcium is elevated a little bit and the Bayer agonist is added, oscillating after-potentials occur as in the case of cardiac glycosides.

In your experiments, the light signal is over approximately at the peak of contraction. This means that the whole metabolic acitivities – splitting of ATP in connection with contractile tension development and in connection with relaxation by re-uptake of calcium into the sarcoplasmic reticulum – is already over at the moment of peak tension. This is in agreement with our finding that relaxation induced by quick release just at the moment of peak tension has no influence on ATP consumption and on the rate of respiration. It is an important finding, that the calcium re-uptake responsible for relaxation has already ended, at the moment of peak tension.

Wier: I am not sure whether we can conclude that. Certainly, the luminescence is back to a low level, but this does not mean that the uptake of calcium is over at that time.

Bayer-Symposium IX
Cardiovascular Effects of Dihydropyridine-Type
Calcium Antagonists and Agonists, 198–215

Voltage-Dependent Modulation of Cardiac Ca-Channels by Dihydropyridines

R. S. Kass, M. C. Sanguinetti, P. B. Bennett, B. E. Coplin, and D. S. Krafte

Introduction

The purpose of this chapter is to discuss recent observations made in this and other laboratories that demonstrate voltage-dependent modulation of Ca-channel currents in cardiac cells by dihydropyridine Ca-channel antagonists and agonists. In order to interpret these observations, the effect of membrane potential on the state of the Ca-channel is first discussed. Then, after reviewing the experimental data that show voltage-dependent changes in drug potency, the results are discussed within the framework of the modulated receptor hypothesis of Hille (1977) and Hondeghem and Katzung (1977) that relates drug-receptor interactions to changes in state of a channel.

The results described in this chapter were obtained from macroscopic current measurements in calf Purkinje fibers and enzymatically-dispersed guinea pig ventricular cells. A standard two-microelectrode voltage clamp arrangement was used to measure membrane current in the Purkinje fiber experiments; the whole cell recording configuration of the patch clamp technique (Hamill et al. 1981) was used to measure currents in the ventricular cells. Studies in which single Ca-channel currents were measured are discussed in the chapter by Hess et al. (pp. 34–55 in this book).

Voltage- and Ca-Mediated Inactivation of Cardiac Ca-Channels

Ca-channels open more frequently when the cell membrane is depolarized from negative resting (or holding) potentials to voltage more positive than −40 mV (see Reuter 1979; Reuter et al. 1982; Kass and Sanguinetti 1984). However, as the duration of the step depolarization is prolonged, many Ca-Channels close, or inactivate. The inactivation process in cardiac Ca-channels is thought to be regulated by cell membrane potential, Ca ions, or both. Interest in distinguishing the mechanisms of inactivation of the cardiac Ca-channel stems, in part, from the suggestion that certain Ca-channel antagonists might interact preferentially with the inactivated state of this channel (Sanguinetti and Kass 1984a; Uehara and Hume 1984; Bean 1984).

When a channel inactivates, it does not conduct ions. Thus an inactivated channel and a drug-blocked channel become indistinguishable: neither allows ion movement across the cell membrane. If a drug were to act by increasing the probability of finding a channel in the inactivated state, it would reduce the number of channels available for ion conduction leading to a decrease in Ca-channel current and subsequent electrical/mechanical activity. Before discussing experimental evidence for this mode of action by dihydropyridine Ca-channel antagonists, it is necessary to review some aspects of the mechanisms that underlie Ca-channel inactivation in cardiac cells.

Evidence for a Voltage-Dependent Process in Heart

Until recently, inactivation of calcium channels in heart, as well as other tissues, was thought to be regulated by a voltage-dependent mechanism similar to that described by Hodgkin and Huxley (1952) for sodium channels in the squid axon. However, results of experiments reported by Eckert et al. (1981) indicate that, at least in molluscan neurons, Ca-channel inactivation can be accounted for by a Ca- (not voltage-) dependent mechanism. In view of this new information, several groups have reevaluated the inactivation process in cardiac Ca-channels to test whether Ca-mediated inactivation exists in these cells.

Inactivation of cardiac Ca-channel currents was first suggested as a voltage-dependent process in experiments carried out in multicellular preparations (see Reuter 1979; Coraboeuf 1980). Ca-dependent action potentials (slow responses), measured in partially depolarized Purkinje fiber strands or in working myocardial muscle, were reduced by voltage depolarizations at voltages more positive than those required to inactivate nerve sodium channels (see Carmeliet 1980; Reuter 1979 for review).

These observations were supported by voltage-clamp experiments in Purkinje fiber bundles (Reuter 1967; Vitek and Trautwein 1971) and other preparations (Rougier et al. 1969; Beeler and Reuter 1970; New and Trautwein 1972). It should be pointed out that measurements of Ca-channel currents in these multicellular preparations were hampered both by problems of voltage non-uniformity and by the overlap of several time- and voltage-dependent membrane currents, but despite these obstacles, the work demonstrated the existence of a Ca-sensitive current at voltages more positive than -40 mV. This suggested that Ca-channels begin to open as depolarizing voltage steps are made more positive than -40 mV, provided the depolarizing step is made from a negative (holding) potential (potentials more negative than -40 or -50 mV).

When a test depolarization was preceeded by a depolarizing prepulse, the amount of Ca-sensitive current measured during the test pulse was reduced. Since prepulse voltage could influence the magnitude of the Ca-sensitive current measured during a test voltage step, this observation suggested that voltage can cause channels that conduct Ca ions to inactivate, or be removed from the pool of channels available for ion conduction during the test voltage step. Using prepulse protocols that were based on sodium channel current studies in nerve, current during the test pulse was measured systematically as a function of prepulse/voltage. The curves that resulted resembled the steady-state inactivation curve for nerve sodium channel currents, except that the half maximal voltage for the Ca current inactivation curve occurs at more positive voltages (near −20 mV).

The time-course of inactivation was difficult to measure in these experiments because it was difficult to separate individual current components measured in response to a single voltage pulse. Nevertheless, several studies using sucrose-gap arrangements found that the time constants of inactivation of Ca-channel current changed with membrane potential, increasing as voltages were made more positive (see Reuter 1979).

The interpretation of these observations, as was the case in nerve sodium channels, was that cardiac Ca-channels inactivate in a voltage-dependent manner. That is, membrane potential causes the inactivation mechanism (gate) to change states. Depolarization results in a change from mostly open to mostly closed inactivation gates. Channels with closed inactivation gates are not available for ion conduction, and thus, are effectively blocked.

Evidence for Voltage- and Ca-Mediated Inactivation in Heart

The reports of Ca-dependent inactivation in neuronal tissue (Eckert et al. 1981; Brown et al. 1981) have stimulated reinvestigation of the nature of Ca-channel inactivation in cardiac cells. This work has been made possible by the introduction of improved techniques: pharmacological separation of time-dependent currents is now possible (Kass et al. 1982; Marban and Tsien 1982) and enzymatic dispersion of cardiac tissue enables voltage-clamp investigations of membrane currents in single cardiac myocytes. The following section reviews some of these recent observations and relates them to the modulation of Ca-channel currents by drugs.

Two observations made by Eckert et al. (1981) are very important to the Ca-mediated inactivation hypothesis: 1) decay of Ca-channel current during a depolarizing voltage pulse is proportional to current amplitude when Ca is the charge carrier and is slowed or absent when Ba or Sr replace Ca; and 2) inactivation produced by a pre-pulse varies with Ca entry during that prepulse. Inactivation that is voltage-mediated is characterized by 1) inactivation rates that are independent of inward current amplitude, and 2) inactivation that persists when Ca is replaced by Ba or Sr in the extracellular solutions (for review, see Tsien 1983).

Marban and Tsien (1981) first raised the possibility of Ca-mediated inactivation in cardiac cells. Since their observation in nystatin-treated Purkinje fibers, others have also provided evidence that Ca-current inactivation in a variety of cardiac cells is, at least in part, Ca-mediated (Hume and Giles 1982; Mentrard et al. 1984; Josephson et al. 1984). The principal evidence for this interpretation has come from the relationship between Ca entry during a conditioning pulse and Ca-current inactivation observed during a subsequent test pulse. This type of relationship was first described by Tillostson (1979) in molluscan neurons. As prepulse voltages are made more positive than approximately +10 mV, peak Ca-

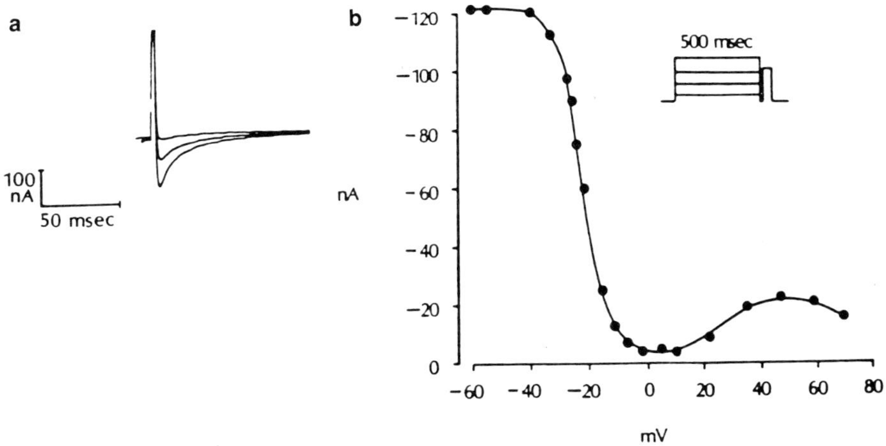

Fig. 1 a, b. Calcium current 500 ms inactivation curve: recovery of current after prepulses to positive potentials. Pulse protocol (*inset*): current was measured during a test pulse to 0 mV that had been preceded by 500 ms conditioning prepulses. A 10 ms return to the holding potential (−63 mV) separated prepulse from test pulse. **a** Current traces recorded at 0 mV after prepulse to −55, −21, and +22 mV (bottom trace to top trace). **b** Plot of peak inward test current against conditioning pulse potential. 5.4 mM Ca Tyrode solution. Preparation 227-1 (Kass and Sanguinetti, unpublished data)

current measured during the subsequent test pulse reaches a minimum and then becomes larger as prepulse voltages are made more positive. This results in a "U-shaped" Ca-current availability curve that is not predicted by previous models for a voltage-dependent inactivation process, although it should be pointed out that certain voltage-dependent schemes can account for such a relationsphip (Chandler and Meves 1970). Kass and Sanguinetti (1984) investigated inactivation of Ca-channel currents in the calf Purkinje fiber (in which outward currents were first blocked by injection of tetrabutylammonium) and found that inactivation could be relieved by very positive prepulses in some of their experiements, but only incompletely and infrequently (Fig. 1). In that study, inactivation kinetics were studied to further test the Ca-mediated inactivation hypothesis.

Figure 2 illustrates one method of measuring the time course of inactivation of Ca-channel current. It shows leak-substracted Ca-currents measured during voltage steps to −8 mV (Fig. 2a) and +14 mV (Fig. 2b) recorded in a calf Purkinje fiber (Kass and Sanguinetti 1984). In each case, current and the best-fit of a two exponential function are superimposed. The decay of inward current was always best fit by functions with two exponential components in the multicellular Purkinje fiber preparation. When Ca is the charge carrier, both time constants are fast ($\tau_1 \leqq 10$ ms; $\tau_2 \leqq 100$ ms), and show little variation with test pulse voltage. Similar results have been found in isolated ventricular cells (Isenberg and Klockner 1982).

Kass and Sanguinetti (1984) found that at some voltages replacement of Ca by Ba or Sr (Fig. 3) greatly slowed the time course of inactivation, but certainly did not prevent the decay of current through the Ca-channel. However, when the

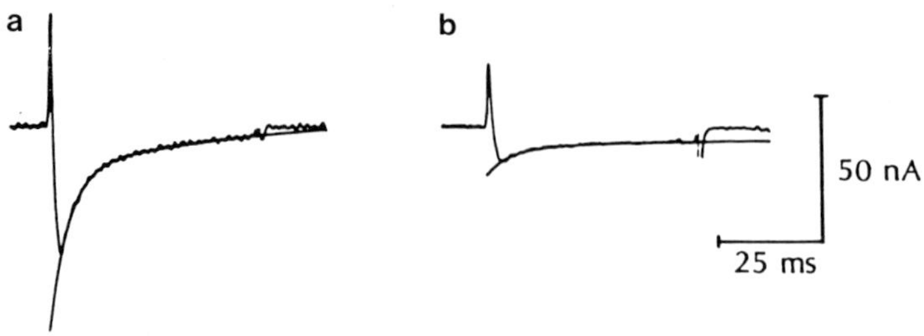

Fig. 2 a, b. Time course of calcium current inactivation during depolarizing voltage pulses. The time-dependence of membrane current was analyzed after subtracting off background current measured in the presence of nisoldipine (10 μM). **a** Current measured in response to a voltage pulse to +14 mV: $\tau_1 = 5$ ms, $\tau_2 = 60$ ms. **b** Current measured in response to a pulse to −18 mV: $\tau_1 = 5$ ms; $\tau_2 = 47$ ms. 5.4 mM Ca, HP = −63 mV. Preparation 292-2 (Kass and Sanguinetti 1984, (by copyright permission of the Rockefeller University Press)

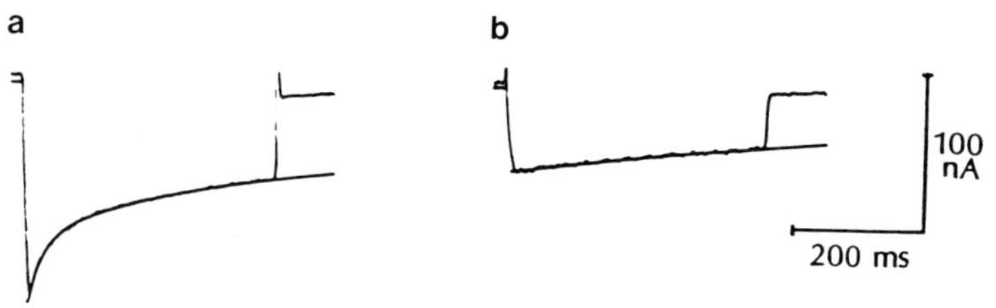

Fig. 3. Time course of Sr current inactivation measured during depolarizing steps. Nisoldipine-sensitive current traces are shown superimposed on curves returned by the fitting routine. **a** Pulse voltage = +18 mV; $\tau_1 = 13$ ms; $\tau_2 = 155$ ms. **b** Pulse voltage = −11 mV; $\tau_1 = 94$ ms; $\tau_2 = 744$ ms. HP = −50 mV. Preparation 301-1. 5.4 mM Sr-Tyrode solution (Kass and Sanguinetti 1984, by copyright permission of the Rockefeller University Press)

inactivation rate was measured over a wide voltage range for Sr and Ba currents both time constants of inactivation were found to be very voltage-dependent. Thus replacement of Ca by Ba or Sr markedly altered the voltage dependence of the onset of inactivation, but had little effect on the time course of recovery from inactivation. This observation raised the possibility that Ca entry during voltage depolarization might cause additional inactivation via a Ca-mediated process and account for the dramatic difference observed between the inactivation rate of Ca and Sr (or Ba) currents during depolarizing pulses.

Furthermore, these experiments show that the inactivation rate of Ca-channel current in the Purkinje fiber is not current-dependent when Sr carries the charge. Figure 4 shows peak inward current and inactivation rate plotted against pulse voltage. The inactivation rates of Ca-channel currents measured during steps to voltages more positive than +5 mV are fast, but independent of the test potential, despite the fact that peak inward current decreases as the voltage steps are made more positive. This argues against a current-dependent inactivation mechanism.

Figure 5 shows similar results obtained in isolated ventricular cells. In the experiment shown in this figure (Krafte and Kass, unpublished data), the inactiva-

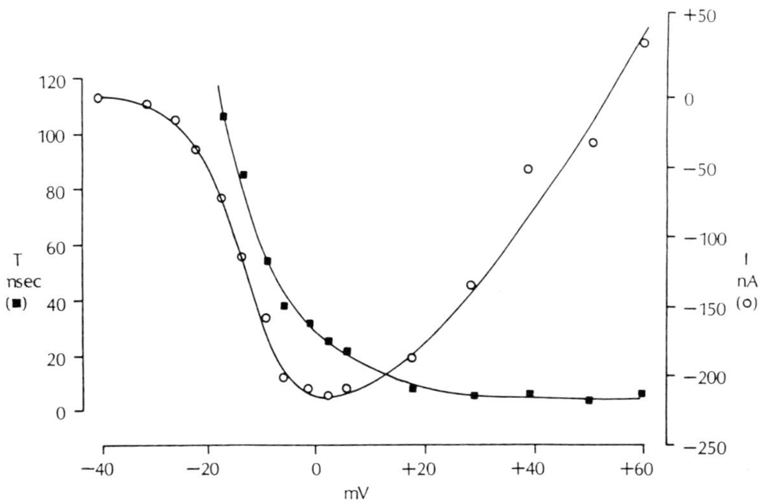

Fig. 4. Sr current inactivation rate is not current-dependent. Peak Sr current was measured by subtraction of background currents [measured in the present of nisoldipine (10 μM)] and plotted against pulse voltage (0). The time course of Sr current decay was determined for each record (see Methods). The fast time constants obtained by this procedure are also plotted against test pulse voltage (■). Preparation 301-3 (Kass and Sanguinetti, unpublished data)

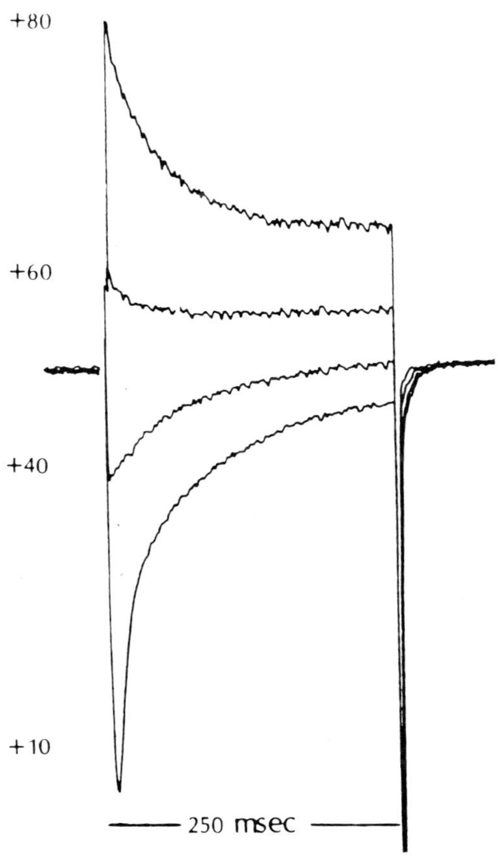

Fig. 5. Membrane current in response to 250 ms depolarizing voltage steps in the isolated guinea pig ventricular myocyte. Membrane potential was held at −50 mV and stepped to the indicated voltages. Peak current became less inward as the test potential became more positive and reversed above +50 mV. The inactivation rate is still significant at +80 mV (Krafte and Kass, unpublished data, 0684E5)

tion rate of Ca current remains very fast even at voltages more positive than the Ca-channel reversal potential. If inactivation of these channels were caused entirely by Ca entry, the inactivation rates would be expected to become slower or non-existent at these voltages.

The simplest interpretation of these results is that Ca-channel current in cardiac cells inactivates via mechanisms that are both voltage-dependent and Ca-dependent. The results obtained in Ba- or Sr-containing solutions may be explained if these divalent cations are unable to substitute for Ca in enhancing inactivation. In this view, Ba (or Sr) currents predominantly reflect a voltage-dependent process whereas Ca currents reflect both voltage- and Ca-mediated mechanisms. If this is the case, then studies that focus on voltage-dependent inactivation of the Ca-channel would be simplified if Ba or Sr replaced Ca in the test solutions. This approach has already been followed in several investigations of Ca-channel modulation by organic compounds (Lee and Tsien 1983; Sanguinetti and Kass 1984a; Hess et al. 1984).

Slow Inactivation

The time constants of the inactivation processes discussed above range from a few ms to hundreds of ms (at 37 °C). Kass and Scheuer (1982) also reported a very slow component of inactivation of Ca-channel current in the calf Purkinje fiber. The time course of the slow process (at 37 °C) is on the order of several seconds and is independent of the divalent charge carrier. Slow inactivation might be particularly important to drug-channel interactions with certain organic compounds because these interactions occur very slowly. A very slow inactivation process has also been observed in isolated ventricular cells (Krafte and Kass, unpublished data).

State-Dependent Modulation of Ca-Channel Current

Pharmacological studies have provided considerable information about the molecular structure of ion channels in the membranes of excitable cells. For example, tetrodotoxin has been used to block, probe, and count Na-channels in nerve and skeletal muscle. Quaternary ammonium compounds have proven to be very effective potassium channel blockers and have been used to investigate the architecture of potassium channels in nerve and skeletal muscle preparations (see Hille 1977; Armstrong 1969). More recently, organic compounds that block Ca-channels in cardiac and smooth muscle cells have been used to probe the structure and function of these channels on the basis of electrophysiological and binding studies (see Schwartz and Triggle 1983). Advances in the characterization of Ca-channel current in recent years can be attributed, in large part, to the discovery of these organic compounds. Modulation of Ca-channel currents by these drugs appears to be strongly affected by the state of the channel (see Sanguinetti and Kass 1984a) and may even be due to modification of the mode of channel gating (Hess et al. 1984).

The remainder of this chapter is a review of the proposed mechanisms of action of organic compounds that have been shown to modify Ca-channel currents in cardiac preparations. The review will focus upon results from voltage clamp studies of isolated cardiac tissue and single cardiac cells, and will emphasize the actions of dihydropyridine derivatives (i.e. nifedipine, nisoldipine) and diarylalkylamine antagonists (i.e. verapamil, D 600, AQA 39).

Mechanisms of Action of Ca-Channel Antagonists

Organic compounds that inhibit Ca-channel currents (Ca-channel antagonists) are effective in micromolar and even nanomolar concentrations, but the potency of these drugs depends upon the conditions under which they are applied, specifically upon stimulation rate and cell resting potential.

Frequency-Dependent Block

Thorough investigation of the mechanisms of action of all organic Ca-channel blockers by voltage clamp techniques has revealed that block of Ca current by each of these compounds is strongly modulated by membrane potential. Consequently, there is frequency (use)-dependent block of contractile activity and Ca current in cardiac tissue by these agents. In each case, inhibition of Ca current is augmented by depolarization, caused either by an increase in the frequency of stimulation, or by changes in resting (or holding) membrane potential. Hyperpolarization reverses Ca current inhibition, presumably by causing a voltage dependent decrease in the affinitiy of the drug for its receptor. An example of use dependent effects of verapamil is illustrated in Fig. 6.

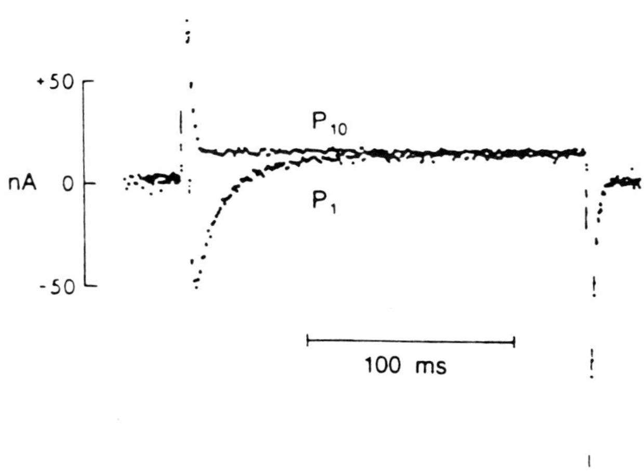

Fig. 6. Pulse-dependent block of Ca-channel current by D 600. Current traces are shown in response to the first (P_1) and tenth (P_{10}) applied from a -40 mV holding potential after a 2 min pulsefree period at -70 mV. Inward current is pronounced during the first pulse but is completely blocked by the tenth pulse. See Kass (1982) for details

Use-dependent block of Ca current results from a drug-induced prolongation of the time required for the channels to recover from the inactivated state. Ca-channels normally recover from inactivation in a biexponential manner and the time constants are dependent upon voltage. D 600 (Pelzer et al. 1982), verapamil (Kohlhardt and Mnich 1978), nisoldipine (Sanguinetti and Kass 1984a), nitrendipine (Lee and Tsien 1983), and diltiazem (Uehara and Hume 1984) all prolong the time required for this recovery process. Fewer channels return to the pool available for conduction during the interpulse interval because the time for recovery from inactivation is prolonged. This results in a cumulative decrease in channels available for conduction with repetitive depolarization. Compounds that exhibit the greatest frequency dependent block (i.e. D 600, verapamil) slow this process to a greater extent than the dihydropyridines (i.e. nifedipine and nisoldipine).

How do Ca-channel antagonists retard the recovery from inactivation of Ca current, and why are some drugs more effective than others in this respect? A plausible explanation is provided by the modulated receptor hypothesis (Hille 1977; Hondeghem and Katzung 1977) proposed to account for the time- and voltage-dependence of local anesthetic block of Na-channels. The model propose that drugs can bind to a site in or near a channel, and that the affinity for this site varies depending upon the state of the channel (i.e. rested, open or inactivated) which in turn is a function of membrane potential. Furthermore, the model assumes that drug-bound channels do not conduct. Thus inactivated and drug-bound channels are indistinguishable electrically: neither conducts. Recovery from "apparent inactivation" in the presence of drug must include a fraction of channels that recover slowly from the drug-bound (and thus nonconducting) condition. This concept has been extended to explain the voltage-dependent interaction of organic Ca entry blockers with the Ca-channel (Hondeghem and Katzung 1984; McDonald et al. 1984).

The model also predicts that ionized drugs can only bind to the channel-associated receptor when a hydrophilic pathway to this site is provided, that is when the channels are in the open state configuration. Thus, drugs are assumed to act at a site within the membrane. Uncharged drugs can reach this receptor either through a hydrophilic pathway or a hydrophobic pathway (via the lipid membrane surrounding the channel). The degree of drug ionization can be calculated based upon the pKa of the compound and pH of the Tyrode solution. At physiological pH, the diarylalkylamines (verapamil, D 600, AQA 39; pKa = 8–9) are highly charged, whereas most dihydropyridines (nitrendipine, nisoldipine, nifedipine; pKa < 3) exist almost exclusively in the neutral state.

The results of voltage camp experiments with Ca-channel blockers support these generalized predictions relating drug ionization to mode of action.

Diarylalkylamine Antagonists: Verapamil and D 600

Several groups have now reported that block by verapamil and related compounds develops only if a train of voltage depolarizations is imposed on the preparation under investigation (Pelzer et al. 1982; Kass 1982; Lee and Tsien 1983;

Sanguinetti and Kass 1984a). Block by these compounds does not develop even at holding potentials as positive as −40 mV in the absence of repetitive depolarization (Sanguinetti and Kass 1984a). These results suggested that Ca-channels must first open before these compounds can block. This suggestion is consistent with the modulated receptor hypothesis because these compounds are nearly fully charged at physiological pH, and experimental evidence for open channel block by these drugs has been provided by Pelzer et al. (1982) and Lee and Tsien (1983).

Although conclusive proof that these drugs bind preferentially to a specific channel state is lacking, it is clear that opening of Ca-channels is a prerequisite to inhibition of Ca-channel current by the diarylalkylamines. In fact it is conceivable that once these drugs gain access to the interior of the channel during activation they then bind preferentially to the inactivated state rather than the open state of the channel.

The rate of onset of Ca-channel block during a train of depolarizing pulses and the steady level of block achieved is increased when the duration of each pulse is prolonged. This characteristic has been observed in voltage clamped ferret papillary muscle (Kanaya et al. 1983) and calf Purkinje fibers (Sanguinetti and Kass 1984a). Assuming that drug-bound channels undergo state transitions in a voltage and time dependent manner, the end result of a prolonged depolarization (or repeated depolarizations of sufficient duration) would be a stabilization of channels in the drug-bound inactivated state. The interaction of verapamil, D 600 and AQA 39 with the Ca-channel can be visualized as occurring via the pathway R→O→O*→I* (McDonald et al. 1984), shown diagramatically below in a scheme first described by Hille (1977) for local anesthetic interaction with Na-channels during a depolarizing event. Here R, O, and I represent Ca-channels in the rested, open and inactivated state respectively, and R*, O*, and I* represent drug-bound channels. Support for such a mechanism also comes from experiments with D 600 that show a large drug-induced hyperpolarizing voltage shift in Ca current availability in isolated frog atrial cells (Uehara and Hume 1984).

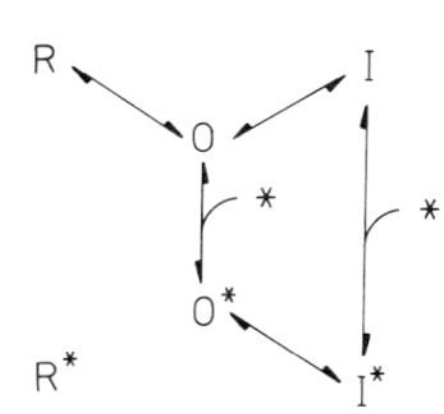

Dihydropyridine Antagonists

Initial voltage clamp studies using nifedipine, nitrendipine and nisoldipine demonstrated that these compounds were potent Ca-channel blockers, but were not characterized by significant use-dependent actions (Tung and Morad 1983; Kass 1982; Bayer and Ehara 1978; Kohlhardt and Fleckenstein 1977). Some studies also suggested that nifedipine did not alter the time course of the recovery from inactivation (Kohlhardt and Fleckenstein 1977), consistent with a lack of use-dependent block, and thus a mode of action independent of channel state. However, more recent investigations have made it clear that these compounds do slow the recovery from inactivation and inhibit Ca-channel currents in a frequency-dependent manner (Lee and Tsien 1983; Uehara and Hume 1984; Sanguinetti and Kass 1984a). Depending on experimental conditions, use-dependent block by the dihydropyridines can be described as mild (Lee and Tsien 1983) or marked (Sanguinetti and Kass 1984a). In the latter case, little or no block is caused by 0.2 μM nisoldipine when the holding potential is hyperpolarized (−70 mV) and the pulses are brief (50 ms) and infrequent (0.1 Hz). However, pulsing at high frequencies (5 Hz) results in considerable (75%) block by the same nisoldipine concentration.

The most dramatic difference between the actions of the diarylalkylamines and the dihydropyridines is that membrane potential markedly modulates block of Ca-channel currents by the dihydropyridines even in the absence of repetitive pulsing. For example, nisoldipine or nitrendipine (0.2 μM) only slightly inhibits Ca-channel current when the membrane potential is held at −70 mV for two min, but almost completely blocks the channels when the holding potential is changed to depolarized (−45 mV) levels (Sanguinetti and Kass 1984a; Fig. 7). As noted previously, no block develops in the presence of verapamil simply by holding the membrane at −45 mV, suggesting that block of Ca-channels by nisoldipine and nitrendipine can develop without the prerequisite of Ca-channels first being in the open state.

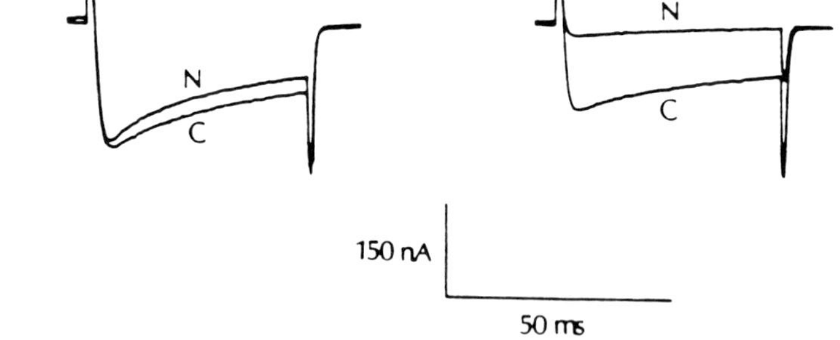

Fig. 7 a, b. Holding potential influences Ca-channel current blockade by nisoldipine. Membrane current in response to voltage pulse to 0 mV applied from −70 mV holding potential (**a**) and −45 mV holding potential (**b**) in the absence (*C*) and presence (*N*) of nisoldipine (200 nM). Pulses were applied after 2 min pulse-free interval at each holding potential. 5.4 mM Sr^{++} Tyrode's solution +10 μM TTX. Preparation 317-1 (Sanguinetti and Kass 1984a, permission of the American Heart Association, Inc.)

What causes the dramatic effects of membrane potential upon Ca-channel inhibition by dihydropyridines? One possibility is that these drugs interact preferentially with channels that are inactivated. If this were the case, then the influence of membrane potential on drug-potency should be predicted by the voltage-dependence of the steady-state inactivation curve for the Ca-channels.

To test for such a possibility, Sanginetti and Kass (1984a) measured the influence of holding potential on Ca-channel block by nisoldipine over a range of voltages. They also varied the length of time the membrane was held at each of these conditioning potentials. The results of these experiments revealed two important aspects of drug-channel interaction by this dihydropyridine. When the conditioning prepulses were brief (500 ms to 1 s), the voltage-dependence of Ca-channel availability was unchanged from drug-free conditions. However, when the duration of the conditioning prepulses was increased to 30 s, the functional form of the relationship between Ca-channel availability and membrane potential was the same in the presence and absence of drug, but in the presence of drug, it was shifted in the hyperpolarizing direction by approximately 19 mV. A drug-induced hyperpolarizing shift in the steady-state inactivation curve is consistent with an interaction between the drug and the inactivated state of the channel (Hille 1977, 1978). However, the drug-induced shift occurs only if conditioning prepulses are sufficiently long. Thus it is possible, that this interaction requires slow inactivation of these channels.

"Apparent dissociation constants" for nisoldipine binding to rested and inactivated channel states were calculated from the data of the experiment shown in Fig. 8. The dissociation constants were 1,340 nM for resting channels and 1 nM for inactivated channels. The calculations were made assuming that nisoldipine binds only to Ca-channels in the rested or inactivated state, using an equation described by Bean et al. (1983) which relates the shift in the steady-state availability curve and the drug concentration to apparent dissociation constants for binding to inactivated and rested state channels. In this computation, slow inactivation was not considered as an additional state for the channel.

A 1,000-fold difference in "apparent binding constants" is the same as the difference previously reported for the discrepancy between the K_d for binding of [^{3}H]-nitrendipine to cardiac membranes (0.1–1.0 nM) and the IC 50 for inhibition of contraction of Ca current of cardiac tissue (Janis and Triggle 1983; Bolger et al. 1983; Ferry and Glossman 1982; Kass 1982). Thus the K_d for binding reflects the affinity of the drugs for depolarized membrane, perhaps specifically to channels that are in the inactivated state.

What causes the contrast between the holding potential modulation of block by the dihydropyridines and the diarylalkylamines? One possibility is the difference in the relative hydrophilicity of these compounds. Nisoldipine and nitrendipine are highly lipophilic, unlike verapamil or D 600, and respond to changes in membrane potential similarly. To determine whether the observed differences in blocking activity of these compounds are due to differences in hydrophilicity or to structural dissimilarities, Sanguinetti and Kass (1984a) studied the influence of membrane potential on the blocking actions of nicardipine. Nicardipine is a dihydropyridine that is 28% ionized at pH 7.4. The results of these experiments showed that nicardipine exhibits an intermediate level of holding potential-de-

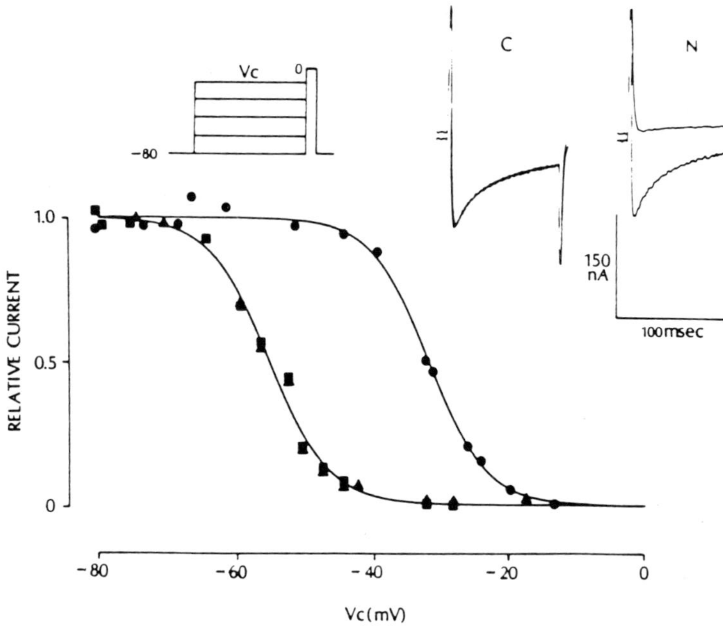

Fig. 8. Effect of nisoldipine on voltage-dependence of Ca-channel current availability. Prepulses (V_C), 30 s in duration, were followed by a 100 ms test pulse (V_T) to 0 mV. Graph shows normalized plot of maximum inward current measured during V_T in the absence (●) and present of nisoldipine (200 nM ▲, 400 nM, ■) vs. V_C. Peak current in presence of nisoldipine was 87% (200 nM) and 77% (400 nM) of that recorded in control. Inset: Pulse protocol and current traces in response to test pulse following 30 s conditioning pulse to −44 mV and −74 mV, control (*C*), nisoldipine (*N*). Curve: best fit of function $(1+\exp(V-V_h)/k)-1$ to data. Control: $V_h=-32$ mV, k=4.1. Nisoldipine: $V_h=-53.4$ mV (200 nM), −55 mV (400 nM), k=4.2 (200 nM), 4.4 (400 nM). 5.4 mM Sr^{2+} Tyrode solution +10 μM TTX. Preparation 339-1 (Sanguinetti and Kass 1984a, by permission of the American Heart Association, Inc.)

pendent block of Ca-channel current. They concluded from this work that dihydropyridines probably interact with Ca-channels via pathway R→0→O*→I* or R→I→I*, depending upon membrane voltage and hydrophilicity of a given compound.

Modification of Surface Charge Can Influence Drug Activity

Observations by Fleckenstein and others (see Fleckenstein 1983 for review) that elevation of extracellular Ca could relieve inhibition of Ca-dependent responses by a variety of drugs in cardiac and smooth muscle contributed to the definition of these drugs as Ca antagonists. Although some recent electrophysiological data (Lee and Tsien 1983) support the interpretation of a form of antagonism between Ca and these drugs, in millimolar concentrations Ca does not antagonize drug binding (Janis and Triggle 1983). In the previous section, results were presented that showed that dihydropyridines exert at least some of their inhibitory actions

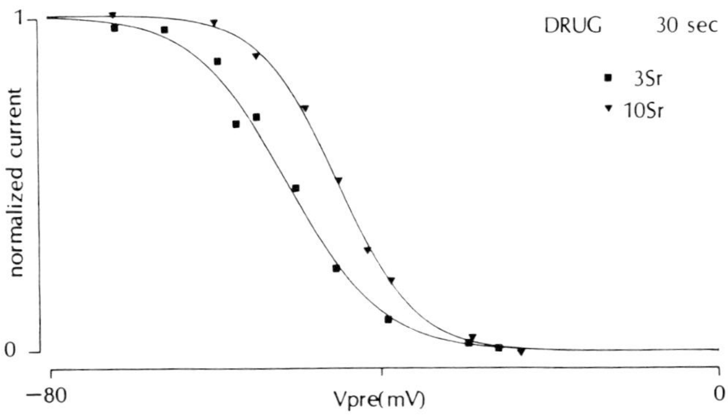

Fig. 9. Elevation of extracellular Sr shifts the relationship between Ca-channel availability and membrane potential. Membrane current was measured during test pulses to 0 mV after 30 s (filled symbols) conditioning prepulses. Normalized current measured in 3 mM Sr (■) and 10 mM Sr (▼) is plotted against prepulse voltage. 200 mM nisoldipine was present during the 30 s prepulse experiments (Kass et al., unpublished data)

on Ca-channel currents by causing hyperpolarizing shifts in the relationship between availability of Ca-channels and membrane potential. We thus considered the possibility that some of the antagonistic effects of Ca and other divalent cations might be due to opposing (depolarizing) shifts in this relationship brought on by changes in negative surface potentials at the outer surface of the sarcolemmal membrane.

The outer surface of cells is thought to have a negative surface charge layer that can be screened or reduced by monovalent and divalent cations (see Hille 1984 for review). This change in surface charge alters the transmembrane electric field and thus can influence voltage-dependent gating. Consequently, elevation of external divalent cation concentration should cause a depolarizing shift in the relationship between steady-state voltage dependent inactivition (availability) and membrane potential as demonstrated in Fig. 9 A. Figure 9 B shows the results of an experiment to test whether this effect exists in the presence of the dihydropyridine nisoldipine. The figure shows steady-state (30 s prepulses) inactivation curves measured in two concentrations of external Sr in the presence of 200 nM nisoldipine. In 3 mM Sr, the half maximal voltage for this relation was determined to be −50 mV, a voltage similar to that previously reported for this drug concentration. When this experiment was repeated in 10 mM Sr, the half maximal voltage was found to be −40 mV, a depolarizing shift of 10 mV.

What does this shift mean in terms of drug inhibition of Ca-channel current? The depolarizing shift in the inactivation curve means that at any given voltage, there is a smalller fraction of channels that are inactivated (and thus not available for ion conduction) in the elevated Sr solution, even though drug concentration remains unchanged. This results in a larger Ca-channel current. This effect is most pronounced at voltages where the inactivation curve changes most steeply as a function of membrane potential (between −60 mV and −40 mV in Fig. 9 B). Since the same depolarizing shift can be seen in the absence of drug, this experiment provides evidence that screening of surface charges by divalent cations can account, at least in part, for their antagonistic actions on the inhibitory effects of dihydropyrine derivatives.

Ca-Channel Agonists

Slight modifications in the structure of nifedipine have led to the discovery of dihydropyridines that increase smooth and cardiac muscle contractility (Schramm et al. 1983). Subsequent studies have shown that one of these compounds, Bay k 8644 increases the magnitude of Ca-channel current (Cohen and Chung 1984; Hess et al. 1984; Sanguinetti and Kass 1984 b). In each study it was noted that

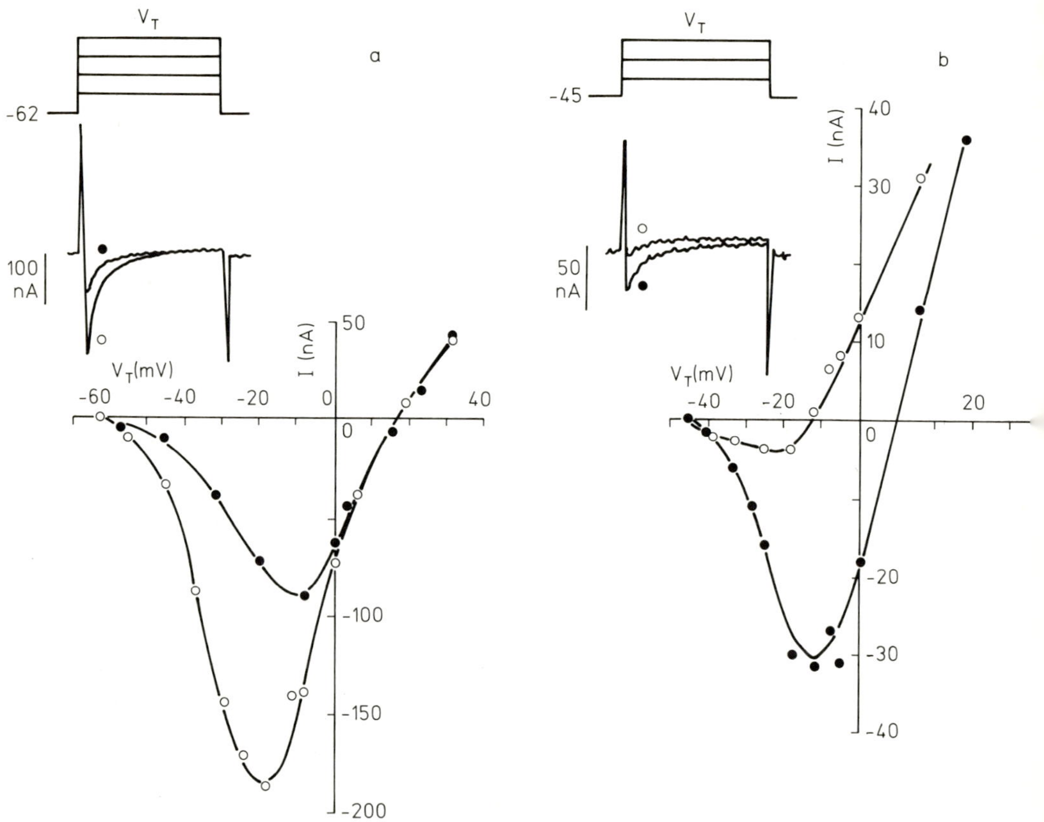

Fig. 10 a, b. Influence of holding potential on the activity of Bay K 8644 (0.5 μM) on membrane current. Membrane current was recorded in response to 100 ms test pulses (*inset*) applied to voltages from a holding potential of −62 mV (**a**) or −45 mV (**b**). The *insets* in both panels show current traces in response to voltage steps to −10 mV from each holding potential in the absence (●) and presence (○) of drug. The graphs show peak inward current plotted against test pulse voltage in the absence (●) and presence (○) of drug, and the curves are hand drawn. The standard modified Tyrode solution consisted of (mM): 150 NaCl, 4 KCl, 5.4 $CaCl_2$, 0.5 $MgCl_2$, 5 glucose, and 10 Tris-HCl buffer (pH 7.4). Preparation 351-1 (Sanguinetti and Kass 1984 b)

the greatest increase in Ca-channel current occurs during weak depolarizations and that current measured during a pulse appears to inactivate more rapidly in the presence of the drug. It has also been reported that inward tail currents measured after repolarization were larger and deactivated more slowly than under drug-free conditions.

The results of studies of the influence of Bay K 8644 on cell-attached patch recordings of single Ca-channel currents are discussed in the chapter by Hess et al. (pp. 34–55 in this book). The studies presented in that chapter show that this drug promotes an indigenous mode of gating (mode 2) that favors long open times for the channel. Sanguinetti and Kass (1984b) found that depending on membrane potential, this compound can either enhance or block Ca-channel currents. Figure 10 shows that holding potential can cause this compound to act either as an agonist or an antagonist. The figure shows Ca currents and peak-inward current/voltage relationships measured in the absence (●) and presence (○) of 0.5 μM Bay K 8644. When currents are measured from a negative holding potential (Fig. 10A), the drug increases Ca current. In the same experiment, when the holding potential is depolarized (Fig. 10B) the drug inhibits currents. Thus a fixed concentration of this compound can either augment or decrease Ca-channel current, depending on the conditions under which it is applied.

Future studies will be needed to determine whether the blocking actions of Bay K 8644 are similar to those of other dihydropyridines, and to determine the relative potencies for excitatory or inhibitory activity on the Ca-channel.

References

Armstrong CM (1969) Inactivation of the potassium conductance and related phenomena caused by quaternary ammonium ion injection in squid axons. J Gen Physiol 54:553–575

Bayer R, Ehara T (1978) Comparative studies on calcium antagonists. Prog Pharmacol 2:31–37

Bean BP (1984) Nitrendipine block of cardiac calcium channels: High-affinity binding to the inactivated state. Proc Natl Acad Sci 81:6388–6392

Bean BP, Cohen CJ, Tsien RW (1983) Lidocaine block of cardiac sodium channels. J Gen Physiol 81:613–642

Beeler GW Jr, Reuter H (1970) Membrane calcium current in ventricular myocardial fibres. J Physiol 207:191–209

Bolger GT, Genog P, Klockowski R, Luchowski E, Siegel H et al. (1983). Characterization of binding to the Ca^{++} channel antagonist, ^{3}H-nitrendipine, to guinea pig ileal smooth muscle. J Pharmacol Exptl Therap 225:291–309

Brown AM, Morimoto K, Tsuda Y, Wilson DL (1981) Calcium current-dependent and voltage-dependent inactivation in Helix Aspersa. J Physiol 320:193–218

Carmeliet E (1980) The slow inward current: non-voltage-clamp studies. In: Zipes DP, Bailex JC, Elharrar V (eds) The slow inward current and cardiac arrhythmias. Martinus Nijhoff, The Hague

Chandler WK, Meves H (1970) Slow changes in membrane permeability and long-lasting action potentials in axons perfused with fluoride solutions. J Physiol 211:707–728

Cohen CJ, Chung M (1984) A nifedipine derivative (Bay K 8644) that increases Ca currents in myocardial cells: a novel positive inotropic agent. Biophys J 45:394a

Coraboeuf E (1980) Voltage clamp studies of the slow inward current. In: Zipes DP, Bailey JC, Elharrar V (eds) The slow inward current and cardiac arrhythmias. Martinus Nijhoff, The Hague, pp 25–95

Eckert R, Tillotson DL (1981) Calcium-mediated inactivation of the calcium conductance in caesium-loaded giant neurones of *Aplysia californica*. J Physiol 314:265–280

Ferry DR, Glossmann H (1982) Evidence for multiple receptor sites within the putative calcium channel. Naunyn-Schmied. Arch Pharmacol 321:80–83

Fleckenstein A (1983) History of calcium antagonists. Circ Res 52:13–116

Hamill OP, Marty A, Neher E, Sakmann B, Sigworth FJ (1981) Improved patch-clamp techniques for high-resolution current recording from cells and cell-free membrane patches. Pflügers Arch 391:85–100

Hess P, Lansman JB, Tsien RW (1984) Different modes of Ca-channel gating behavior favoured by dihydropyridine Ca agonists and antagonists. Nature 311:538–544

Hille B (1977) Local anesthetics: Hydrophilic and hydrophobic pathways for the drug-receptor reaction. J Gen Physiol 69:497–515

Hille B (1978) Local anesthetic action on inactivation of the Na-channel in nerve and skeletal muscle. Possible mechanisms for antiarrythmic agents. In Morad M (ed) Biophysical aspects of cardiac muscle. Academic Press, New York, pp 55–74

Hille B (1984) Modifers of gating. In: Ionic channels of excitable membranes. Sinauer Associates, Sunderland Ma, pp 316–326

Hodgkin AL, Huxley AF (1952) A quantitative description of membrane current and its application to conduction and excitation in nerve. J Physiol 117:500–544

Hondeghem LM, Katzung BG (1977) Time- and voltagedependent interactions of antiarrhythmic drugs with cardiac sodium channels. Biochem Biophys Acta 472:373–398

Hondeghem LM, Katzung BG (1984) Antiarrhythmic agents: The modulated receptor mechanism of action of sodium and Ca-channel blocking drugs. Ann Rev Pharmacol Toxicol 24:387–423

Hume JR, Giles W (1982) Turn-off a TTX-resistant inward current "i_{Ca}" in single bullfrog atrial cells. Biophys J 37:240 a

Isenberg G, Klockner U (1982) Calcium currents of isolated bovine ventricular myocytes are fast and of large amplitude. Pflugers Arch 395:30–41

Janis RA, Triggle DJ (1983), New Developments in Ca^{2+} channel antagonists. J Med Chem 26:775–785

Josephson IR, Sanchez-Chapula J, Brown AM (1984) A comparison of calcium currents in rat and guinea pig single ventricular cells. Circ Res 54:144–156

Kanaya S, Arlock P, Katzung B, Hondeghem LM (1983) Diltiazem and verapamil preferentially block inactivated cardiac calcium channels. J Molec Cell Cardiol 15:145–148

Kass RS (1982) Nisoldipine: a new, more selective calcium current blocker in cardiac Purkinje fibers. J Pharm Exp Ther 223:446–456

Kass RS, Sanguinetti MC (1984)M Inactivation of Ca-channel current in the calf cardiac Purkinje fiber: Evidence for voltage and Ca-mediated mechanisms. J Gen Physiol 84:705–726

Kass RS, Scheuer T (1982) Slow inactivation of calcium channels in the cardiac Purkinje fiber. J Molec Cell Cardiol 14:615–618

Kass RS, Scheuer T, Malloy KJ (1982) Block of outward current in cardiac Purkinje fibers by injection of quaternary ammonium ions. J Gen Physiol 79:1041–1063

Kohlhardt M, Fleckenstein A (1977) Inhibition of the slow inward current by nifedipine in mammalian ventricular myocardium. Nauny-Schmiedeberg's Arch. Pharmacol 298:267–272

Kohlhardt M, Mnich Z (1978) Studies on the inhibitory effect of verapamil on the slow inward current in mammalian ventricular myocardium. J Molec Cell Cardiol 10:1037–1052

Lee KS, Tsien RW (1983) Mechanism of calcium channel block by verapamil, D 600, diltiazem, and nitrendipine in single dialyzed heart cells. Nature 302:790–794

Marban E, Tsien RW (1981) Is the slow inward calcium current of heart muscle inactivated by calcium? Biophys J 33:143 a

Marban E, Tsien RW (1982) Effects of nystatin-mediated intracellular ion substitution on membrane currents in calf Purkinje fibres. J Physiol 329:569–587

McDonald TF, Pelzer D, Trautwein W (1984) Cat ventricular muscle treated with D 600: characteristics of calcium channel block and unblock. J Physiol 352:217–241

Mentrard D, Vassort G, Fischmeister R (1984) Calciummediated inactivation of the calicum conductance in cesium-loaded frog heart cells. J Gen Physiol 85:105–131

New W, Trautwein W (1972) Inward membrane currents in mammalian myocardium. Pflugers Arch 334:1–23

Pelzer D, Trautwein W, McDonald TF (1982) Calcium channel block and recovery from block in mammalian ventricular muscle treated with organic channel inhibitors. Pflug Arch 394:97–105

Reuter H (1967) The dependence of slow inward current in Purkinje fibres on the extracellular calcium concentration. J Physiol 192:479–492

Reuter H (1979) Properties of two inward membrane currents in the heart. Ann Rev Physiol 41:413–424

Reuter H, Stevens CF, Tsien RW, Yellow G (1982) Properties of single calcium channels in cardiac cell culture. Nature 297:501–504

Rougier O, Vassort G, Garnier D, Gargouil YM, Coraboeuf E (1969) Existence and role of a slow inward current during the frog atrial action potential. Pflugers Arch 308:91–110

Sanguinetti MC, Kass RS (1984a) Voltage dependent block of calcium channel current in the calf cardiac Purkinje fiber by dihydropyridine Ca-channel antagonists. Circ Res 55:336–348

Sanguinetti MC, Kass RS (1984b) Regulation of cardiac calcium channel current and contractile activity by the dihydropyridine Bay K 8644 is voltage dependent. J Molec Cell Cardiol 16:667–670

Schramm M, Thomas G, Towart R, Frankowiak G (1983) Novel dihydropyridines with positive inotropic action through activation of Ca^{2+} channels. Nature 303:535–537

Schwartz A, Triggle DS (1983) Cellular action of calcium channel blocking drugs. Ann Rev Med 35:325–339

Tillotson D (1979) Inactivation of Ca conductance dependent on entry of Ca ions in molluscan neurons. Proc Natl Acad Sci 76:1497–1500

Tsien RW (1983) Calcium channels in excitable cell membranes. Ann Rev Physiol 45:341–358

Tung L, Morad M (1983) Electrophysiological studies with Ca^{2+} entry blockers. In: Merrill GF, Weiss HR (eds) Ca^{2+} entry blockers, adenosine, and neurohumors. Urban & Schwarzenberg, Baltimore

Uehara, A, Hume JR (1984) Interactions of organic Ca-channel antagonists with Ca-channels in isolated frog atrial cells: test of a modulated receptor hypothesis. Biophys J 45:50a

Vitek M, Trautwein M, Trautwein W (1971) Slow inward current and action potential in cardiac Purkinje fibres. The effect of Mn ions. Pflugers Arch 323:204

Discussion

(pp. 198–215)

Glossmann: Do you think there might be a possibility that depending on voltage the conformation of the channel is changed in such a way that the symmetry is changed?

Kass: This could be the case. In fact, such a conformational change has been suggested by Hille in his modulated receptor hypothesis.

Glossmann: Then I should add that Bay K 8644 is a chiral compound.

Bevan: Vascular contraction in response to stretch, is dependent upon external calcium. This contraction is potentiated by Bay K 8644. However, if we partially deplarize the tissue with potassium, the effect of this compound seems to change to antagonism.

Kass: Without measuring the membrane current I would hesitate to call it the same, but certainly your finding is consistent with ours.

Fleckenstein: You reported that the duration of the action potential's plateau was strongly reduced if the stimulation-frequency was increased in the presence of verapamil. But in the presence of nifedipine the change was relatively small. This effect has also been observed by many other investigators.

Kass: In fact the action potentials I showed were from a report by Bayer et al. (Prog Pharm 5:53–84, 1982) and not from my own work.

Fleckenstein: In partially depolarized papillary muscles (by increasing potassium concentration up to 19 mmol/l) we found a similar reduction of the duration of the calcium-mediated action potential after increasing the stimulation frequency both with verapamil and nifedipine: The big difference which is found in fully polarized preparations disappeared. I have no explanation for this difference between the fully polarized preparation and the partially depolarized preparation in which we have a pure calcium-dependent action potential.

Kass: What concentration of nifedipine did you use?

Fleckenstein: 1,5 to 3×10^{-6}mol/l.

Kass: That is actually quite a high concentration. According to our results you would have considerable rested-state block at these concentrations, and thus not much frequency dependence at all. Therefore I cannot explain your observations in terms of our results.

Bechen: In your clamp records, there was no accelerated inactivation of the clamp current. Is the rate of inactivation during a single voltage pulse speeded up by nisoldipine?

Kass: There is some speeding of inactivation during a single pulse by nisoldipine but really not to a great extent. The major effects of voltage on nisoldipine-block take longer time to develop. Each of these test pulses was about 50 milliseconds long, which is very brief compared to the time constant for drug-block to develop or to be removed which is on the order of seconds.

Godfraind: Have you tested the effect of dihydropyridines other than nisoldipine on the inactivation curve?

Kass: We have the same results with nitrendipine, nifedipine and with nicardipine, but nicardipine appears to need the channel first to be opened before it can be fully effective. We suggest that this characteristic is related to the degree of ionization of this drug at physiological pH.

Hess: Is the activation by Bay K 8644 then due to binding to the open channels and not to the resting channels?

Kass: We have not done experiments that measure possible state-dependent binding of Bay K 8644. We have simply found that membrane potential can switch the modulating activity of this drug from agonist to antagonist. Future work will be addressed towards the question of state-dependent binding.

Hess: Bay K 8644 probably has its highest affinity to the channel when it is in its open mode. We think the transitions between those modes are slow in comparison to the transitions between closed and open states.

Bayer-Symposium IX
Cardiovascular Effects of Dihydropyridine-Type
Calcium Antagonists and Agonists, 218–232

Effects of the Calcium Agonistic Dihydropyridine Bay K 8644 on the Heart

R. GROSS, M. BECHEM, M. KAYSER, M. SCHRAMM, R. TANIEL, and G. THOMAS

Introduction

Besides their well documented therapeutic value the organic Ca^{2+}-antagonists contributed a great deal to basic sciences since they triggered investigations leading to a better understanding of membrane physiology. Recently, it was shown that minor changes to the nifedipine molecule (Fig. 1) lead to dihydropyridine-derivatives with pharmacological properties just opposite to the classical calcium antagonistic dihydropyridines: Bay K 8644 (methyl 1,4-Dihydro-2, 6-dimethyl-3-nitro-4-(2-trifluoromethylophenyl)- pyridine-5-carboxylate) is a calcium agonistic dihydropyridine which increases calcium influx into the cell (Schramm et al 1983; Meyer et al. 1985) and by this mechanism increases force of contraction both of smooth and of heart muscle. Apart from offering a new tool for basic research it may introduce a new class of potent positive inotropic drugs. This report is to summarize findings with Bay K 8644 as obtained both in vivo and in vitro with respect to its effects on the heart.

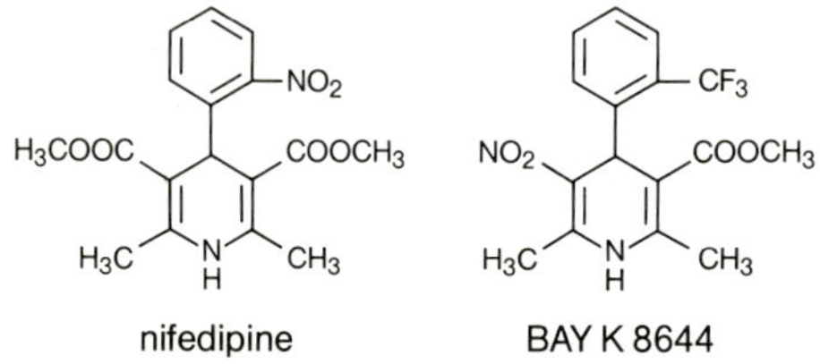

Fig. 1. Chemical structure of nifedipine and Bay K 8644

Material and Methods

1 In Vitro-Studies

1.1 Isolated Atria

Left atria of the guinea-pig heart were suspended in organ baths containing 100 ml Krebs-Henseleit solution (118 mmol/l NaCl, 4.8 mmol/l KCl, 1.2 mmol/l

KH_2PO_4, 1.2 mmol/l $MgSO_4$, 25 mmol/l $NaHCO_3$, 0.013 mmol/l EDTA (ethylenediaminetetraacetic acid disodium salt, 10 mmol/l glucose, 1.8 mmol/l $CaCl_2$) maintained at 30 °C and oxygenated with 95% O_2+5% CO_2 (pH 7.4). Resting tension was adjusted to 0.5 to 1.0 g. The atria were electrically stimulated (1 Hz, 2 ms, 16 V square wave), isometric force of contraction was measured with Statham UC 2 strain gauges and recorded with a penwriter (Hellige, West Germany).

1.2 Isolated Perfused Hearts

Hearts of adult guinea-pig (200–250 g) were perfused according to Langendorff (Langendorff 1895) as modified by Opie (1965) at 32 °C in a non-recirculating system. The perfusion medium was filtered Krebs-Henseleit solution as above but with only 1.2 mmol/l $CaCl_2$. The hearts were perfused at a constant volume rate. A latex balloon filled with saline and connected to a pressure transducer (Statham) via a metal cannula, was inserted into the left ventricular cavity to measure the isovolumetric contractions of the left ventricle and heart rate. A second pressure transducer was connected to the aortic cannula in order to record perfusion pressure. Drug solutions were infused into the aortic cannula at a rate of 1% of the total flow rate.

1.3 Papillary Muscle

Papillary muscles with diameters less than 1 mm of the right ventricle of guinea-pig hearts were mounted vertically into an organ bath containing 100 ml of Krebs-Henseleit solution (composition as above with 1.8 mmol/l $CaCl_2$) maintained at 30 °C. Resting tension was adjusted to 0.2 to 0.4 g and the muscles were stimulated with square wave pulses (0.5 ms, 4 Volt). Force of isometric contraction was measured with Statham UC 2 strain gauges and recorded on a tape recorder. The muscles were driven at least for 1 h at a stimulation rate of 1 Hz for equilibrium.

1.4 Lubrol-WX-Treated Glycerol Extracted Cardiac Muscle

Trabeculae septomarginales of the pig heart were chemical skinned as described previously (Herzig et al. 1981): they were treated with detergent containing glycerol solution (50% glycerol, 20 mmol/l imidazole, 10 mmol/l Na-azide, 0.5% lubrol-WX, 2 mmol/l dithioerythritol, pH 7.3) for 24 h at 4 °C. The fibres were stored at −20 °C in the same solution but without lubrol until the time of experiment. Bundles of these fibres with diameters of 0.1–0.2 mm were mounted horizontically on an isometric force transducing device and immersed into 1 ml of relaxing solution (12 mmol/l $MgCl_2$, 30 mmol/l imidazole, 5 mmol/l EGTA [ethylene glycol-bis (β-aminoethylester) N, N, N′, N′-tetra acetic acid) 5 mmol/l Na-azide as well as 10 mmol/l ATP, 10 mmol/l creatine phosphate, and creatine kinase (25 U ml, Boehringer, Mannheim FRG), as ATP reconstituting system. The pH of the solution was adjusted to 6.7 with KOH and ionic strength to 0.14 with KCl. The fibres were stretched in relaxing solution until resting tension was just noticeable. Contraction was induced by calcium-EGTA containing activation solution.

The calcium concentration was calculated using an apparent K_D value for calcium-EGTA of 1.5×10^{-6} at pH of 6.7. Test substances were dissolved in DMSO and applied in 10 μl aliquots (1% of bath volume). The controls also contained 10 μl DMSO/ml.

1.5 Saponin-Treated Cardiac Muscle

Trabeculae of guinea-pig hearts were mounted on an isometric force transducing device and immersed into Tyrode solution containing 2.53 mmol/l calcium and 3 mmol/l EGTA. They were immersed into saponin (100 μg/ml) containing relaxing solution (see above) for 15 min. After washing free of saponin by relaxing solution the fibres were loaded with "activation solution" (6 μmol/l free Ca^{2+}) for 7 min and then again immersed into relaxing solution. The EGTA concentration was reduced to 0.2 mmol/l before testing for calcium release with Bay K 8644 or caffein in order to avoid trapping of released calcium.

For all in vitro studies Bay K 8644 was dissolved in DMSO (dimethylsulfoxide) and appropriate solutions for injection in the organ bath or the perfusate were prepared by dilution with 0.9% NaCl. Although Bay K 8644 proved to be less light-sensitive than nifedipine, care was taken to protect the solutions from day light using sodium vapour lamps and by covering syringes, organ baths and infusion lines by aluminum foil.

2 In Vivo-Studies

2.1 Anaesthetized Dogs

Male and female mongrel dogs weighing 20–30 kg were anaesthetized with 30 mg/kg body weight i.v. of sodium pentobarbital. The animals were intubated and mechanically ventilated (Engstroem 300 respirator Solna, Sweden). Respiration was monitored with a CO_2-Analyzer (Datex CD 101, Helsinki, Finnland). Arterial pressure was measured with a Statham pressure transducer. A catheter tip manometer (Millar Micro Tip, Houston, Texas, USA) was placed in the left ventricle via the left carotid artery for registration of left ventricular pressure and LV (dP/dt).

A left thoracotomy was performed and an electromagnetic flow probe (Gould Statham, Oxnard, California, USA) was put around the ascending aorta to measure the cardiac output. Total peripheral resistance was calculated continuously by dividing mean arterial pressure by cardiac output with an analogue computer (ifd, Mülheim/Ruhr, West Germany). Another electromagnetic flow probe was put around the origin of the left circumflex artery for measuring coronary blood flow. A continuous i.v. infusion of sodium pentobarbital with an infusion rate of 1–2 mg/kg/min was adjusted to depress LV $(dP/dt)_{max}$ to approximately 1,000 mmHg/s. For the dose-response curves cardiac output was measured by the dye-dilution technique (Schwarzer TVS 4000 Munich, West Germany).

2.2 *Anaesthetized Rhesus Monkeys*

9 rhesus monkeys of either sex (body weight 5.2±0.4 kg) were anaesthetized by injection of 30 mg/kg barbiturate (Nembutal) followed by a continuous infusion of 3 mg/kg/h and artificially ventilated (Pulmomat, Draeger, Lübeck, West Germany) through a tracheostomy with a mixture of 50% O_2 and 50% N_2O. A catheter tip manometer (Millar Micro Tip, Houston, Texas, USA) was placed into the left ventricular cavity via the right carotid artery. Aortic pressure was measured via a Tygon catheter (Norton Industries, USA) fed into the left brachial artery and advanced into the thoratic aorta by an extracorporal pressure transducer (CP-01, Century Technol. Inglewood, USA). After a left thoracotomy in the IV intercostal space a precalibrated flow probe (Zepeda Instr., Seattle, USA) of appropriate size (6 or 7 mm i.d.) of an electromagnetic flow meter (SWD-4F, Zepeda Instr., Seattle, USA) was placed around the ascending aorta close to its root for measuring aortic blood flow. Pressure recordings were obtained using bridge amplifiers (DCB-4B, ifd, Mülheim, West Germany), mean values and derivatives (dP/dt) were on-line calculated by an analogue computer (ACl, ifd, Mülheim, West Germany). Heart rate was derived (FR 4, ifd) from the left ventricular pressure signal. Stroke volume was numerically calculated from cardiac output and heart rate. All variables were recorded on a 8 channel oscillographic recorder (Gould 2800, Cleveland, USA). The evaluated data were taken at the time of maximal response in LV $(dP/dt)_{max}$.

2.3 *Conscious Dogs*

Under sterile conditions and using usual surgical procedures in 11 mongrel dogs of either sex (body weight 20–32 kg) a left thoracotomy in the fifth intercostal space was performed. A tygon catheter was placed into the thoracic aorta (Herd and Barger 1964), and fixed to the adventitia by a small teflon pledget. After blunt dissection of the aorta ascendens an electromagnetic flow probe of appropriate size (Zepeda Instr., Seattle, USA) was implanted close to the aortic root. A precalibrated miniature pressure transducer (P6 or P7, Konigsberg Instr., Pasadena, USA) was implanted into the left ventricle via the left atrial appendage (Groß et al. 1979). Epicardial pacing electrodes were sutured to the base of the right ventricle. The thoracotomy was closed in layers. All catheters and leads were subcutaneously led to the neck of the animal and brought out there. After surgery the animals were treated with antibiotics (Mezlocilline 2 g/die, Bayer AG, West Germany) and allowed to recover for at least 2 weeks. Successful experiments could be performed in 9 dogs. All hemodynamic parameters were continuously recorded on an oscillographic recorder (Gould 2800, Cleveland, Ohio, USA). Simultaneously, all directly measured hemodynamic variables were digitized (PCM-system, K 1180, Kayser Threde, München, West Germany) and stored on tape recorder (Technics Autoreverse, RS 1700, Matsushita Electronics, Osaka, Japan).

For all in vivo experiments, Bay K 8644 was dissolved in "placebo solution" (60 g glycerol, 100 g H_2O, polyethyleneglycol 400 ad 1129 g) and administered via a peripheral vein.

Results and Discussion

Anaesthetized Dogs

Injection of 30 μg/kg b.w. Bay K 8644 into anaesthetized dogs causes total peripheral resistance to increase, accompanied by a rise of blood pressure and left ventricular peak pressure. LV $(dP/dt)_{max}$ increases and peak aortic blood flow velocity in face of increasing blood pressure is diminished. Probably due to the depth of anaesthesia chosen in this preparation heart rate does not change. Central venous pressure does not show any significant change. Shortly after injection

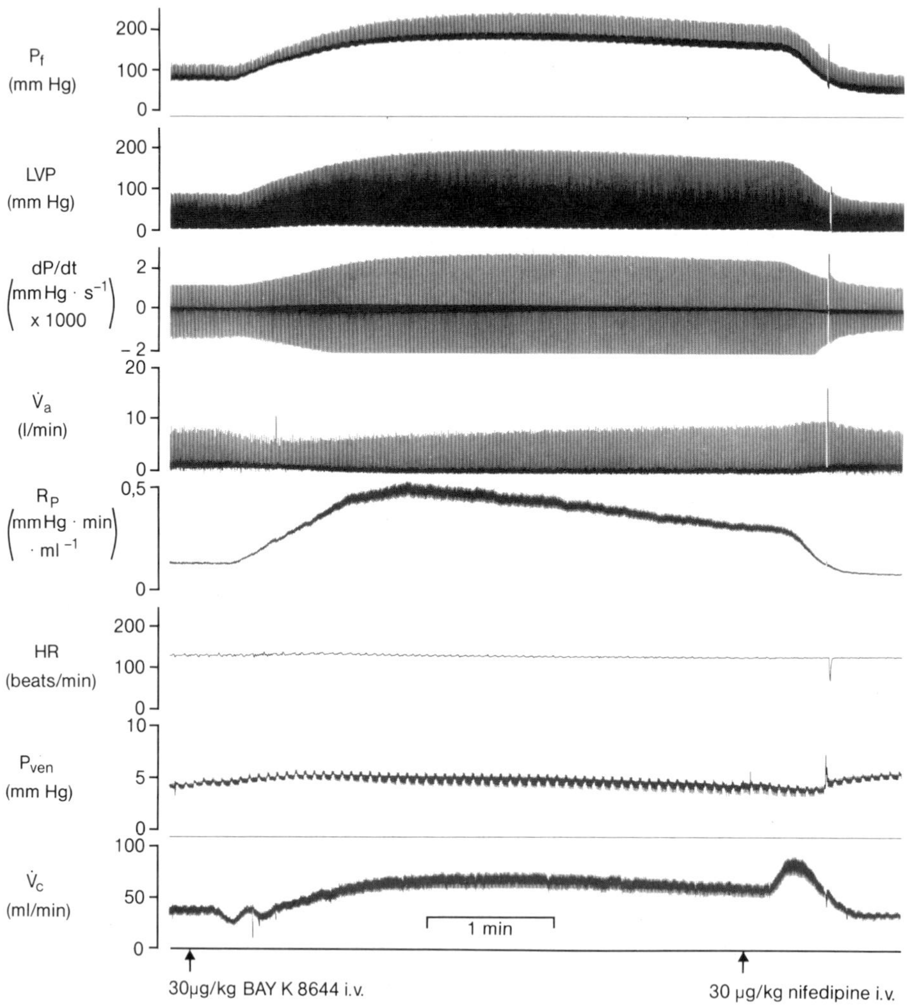

Fig. 2. Effects of intravenous injection of Bay K 8644 and subsequent injection of Nifedipine on arterial blood pressure (P_f), left ventricular pressure (*LVP*), rate of rise of left ventricular pressure (*dP/dt*), aortic flow, ($\dot{V}_a$), peripheral resistance (R_p), heart rate (*HR*), central venous pressure (P_{ven}), and mean coronary blood flow ($\dot{V}_c$)

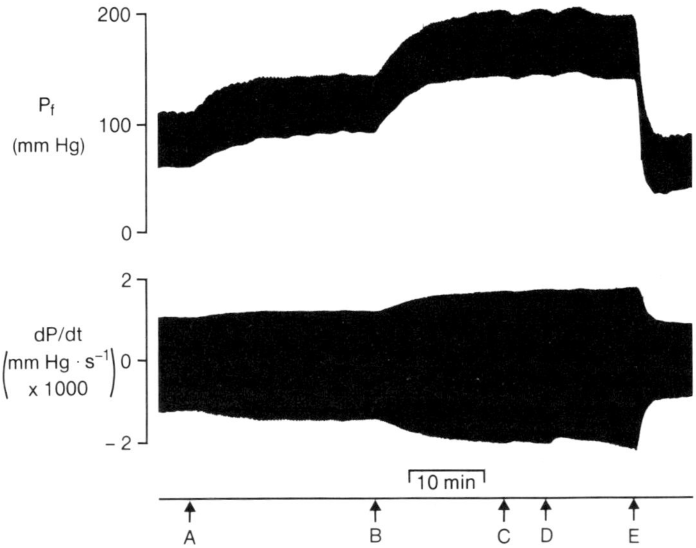

Fig. 3. Influence of Bay K 8644 on arterial blood pressure (P_f), and rate of rise of left ventricular pressure (*dP/dt*). *A:* Start of infusion of Bay K 8644 at a rate of 1 µg/kg/min. *B:* Increase of infusion rate to 3.8 µg/kg/min. *C:* Intravenous injection of 0.5 µg/kg propranolol. *D:* Intravenous injection of 0.5 mg/kg phentolamine. *E:* Intravenous injection of 30 µg/kg nifedipine

there is a transient fall of coronary blood flow despite the concomitant increase of driving pressure which is followed by a probably metabolically mediated coronary vasodilation and increase in blood flow. Injection of 30 µg/kg nifedipine i.v. completely counteracts all these changes (Fig. 2). The positive inotropic and vasoconstrictive effects of Bay K 8644 are not mediated by adrenergic mechanisms since the blood pressure rise and the increase of LV $(dP/dt)_{max}$ elicited by a continuous infusion of Bay K 8644 cannot be blocked by i.v. injection of either 0.5 mg/kg propranolol or 0.5 mg/kg phentolamine. In contrast to this, i.v. injection of 30 µg/kg nifedipine completely abolishes both the inotropic and vascular effects of Bay K 8644 (see Fig. 3).

In Fig. 4–6 dose-response-curves are given for the hemodynamic effects of Bay K 8644 as means obtained in 5 dogs under deep pentobarbital anaesthesia. Threshold dose for blood pressure effects (both mean and systolic) is 3 µg/kg, maximal effects are observed with 100 µg/kg. At this dose, systolic pressure rises up to 260 mm Hg. With higher doses serious arrhythmias occurred except for 2 dogs in which 300 µg/kg could be tested. As mentioned before, probably due to the depth of anaesthesia there is no change of heart rate over the whole dose range tested. LV $(dP/dt)_{max}$ also dose-dependently rises from a resting value of about 1.000 mm Hg/s up to more than 6.000 mm Hg/s, i.e. by about 500–600%. Since cardiac output and stroke volume do not change (Fig. 6) the pumping performance of the heart can only be read from the increased stroke work.

In anaesthetized rhesus monkeys intravenous injection of 1 to 30 µg/kg Bay K 8644 causes a dose-dependent increase of systolic arterial blood pressure and

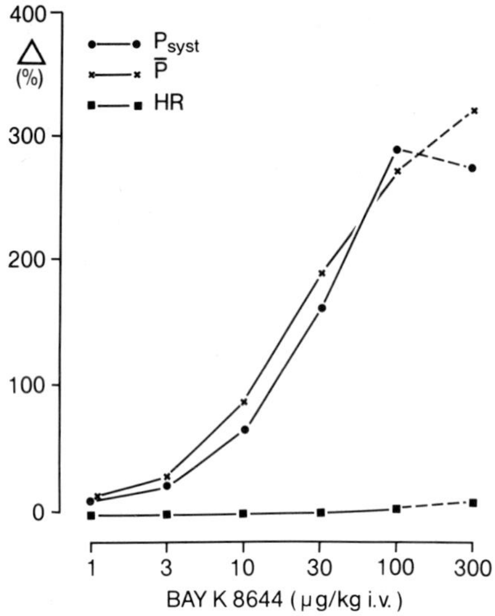

Fig. 4. Dose-response curves to Bay K 8644 with respect to systolic flow and pressure (P_{syst}), mean arterial pressure ($\bar{P}$) and heart rate (*HR*) plotted as percent change relative to resting values. Means of 5 experiments (at 300 μg/kg: n = 2)

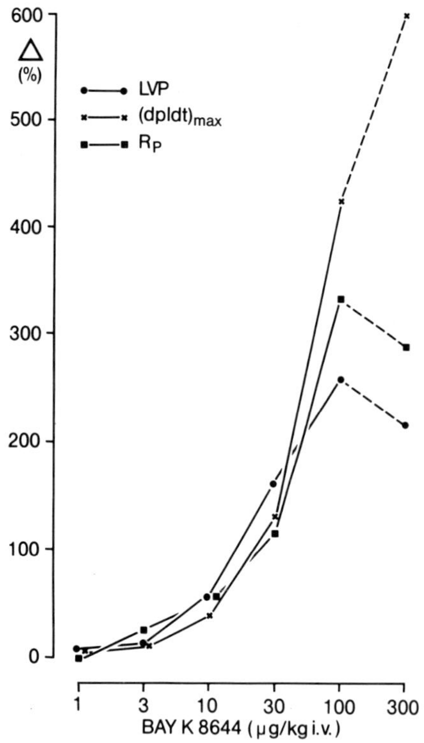

Fig. 5. Dose-response curves to Bay K 8644 with respect to the left ventricular pressure (*LVP*), maximal rate of rise of left ventricular pressure [$(dP/dt)_{max}$] and peripheral resistance (R_p) plotted as percent change relative to resting values. Means of 5 experiments (at 300 μg/kg: n = 2)

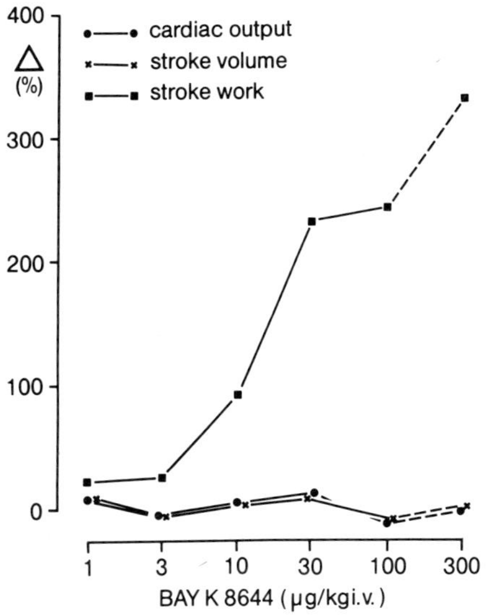

Fig. 6. Dose-response curves to Bay K 8644 with respect to cardiac output, stroke volume and stroke work plotted as percent change relative to resting values. Means of 5 experiments (at 300 μg/kg: n = 2)

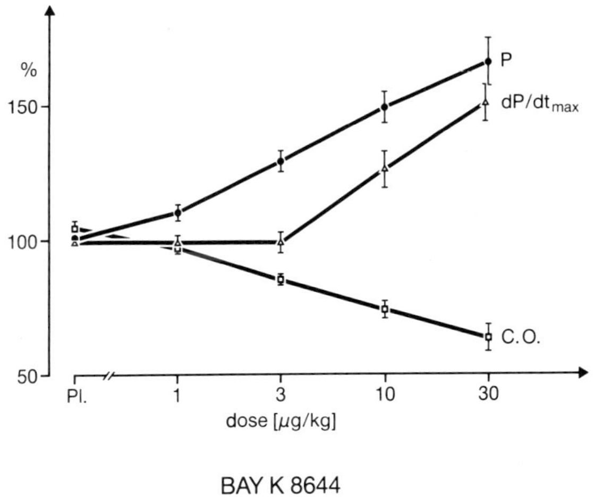

Fig. 7. Dose-response curves for systolic blood pressure (*P*), maximal rate of rise of left ventricular pressure (*dP/dt*), and cardiac output (*C.O.*) as means with their standard errors measured in 9 anaesthetized rhesus monkeys after intravenous injection of Bay K 8644. Given are the variables relative to their control values. *Pl.*: solvent control

LV $(dP/dt)_{max}$ to about 150% of control which amounts to 121 ± 10 mm Hg and 2.900 ± 262 mm Hg/s, respectively. Since for cardiac output the early minimum after injection was evaluated there is a dose-dependent transient fall which is mainly due to a reflex drop in heart rate (Fig. 7).

In isolated guinea-pig atria the effects of addition of 280 nM/l Bay K 8644 on extent and shape of contraction resemble those of an increase in extracellular Ca^{2+}-concentration. In accordance with the competitive antagonism between this Ca^{2+}-agonistic dihydropyridine and the Ca^{2+}-antagonistic dihydropyridines (Towart et al. 1985) Bay K 8644 leads to just the opposite effects of nifedipine (Fig. 8) but obviously different from the results obtained with catecholamines, as exemplified by the different time to peak tension and relaxation velocity (Fig. 8).

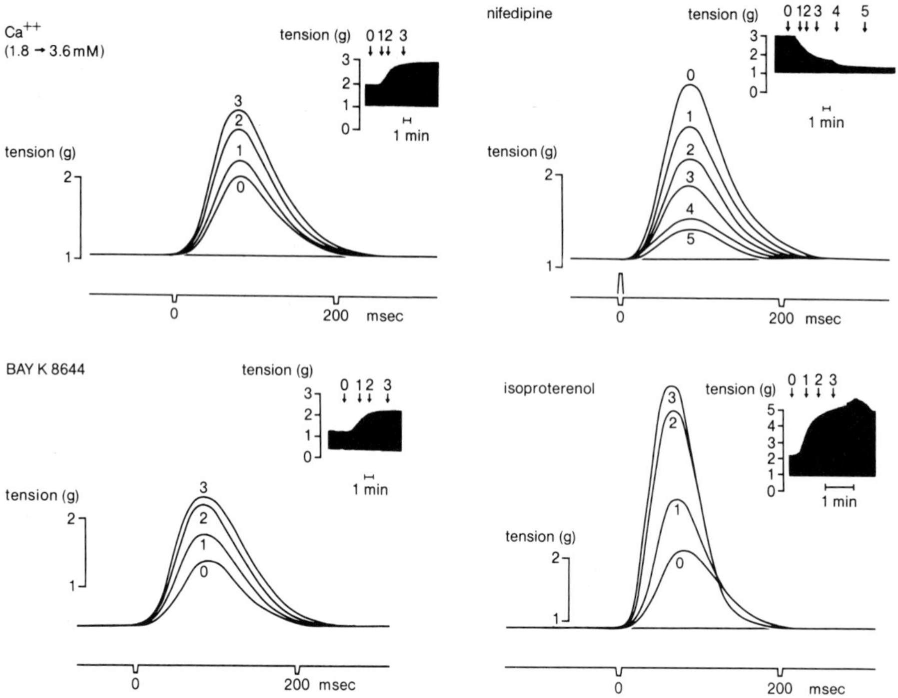

Fig. 8. Effects of increasing Ca^{2+}-concentration (*upper left panel*), adding of 280 nmol/l nifedipine (*upper right panel*), 280 nmol/l Bay K 8644 (*lower left panel*), and 300 nmol/l isoproterenol (*lower right panel*) to the bathing solution on twitch tension of guinea-pig atria. The numbers on top of the traces represent the time after application (see the inset slow traces). Stimulation frequency = 1 Hz

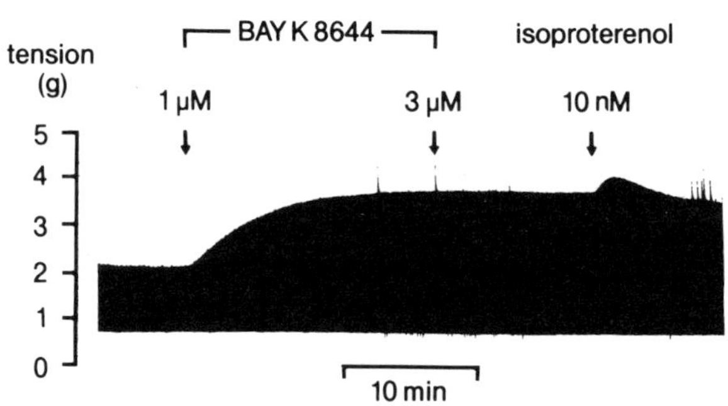

Fig. 9. Effect of 1 μmol/l and 3 μmol/l Bay K 8644 on twitch tension of a guinea-pig atrium and of the additive effect of 10 nmol/l isoproterenol. Stimulation frquency = 1 Hz

The positive inotropic effects of Bay K 8644 and of catecholamines are additive since force of contraction of isolated guinea-pig atria can be further increased by addition of 10 nM/l isoproteronol on top of a supramaximal concentration of Bay K 8644 of 3 μmol/l (Fig. 9). This indicates that the mechanisms by which Bay K 8644 increases force of contraction differ from that of catecholamines. The positive inotropic effect of Bay K 8644 in isolated guinea-pig papillary muscles is shown in Fig. 10. 280 nM/l Bay K 8644 lead to an increase of isometric force

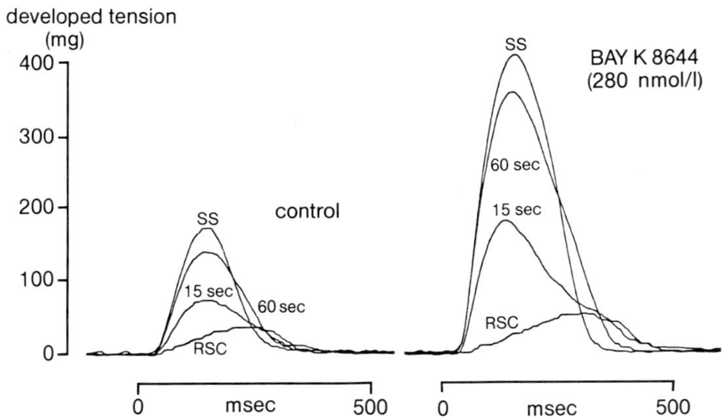

Fig. 10. Development of force of contraction of a guinea-pig papillary muscle after 15 min rest from the rested-state contraction (*RSC*), 15 s, 60 s after start of stimulation of the "steady-state" contraction (*SS*) under control conditions (*left panel*) and under the influence of 280 nmol/l Bay K 8644 (*right panel*). Stimulation frequency: 1 Hz

of contraction under steady state conditions (stimulation frequency 1 Hz) by 165%. Under rested-state conditions there is a clear prolongation of the duration of contraction in presence of Bay K 8644. This finding is in good agreement with the action potential prolonging effect (Thomas et al. 1985a) and the increased Ca^{2+}-influx into the cells (Towart et al. 1985) brought about by the compound. Since the rested-state contraction of a guinea-pig papillary muscle depends to a higher degree on transmembrane Ca^{2+}-influx as compared to steady-state conditions (Seibel et al. 1978) and this transmembraneous Ca^{2+}-influx needs obviously longer time to give rise to cytosolic Ca^{2+} as compared to Ca^{2+}-release from the sarcoplasmic reticulum, the maximal peak of developed force occurs later. The compound not only increases the height of rested-state contraction but also maintains rested-state contractions for a longer time as compared to control (Fig. 10). It is only for a couple of beats until the intracellular stores are refilled by the Ca^{2+} having flown in and the steady-state effect is observed. The time course of development of the early contraction peak after a resting-state contraction favours the idea that the refilling of the stores happens faster, probably due to the higher amount of Ca^{2+} flowing into the cell during the first beats after resting-state contraction.

In order to test whether in addition to the meanwhile known effects on the sarcolemmal membrane Bay K 8644 might have effects on the contractile elements themselves, or the sarcoplasmic reticulum, experiments were performed in skinned fibres. Over the whole concentration range from 3×10^{-8} to 3×10^{-5} mol/l there was no effect of half maximally contracted glycerol-lubrol treated fibres (see Fig. 11) nor was there any shift in the Ca^{2+}-sensitivity curve of these preparations under the influence of 1 µmol/l Bay K 8644 (see Fig. 12). This finding of a lack of effect of Bay K 8644 on the contractile elements themselves, however, does not rule out an effect of the compound on the intracellular Ca^{2+}-stores as the glycerol/lubrol treatment certainly also destroys the integrity of the sarcoplasmic

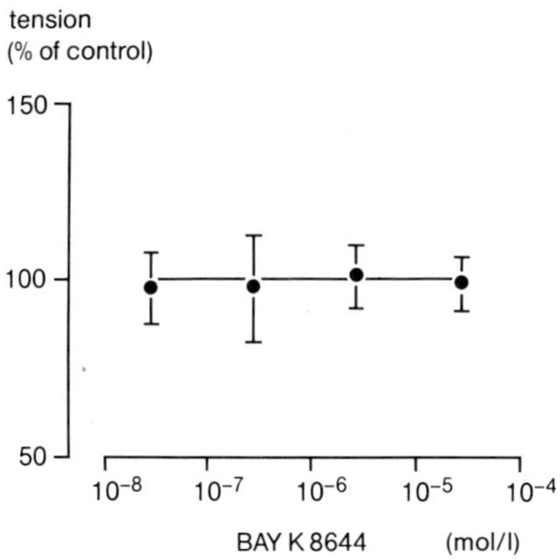

Fig. 11. Dose-response curve to Bay K 8644 for the calcium induced force of contraction of skinned cardiac fibers. Means with their standard errors from 4 fibres (Thomas et al. 1985 b)

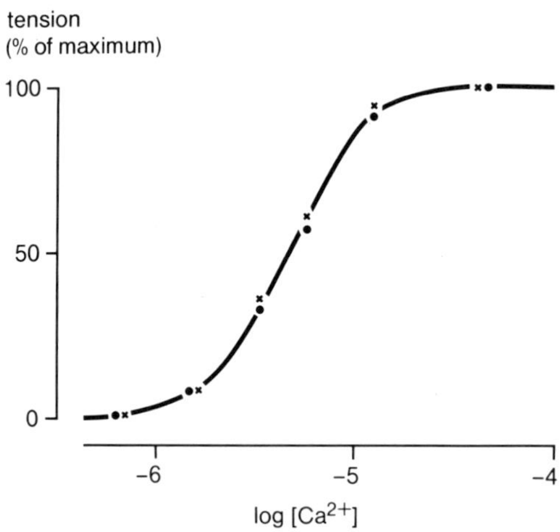

Fig. 12. Calcium-sensitivity curves of a skinned cardiac fiber in presence (x) and absence (●) of 1 μmol/l Bay K 8644 (Thomas et al. 1985 b)

reticular membranes. In saponin-treated guinea-pig trabeculae Bay K 8644 did not exhibit a "caffein-like" effect (Thomas et al. 1985 b). These findings provide further evidence for a mere action on the sarcolemmal membrane as the basic mechanism for the inotropic effect of Bay K 8644.

The dose-response curves for the isovolumetrically developed maximal pressure, the coronary perfusion pressure, and heart rate of the isovolumically perfused isolated guinea-pig heart are given in Fig. 13 as percentage of the maximal drug effect. Both perfusion pressure and left ventricular pressure increase dose dependently starting at a concentration of 10^{-9} mol/l. A maximal effect is obtained at 10^{-7} mol/l. The increase of perfusion pressure resembles the coronary vasoconstricting effect observed in anaesthetized dogs (Fig. 2). One decade higher concentrations increase heart rate. The maximal increase in heart rate amounts to about 20% of resting heart rate.

In conscious dogs there is – in contrast to the effects shown in deeply anaesthetized dogs – a high vagal tone which is reflexely further activated by pharmacologically mediated pressure rises (Scher et al. 1972). Bay K 8644 dose depen-

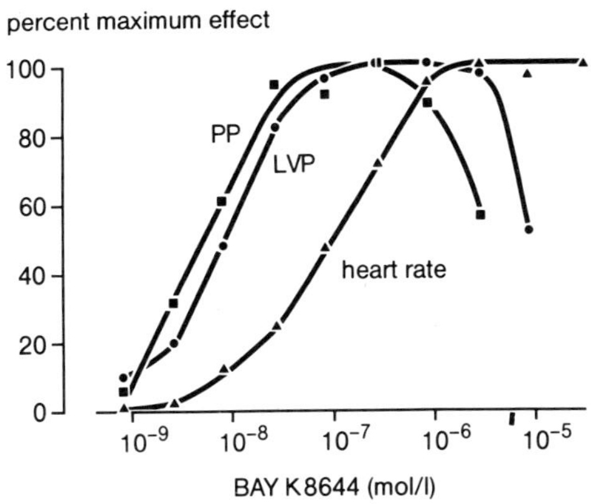

Fig. 13. Dose-response curves to Bay K 8644 with respect to perfusion pressure (*PP*), left ventricular pressure (*LVP*), and heart rate in the isovolumically perfused isolated guinea-pig heart. Each point is a mean value of 4 observations

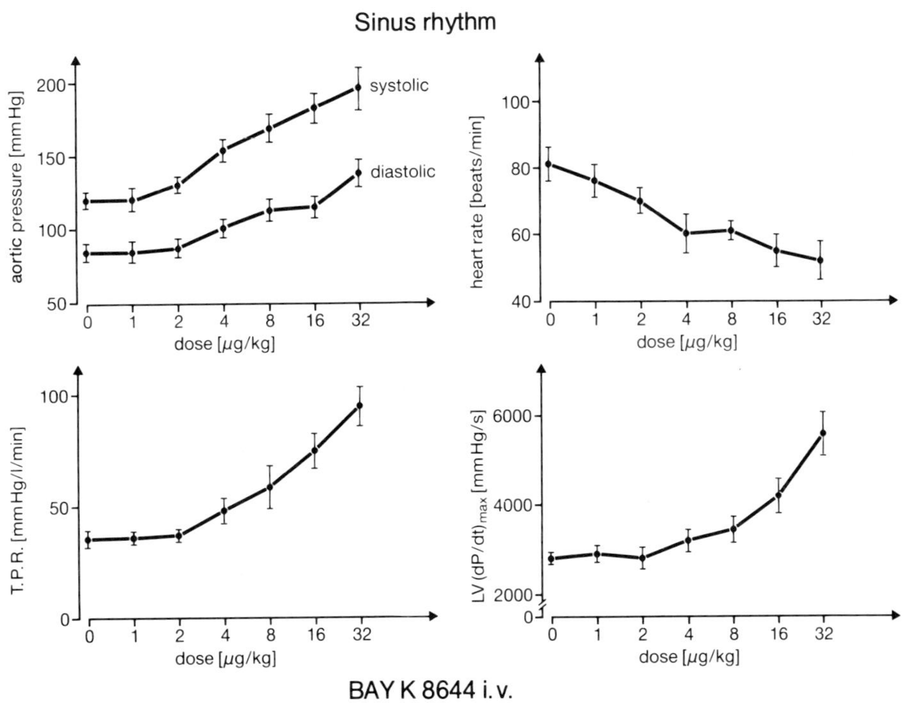

Fig. 14. Dose-response curves for Bay K 8644 i.v. in 7 conscious dogs. Given are the means with their standard errors at the time of the maximal effect in rate of rise of left ventricular pressure

dently increases both systolic and diastolic blood pressure beginning at 2 μg/kg i.v. up to 196 ± 15 mm Hg systolic and 138 ± 9 mm Hg distolic at 32 μg/kg i.v. Concomitantly, there is a drop in heart rate from a resting value of 82 beats/min down to 50 beats/min at 32 μg/kg i.v. (Fig. 14). This fall in heart rate cannot be attributed to a direct drug action since Bay K 8644 per se has a positive chronotropic effect (Fig. 13). The fall in heart rate, therefore, is probably mediated by a baroreceptor reflex counterregulation. Due to its vasoconstricting effects (Schramm et al. 1983; Towart et al. 1985) total peripheral resistance dose-dependently increases to values more than double the resting value. LV $(dP/dt)_{max}$ dose-dependently rises from resting values of 2.800 ± 150 mm Hg/s up to 5.600 ± 500 mm Hg/s at 32 μg/kg i.v.

In order to circumvent the known influence of heart rate on rate of rise of LV pressure (Furnival et al. 1970) experiments were performed in which heart rate was kept constant by right epicardial pacing at a rate of 150 beats/min. The dose response curves of these experiments are given in Fig. 15. There is a dose-dependent increase in LV $(dP/dt)_{max}$ and in arterial blood pressure which is slightly higher as compared to the results obtained at spontaneous sinus rhythm. Starting from a resting value of 2.900 ± 200 mm Hg/s LV $(dP/dt)_{max}$ increases up to 6.100 ± 800 mm Hg/s, blood pressure, rises from 130 mm Hg to 216 mm Hg (systolic) and from 100 to 162 (diastolic) as an average from data obtained in 5 dogs with their hearts paced at 150 beats/min. The transient drop in LV $(dP/dt)_{max}$ observed shortly after injection of Bay K 8644 occurs only in experiments in which heart rate is reflexely diminished but not in experiments with constant heart rate. This finding supports the idea that this transient fall is not due to the coronary constricting effect of the compound (Schramm et al. 1983) but rather is related to heart rate changes.

Since LV $(dP/dt)_{max}$ is only one parameter of inotropism, which can under certain conditions lead to misinterpretations and depends on many variables (see above, Furnival et al. 1970; Wallace et al. 1963), it was tried to abstract from these influences and to obtain ventricular function curves (Sarnoff and Mitchell 1962) in conscious dogs at a constant heart rate of 150 beats/min. Stroke work under control conditions amounts to 0.34 Nm at 4 mm Hg left ventricular end-diastolic

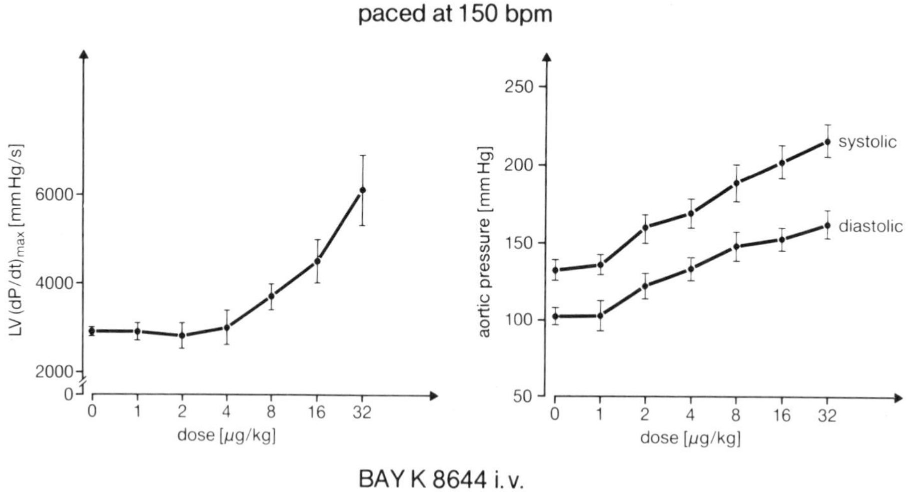

Fig. 15. Dose-response curves for Bay K 8644 i.v. in 5 conscious dogs with their hearts paced at 150 beats/min. Given are the means with their standard errors at the time of the maximal effect rate of rise of left ventricular pressure

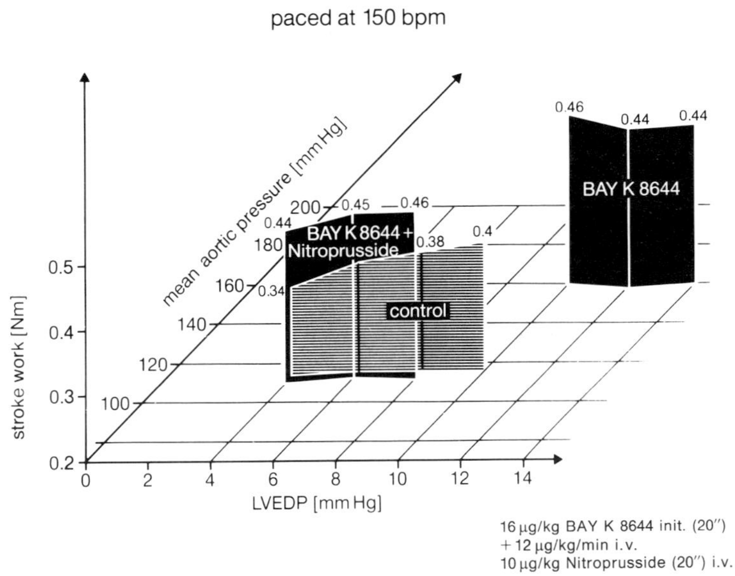

Fig. 16. Ventricular function curves in a conscious dog at rest (control), under the influence of Bay K 8644 i.v., and under the combined influence of Bay K 8644 i.v. and nitroprusside i.v.

pressure and 115 mm Hg mean aortic pressure. By spontaneous changes in preload and heart rate it reaches 0.40 Nm at 10 mm Hg left ventricular enddiastolic pressure. By injection of 16 µg/kg Bay K 8644 i.v. during 20 s followed by a continuous infusion of 12 µg/kg/min i.v. a steady-state is reached: the ventricular function curve is shifted to the upper right. Stroke work increases to 0.46 and 0.44 Nm at LVEDP between 10 and 14 mm Hg but against a mean aortic pressure of 160 mm Hg. In order to abstract from the effects of aortic pressure on stroke work, during the steady-state of drug action an i.v. injection of 10 µg/kg sodium nitroprusside was given over 20 s, a dose appropriate to bring mean aortic blood pressure back to its resting value (Fig. 16). At matched left ventricular end-diastolic pressures stroke work was clearly increased by 21% to 29% indicating that Bay K 8644 enables the heart to perform a higher work with the same preload and against the same aortic pressure: the ventricular function curve lies well above control as evidence of the positive inotropic effect.

In summary, Bay K 8644 is a new positive inotropic and vasoconstrictive compound which differs in many respects from other inotropic substances, both in structure and in its cellular mechanism. Since this compound induces a new mechanism, it seems to be an interesting pharmacological tool. It also shows that the class of dihydropyridines is obviously able to truly modulate Ca^{2+}-influx into the cell. Moreover, it offers a novel mechanism of positive inotropic drug action which could lead to the development of powerful drugs for the treatment of congestive heart failure.

References

Furnival CM, Linden RJ, Snow HM (1970) Inotropic changes in the left ventricle: the effect of changes in heart rate, aortic pressure and end-diastolic pressure. J Physiol 211:359–387

Gross R, Kirchheim K, von Olshausen K (1979) Effect of Nimodipine on coronary and systemic hemodynamics in the conscious dog. Arzneim Forsch/Drug Res 29:1361–1368

Herd JA, Barger J (1964) Simplified technique for chronic catheterization of blood vesssels. J Appl Physiol 19:791–792

Herzig JW, Köhler G, Pfitzer G, Rüegg JC, Wölffle G (1981) Cyclic AMP inhibits contractility of detergent treated glycerol extracted cardiac muscle. Pflügers Arch 391:208–212

Langendorff O (1895) Untersuchungen am überlebenden Säugetierherzen. Pflügers Arch Ges Physiol 6:291–332

Meyer H, Wehinger E, Bossert F, Böshagen H, Franckowiak G, Goldmann S, Seidel W, Stoltefuß J (1985) Chemistry of 1,4-Dihydropyridines. This volume.

Opie L (1965) Coronary flow rate and perfusion pressure as determinants of mechanical function and oxidative metabolism of isolated perfused rat heart. J Physiol 180:529–541

Sarnoff SJ, Mitchell JH (1961) The control of the function of the heart. In: Handbook of Physiology, Circulation, Sec 2, Vol 1. Amer Physiol Soc, Washington

Scher AM, Ohm WW, Bumgarner K, Boynton R, Young AC (1972) Sympathetic and parasympathetic control of heart rate in the dog, baboon and man. Fed Proc 31:1219–1225

Schramm M, Thomas G, Franckowiak G (1983) Novel dihydropyridines with positive inotropic action through activation of Ca^{2+} channels. Nature 303:535–537

Seibel K, Karema E, Takeya K, Reiter M (1978) Effect of noradrenaline on an early and a late component of the myocardial contraction. Naunyn-Schmiedeberg's Arch Pharmacol 305:65–74

Thomas G, Chung M, Cohen CJ (1985a) A dihydropyridine (Bay K 8644) that enhances calcium currents in myocardial cells: a new type of positive inotropic agents. Circ Res 56:87–96

Thomas G, Gross R, Pfitzer G, Rüegg JC (1985b) The positive inotropic dihydropyridine Bay K 8644 does not affect calcium sensitivity or calcium release of skinned cardiac fibres. Naunyn Schmiedeberg's Arch Pharmacol 328:378–381

Towart R, Kazda S, Lamp B, Thomas G, Schramm M (1985) Effect of dihydropyridine calcium channel modulators on isolated peripheral and cerebral vessels. This volume

Wallace AG, Skinner JR NS, Mitchell JH (1963) Hemodynamic determinants of the maximal rate of rise of left ventricular pressure. Am J Physiol 205:30–36

Discussion

(pp. 218–232)

Godfraind: Can you explain why the additive action of isoprenaline and BAY K 8644 was not sustained?

Groß: It might be that there was a fast degradation by oxidation of the catecholamine. We tried to do further experiments with different dosages of isoproterenol but there was the problem that due to arrhythmias reliable measurements of tension were not possible for the whole dose range.

Brown: I am interested to see that you see no change in sinus rhythm. Does that mean that these compounds do not affect the slow inward current driving the pacemaker at all? If so, why is this current resistant?

Groß: In the deeply anaesthetised dog, there is no heart-rate effect, but there is a clear-cut effect on the sinus node itself: the compound has positive chronotropic activity as shown by dose-response curves of a Langendorff preparation at spontaneous sinus rhythm. However, in a conscious dog with an active baro-reflex counterregulation you even get a decrease in hart rate. This is comparable to the effect when you inject noradrenaline into conscious dogs: You have a direct positive chronotropic action which is reflexely counteracted. From the mechanism of action of BAY K 8644 and what we learned about the Ca^{2+}-channels we would expect a positive chronotropic action and we do see it.

Graefe: What was the absolute increase in heart rate you have observed in the Langendorff preparation? The second question is: You stressed that the drug-induced decrease in heart rate in vivo is a consequence of the increase in blood pressure and triggered by the baroreflex mechanism. Have you seen any increase in heart rate in vivo after pretreatment with atropine?

Groß: We did not perform the experiment with atropine in the conscious dog but in anaesthetised dogs pretreated with atropine we see no change in heart rate. The maximal increase of heart rate in the Langendorff heart was about 20% of the resting heart rate.

Kadowitz: I was very surprised by the effects of the calcium agonist and its lack of effect on cardiac output. I understand that in the deeply anaesthetised dog you did have a very large increase in systemic arterial pressure, so impedance is increased, but in the conscious animal there was a very modest increase in systemic arterial pressure and I also understand that you had a bradycardia. Now, in the paced animal I would have expected to see you unmask an effect on cardiac output and all agents that are used in the treatment of congestive heart failure increase cardiac output. What happened after you unloaded the animal with nitroprusside: You should have unmasked an increase in cardiac output and stroke volume under these conditions.

Groß: From the experiments with ventricular function curves under nitroprusside you can read an increase in stroke work at constant heart rate, same preload against the same aortic pressure, hence a rise in stroke volume.

Kadowitz: It is just hard for me to believe that in a heart that has normal characteristics that the impedance could really affect stroke volume that much. Although Dr. Warltier tells me that he has seen similar data. There must be something else going on with this Ca^{2+}-agonist that we don't fully understand. We don't see it with catecholamine inotropic stimulation or even digitalis which produces an increase in the total peripheral resistance in these preparations. Dr. Schwartz proposes us a mechanism: coronary vasoconstriction.

Groß: If you look at the time course, shortly after the injection there is a diminution of LV (dP/dt) min which is an estimate for an ischemic reaction. And there is a transient decrease of stroke volume. After this minimum both increase again.

Warltier: There is another explanation for the effects on heart rate that you see between conscious and anaesthetised animals. In conscious animals when we give a bolus of BAY K 8644, we see a nice reflex bradycardia as well. During constant infusion of this drug, however, we see absolutely no change in heart rate, and this is quite different from the prominent reflex bradycardia one gets with equipressor infusions of a drug like phenylephrine. So I do not think it is just simply due to the effects of anesthesia. When we have concomitant nitroprusside to control mean arterial pressure during BAY K 8644 we expected to possibly see an increase in heart rate if the drug had direct effects. We did not observe this.

Groß: Also with constant infusion, or oral administration of the drug we see a reflex bradycardia.

Taira: How did BAY K 8644 affect myocardial oxygen consumption in anaesthetised dogs and unanaesthetised dogs with nitroprusside infused.

Groß: We did not measure oxygen consumption in conscious dogs. Dr. Schramm found that in anaesthetised dogs without nitroprusside oxygen saturation in the coronary sinus decreased. This could be due to two effects, both vasoconstriction and increase of consumption.

Scriabine: I wonder what is the explanation for the secondary increase in coronary blood flow after BAY K 8644. Is that really a metabolic effect? Wouldn't you consider a possibility that this increase in coronary blood flow is an evidence of Ca^{2+}-antagonist action of BAY K 8644 on coronary vessels?

Groß: We see a transient coronary constriction at the beginning of the injection. If the secondary increase would be due to a Ca^{2+}-antagonistic effect of high doses of the drug as observed in isolated tissue, then increasing the dose should abolish the transient constriction at the beginning and depress the positive inotropic effect, too. Since both are still there, this explanation seems unlikely.

Nayler: We have heard a lot about the effects of these drugs on peripheral resistance and peak developed tensions. What happened to the biochemistry of the heart muscle.

Groß: We have not measured this.

Nayler: What happens to the regional distribution of flow? It is allright to say coronary flow goes up or down, but what happened to the regional distribution?

Groß: We didn't measure regional flow distribution.

Scriabine: What is the mechanism of ventricular arrhythmias after toxic doses of BAY K 8644? Are these effects due to a direct effect of Ca^{2+} entry leading to Ca^{2+} overload or can catecholamine release may also be involved?

Groß: They might both be involved. In isolated organs at high concentrations arrhythmias occur, this is in favour of a direct drug-effect. We have no data so far on catecholamine release.

Fleckenstein: Under the influence of the Ca^{2+}-agonist there is probably in most cases a mixed effect of direct Ca^{2+} influx promotion and Ca^{2+} influx promotion by beta-receptor stimulation because the catecholamine release is also Ca^{2+} mediated. Experiments on isolated preparations – especially electrophysiological ones – are in most cases clearer than those carried out in the whole animal which very often resembles a black box. You have stimulated an extended and interesting discussion. Thank you very much.

Bayer-Symposium IX
Cardiovascular Effects of Dihydropyridine-Type
Calcium Antagonists and Agonists, 236–247

Myocardial Effects of Dihydropyridines in Patients

P. G. HUGENHOLTZ, J. W. DE JONG, and P. W. SERRUYS

Introduction

Of the many possible applications of the dihydropyridines in clinical cardiology, I have chosen to talk only about conditions in which acute cardiac ischemia is present. This the more so since Lichtlen (1984) and Buhler (1984), respectively, will talk about the effects of these compounds on the coronary vasculature and on the peripheral vasculature in hypertension.

Acute myocardial ischemia in humans occurs often, perhaps more often than suspected, since some authors claim that 80% of all ischemic episodes may be asymptomatic. However, four ischemic conditions present themselves to the clinician during which a patient happens to be well instrumented, can be carefully monitored and is able to provide us with a set of data from which the evidence for cardiac protection with dihydropyridines can be deduced.

These are respectively: patients requiring acute cardiovascular surgery going on or off cardiopulmonary bypass, intermittent acute coronary obstruction such as seen during the percutaneous transluminal angioplasty (PTCA) procedure, observations with acute unstable angina pectoris in patients already in the coronary care unit, and finally in those individuals who in the first hours after onset of symptoms for acute myocardial infarction undergo a procedure with desobstruction of the coronary artery thrombus, for example, with intracoronary streptokinase. The latter for lack of space cannot be disucssed. All four conditions have in common not only that relevant observations can be made but they offer the clinician the chance of treating his patients with the dihydropyridines where their cardioprotective, in addition to other, effects are most desired. These are situations where the drug can be given prior to or immediately after the onset of ischemia and they also provide circumstances where the effects of these drugs on the coronary circulation itself or on peripheral arterial resistance are minor or can be ignored, since both are more or less bypassed as a result of the intervention. By way of contrast, current trials where these drugs have been given to patients with fully developed myocardial infarction will be briefly discussed since they provide equally strong arguments to consider this application a contraindication to the use of these drugs.

It is a very logical concept that a cardiac cell threatened by oxygen shortage should be induced to reduce its metabolic activity to enhance its chances for survival. The same goes for the surrounding cardiac tissues. Indeed, the currently accepted rationale for the use of beta-adrenoceptor antagonists is that these drugs inhibit the positive chronotropic and inotropic effects of excessive sympathetic stimulation and thus reduce oxygen consumption. Experimental evidence recently presented by Saxena (1983) indicates that overall transmural bloodflow to the ischemic zone may or may not increase after beta-blocker therapy but that there is usually a redistribution of flow in favor of the endocardium where the effects of ischemia would be earliest noted. Mechanisms for this favourable redistribution are: the increase in the diastolic filling period and changes in autoregulation of the vasomotor tone. On the other hand, beta-blockers have been shown to increase coronary vasomotor tone and thus to reduce coronary flow. As far as calcium antagonists go, experimental evidence gathered from nifedipine, verapamil and diltiazem, strongly confirms their primary dilatory action on the epicardial coronary arteries so that coronary flow is markedly increased, including collateral bloodflow as well as the capillary bloodflow in the ischemic region (Verdouw et al. 1981). It therefore seems attractive to recommend in incipient ischemic states, a combination of beta-blockers and calcium antagonists.

Schmutzler (1981), Dargie et al. (1981), Verdouw et al. (1983). De Jong et al. (1983), as well as Vanhaleweyk et al. (1983) and Wolffenbuttel and Verdouw (1983) have demonstrated in the animal that various combinations have greater efficacy in reducing the ischemic state than a beta-blocker or calcium antagonist can achieve alone. We have repeatedly argued that their combination apart from being synergistic could reduce their respective (unwanted) side-effects (Hugenholtz et al. 1983).

The unique cardioprotective effects of the calcium antagonists in reducing excessive calcium influx, thus avoiding the early disruption of the intracellular apparatus, have major attractions. In a 1982 review on pharmacological salvage of myocardium, Lange and Sobel wrote: "During the past decade, efforts to limit the extent of myocardium exhibiting infarction once ischemia has been initiated, have focused on manipulation of myocardial oxygen supply and demand as well as on the process of injury itself. Interventions or promises range from the conventional, moderate increase in inspired oxygen content to the administration of hyaluronidase or intracoronary thrombolysis to augment the oxygen supply, the use of beta-adrenergic blocking drugs and nitroglycerine to diminish demand, and the administration of calcium antagonists and prostaglandin synthesis inhibitors to limit the injury process. The ultimate effects on infarct size and long-term mortality have yet to be established unequivocally for any of these approaches in the clinical setting of an acute myocardial infarction, but significant preservation of ischemic myocardium with cardioplegia and with administration of nifedipine during coronary artery bypass surgery have been documented." They conclude "Several prospective large scale blinded random sample selection clinical trials are currently in progress. Their results should definitively elucidate the clinical utility of specific interventions and should help to further improve the management of patients with ischemic heart disease." Unfortunately, by now, mid 1984, only few of these trials have been published and some have addressed the wrong clinical population, in my view, since they concentrate on myocardial infarction, after this has been established.

Coronary bloodflow is capable of autoregulation, rising in situations with increasing O_2 demand and falling with reduced O_2 demand. This adjustment is achieved by means of appropriate alterations in coronary vascular resistance via various, mainly humoral, factors. A primary increase in vascular tone, with a reduction in coronary artery lumen is therefore highly unfavourable. Furthermore, as the major part of the coronary bloodflow through the myocardium occurs during diastole its duration and the aortic diastolic pressure level determine the adequacy of perfusion. Tachycardia which encroaches upon diastole tends to reduce coronary bloodflow as does decreased arterial perfusion pressure in the distal coronary circulation, such as may occur with coronary stenoses. Consequently, reduced aortic pressure, increased left ventricular filling pressure, and tachycardia all are to be avoided as they will reduce supply even further. In fact, nifedipine, if given orally or sublingually in adequate doses, will achieve these three effects rather quickly, all of which are unfavourable, but it will increase coronary artery flow. All of these provide arguments to give this drug early for cardioprotection, preferably through the intra-coronary route. On the other hand, myocardial oxygen consumption varies also with the contractile state of the myocardium, the heart rate, the wall tension, and the duration of contraction. Wall tension or wall stress is determined by afterload which reflects the prevailing aortic pressure and the ventricular muscle mass. Where there is an enhancement of contractile state, such as with an increased heartrate, or with elevated aortic systolic pressure, or when there is an increase in preload, such as with an elevated left ventricular diastolic filling pressure or diastolic volume, myocardial oxygen demand must increase further unbalancing an already primarily disturbed balance between supply and demand. Here again, calcium antagonists will be able to exert a favourable influence.

Parratt summarizes all these considerations in an excellent review of the subject in 1983, when he says: "On theoretical grounds there appear two possible approaches:

1) attempts to prevent infarction in patients who are most at risk such as those with unstable angina or who undergo reinfarction after having suffered an earlier ischemic tissue damaging event.
2) Attempts to reduce the most serious consequences of ischemia such as the suppression of life-threatening ventricular arrhythmias and limiting the extent and severity of myocardial and coronary vascular ischemic damage, preferably by combination of anti-ischemic therapy and rapid coronary arterial reperfusion. The main point of giving drugs in this situation would therefore be to buy time until bloodflow can be reestablished either by aggressive means such as thrombolysis or through the natural expansion of the collateral circulation."

I would strongly support these comments as they are the basic philosophy with which clinicians currently should operate in this field. Rather than to concentrate on effects to study the effects of the dihydropyridines on patients in whom myocardial infarction has already been established, under which circumstances these drugs can be expected to be as inefficacious as are nitroglycerine, nitroprusside and other powerful vasodilators one should refocus on those conditions where timely (if not prophylactic) use of these drugs is still possible. Evidence provided by Muller et al. (1984) has recently shown the uselessness of treating myocardial infarction with nifedipine.

Acute Ischemia During Open Heart Surgery

During open heart surgery there are short periods during which the bloodsupply through the heart has to be stopped such as for example during cannulation. Also during the usual induction of hypothermia and the subsequent rewarming period, there are transient disturbances in oxygen demand and supply. Whilst the overall myocardial damage, induced by the use of the cardiopulmonary bypass procedure, is restricted through cooling and the induction of electromechanical arrest, there is, during most various cardiovascular surgery procedures, evidence for the release for cardiac enzymes; other signs indicating frank myocardial infarction occur in 5 to 10% of all cases. Serruys et al. (1980) in our laboratory have shown that, when regional epicardial movements during systole are carefully measured, normal contractile behaviour in areas not even directly affected by the surgeons knife, fails to return to normal until six weeks after the procedure. Apparently, there are several periods during the procedure of open heart surgery that the myocardium can suffer considerable damage. Perhaps the most obvious of these occurs during reperfusion. Whilst such damage is difficult to demonstrate in terms of outright mortality, except perhaps in patients with multi valvular disease with severely damaged hypertrophic and dilated hearts, as shown by Clark et al. (1979), it is very plausible that if more subtle measurement techniques could be provided, significant damage in the otherwise healthy myocardium could be demonstrated as a consequence of "uncomplicated" open heart surgery. In fact, in his presidential address, entitled "Intellectual creativity in thoracic surgeons" Spencer (1983) discussed several major breakthroughs in cardiovascular surgery over the past 30 years. One of these topics relates on the preservation of cardiac function and he points to the need for further improvements in this area. Buckberg et al. (1975) asked themselves therefore a different question: "Why should a heart which did not need pharmacological or mechanical support before operation require these interventions after the cardiac lesion has been corrected?". In earlier studies from our laboratory Brower et al. (1982) showed that when intermittent clamping of the aorta, a technique previously frequently used, was compared to potassium cardioplegia, the results were considerably more damaging to myocardial contractility. In fact, the amount of creatine kinase released was three times as high as with the former technique. Furthermore, Van der Vusse et al. (1984) has recently shown that when ATP, creatine phosphate and glycogen content are measured in human myocardial biopsies at the time of surgery (as markers for the efficacy of cardioprotection during the aorto-coronary bypass surgery), continuous aortic cross clamping with multidose St. Thomas cardioplegia did not result in any change in the above indicators. By contrast hypothermic intermittent cross clamping resulted in a significant reduced tissue content of these markers of myocardial energy supply.

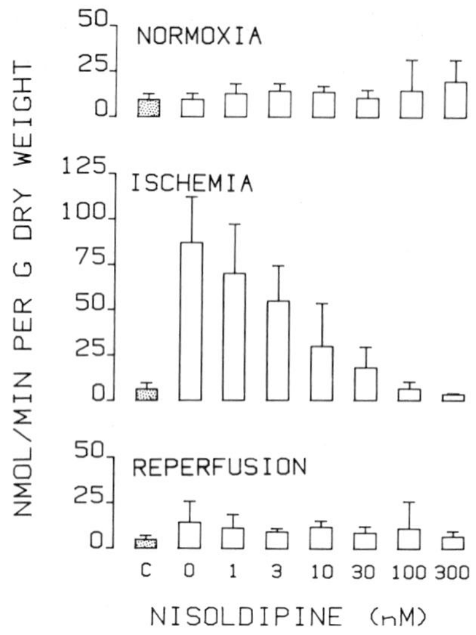

Fig. 1. In an isolated ratheart (Langendorff preparation) the effect of increasing dosis of nisoldipine was such that the release of ATP derivatives was shown to be completely suppressed at the highest levels. The preparation was rendered ischemic for 15 min, during which a massive release of purine derivatives was seen under control circumstances (*C*). Nisoldipine was given 15 min prior to the experimental ischemic episode (De Jong et al. 1984)

De Jong (1985) in a recent overview has argued on the basis of strong evidence from his own laboratory and from other studies that the rapid breakdown of high-energy phosphate can be interrupted when verapamil, nifedipine, diltiazem or nisoldipine are given prior to the induction of ischemia. Furthermore, the efficacy of nifedipine and nisoldipine was demonstrated by his group to be dose dependent (Fig. 1; De Jong et al. 1982). Accordingly he recommends that the current habit to protect the myocardium by means of electro mechanical arrest via potassium cardioplegia with reduction in energy consumption through hypothermia should be strongly supported. In fact, since the regulation of calcium transport is the main factor, combining arrest with reduced O_2 consumption, the timely use of calcium antagonists presents itself strongly as an added feature. Yet, only two clinical studies have been reported which support the experimental evidence provided by others. Clark et al. (1983) report the beneficial effects of nifedipine in a large scale trial of patients undergoing open heart surgery, whilst recently lidoflazine was shown by Flameng et al. (1983) to have a strong protective effect in extensive aorto coronary artery bypass grafting. In the latest study evidence also was provided through electronmicroscopy. Clearly then in this, potentially immensely important, area of application, insufficient studies with the use of calcium antagonists have been reported so far and it is to be welcomed that there are ongoing studies (Hauf et al. 1984).

Intermittent Ischemia in the Catheterisation Laboratory and the Coronary Care Unit

A perhaps still more subtle form of induced ischemia in humans occurs during the percutaneous transluminal angioplasty procedure. Here, ischemia is willfully induced by inflation of a cuff balloon around an intra coronary catheter in an effort to dislodge, compress or tear the atheromatous plaque. As the indications for such a non surgical desobstruction of coronary artery stenosis are expanding and the number of vessels, which will be "treated" is increasing, the total time that the myocardium distal to the intentional obstruction may become ischemic, will equally become longer. Occlusion times of up to 10 min have now been reported.

Initially after an occlusion, that is to say within 10 to 15 seconds the coronary sinus efflux will contain increasing amounts of H^+-ions and shortly afterwards K^+-ions. These are the first substances to leak from the cell during ischemia. They are shortly thereafter followed by lactate and the various break down products of the high energy phosphate metabolism, such as hypoxanthine. At approximately this time the regional myocardial contraction diminishes, and eventually ceases. In effect, within 28 beats after the onset of total occlusion, mechanical action of that particular regional segment can be demonstrated to have ceased. Recently Serruys et al. (1984a, b) reported that regional anaerobic metabolism is reversible, provided this interval is short. They studied 10 patients in whom transient transluminal occlusion lasting for 30 to 65 s was repeated between 2 and 7 times. To assess the extent of ischemia in the area perfused by the left anterior descending artery, coronary sinus and great cardiac vein flow were measured during each transluminal occlusion period. Differences between the aortic and great coronary vein concentrations of lactate and hypoxanthine, as the most readily measurable catabolite of adenosine monophosphate, were determined prior to the PTCA procedure, 5 to 15 s after each occlusion and 15 min after completion of the procedure, as shown in Table 1 and Fig. 2–5. These shortlived occlusions leading to glycolysis and an excess of ATP breakdown are apparently reversible. When the same group looked at the effect of repeated trans luminal occlusion on global and regional left ventricular chamber stiffness, they found that global stiffness was transiently increased and furthermore that regional stiffness in the ischemic zone, induced by the angioplasty procedure, remained augmented up to 15 min after the procedure. Severe regional changes in relaxation (Serruys et al. 1984a), are an early sign of dysfunctioning of the ventricle, presumably because of a disturbance in calcium transport (Table 2). These data indicate that the boundary between reversible and irreversible damage may occur approximately

Table 1. Myocardial release of hypoxanthine and lactate during repeated coronary angioplasty in 10 patients (Serruys et al. 1984b)

	Pre PTCA	TO peak data	TO pooled data	Post PTCA
CSF ml/min	154	–	115★	169
GCVF ml/min	85	–	56★	96
A-GCV-LC mmol/l	+ 0.12	−0.88★	− 0.47★	+ 0.11
A-GCV-Hx µmol/l	+ 0.23	−3.13★	− 1.34°	+ 0.25
		°p<.01	★p<.005	

PTCA = percutaneous transluminal angioplasty; CSF = coronary sinus flow; GCVF = great coronary vein flow; A = arterial; LC = lactate; Hx = hypoxanthine; TO = transluminal occlusion

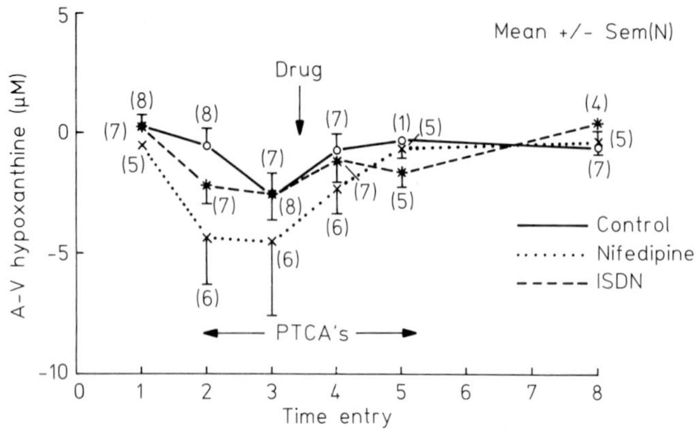

Fig. 2. The level of myocardial hypoxanthine efflux from the coronary sinus is measured just before (*1*), after the first (*2*) and second (*3*) PTCA. When nifedipine or isosorbide dinitrate is given before the third PTCA (*4*) there is no release of hypoxanthine although in the average of 6 experiments before nifedipine there had been marked hypoxanthine production during the first (unprotected) PTCA. It should be noted that the release of hypoxanthine was also less in the control group, presumably because of recruitment of collateral flow. (*5*) = fourth PTCA; (*8*) = 15 min after last PTCA

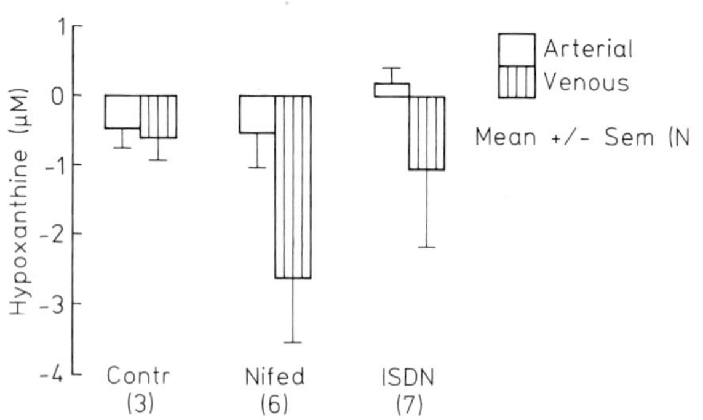

Fig. 3. The data from the second series of patients studied during PTCA restated to show the difference of arterio-venous hypoxanthine levels in control and treatment patients by subtracting the level of the first and the second determination averaged from that obtained during the third PTCA. It can now be shown that the greatest reduction in hypoxanthine release is obtained by nifedipine pretreatment.

15 min after interruption of blood flow in the human situation. These data correspond to those reported by Jennings et al. (1975) and Schaper (1983) for experimental ischemia induced in animals. A number of years ago Nayler and Poole-Wilson (1981) had already indicated that either during experimental interruption of blood supply or during a cardiopulmonary bypass procedure, relatively short-lived periods of ischemia, varying between 15 and 60 min, could induce permanent damage to the intracellular cardiac metabolism. They also demonstrated in eloquent experiments that the prior adminstration of calcium antagonists and or beta-blockers could protect cells, rendered ischemic under those circumstances, completely.

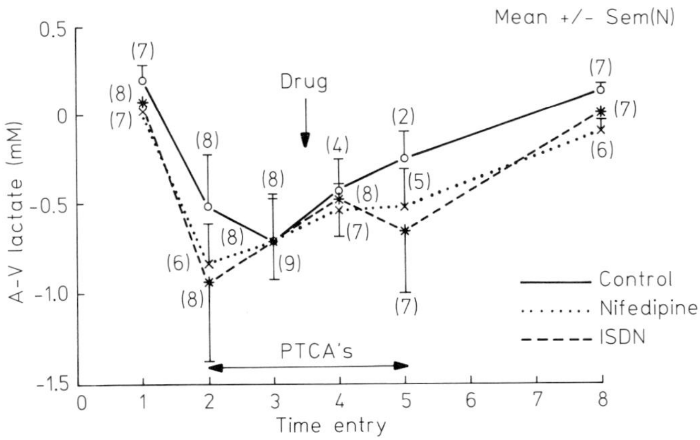

Fig. 4. Myocardial lactate efflux after and during PTCA. Explanation as in legend of Fig. 2. There is no obvious difference between control or nifedipine or isosorbide dinitrate pretreated patients

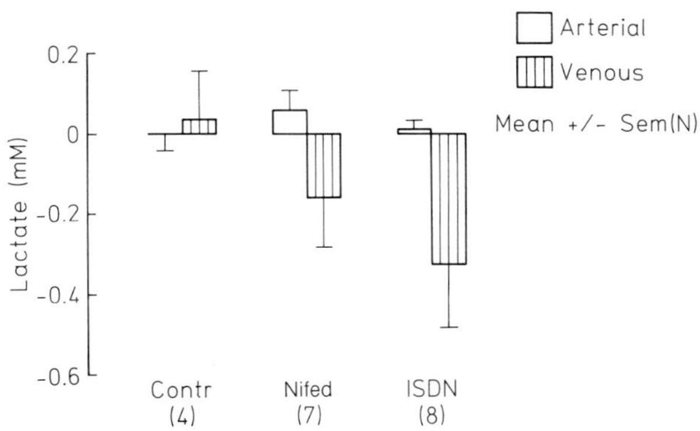

Fig. 5. For lactate the greatest reduction in production is achieved with isosorbide dinitrate

Table 2. Hemodynamic changes before (pre), during occlusion of 20 and 50 seconds duration and after 15 min. Note how there is a rapid increase in end-diastolic pressure which returns to normal afterwards. In contrast, the stiffness parameters βV, βL IZ, and βL BZ remain abnormal. An example of a "stunned" myocardium (Serruys et al. 1984c)

	Pre	20 s occl	50 s occl	Post
EDP (mmHg)	19.6	22.3	30.0*	19.0
EDVI (ml/m^2)	78	82	87	85
βV (ml/m^2)	0.023	0.065*	0.065*	0.044
βL IZ (cm)	3.1	5.6*	5.4	6.5*
βL BZ (cm)	2.8	6.6*	7.6*	5.9
βL NIZ (cm)	4.0	5.0	5.5	3.6

* Denotes a significant difference, $p<0.05$
EDP = left ventricular end-diastolic pressure; EDVI = end-diastolic volume index; β = constant of global (or regional) chamber stiffness; V = volume; L = length; IZ = ischemic zone; BZ = border zone; NIZ = non-ischemic zone

It would appear therefore that dihydropyridines, in particular during the phase when reperfusion takes place, whether after open heart surgery or balloon dilatation, will find their "Finest Hour" (Churchill 1948). With rewarming the protection from hypothermia has been removed. With reperfusion the necessary potassium excess will be washed out, oxygen returns through the reestablished blood flow to the cell and, in the first instance, the cells in the vascular wall are threatened with the socalled "calcium paradox". In fact, in surgical conditions as well, the vasculature will have been induced to excessive high concentrations of potassium leading to further vascular stiffness while during PTCA such potassium excess will automatically follow. Since under experimental conditions, Fleckenstein (1983) has indicated that calcium antagonists are particularly effective in reducing spasm induced by potassium, it would appear most important to administer these drugs early on. Whether the dihydropyridines exert their beneficial influence primarily through their action on the vascular wall or primarily through their action on myocardial tissue will ultimately remain a moot point in the individual case.

Unstable Angina Pectoris in the Coronary Care Unit

In unstable angina pectoris, there is relatively little definite information in the literature regarding the exact mechanism of action of calcium antagonism. This is readily explicable because of the uncertainties surrounding the causes of unstable angina pectoris. Despite emphasis on the role of coronary artery spasm, recently reemphasized by three excellent books (Opie 1984; Stone and Antman 1983; Fleckenstein 1983) it has still not been generally accepted that this occurs more than in a relatively few cases. The general assumption is more that fixed organic stenosis through atherosclerotic involvement of the arterial wall with increased tonus of the uninvolved parts of the wall is the usual cause. Although it is now known that obstruction is not always concentric and, indeed, frequently may be eccentric, the concept of fixed stenosis has remained. In the majority of patients with unstable angina, however, the anatomical situation probably lies between fixed stenosis and frank spasm. Particularly when excentric lesions are present which leave part of the circumference of the vascular wall intact (or hypersensitive), vasoconstrictive stimuli may cause marked changes in the tone of that part of the vessel wall and thus influence the coronary blood flow to reduce blood supply.

Several authors have now demonstrated spontaneous changes in coronary vascular resistance independent of identifiable changes in myocardial metabolic demand. During exercise just as with mental stress or inhalation of cold air, such vasoconstrictive reactions may occur and be an explanation both for the "walk through phenomenon" (being a spontaneous reduction in tone), mental adaptation and for the action of calcium antagonists.

The hypothesis has also been put forward that there is a subset of patients with angina with inappropriate vasoconstriction, which may worsen with beta-adrenergic blockade. In fact, Yasue et al. (1976, 1979) have specifically argued against beta-blockers in these individuals, as they showed that beta-blockers may induce vasoconstrictive action. Since in our unstable angina patients who had remained unresponsive during 8 h of beta-blockade (Hugenholtz et al. 1981), the response to nifedipine was so consistent (and just as effective as had been pain relief by intraaortic balloon pumping in our previous experience with the same kind of patients), there is little doubt that nifedipine was the critical agent. Several authors state that there now might very well be a preference for the use of Ca^{2+} antagonists over beta-blockade in patients suspected of having abnormally increased coronary vasomotor tone (Muller et al. 1984).

This concept of disturbed dynamic coronary obstruction in the presence of "normal" or mildly diseased coronary arteries implies a direct role for coronary vasodilators in patients with any form of angina pectoris, even when frank coronary spasm is absent. Also implicit in the hypothesis is the concept that the dynamic and fixed components may contribute variably to the degree of obstruction in different patients. It should not be surprising therefore that in patients with largely fixed obstructions, benefit will mainly come from attemps to lower myocardial O_2 utpake with beta-blocking agents while in those with mainly vasomotor derangement will benefit primarily from calcium antagonists and nitrates.

It is clear that in unstable angina the primary action of the dihydropyridines lics in their vasodilating action. However, we have argued before (Hugenholtz et al. 1982) that when repeated episodes of interruption of vascular supply have caused biochemical derangements, a state of "stunned" myocardium occurs. The region is mechanically inactive but still viable and, it is here that the dihydropyridines would have their most exciting application because the cellular "cardioprotective" element comes into play.

Myocardial ischemia in the first steps of its generation is essentially a regional phenomenon. If bloodflow, however modest, with respect to local demand, becomes inadequate regional myocardial ischemia will occur and contractile function of those ischemic cells will be rapidly lost. As repeatedly observed at cardiac catheterization, myocardial abnormalities such as dyskinesia may take place in a given region, with the ischemic segment becoming stiffer, in turn leading to increased enddiastolic pressure and volume and thus worsening the situation. Such a rise in left ventricular diastolic pressure would, by itself, tend to worsen ischemia, via an increase in myocardial oxygen demand and by reduction in oxygen supply through the (compressed) capillary bed. This can become the starting round of another bout of increasing ischemia. If then also pain occurs, symphathetic stimulation of nerve endgings will lead to the further release of catecholamines, which, as Nayler (1984) has shown in this symposium, already are leaking from the cardiac cell within a few minutes of ischemia. All these tend to increase the existing tachycardia and will further raise bloodpressure thus increasing afterload. There now is further adverse influence on myocardial oxygen supply while demand increases and this will contribute to a mulitplier effect, a vicious circle. Again, the dihydropyridines may break this cycle.

If, on the other hand, during the course of ischemia, an increase in oxygen supply resulting from reduced coronary vascular resistance and increasing aortic pressure closes the oxygen demand-supply gap by homeostatic mechanisms, myocardial cells will recover their function and become less stiff. The left ventricular diastolic pressure in turn will fall and help further to ameliorate the ischemia. It is likely that many ischemic episodes observed on the coronary care unit or on Holtermonitoring, but not reported by the patient, will follow this course. Stated concisely: this series of events suggests that ischemia either tends to deepen and spread due to secondary hemodynamic effects of the ischemia or that an interference with this circular sequence may lead to recovery along a similar course but in the opposite direction. The outcome in any particular episode will therefore not only depend on natural capacity of the human system to correct its derangements, but also on the timely therapeutic interventions instituted by the physician. It is here that the dihydropyridines will find their optimal application.

References

Brower RW, Jong JW de, Haalebos M, Simoons ML, Bos A vd, Jong DS de, Bos E, Hugenholtz PG (1982) Evaluation of cardioplegia in coronary artery bypass graft surgery. In: Just H, Tschirkov A, Schlosser V (eds) Kalziumantagonisten zur Kardioplegie und Myokardprotektion in der offenen Herzchirurgie. Thieme, Stuttgart, p 69

Buckberg GD, Olinger GN, Mulder DG, Maloney Jr JV (1975) Depressed postoperative cardiac performance. Prevention by adequate protection during cardiopulmonary bypass. J Thorac Cardiovasc Surg 70:974

Buehler H (1984) In these proceedings

Churchill W (1948) The gathering storm. Publication Company, Boston

Clark RE, Magovern GJ, Christlieb, IY, Boe S (1983) Nifedipine cardioplegia experience: results of a 3-year cooperative clinical study. Ann Thorac Surg 36:654

Clark RE, Christlieb IY, Henry PD, Fisher AE, Nora JD, Williamson JR, Sobel BE (1979) Nifedipine: a myocardial protective agent. Am J Cardiol 44:825

Dargie HJ, Lynch PG, Krikler DM, Harris L, Kirkler S (1981) Nifedipine and propranolol: a beneficial drug interaction. Am J Med 71:676

Flameng W, Borgers M, Van der Vusse GJ; Demeyere R, Vandermeersch E, Thone F, Suy R (1983) Cardioprotective effects of lidoflazine in extensive aorta-coronary bypass grafting. J Thorac Cardiovasc Surg 85:758

Fleckenstein A (1983) Calcium antagonism in heart and smooth muscle. Wiley, New York

Hauf E (1984) Personal communications

Hugenholtz PG, Michels HR, Serruys PW, Brower RW (1981) Nifedipine in the treatment of unstable angina, coronary artery spasm and myocardial ischemia. Am J Cardiol 47:163

Hugenholtz PG, Michels HR, Serruys PW, Simoons ML (1982) What is preferable in unstable angina, beta-blockade or calcium inhibition? Hart Bull 13:171

Hugenholtz PG, Verdouw PD, Jong JW de, Serruys PW (1983) Nifedipine for angina and acute myocardial ischaemia. Postgrad Med J (Suppl 2) 59:40

Jennings RB, Ganote CE, Reimer KA (1975) Ischemic tissue injury. Am J Pathol 81:179

Jong JW de (1985) Calcium antagonisten en cardioplegie. Hart Bull 16:4

Jong JW de, Harmsen E, Tombe PP de, Keijzer E (1982) Nifedipine reduces adenine nucleotide breakdown in ischemic rat heart. Eur J Pharmacol 81:89

Jong JW de, Harmsen E, Tombe PP de, Keijzer E (1983) Energy conservation in ischemic rat heart by nifedipine plus propranolol. Eur Heart J (Supp C) 4:25

Jong JW de, Huizer T, Tijssen JGB (1984) Energy conservation by nisoldipine in ischaemic heart. Br J Pharmacol 83:943

Lange LG, Sobel BE (1982) Pharmacological salvage of myocardium. Ann Rev Pharmacol Toxicol 22:115

Lichtlen P (1984) In these proceedings

Muller JE, Morrison J, Stone PH, Rude RE, Rosner B, Roberts R, Pearle DL, Turi ZG, Schneider JF, Serfas DH, Tate C, Scheiner E, Sobel BE, Hennekens CH; Braunwald E (1984) Nifedipine therapy for patients with threatened and acute myocardial infarction: a randomized, double blind, placebo-controlled comparison. Circulation 69:740

Muller JE, Turi ZG, Pearle DL, Schneider JF, Serfas DH, Morrison J, Stone PH, Rude RE, Rosner B, Sobel BE, Tate C, Scheiner E, Roberts R, Hennekens CH, Braunwald E (1984) Nifedipine and conventional therapy for unstable angina pectoris: a randomized double blind comparison. Circulation 69:728

Nayler WG (1984) In these proceedings

Nayler WG, Poole-Wilson P (1981) Calcium antagonists: definition and mode of action. Bas Res Cardiol 76:1

Opie LH (1984) Calcium antagonists and cardiovascular disease. Raven Press, New York

Parratt JR (1983) Pharmacological agents to aid the clinician in combating myocardial ischemia. Eur Hear J (Suppl D) 4:91

Saxena PR (1983) Beta-adrenoceptor antagonists and blood flow to the jeopardized myocardium. Eur Heart J (Suppl D) 4:101

Schaper W (1983) Natural defense mechanisms during ischemia. Eur Heart J (Suppl D) 4:73

Schmutzler H (1981) Possibilities and perspectives of combination therapy. Adalat and beta-blockers. In: Coronary heart disease – calcium antagonist Adalat, a worldwide success. Bayer, Leverkusen, p 87

Serruys PW, Brower RW, Katen HJ ten, Meester GT (1980) Recovery from circulatory depression after coronary artery bypass surgery. Eur Surg Res 12:369

Serruys PW, Wijns W, Brand M vd, Meij S, Slager C, Schuurbiers JCH, Hugenholtz PG, Brower RW (1984a) Left ventricular performance, regional blood flow, wall motion, and lactate metabolism during transluminal angioplasty. Circulation 70:25

Serruys PW, Wijns W, Zeegers E, Brand M vd, Feyter P de, Jong JW de (1984b) Myocardial release of hypoxanthine and lactate during PTCA: a quickly reversible phenomenon. Circulation (Suppl 2) 70:II–299 (Abstr)

Serruys PW, Wijns W, Grimm J, Slager CJ, Hess OM (1984c) Effects of repeated transluminal occlusions during angioplasty on global and regional left ventricular chamber stiffness. Circulation (Suppl 2) 70:II–348 (Abstr)

Spencer FC (1983) Intellectual creativity in thoracic surgeons. J Thorac Cardiovasc Surg 86:163

Stone PH, Antman EM (1983) Calcium channel blocking agents in the treatment of cardiovascular disorders. Futura Publishing, Mount Kisco, New York

Vanhaleweyk GLJ, Serruys PW, Hugenholtz PG (1983) Antianginal electrophysiologic and hemodynamic effects of combined beta-blocker/calciumantagonist therapy. Eur Heart J (Suppl D) 4:117

Verdouw PD, Hartog JM, Cate FJ ten, Schamhardt HC, Bastiaans OL, Bremen RH van, Serruys PW, Hugenholtz PG (1981) Effects of nifedipine on the recovery of regional myocardial performance during reperfusion of ischemic myocardium. Prog Pharmacol 4:91

Verdouw PD, Wolffenbuttel BHR, Cate FJ ten (1983) Nifedipine with and without propranolol in the treatment of myocardial ischemia: effect on ventricular arrhythmias and recovery of regional wall function. Eur Heart J (Suppl C) 4:101

Vusse GJ van der, Coumans WA, Veen E vd, Drake AJ, Flameng W, Suy R (1984) ATP, creatine phosphate and glycogen content in human myocardial biopsies: markers for the efficacy of cardioprotection during aorto-coronary bypass surgery. Vasc Surg 18:127

Wolffenbuttel BHR, Verdouw PD (1983) Nifedipine and myocardial performance in the presence and absence of beta-blockade with propranolol. Arch Int Pharmacol Ther 266:83

Yasue H, Touyama M, Kato H, Tanaka S, Akiyama F (1976) Prinzmetal's variant form of angina as a manifestation of alpha-adrenergic receptor-mediated coronary artery spasm: documentation by coronary arteriography. Am Heart J 91:149

Yasue H, Omote S, Takizawa A, Nagao M, Miwa K, Tanaka S (1979) Circadian variation of exercise capacity in patients with Prinzmetal's variant angina: role of exercise induced coronary arterial spasm. Circulation 59:938

Discussion

(pp. 236–247)

Schwartz: The goal in treating angina pectoris is to use concentrations of these drugs that produce a modest drop in afterload, but certainly an increase in coronary flow without "steal". But the goal in preventing the heart against ischemic-induced damage is, perhaps, much more complicated with membrane and intracellular effects probably playing important roles. I wonder, therefore, if the clinical trials are employing dose ranges of the calcium antagonists that are consistent with the beneficial effects that have been observed in the animal studies.

Hugenholtz: I tried to concentrate on the cardioprotective aspects of these drugs in ischemia. Usually there must be a mixed effect: A coronary dilating effect, a decrease in afterload and better capillary blood supply, better oxygenation, overall with less work, all these things must be synergistic. I have taken the additional cardioprotective effect in situations where that will be the dominant one. Take the PTCA situation: I do not think that here afterload is a relevant matter. Because you have a temporary interruption of blood supply. There you clearly would like to have an immediate protective effect, as the dominant one, I think the same thing goes on with the streptokinase patients because there will be reperfusion damage. Again a peripheral unloading might be effective, but what I want to see is what happens immediately after you throw the oxygen supply back in. There you cause the temporary calcium overload. I hope, I drew your attention to that kind of clinical application. In the general treatment of angina in all forms and in the general approach of a physician to how these drugs work he can never separate the three main effects. And if there were a drug that could select really one and not the others, I would be very happy, too. We do feel that nisoldipine in doses that already have a profound effect on phosphate metabolism, has less effect on vasodilation than nifedipine has. Whether nisoldipine will be the ideal drug that only takes on one aspect of the whole spectrum, I cannot tell.

Fleckenstein: In one of these studies you mentioned a dose of 120 mg nifedipine was given to the patients. Wouldn't coronary perfusion pressure be too much reduced with such huge doses? We know from dog experiments in which the coronary arteries were ligated that with high doses of nifedipine the situation became even worse because perfusion pressure was diminished too much while with smaller doses one could decrease the extension of the infarcted zone.

Hugenholtz: I couldn't argue with you. At the time these studies were done, they were supported by another branch of the American pharmaceutical industry namely Pfizer. And I have the feeling that this had much to do with the dose chosen. When I heard that dose I was absolutely flabbergasted; 120 mg nifedipine in a patient known to have a myocardial infarction, is to ask for difficulties. But that whole study was done as is so often the case under certain pressures from different sides and for different reasons. It leaves you with a bad taste because of design errors, just as for the verapamil study.

Fleckenstein: You mentioned this negative Danish verapamil study there are also some objections to its design.

Hugenholtz: Yes, that is right.

Kadowitz: Would you have some concerns about what you are actually measuring by measuring a cardiac vein effluent and coronary sinus effluent because of the inaccuracy of the method. Once you apply a PCTA or streptokinase, then the distribution of flow can change.

Hugenholtz: First of all we never measure the coronary blood flow in patients who receive thrombolytic treatment, it is strictly related to the percutaneous transluminal angioplasty protocol. Second, the measurement is known to have its inaccuracies, but these are relative measurements and we have never taken them like absolute values. We see changes as they occur when we occlude and desobstrue and from this we know that we are in the venous vessel draining the artery that has been occluded. You are right, the method is incomplete, but I know no better one I can use in the human.

Kadowitz: You use 4 separate PCTA's in a patient? You do this in order to get a certain amount of the flow restoration or obstruction reduction?

Hugenholtz: We go up to 11 successive dilation attempts. As you inflate the balloon, you interrupt blood flow. This is why I think the drug will have an increased use if we could trust them to act. After 45 to 60 s, you must deflate since you want to reperfuse intermittently. So if you then revisualize the vessel and see that you have not properly desobstructed, you reinflate the balloon a second time. We are not inflating it simply for the experiment; it is because on average patients require up to 5 dilatations each of a period of just under a minute before you have sufficient reduction at the site of the obstruction.

Kadowitz: What do you do with the patients that don't have successful PCTA, do they improve from the calcium entry blockade treatment?

Hugenholtz: No, once you have decided – in most hospitals in Europe together with the cardiac surgeon – that the patient is a candidate, the indication is first and foremost whether you can reach the site with the balloon dilatation catheter. By definition this means that it must be nowadays either proximal or in the middle of the vessel. Secondly it must be a lesion of which the surgeon says: Why don't you do it because you can get it done quicker or better. This minor operation takes exactly two days of the patient's morbidity instead of a month and that at a third of the price. In practice there are something like 15% in whom we fail. The converse also happens: We had a number of patients in whom a dilatation was done when their bypass didn't work. So it is a technique which goes hand in hand with the surgeons. PTCA opens up a whole lot of situations where you induce ischemia willfully, in the hope that you won't do any more damage than the good you expect to achieve. This is where this drug should be used far more aggressively in a prophylactic manner selectively in the coronary systems.

Godfraind: Do you suppress drug pretreatment or do you think that if somebody is nicely on beta-blocker, you would suppress beta-blocker to go on a trial with dihydropyridines?

Hugenholtz: Let me define where we want to use the Ca^{2+}-antagonist for. Our trial with 650 patients in the Netherlands for unstable angina has been so designed that patients who were on drugs other than a beta-blocker, would be stopped under the assumption that if they came in with unstable angina then that drug was not very good for them. If they were on beta-blockers we would continue with that beta-blocker because the slow washout and the urgency of treatment and add whatever the protocol called for. In trials for infarction or the prestages of infarction we clearly would discontinue all therapy because it has already proven to be ineffective. In stable angina pectoris you should such a patient stop him from being on bad therapy for several reasons: You in fact don't know whether he was taking it. Many patients upon becoming asymptomatic stop their medication. So the history is extremely unreliable. This is a complex answer to a complex question.

Session IV: Effects on Smooth Muscle

Chairman: C. VAN BREEMEN

Bayer-Symposium IX
Cardiovascular Effects of Dihydropyridine-Type
Calcium Antagonists and Agonists, 252–256

Effect of Dihydropyridines on Visceral Smooth Muscle

L. MISSIAEN, J. EGGERMONT, B. HIMPENS, and R. CASTEELS

The primary role of calcium ions as an intermediary in the regulation of excitation-contraction coupling is still accepted. Our present views on the cytoplasmic calcium, the intracellular stores of this ion and its regulation are based on indirect experimental evidence. The dimensions of smooth muscle cells and the complex structure of tissues composed of such cells have only allowed in a few instances to visualize cellular Ca compartments [1]. Recently the changes of cytoplasmic calcium concentration have also been investigated using the bioluminiscent calcium indicator aequorin [2, 3]. The various experimental results obtained in studying smooth muscle cells suggest that these cells have an intracellular store from which calcium can be released and that a maintained contraction depends on a continuous supply of calcium from the external medium [4, 5]. Also the amplitude of these force developments is determined by the external calcium concentration. The cells could be considered as a one-way system with calcium flowing into the cells and being extruded out of the cell. The recycling of calcium between the cytoplasm and the cellular calcium store, as observed in skeletal muscle fibres is probably only poorly developed in smooth muscle. In Ca-free medium a single supramaximal stimulus with an agonist induces only a transient contraction and a second application of the stimulus during a maintained exposure to Ca-free medium is neither accompanied by a second phasic contraction nor by a release of Ca from the tissue.

The entry of external Ca^{2+} across the plasma membrane is therefore not only essential for the maintenance of a force development but also for a direct or indirect refilling of the intracellular Ca stores [6]. One could speculate that the cytoplasmic Ca concentration is determined by the interplay of this Ca influx and the Ca-extrusion and that a reduction of the force development of the cells could be due either to a decreased influx or to an increased efflux. There is as yet no conclusive evidence that the force development could be modulated by the latter mechanism, although it has been claimed that some agonists could modulate the Ca extrusion by interacting with the Ca Mg ATPase of the plasma membrane [7].

One of the main pharmacological approaches to reduce smooth muscle contraction remains therefore the use of substances which limit the passage of Ca across the so-called Ca channels [8]. That such channels exist is again accepted on the basis of indirect evidence and by analogy with other excitable tissues. There has not been up till now any recording of the Ca currents through single channels of smooth muscle cells as obtained in several other types of cells. The classification of Ca channels in two subgroups, the receptor operated channels and the voltage-dependent ones although attractive, remains hypothetical [9]. An important argument in favour of this classification is the finding that the organic Ca antagonists reduce the increase by K-depolarization of the Ca-entry and the force development induced in vascular smooth muscle to a larger extent than the increases elicited by the action of agonists at the membrane [5, 10, 11]. This idea of two types of Ca channels has also been extrapolated to visceral smooth muscle, although it has been reported that Ca antagonists inhibit similarly the increased force development induced in some visceral smooth muscle by K-depolarization and by agonist action [12, 13].

In the present report we describe some data obtained during a study of the interactions of the dihydropyridines, Bay K 8644 [14] and nitrendipine with the force development of two types of visceral smooth muscle. This study is only part of an investigation which has to include ^{45}Ca exchange, measurement of transmembrane potential and changes of the cytoplasmic Ca^{2+} concentration. A direct measurement of this latter unknown parameter, is essential for an understanding not only of the functional effects of the dihydropyridines but also of the excitation-contraction coupling in smooth muscle.

Methods

Strips of smooth muscle (length 7–10 mm; diameter 0.3–0.5 mm) were dissected from the ileum of guinea-pig (300–400 g) and from the myometrium of Wistar rats (150–200 g). The tissues were immediately transferred to warmed and oxygenated Krebs solution, mounted isometrically in a chamber of 1 ml volume and superfused at a rate of 3–4 ml/min. The Krebs solution contained (mM) Na, 135.5; K, 5.9; Ca, 1.5; Mg, 1.2; Cl, 143.8; glucose, 11.5 and was buffered with 11.6 mM Na-Hepes in order to avoid pH changes as a function of temperature.

The experiments were either performed at 20 °C or at 35 °C. The lower temperature was used to reduce spontaneous activity. The $[Ca^{2+}]_0$ was reduced to 0.2 mM for experiments with Bay K 8644 in order to avoid maximal activation of the contractile proteins during application of this inotropic substance. For experiments with nitrendipine 1.0 mM Ca^{2+} was used throughout. All experiments in which dihydropyridines were used, were performed under Na-light. K-rich solutions were prepared by replacing NaCl by an equivalent amount of KCl and as stimulating agonists we used carbachol and oxytocin.

Results

Ileal smooth muscle is characterized by spontaneous spike discharge and an intracellular calcium store which is very rapidly depleted in Ca-free medium as also observed for taenia coli [15]. We have previously observed that although reducing the temperature to 20 °C inhibits the spontaneous spike discharge, this procedure makes the aspecific desensitization much more pronounced after carbachol stimuli [16]. We have therefore performed these experiments at 35 °C and at 0.2 mM Ca^{2+} for the experiments with Bay K 8644 and at 1 mM Ca^{2+} for those with nitrendipine. 10^{-8} Bay K 8644 increased the force development induced by increasing $[K]_o$ and carbachol concentrations similarly. Also the inhibitory action of 10^{-8} M nitrendipine on the force development induced by K-rich solutions and different carbachol concentrations was very similar. These findings are compatible with the hypothesis that there is only one single type of Ca channel in this visceral smooth muscle. However as pointed out by Ichida et al. [13] several other possible explanations can be given for the same sensitivity to Ca antagonists and Ca-agonists.

The myometrium of the rat has been investigated at two different hormonal conditions. Oestrogen dominated myometrium was obtained from non-pregnant rats during oestrus, as determined by vaginal smear, while progesterone dominated myometrium was isolated from rats at day 13 of pregnancy.

These experiments on myometrium were performed at 20 °C in order to reduce the spontaneous spike discharge and the concomitant phasic force development. In contrast with our observations in ileum [16] this lowering of the temperature did not induce in the myometrium the aspecific desensitisation. In these experiments on myometrial strips, the results obtained with K-rich solutions should be interpreted with caution because this type of stimulation not only affects smooth muscle cells directly, but it can in addition release transmitters from the different types of nerve fibres present in this tissue. Also the possibility of a release of histamine from Mast cells or a modification of the prostaglandin production has not been excluded.

We will first describe the data, which we have obtained on the myometrial strips isolated at day 13 of the pregnancy and which can be considered as progesterone dominated.

The tissues were quiescent at 20 °C, 5.9 mM $[K^+]_o$ and 0.2 mM $[Ca^{2+}]_o$, but on increasing $[K^+]_o$ to 11.8 mM, phasic contractions appeared. From 23.6 mM $[K^+]_o$ onwards the tension response was maintained. Repeating the same type of K-depolarizations but in the presence of 10^{-4} M atropine resulted in a significant reduction of the force development, suggesting that part of the contraction occuring during K-depolarization is due to a stimulation of cholinergic nerve fibres.

Adding 10^{-7} M Bay K 8644 to the perfusing solution induced at 5.9 and 11.8 mM $[K^+]_o$, spontaneous phasic contractions of high amplitude. A further increase of $[K^+]_o$ elicited a tonic force development which was 1.5 to 2.0 times higher than in the controls. Bay K 8644 increased similarly the force development caused by oxytocin (30 mU–0.3 mU/ml) and carbachol (10^{-3} M–10^{-6} M).

In the experiments in which the effect of 2×10^{-10} M nitrendipine was studied we used 1.0 mM $[Ca^{2+}]_o$. The pattern of force development induced by K-rich solution, carbachol and oxytocin was decreased to the same extent for all stimulations.

The oestrogen dominated myometrium was not spontaneously active at 20 °C and 0.2 mM Ca^{2+}. The preparations were stimulated again with K-rich solutions carbachol and oxytocin in the absence and in the presence of 10^{-7} Bay K 8644. The increase of the force development by this dihydropyridine compound in these oestrogen dominated cells was much less than in the progesterone dominated ones. In the presence of 10^{-7} M Bay K 8644 the force development often appeared with a prolonged delay after the exposure of the tissue to carbachol. It is possible that this phenomenon could be due to an inhibitory action of Bay K 8644, as has also been observed in other tissues at higher concentration [17]. An unexspected observation was than on washing out this substance, the mechanical response to stimuli with carbachol and oxytocin became larger than in the presence of Bay K 8644.

The action of 2×10^{-8}M nitrendipine on the force development of oestrogen dominated myometrium varied as in some vascular smooth muscle according to the type of stimulus. The contractions elicited by K-depolarization, were inhibited to a larger extent than those caused by carbachol and oxytocin.

Conclusions

These preliminary results suggest that the hormonal status of the animal could exert an effect on the Ca channels of the membrane of myometrial cells. The progesterone dominated myometrium of the pregnant rat seems to have Ca channels which are similar with those of ileal smooth muscle. The enhancing action of Bay K 8644 and the inhibitory action of nitrendipine are not different for stimulation by K-rich medium or by the agonists carbachol and oxytocin. In oestrogen dominated myometrium 10^{-8}M Bay K 8644 exerts a weak action on all stimuli and seems even to exert an inhibitory action on the frequency of the phasic contraction. It is not possible to explain the increase of the force development after washing out Bay K 8644. The inhibitory effect of nitrendipine on the oestrogen dominated myometrium is more pronounced for stimulation by K-depolarization than for stimuli with agonists. This observation is reminiscent of the more selective action of Ca blocking agents in some vascular smooth muscle tissues on contractions induced by K-depolarization than on those elicited by noradrenaline [5, 10, 11].

More detailed analysis of the interaction of Bay K 8644 and of nitrendipine with the excitation-conctraction coupling in myometrium and ileum is required before drawing conclusion on the effect of hormones on the number of Ca channels and on the nature of those Ca channels. The proposed distinction between receptor-operated channels and voltage dependent ones remains unsettled. Moreover it is doubtfull whether information on the differential action of Ca blocking agents on force development by K-depolarization or by agonists is sufficient to determine the nature of Ca-channels. It should also be pointed out that as shown by Morgan and Morgan [2, 3] the amplitude of the force development can not any longer be considered as an estimate of the cytoplasmic calcium concentration. A better understanding of the intracellular regulation of the force development and its relation to the cytoplasmic Ca^{2+} concentration and the Ca-influx is necessary before we can fully understand the action of the dihydropyridines.

References

1. Devine CE, Somlyo AV, Somlyo AP (1971) Sarcoplasmic reticulum and excitation-contraction coupling in mammalian smooth muscle. J Cell Biol 52:690–715
2. Morgan JP, Morgan KG (1982) Vascular smooth muscle: The first recorded Ca^{2+} transients. Pflugers Arch 395:75–77
3. Morgan JP, Morgan KG (1984) Stimulus-specific patterns of intracellular calcium levels in smooth muscle of ferret portal vein. J Physiol 351:155–167
4. Droogmans G, Raeymaekers L, Casteels R (1977) Electro- and pharmacomechanical coupling in the smooth muscle cells of the rabbit ear artery. J Gen Physiol 70:129–148
5. Casteels R, Droogmans G (1981) Exchance characteristics of the noradrenaline-sensitive calcium store in vascular smooth muscle of rabbit ear artery. J Physiol 317:263–279
6. Casteels R, Droogmans G, Raeymaekers L, Wuytack F (1982) Ca-exchange and transport in vascular smooth muscle cells. In: Yoshida H, Hagihara Y, Ebashi S (eds) Advances in pharmacology and therapeutics II, vol 3. Pergamon Press, Oxford New York, pp 71–79
7. Soloff MS, Sweet P (1982) Oxytocin inhibition of $(Ca^{2+}+Mg^{2+})$-ATPase activity in rat myometrial plasma membranes. J Biol Chem 257:10687–10693
8. Fleckenstein A, Tritthart H, Doring HJ, Byon YK (1972) Bay a 1040 – ein hochaktiver Ca^{++}-antagonischer Inhibitor der elektro-mechanischen Koppelungsprozesse im Warmblutermyokard. Arzneim Forsch 22:22–33
9. Bolton TB (1979) Mechanisms of action of transmitters and other substances on smooth muscle. Physiol Rev 59:607–718
10. van Breemen C, Hwang OK, Meisheri KD (1981) The mechanism of inhibitory action of diltiazem on vascular smooth muscle contractility. J Pharmacol Exp Ther 218:459–463
11. Godfraind T (1983) Actions of nifedipine on calcium fluxes and contraction in isolated rat arteries. J Pharmacol Exp Ther 224:443–450
12. Casteels R, Login IS (1983) Reserpine has a direct action as a calcium antagonist on mammalian smooth muscle cells. J Physiol 340:403–414
13. Ichida S, Moriyama M, Terao M (1984) Characteristics of Ca influxes through voltage- and receptor-operated Ca channels in Uterine smooth muscle. J Pharmacol Exp Ther 228:439–445
14. Schramm M, Thomas G, Toward R, Franckowiak G (1983) Novel dihydropyridines with positive inotropic action through activation of Ca^{2+} channels. Nature 303:535–537
15. Casteels R, Raeymaekers L (1979) The action of acetylcholine and catecholamines on an intracellular calcium store in the smooth muscle cells of the guinea-pig taenia coli. J Physiol 294:51–68
16. Himpens B, Droogmans G (1984) Relation between intracellular Na concentration and desensitization in smooth muscle of ileum and taenia coli of the guinea-pig. Arch Int Pharmacol Pharmacodyn (in press)
17. Grupp G, Grupp IL, Dube GP, Schwartz A (1984) Effects of dihydropyridine Ca^{2+} agonist Bay K 8644 on porcine coronary artery and isolated rat hearts. Cell Calcium 5:313 (abstract E5)

Discussion

(pp. 252–256)

Fleckenstein: Visceral smooth muscle including the uterus are activated by Ca^{2+}-mediated spike potentials. This bioelectric activity is in all cases more sensitive to Ca^{2+}-antagonists than is excitation-contraction-coupling. Thus, we have always a superposition of 2 effects by Ca^{2+}-antagonists in visceral smooth muscle: First suppression of the Ca^{2+}-dependent spike activity and second blockade of excitation-contraction-coupling. Have you any observations on the effects of the Ca^{2+}-agonist on spike discharge of visceral smooth muscle preparation? Just opposite to the effects o Ca^{2+}-antagonists – the Ca^{2+}-agonist should stimulate first Ca^{2+}-carried spike discharge and second excitation-contraction-coupling.

Casteels: In this first series of experiments we have tried to determine some of the properties of the tissues. In a second stage we want to find out the effects of the dihydropyridines on the electrophysiological properties of the cells. However, these experiments have proved to be much more complicated that we originally thought and caused some delay of our electrophysiological analysis.

Cauvin: I just wanted to make a comment about the electrophysiology in this tissue. Tom Bolton found that in voltage-clamped cells from the guinea-pig ileum the depolarization produced by carbachol actually depends upon Ca^{2+}-entry. Therefore, whether or not there is a genuine electro-mechanical coupling versus pharmaco-mechanical coupling is really not clear.

Casteels: Yes, I fully agree. From the point of view of the Ca^{2+}-channels in smooth muscle there is too much theory and insufficient experimental evidence to know exactly how Ca^{2+}-channels are regulated in these tissues.

Van Breemen: You find that on oestrogen domination you have a decrease in the sensitivity of the carbachol-induced contractions to nitrendipine. In the smooth muscle of the rabbit aorta and other tissues we found no inverse correlation between the sensitivity of Ca^{2+}-antagonists and the amount of intracellular release of Ca^{2+}. Is there a change in the intracellular agonist-releasable Ca^{2+} upon estrogen treatment?

Casteels: We have started only for the progesterone-dominated myometrium the study of the cellular Ca^{2+} stores. These tissues lose Ca^{2+} more rapidly than most vascular tissues and the rate of re-filling of this store is similar to its rate of depletion. Obviously, this aspect must be further investigated.

Scriabine: Do your experiments on myometrium suggest that BAY K 8644 may have labourinducing (oxytocic) activity? Nitrendipine and other Ca^{2+}-antagonists were reported to delay premature labour. Can we expect an opposite effect with the agonist? The second question is whether you saw a specificity of the agonist for either uterine or intestinal musculature?

Casteels: One cannot easily extrapolate from rat myometrium to the human one. Regarding your second question, I can only tell you that the sensitivity of the ileum for the dihydropyridines is larger than of the myometrium.

Bayer-Symposium IX
Cardiovascular Effects of Dihydropyridine-Type
Calcium Antagonists and Agonists, 259–269

Effects of Ca^{2+} Antagonists on Isolated Rabbit Mesenteric Resistance Vessels as Compared to Rabbit Aorta

C. CAUVIN and C. VAN BREEMEN

Introduction

We have reported (Cauvin et al. 1984a) that norepinephrine-(NE-)activated rabbit mesenteric resistance vessels are far more sensitive to inhibition by diltiazem than are aortae. Not only are the contractions far more sensitive to diltiazem, but also the NE-stimulated $^{45}Ca^{2+}$ influx. Activation with 80 mM K^+, on the other hand, is similar in its diltiazem sensitivity in the two vessel types. We have now extended our studies to include three other Ca^{2+} antagonists (CAts): D600, and the two dihydropyridines, nisoldipine and PY108-086. We have hypothesized previously (Cauvin et al. 1984a) that the high sensitivity of the NE-activated mesenteric resistance vessels to diltiazem may be related to their relative lack of agonist-induced release of intracellular Ca^{2+}. We have attempted to further investigate this possibility and to study other possible theoretical reasons why Ca^{2+} influx stimulated by NE in the rabbit mesenteric resistance vessels is more sensitive to CAts than is that in the aorta.

Methods

Measurements of tension, ^{45}Ca influx and membrane potential (E_m) in the rabbit aorta and mesenteric resistance vessels have been described previously (van Breemen et al. 1981; Cauvin and Malik 1984; Cauvin et al. 1984a, b).

Results and Discussion

The rabbit mesenteric resistance vessels have proven to be remarkably sensitive to all the CAts we have studied thus far. Table 1 lists the IC_{50}'s for inhibition by nisoldipine, PY108-086, diltiazem, and D600 of NE and 80 mM K^+-induced peak contractions and ^{45}Ca influx in the rabbit aorta and peak contractions in

Table 1

	IC_{50}'s – Inhibition of tonic contractions			
	Aorta		Mesenteric resistance vessels	
	80 mM K^{+a}	10^{-5} M NE[b]	80 mM K^+	10^{-4} M NE
Nisoldipine	2×10^{-9} M	$>10^{-3}$ M	2×10^{-9} M	10^{-10} M
PY 108–068	10^{-10} M	$\gg10^{-3}$ M	2×10^{-8} M	2×10^{-9} M
Diltiazem	5×10^{-7} M	$>10^{-3}$ M	6×10^{-7} M	10^{-8} M
D600	2×10^{-7} M	$>10^{-3}$ M	3×10^{-7} M	2×10^{-8} M
	IC_{50}'s – inhibition of ^{45}Ca influx (90 s) Aorta			
	80 mM K^+		10^{-5} M NE	
Nisoldipine	1×10^{-9} M		10^{-7} M	
Diltiazem	3×10^{-7} M		3×10^{-4} M	
D600	2×10^{-7} M		10^{-5} M	

[a] 3 mM Phentolamine was added to all high K^+ solutions
[b] 10^{-5} M propranolol was added to all NE containing solutions

the mesenteric resistance vessels. For each of the CAts, the IC_{50}'s for inhibition of 80 mM K^+-induced contractions are nearly the same in the two vessels, with the exception of the PY108-086. This dihydropiridine appears to be a more potent inhibitor of K^+contractions in the aorta. The dose-response curves for diltiazem, D600, and nisoldipine inhibition of 80 mM K^+-induced contractions of the rabbit aorta are virtually identical to those for inhibition of stimulated $^{45}Ca^{2+}$ influx. (Loutzenhiser and van Breemen 1983a). Similarly, the dose-response curves for diltiazem inhibition of 80 mM K^+-induced contraction closely parallel those for inhibition of stimulated $^{45}Ca^{2+}$ influx in the mesenteric resistance vessels (Fig. 1; Cauvin et al. 1984a). These results are to be expected, because 80 mM K^+-induced contractions are completely dependent upon stimulated Ca^{2+} entry; thus, inhibition of 80 mM K^+-induced contraction should coincide with inhibition of stimulated $^{45}Ca^{2+}$ influx. Therefore, the IC_{50}'s for nisoldipine, PY108–086, diltiazem, and D 600 inhibition of 80 mM K^+-induced activation should accurately reflect the relative binding affinities of these compounds for the potential sensitive Ca^{2+} channels (PSC) in these vessels. It appears that nisoldipine has the highest affinity for the PSCs, followed by PY108-086, followed by diltiazem and D600, which are of about the same affinity for the PSCs.

The IC_{50}'s for CAt inhibition of NE-induced contractions in the aorta and mesenteric resistance vessels are enormously different (Table 1). Nisoldipine, PY108-086, diltiazem and D600 are each four to five orders of magnitude more potent in inhibiting NE-induced contractions of the resistance vessels as compared to those of the aorta (Table 1). The order of potency of the CAts in inhibiting the NE-induced contractions in the resistance vessels is the same as it is for

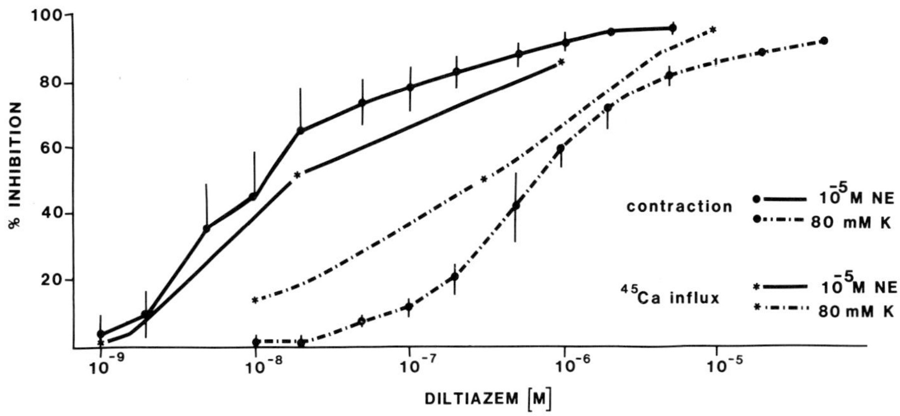

Fig. 1. Inhibition by diltiazem of 10^{-5} M norepinephrine-(*NE*)induced and 80 mM K-induced contractions and stimulated ^{45}Ca influx in mesenteric resistance vessels. Each point on contraction curves represents the mean ± SEM for 4–5 experiments. Each point on ^{45}Ca influx curves represents the mean for at least 3 tissues each from 3 to 4 rabbits. Standard errors of mean ^{45}Ca influx values were in all cases less than 10% of the mean. (Reprinted with premission from Cauvin et al. 1984a)

80 mM K^+-induced contractions; i.e., nisoldipine > PY108-068 > diltiazem ≅ D600. The ^{45}Ca influx stimulated by NE in the rabbit aorta is more sensitive to CAt inhibition than is the NE contraction of that vessel, but still is approximately one thousand times less sensitive to the CAts than are the NE contractions in the resistance vessels. The much greater CAt sensitivity of the NE-induced contractions in the mesenteric resistance vessels as compared to aorta is not surprising, since we have shown that the contraction induced by NE in the rabbit mesenteric resistance vessels is nearly completely dependent upon extracellular Ca^{2+} (Cauvin et al. 1984a), while that in the aorta utilizes intracellularly released Ca^{2+} as well, and these CAts do not inhibit the release of intracellular Ca^{2+} (Saida and van Breemen 1982a, b). This lack of effect by CAts on intracellular Ca^{2+} release accounts, in part, for the disparity between IC_{50}'s for CAt inhibition of contraction and ^{45}Ca influx stimulated by NE in the aorta, and accounts for the vast differences in IC_{50}'s for CAt inhibition of NE contraction in the two vessels. However, we have also compared the diltiazem inhibition of ^{45}Ca influx stimulated by NE in the two vessels and found that the ^{45}Ca influx stimulated by 10^{-5} M NE in the resistance vessels is also four orders of magnitude nore sensitive to inhibition by diltiazem than is that in the aorta (Cauvin et al. 1984a). Moreover, the diltiazem inhibition of NE-stimulated ^{45}Ca influx closely correlates with its inhibition of contraction in the resistance vessels (see Fig. 1). Such a close correlation between inhibition of contraction and $^{45}Ca^{2+}$-influx is likely to occur also for the other CAts. If so, it would suggest that the high sensitivity of NE-contractions in these vessels is not only due to their relative lack of intracellular Ca^+ release for contraction by NE, but also may be largely due to the high sensitivity of their NE-activated Ca^{2+} influx pathways(s). In fact, these vessels represent one of the rare examples where activation of the vessels with an agonist

is actually more sensitive (by about one order of magnitude) to CAt inhibition than is that induced by high K^+ depolarization (see Table 1 and Fig. 1).

In an attempt to determine why NE-activated Ca^{2+} entry in the mesenteric resistance vessels is so much higher in CAt sensitivity than is that in the aorta, we have looked for possible differences in the mechansims(s) of NE activation of Ca^{2+} entry in the two vessels. One hypothesis holds that α_2-adrenoceptor activation generally demonstrates a much higher sensitivity to CAts than does α_1-activation (van Zwieten et al. 1983 a, b), although recently new α_2-adrenoceptor agonists have been studied which also produce contractions in the pithed rat that are very insensitive to CAts (van Zwieten and Timmermans, to be published). We have, therefore, decided to study the α-adrenoceptor subtypes(s) activated by NE in the aorta and mesenteric resistance vessels. We conjectured that perhaps NE activated α_1-adrenoceptors in the aorta and α_2-adrenoceptors in the resistance vessels, and that perhaps this could explain the high selectivity of CAts for the resistance vessels. We have reported that α_1-adrenoceptors in the rabbit aorta mediate NE stimulation of $^{45}Ca^{2+}$ influx, intracellular Ca^{2+} release, and the resultant contraction (Cauvin et al. 1982; and see Table 2). This conclusion was reached because the α_1-selective antagonist prazosin was approximately three orders of magnitude more potent in inhibiting these processes in the aorta than was the α_2-selective yohimbine (see Table 2). The EC_{50}'s for prazosin and yohimbine inhibition of peak NE-contraction in the rabbit mesenteric resistance vessels (see Table 2) indicate that prazosin is nearly three orders of magnitude more potent than yohimbine in inhibiting NE contractions in the mesenteric resistance vessels as well. These data indicate that NE-activation of these vessels is mediated through α_1-adrenoceptors. Therefore, the high CAt sensitivity of these vessels when activated by NE does not appear to be due to the activation of α_2-adrenoceptors by NE.

The inhibitory effects of the CAts and of the selective α-adrenoceptor antagonists in the mesenteric resistance vessels were measured at the peak of NE-induced tonic tension, which generally occurred at 3–5 min after introduction of NE. However, the NE-induced contractions often exhibited a very rapid phasic component an example of which is shown in Fig. 2 (1st contraction). The nature of this phasic contraction interested us, because it is generally assumed that such phasic contractions are due to the release of intracellular Ca^{2+}, yet we have found little or no contraction in these vessels by NE after 5–10 min in Ca^{2+}-free solution (Cauvin et al. 1984 a). Also, we noted in many experiments that the CAts were

Table 2

	IC_{50}'s for inhibition of maximal NE[a] contraction	
	Aorta	Mesenteric resistance vessels
Prazosin	2×10^{-8} M	10^{-7} M
Yohimbine	8×10^{-6} M	5×10^{-5} M

[a] The maximally effective concentrations of norepinephrine (NE) were 10^{-5} M in the aorta and 10^{-4} M in the resistance vessels

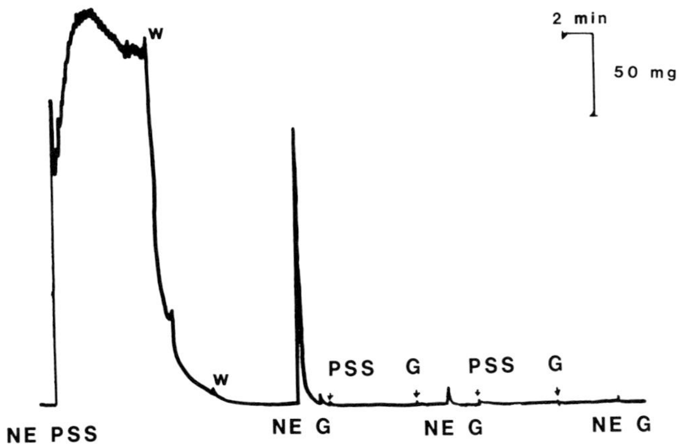

Fig. 2. Representative tracing of a NE (10^{-4} M)-induced contraction in normal physiological saline solution (*PSS*), and after 0, 2, and 4 min in Ca^{2+}-free solution contraining 2 mM EGTA (*G*)

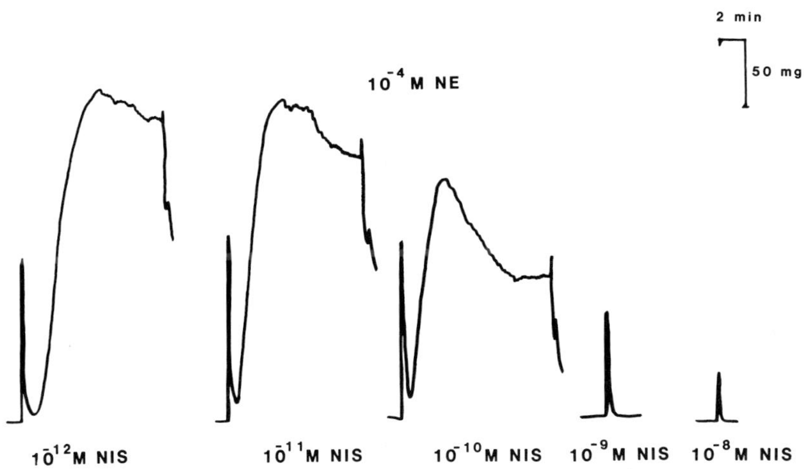

Fig. 3. Representative tracing of NE (10^{-4} M)-induced contractions after increasing concentrations of nisoldipine (NTS). The phasic contraction is more resistant to inhibition than the tonic

capable of inhibiting this phasic contraction quite potently. Figure 3 shows that nisoldipine inhibits such a phasic contraction by NE by about 70% at 10^{-8}M; it completely blocked the tonic contracture, however, at 10^{-9}M. 10^{-8}M nisoldipine certainly has no effect on intracellular Ca^{2+} release in the superior mesenteric artery (Saida and van Breemen 1983 b), so we assumed that it must inhibit this phasic contraction by inhibiting NE-stimulated Ca^{2+} entry. Thus, we hypothesized that the rapid NE-induced phasic contraction of the mesenteric resistance vessels may be supported largely by an extracellular Ca^{2+} source.

Figure 2 shows an experiment that supports this conclusion. The vessels were contracted by NE in normal physiological saline, then the contraction was repeated after various times of incubation (0,2 and 4 minutes) in Ca^{2+}-free PSS containing 2 mM EGTA (G). This experiment shows that at time zero, when the tissues are placed into NE and G simultaneously, that there is some loss of the phasic contraction, but that the tonic contraction is completely abolished in the Ca^{2+}-free PSS. After 2 min incubation in G, introduction of NE produced a very little phasic contraction, and after 4 min in G, the phasic contraction was abolished. This experiment suggests that the phasic NE-contraction may well be due to rapid influx of extracellular Ca^{2+}, since the Ca^{2+} pool which supports this contraction is virtually lost within 2 min in Ca^{2+} free solution. However, we have found a large degree of variability in the time that it takes for the Ca^{2+}-free solution to abolish the NE contraction. This phasic contraction in PSS averages $60 \pm 10\%$ of the maximum tonic tension, and at time zero in G it averages $35 \pm 10\%$. This observation suggests that a large part of the phasic contraction must be due to Ca^{2+} entry. The $t_{1/2}$ for the subsequent loss of the phasic contraction in Ca^{2+}-free solution is 4.5 minutes. In contrast, in the aorta, this $t_{1/2}$ is 20 min, and the amplitude of the response to NE after 10 min in Ca^{2+} free solution is about 80% of maximum (Leyten and van Breemen, in press). A Ca^{2+} pool with a $t_{1/2}$ of 4.5 min may be either a labile intracellular pool or an extracellularly bound pool. Loutzenhiser and van Breemen (1983b) have shown that activation of the rabbit aorta with the prostaglandin analog U44069 involves the release of an extracellularly bound Ca^{2+} pool and subsequent rapid entry of Ca^{2+} from this pool into the tissue. It is possible that a similar phenomenon occurs with agonist activation of the mesenteric resistance vessels. This possibility requires further investigation. It is interesting to note that contraction of these vessels with 80 mM K^+ (plus 3 μM phentolamine) also produces a rapid phasic contraction that is completely dependent upon extracellular Ca^{2+} (i.e., it disappears at time zero in Ca^{2+} free solution). Also, the high K^+ more often than not gave little or no tonic contraction in Ca^{2+}-containing PSS. This may be due to rapid inactivation of PSCs in these vessels (another possibility which requires further investigation).

Another hypothesis that has been forwarded as possibly accounting for the higher CAt sensitivity of NE-activated mesenteric resistance vessels as compared to aorta is that the NE may activate PSCs in the former, but in the latter it may open less sensitive receptor activated Ca^{2+} influx pathways. The existence in smooth muscle of receptor-activated Ca^{2+} influx pathways distinct from PSCs had been hypothesized several years ago (van Breemen et al. 1979; Bolton 1979). We have established two criteria supporting the existence of such pathways in the rabbit aorta: 1) $^{45}Ca^{2+}$ influx through PSCs and through the receptor operated $^{45}Ca^{2+}$ influx pathways can be selectively inhibited by CAts (see Cauvin et al. 1983 for review); and 2) the $^{45}Ca^{2+}$ influx stimulated by maximally activating with NE is additive to that stimulated by 80 mM K^+ (Meisheri et al. 1981). A third criterion that would support this hypothesis would be selective activation of distinct Ca^{2+} entry mechanisms by receptor occupation and membrane depolarization. We have examined this last criterion using electrophysiological measurements. We have found, indeed, that NE does not depolarize the rabbit aorta (Fig. 4). Since we know that NE stimulates $^{45}Ca^{2+}$ influx in this vessel, it must do so through an influx pathway that does not require depolarization for activation.

The picture is not as clear, however, in the mesenteric resistance vessels, which do depolarize in response to NE in a dose-dependent manner (Figure 4). The de-

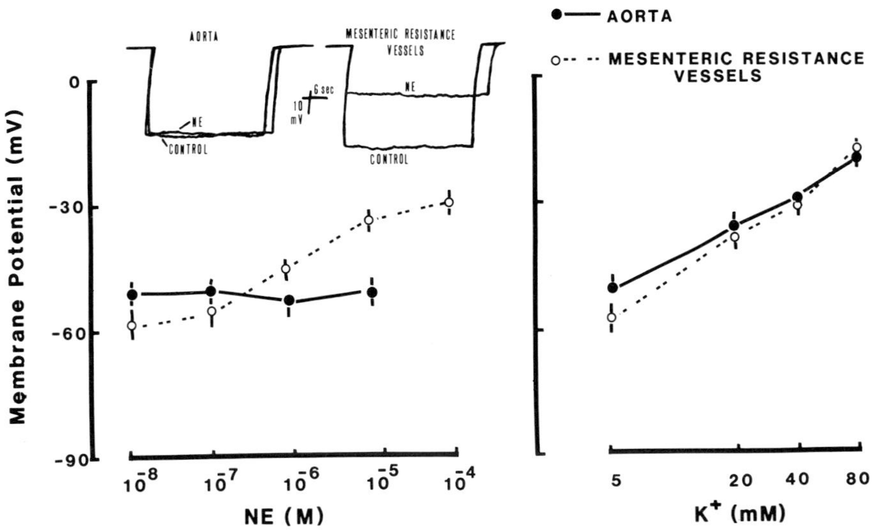

Fig. 4. Concentration-response curves for norepinephrine (NE)-and potassium (K^+)-induced changes in membrane potential in isolated rabbit rabbit aorta and mesenteric resistance vessels. Values are expressed as means ± SEM, and represent at least 5 determinations per animal for at least 5 animals The *insert at top left* shows representative tracings of membrane potentials recordings from the two vessel types. The membrane potentials recorded from tissues during steady state NE contractions are superimposed upon those recorded from tissues during steady state NE contractions are superimposed upon those recorded from tissues resting in PSS. (Reprinted with permission from Cauvin et al. 1984)

gree of depolarization was from a resting potential of -57 ± 2 mV to -30 ± 0.5 mV with 10^{-4}M NE, as compared to -18 ± 3 with 80 mM K^+ (Fig. 4, Table 3). At first we concluded that NE must open PSCs in this vessel; however, further experiments brought this conclusion into question. We observed, for example, that NE was capable of eliciting virtually the same degree of contraction and stimulated $^{45}Ca^{2+}$ influx in a preparation that was already depolarized with 80 mM K^+ as it did in a normal polarized tissue (Table 3). This NE activation of already depolarized tissues occurred in the absence of further depolarization. Moreover, while 10^{-5}M diltiazem had no effect of resting membrane potential or on 80 mM K^+induced depolarization, it completely prevented NE-induced de-

Table 3. Membrane potentials (E_m) in mesenteric resistance vessels

Control (PSS)	-57 ± 2
NE (10^{-4} M)	-30 ± 0.5
80 mM K^+	-18 ± 3
80 mM K^+ plus 10^{-4} m NE	-19 ± 3
PSS + 10^{-5} M diltiazem	-58 ± 1
NE (10^{-4} M) + diltiazem	-29 ± 2

polarization (Table 3). Since this concentration of diltiazem prevents NE-stimulated Ca^{2+} entry in these vessels, we concluded that the NE-depolarization may be secondary to Ca^{2+} entry, rather than the cause of the Ca^{2+} entry. Therefore, it appears likely that NE activates a receptor-operated Ca^{2+} influx pathway in these vessels as well as in the aorta, and that these influx pathways differ markedly in their CAt sensitivity.

We have hypothesized that the CAt sensitivity of the NE-activated Ca^{2+} influx pathway may be inversely related to the degree to which NE releases intracellular Ca^{2+}; i.e., that the agonist-releasable intracellular Ca^{2+} pool (ARC) may modulate the sensitivity of the agonist-activated Ca^{2+} entry mechanism to CAts (Cauvin et al. 1984a). Our reasons for this hypothesis were two-fold: 1) The great difference in CAt sensitivity of NE-activated Ca^{2+} influx between the mesenteric resistance vessels and the aorta is inversely correlated with the degree to which NE releases an ARC in the vessels; and 2) the CAt sensitivity in the rabbit aorta decreases with increasing [NE]s, which also release Ca^{2+} from the ARC to an increasing degree (van Breemen et al. 1982). With diltiazem, for example, there is over a hundred fold increase in the IC_{50} for inhibiting ^{45}Ca influx when one compares a 30% effective [NE] to a 90% effective [NE] (Fig. 5). Such a difference in diltiazem sensitivity of NE-stimulated ^{45}Ca influx with increasing level of NE activation does not occur in the resistance vessels, where increasing levels of activation with NE are not associated with appreciably increasing release of intracellular Ca^{2+} (Fig. 5).

Direct support of this hypothesis, however, has been difficult to obtain. We have tried to examine the diltiazem sensitivity of $^{45}Ca^{2+}$ influx stimulated in the

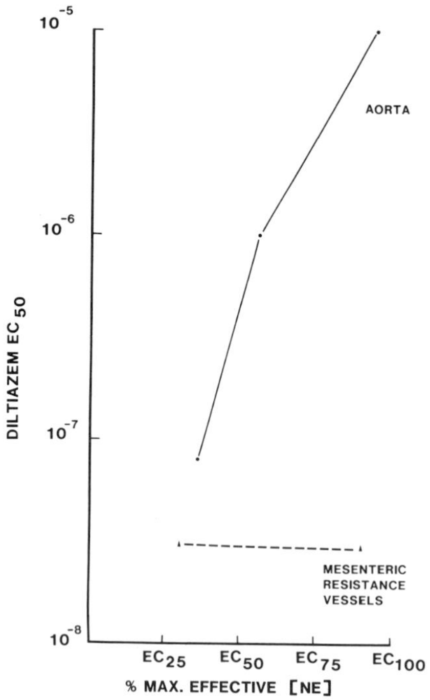

Fig. 5. The half maximally effective diltiazem concentration (*ordinate*) in inhibiting ^{45}Ca influx stimulated by the various percent maximally effective concentrations of norepinephrine (*abscissa*) in isolated rabbit aorta and mesenteric resistance vessels. (Reprinted with permission from Cauvin et al. 1984)

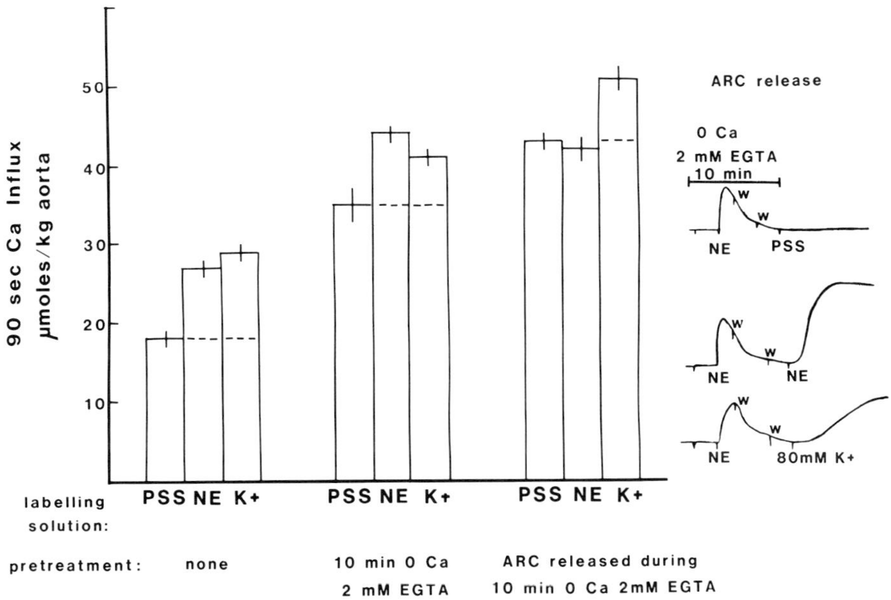

Fig. 6. ^{45}Ca influx into aortic smooth muscle was measured in PSS, PSS+10^{-5} M NE OR 80 mM K PSS after the pretreatments indicated beneath. Agonist releasable CA (*ARC*) was removed from the cells during a 2 min exposure to 10^{-5} M NE after 3 min in Ca free PSS. The tissues were then left in the Ca free PSS for 5 min. The contractions accompanying this last procedure are illustrated on the *far right*. (Reprinted with permission from Cauvin et al. 1984)

rabbit aorta by 10^{-8}M NE (which is quite sensitive as can be seen in Fig. 5) under conditions where the ARC was released by 10^{-5}M NE 5 minutes before the influx measurement. We have found, however, that the intracellular NE-releasable Ca^{2+} pool appears to be involved in the activation of the receptor operated Ca^{2+} influx pathway because, once it has been released, this pathway appears to be incapable of further activation. Figure 6 shows an experiment in which $^{45}Ca^{2+}$ influx was measured in rabbit aortic rings under control conditions, under conditions where the rings were preincubated for 10 min in 0 Ca 2 mM EGTA, and under the same condition except that a 3 min exposure to NE was additionally used to release the ARC. Under normal conditions, (left panel) 10^{-5}M NE and 80 mM K^+ similarly stimulated $^{45}Ca^{2+}$ influx. When the tissues were treated for 10 min in O Ca 2 mM EGTA (middle panel), the basal Ca^{2+} entry into the tissues markedly increased, but this increase did not prevent subesquent opening of PSCs activation of the receptor-operated Ca^{2+} entry mechanism. However, when the ARC was additionally released by NE in O Ca 2 mM EGTA (right panel), the basal Ca^{2+} entry was further increased, but the subsequent addition of 10^{-5}M NE was incapable of stimulating $^{45}Ca^{2+}$ influx above the control. 80 mM K^+, however, could still stimulate $^{45}Ca^{2+}$ influx under these conditions, suggesting that PSCs could still be activated under these conditions. It appears therefore, that the release of intracellular Ca^{2+} is involved in the activation of Ca^{2+} entry by NE and that rebinding of this Ca^{2+} pool may be involved in its subsequent inactivation. This experiment has provided us with this interesting conclusion, but it has not enabled us to test our original hypothesis; i.e., that the release of intracellular Ca^{2+} makes the receptor activated Ca^{2+} entry pathway less sensitive to CAts. In fact, since $^{45}Ca^{2+}$ influx cannot be stimulated by NE after release of the ARC, we appear to be unable to test the hypothesis directly. However, further observations using other agonists, CAts and blood vessels may help to determine whether our hypothesis of negative modulation of the CAt sensitivity of the receptor operated Ca^{2+} entry mechanism by intracellular Ca^{2+} release can be generalized.

Conclusion

From our studies in isolated rabbit aorta and mesenteric resistance vessels, we have concluded that NE is capable of pharmacomechanical coupling in these vascular smooth muscles. We have provided strong evidence in support of the hypothesis of distinct receptor operated and potential sensitive Ca^{2+} influx pathways in these two vessel types. Finally, the CAt sensitivity of the receptor operated Ca^{2+} entry mechanism appears to be different in the two vessel types and to vary within the aorta depending on the [NE], the greatest CAt sensitivity being associated with the least release of intracellular Ca^{2+} by NE. These observations have led us to hypothesize that intracellular Ca^{2+} release by agonists may decrease the CAt sensitivity of the receptor activated Ca^{2+} influx pathway; however, direct support for this hypothesis appears to be very difficult to obtain. Hence, further indirect support will be needed before this generalization can be made.

Acknowledgement. This work was supported by NIH grants HL29467 and HL30412 and the Florida Affiliate of the American Heart Association. Thanks to Libby Blasdel for typing the manuscript.

References

Bolton T (1979) Mechanisms of action of transmitters and other substances on smoth muscle. Physiol Rev 59:607–718

Cauvin C, Saida K, van Breemen C (1984) Extracellular Ca dependence and diltiazem inhibition of contraction in rabbit conduit arteries and mesenteric resistance vessels. Blood Vessels 21:23–31

Cauvin C, Lukeman S, Cameron J, Hwang O, Meisheri K, Yamamoto H, van Breemen C (1984) Theoretical bases for vascular selectivity of Ca^{2+} antagonists. J Cardiovasc Pharmacol 6:S630–S638

Cauvin C, Loutzenhiser R, Hwang O, van Breemen C (1982) α-$_1$-adrenoceptors induce Ca influx and int racellular Ca release in isolated rabbit aorta. Eur J Pharmacol 84:233–235

Leyten PAA, van Breemen C (to be published) The effects of caffeine on the noradrenaline-sensitive calcium store in rabbit aorta. J Physiol

Loutzenhiser R, van Breemen C (1983) Mechanisms of stimulated Ca^{2+} influx and consequences of Ca^{2+} influx inhibition. In: Merrill GF, Weiss HR, Scriabine A (eds) Symposium on Ca^{2+} Entry Blockers, Adenosine and Neurohumors. Urban & Schwarzenberg, München Wien Baltimore, pp 73–91

Loutzenhiser R, van Breemen C (1983) Involvement of extracellularly bound calcium in the activation of arterial smooth muscle. Blood Vessels 20:295–305

Meisheri KD, Hwang O, van Breemen C (1981) Evidence for two separate Ca^{2+} pathways in smooth muscle plasmalemma. J. Memb. Biol. 59:19–25

Saida K, van Breemen C (1983) Inhibiting effect of diltiazem on intracellular Ca^{2+} release in vascular smooth muscle. Blood Vessels 20:105–108

Saida K, van Breemen C (1983) Mechanism of Ca^{2+} antagonist induced vasodilation; intracellular actions. Circ. Res. 52:137–142

van Breemen C, Hwang O, Meisheri K (1981) The mechanism of inhibitory action of diltiazem on vascular smooth muscle contractility. J. Pharmacol. Exp. Ther. 218:459–463

van Breemen C, Aaronson P, Loutzenhiser R (1979) Na^+, Ca^{2+} interactions in mammalian smooth muscle. Pharm. Reviews 30(2):167–208

van Breemen C, Hwang O, Cauvin C (1982) Ca antagonist inhibition of norepinephrine stimulated Ca influx in vascular smooth muscle. In: Godfraind, Albertini A, Paoletti R (eds) Calcium modulators. Elsevier Biomedical Press, Amsterdam, pp 185–198

van Zwieten PA, van Meel JCA, Timmermans PBMWM (1983a) Functional interaction between calcium anatagonists and the vasoconstriction induced by the stimulation of postsynaptic α_2-adrenoceptors. Circulation Research/Suppl. I, Calcium Channel Blocking Drugs. 52:177–180

van Zwieten PA, van Meel JCA, Timmermans PBMWM (1983b) Pharmacology of calcium entry blockers, interaction with vascular alpha-adrenoceptors. Hypertension 5 (Suppl II):18–117

van Zwieten PA, Timmermans PBMWM (to be published) Calcium dependency of vasoconstriction mediated by $alpha_1$ and $alpha_2$ adrenoceptors. J. Cardiovasc Pharmacol.

Discussion

(pp. 259–269)

Thomas: Are your observations on the initial phasic response compatible with the Ca^{2+}-induced Ca^{2+}-release?

Cauvin: I haven't studied Ca^{2+}-induced Ca^{2+}-release in this tissue. In the mesenteric artery we have evidence for Ca^{2+}-induced Ca^{2+}-release. However, in the mesenteric resistance vessels after 1 minute in Ca^{2+}-free solution, virtually 60–70% of that phasic component of contraction is gone. This kind of a time period period probably does not have a lot to do with an intracellular Ca^{2+}-pool. If there was Ca^{2+}induced Ca^{2+}-release it may be that the rapidly entering extracellular Ca^{2+} induces Ca^{2+}-release, but it is probably not an intracellular Ca^{2+}-pool in these vessels which then further triggers release of Ca^{2+} from the sarcoplasmic reticulum.

Thomas: You suggest that EGTA might induce a leaky state, which is very compatible with work on the cardiac muscle. Does under those leaky conditions a Ca^{2+}-antagonist interfere with the increased influx?

Cauvin: The increased Ca^{2+}-influx caused by EGTA treatment in the rabbit aorta is approximately as sensitive to Diltiazem as is Ca^{2+}-influx stimulated by norepinephrine under normal conditions.

From the audience: Could we conclude from there that EGTA does not make holes in the membrane, but rather affects the channel?

Cauvin: I think it probably increases the membrane permeability in general.

Kazda: How rapid is the phasic response restored after giving calcium into the bath again? Does the first challenge provoke the phasic contraction, already?

Cauvin: Yes, it does. I you readminister Ca^{2+} in the resistence vessels after incubation in Ca^{2+}-free solution with EGTA and norepinephrine you get a very rapid contraction.

Fleckenstein: I think that one of the most important findings you have presented is the high calcium dependence of the contractility of the resistance vessels and the very high sensitivity of these particular vessels to calcium antagonists. You used first of all noradrenaline in order to show this. We have studied years ago reactions of these resistance vessels by increasing the intravascular pressure and by direct stretch: Your findings fit very well our earlier experiments. Since there is indirect evidence that the stretch depolarizes smooth muscle under our experimental conditions, in our experiments certainly not a receptor-operated channel was involved, but probably a voltage-dependent channel.

Van Breemen: We should have this discussion after Dr. Bevan's talk.

Hess: I have a general comment on receptor-operated channels. I do not think that the fact that you do not see depolarization with noradrenaline is sufficient evidence for an channel that it not voltage-sensitive, because there are at least two ways to get calcium current in a potential sensitive channel. You can do it by depolarization (e.g. with potassium) but you could also change channel-gating to more negative potentials, for instance by shifting the activation curve. That is not without precedent: in fact it happens with agents like adrenaline or BAY K 8644 in the heart. Before concluding that there is a non voltage-gated receptor-operated channel, we ought to consider this possibility.

Cauvin: If you make the assumption that norepinephrine simply changes the gating of voltage sensitive channel then you would have also to assume that the depolarization opens a different gate, because the calcium influx when add norepinephrine and potassium together in the aorta is completely additive. Thus, if one would assume that potassium depolarization would maximally activate a potential sensitive channel, then you would have to conclude that the norepinephrine would opten that same channel to a greater extent. Electrophysiological data generally show that it is not increased conductance but increased in open time which increases overall current through channels.

Hess: It is in the open probability, but over a limited voltage range you might increase the probability by the same factor.

Brown: Did the EDTA solution contract these tissues, because you have a massive calcium influx?

Cauvin: The calcium which goes into those tissues replaces the stores that have been depleted by EGTA. Under the conditions of activation with potassium there is a delay in contraction because it takes some time to fill up the intracellular stores before Ca^{2+} reaches the myofilaments. With norepinephrine there is a very short delay and then contraction is like normal. These results are explained by intracellular buffering mechanisms.

Casteels: Is one of the main difference between your mesenteric arteries and the aorta not that mesenteric arteries can produce spikes while the aorta does not?

Cauvin: They can spike. They can also rhythmically contract.

Casteels: Can the depolarization observed during exposure to norpinephrine be prevented by diltiazem? If, after a depolarization by norepinephrine, this agonist is washed out, do the cells hyperpolarize? Such an observation would suggest an electrognic Na-extrusion due to a preceding Na-accumulation.

Cauvin: We did check this, and the depolarization appears to be diltiazem sensitive.

Bayer-Symposium IX
Cardiovascular Effects of Dihydropyridine-Type
Calcium Antagonists and Agonists, 272–287

Effect of Dihydropyridine Calcium Channel Modulators on Isolated Peripheral and Cerebral Vessels

R. TOWART, S. KAZDA, B. LAMP, G. THOMAS, and M. SCHRAMM

The pioneering work by Fleckenstein and his group [1, 2] has firmly established the concept of the calcium antagonistic drugs. The most potent and specific calcium antagonists are the dihydropyridines (DHP) [3, 4] such as nifedipine and its analogues nitrendipine and nimodipine. Their actions have been discussed in numerous recent reviews, and are the subject of this volume.

A major advance in the pharmacology of drugs acting on the calcium channel was the discovery, first by Schramm in 1981 [5], and then independently by others (eg. [6, 7]) that certain structural analogues of nifedipine have marked *positive* inotropic effects. The structural similarity of the prototype calcium agonist, BAY K8644, to the "classical" DHPs, and the mutual antagonism between the two compounds (see [8]) suggested to us that BAY K8644 bound to the DHP binding site in the calcium channel, but *increased* rather than decreased the influx of calcium ions. This inital hypothesis has turned out to be substantially correct, and the studies of, *inter alia,* Triggle, Glossman, Hess, Schwartz and Janis reported elsewhere in this volume have examined these phenomena in detail in various tissues.

We here review our own studies on peripheral and cerebral vascular smooth muscle. They show convincingly that the effects of BAY K8644 are confined to the plasma membrane, that the interactions between BAY K8644 and classical DHP's are mutually competitive, that BAY K8644 constricts vascular smooth muscle by increasing the influx of calcium ions, and that cerebral vessels are more sensitive to the effects of DHP calcium agonists and antagonists than peripheral vessels.

Methods

Isolated Rabbit Aorta. Initial experiments were carried out using rabbit aortic strips as described [9]. Later experiments were performed using rabbit aortic rings [10].

"Skinned" Muscle. Rings of rabbit aorta were treated with Triton X-100 according to the method of Ruegg et al. [11].

Isolated Rabbit Saphenous and Basilar Arteries. Rings of rabbit saphenous and basilar arteries were prepared as described [12] using the method of Towart [13].

Calcium Influx Studies. Calcium influx into rings of rabbit aorta was measured with the "lanthanum" method (see [10, 14]).

Drugs and Solutions. BAY K8644 (methyl, 1,4-dihydro-2,6-dimethyl-3-nitro-4-(2-trifluoromethylphenyl)-pyridine-5-carboxylate), was prepared by Dr. G. Franckowiak (Bayer Research Laboratories). Nifedipine and nimodipine were prepared by Bayer Research Laboratories. All DHPs were dissolved initially in dimethylsulphoxide (DMSO), and diluted further in isotonic saline; dilutions and experiments were performed under sodium vapour lighting to prevent photodecomposition. Where not otherwise indicated DMSO solvent control experiments were carried out in parallel, and indicated no vehicle effects. Experiments were carried out using a modified Tyrode's solution for the studies with aorta (see [9]), or Kreb's solution for the comparisons of peripheral and cerebral vessels (see [12]).

Results and Discussion

Interactions of BAY K8644 with Calcium Antagonists. In vivo BAY K8644 reliably increases blood pressure and the force of cardiac contraction (see [15, 16, 8]). It was therefore surprising that the compound had *no effect* on the (non-depolarised) isolated rabbit aortic strip [9] or on the isolated saphenous artery (see Fig. 7b). We therefore compared the effects of BAY K8644 on contractions of the aorta induced by noradrenaline or by potassium. BAY K8644 had little effect on the noradrenaline-induced contractions [9]; likewise the classical DHP calcium antagonists have little effect on noradrenaline-induced contractions of the aorta [17–19]. However BAY K8644 shifted the dose-response curve to potassium to the left ([9] and Fig. 1). Thus the addition of small amounts of potassium (e.g. 15 mM) were subthreshold for contraction in the absence of BAY K8644, but produced near-maximal contractions in its presence. The lack of effect of BAY K8644 in non-spontaneously active tissue, and the requirement of a modest depolarisation for activity has since been observed by other workers in other systems e.g. Ca uptake by NG 108-15 cells [20], Ca uptake and amine release by adrenal medulla [21] and amine release by PC12 phaenochromocytoma cells [22]. In contrast, tissues which *do* show spontaneous activity, e.g. isolated cardiac preparations [23, 15, 24], certain vascular smooth muscle (e.g. rabbit basilar arteries, see below) or certain secretory tissue (e.g. GH_4C_2 pituitary cells [25]) are affected directly by BAY K8644 *without* the need for depolarisation. The implication of this finding is that BAY K8644, and probably classical DHP calcium antagonists, affect the voltage-sensitive calcium channel in its active or inactivated state, but do not affect it in its resting state. Similar evidence has been obtained in cardiac preparations by various workers using classical DHPs (e.g. [26, 27]) or BAY K8644 [28].

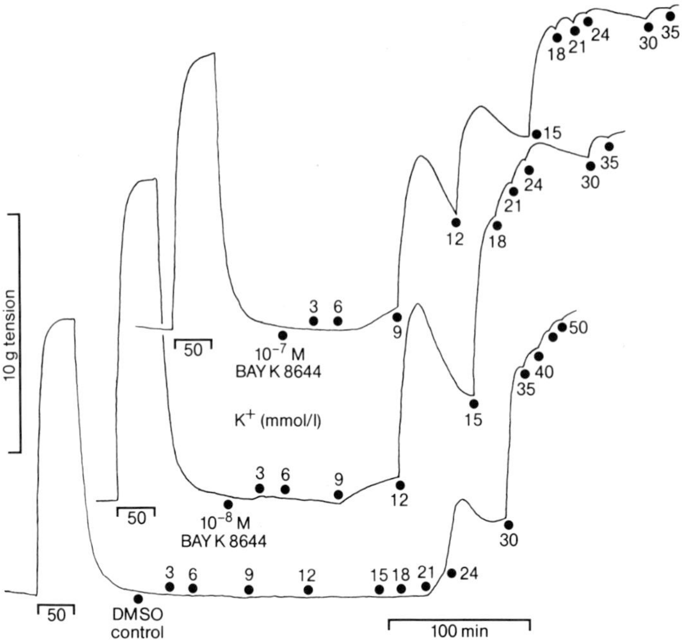

Fig. 1. Effects of BAY K8644 on K^+-induced contractions of rabbit aortic rings. A control contraction was induced by addition of 50 mM KCl (*left*). BAY K8644 10^{-7} M (*top*), 10^{-8} M (*middle*) or DMSO solvent control (*bottom*) was given, and KCl was added incrementally. The figures represent the total K^+ (in mM) added

The practical implication of adding quantities of potassium subthreshold for conctraction is that it allows concentration-response curves for BAY K8644 to be carried out in vessels apparently unresponsive ot the compound (see Figs. 2 and 7c). In adition it allows the investigation of interactions between BAY K8644 and classical calcium antagonists. Figure 3 compares the effect of the DHP nifedipine and the non-DHP calcium antagonist diltiazem on the contractions of the aorta induced by BAY K8644. Note that the DHP calcium antogonist nifedipine shifts the curve concentration-dependently to the right, indicative of competitive antagonism (Fig. 3a) whereas the inhibition due to diltiazem is non-competitive (Fig. 3b). Similar findings of competitive interactions of BAY K8644 and DHP calcium antagonists, and non-competitive inhibition by non-DHP calcium antagonists have been reported by Spedding using taenia-coli [29] and by Miller's group using NG108-15 cells [20]. The competitive nature of the interactions between BAY K8644 and other DHPs suggested to us that BAY K8644 acted by binding to the now well-characterised DHP binding site (see Glossmann, Janis etc., this volume). Since the pharmacological experiments shown in Fig. 3 were completed, various groups have indeed shown that BAY K8644 displaces DHPs from the DHP receptor, and that ^{3}H-BAY K8644 binds to the DHP receptor [30–32].

Effects of BAY K8644 on Calcium Movements. We examined the effects of BAY K8644 on calcium movements using both direct and indirect methods. The

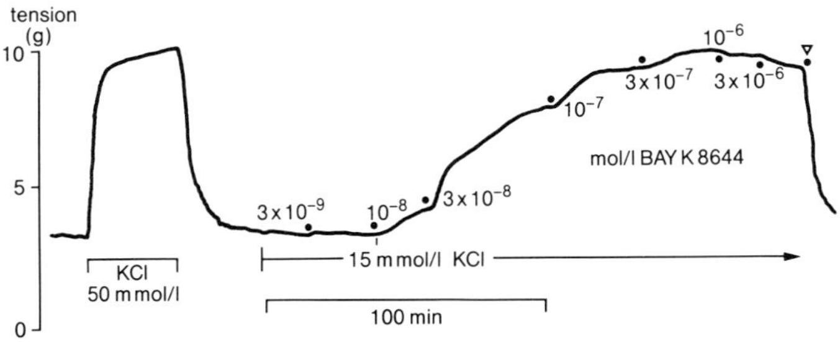

Fig. 2. Addition of 15 mmol/l K^+ to an isolated rabbit aortic ring caused no contraction. This concentration of K^+ was still subthreshold for contraction (cf. Fig. 1). However, the strip was now concentration-dependently contracted by the addition of BAY K8644. ▽ represents washing

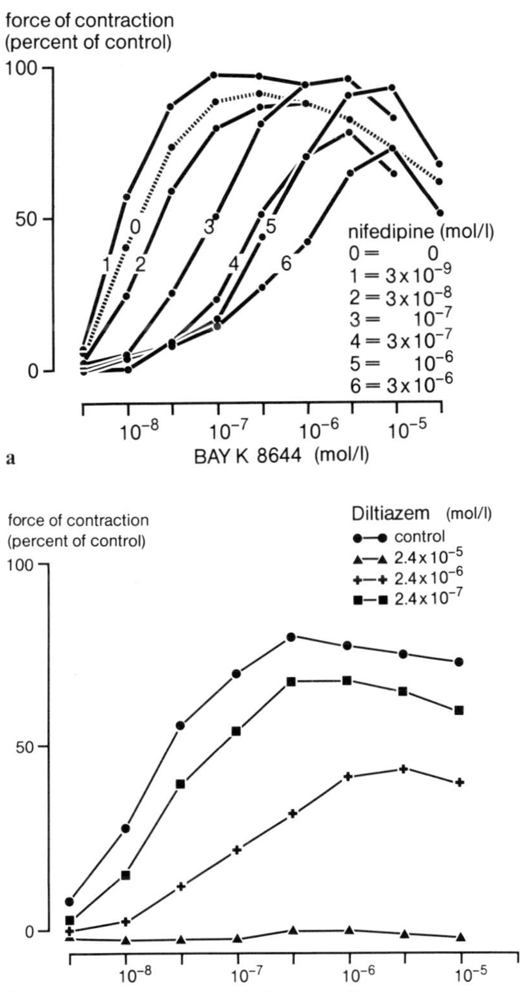

Fig. 3. Effects of the DHP calcium antagonist nifedipine (**a**), and the non-DHP calcium antagonist diltiazem (**b**) on the concentration-response curve of BAY K8644. After a control contraction (50 mm KCl) rabbit aortic rings were partly depolarised by addition of 15 mM K^+. DMSO or nifedipine (**a**), or saline or diltiazem (**b**) were added, and a single concentration-response curve to BAY K8644 was performed. Each point is the mean of at least three observations, and contraction is expressed as % of the previous control contraction. Note that the non-DHP diltiazem antagonises the effect of BAY K8644 non-competitively. **a** from Schramm et al. [15] by permission of Nature

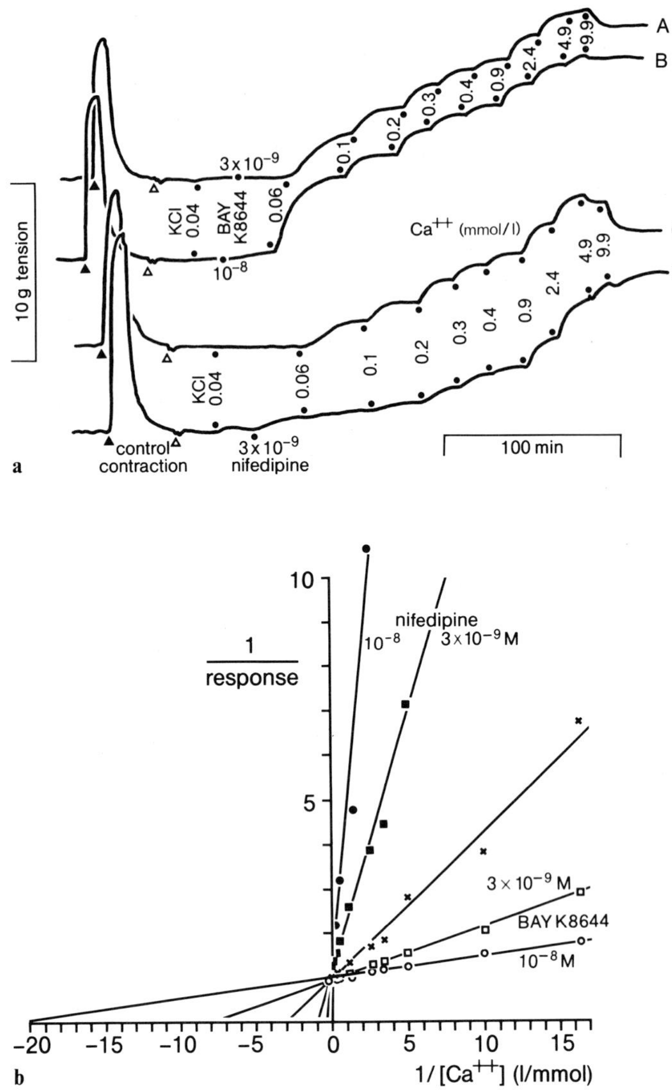

Fig. 4a, b. Effects of increasing Ca-concentrations on contraction of depolarised rabbit aortic rings. **a** Original registration of a single experiment. At control contractions were performed by addition of 80 mM KCl and 5 mM $CaCl_2$. After 10 min the rings were washed with Ca^{++}-free solution containing 1 mM EDTA. A Ca^{++}-free solution *without* EDTA was substituted at △. The effectiveness of the calcium withdrawal is shown by the lack of contractile effect of the addition of 40 mM KCl (●). 20 min later BAY K8644 (3×10^{-9} M, curve A; 10^{-8} M, curve B), nifedipine (3×10^{-9} M, curve D), or DMSO solvent control (curve C) was added. After a further 30 min calcium was added incrementally up to a total concentration of 9.9 mM. **b** The cumulated results of the experiments described above were plotted as a double reciprocal diagram. All effects were normalised to $1.11 \times$ control contraction, as in the control experiments the maximal contractions under cumulative Ca^{++} concentrations were 11% higher than the control contractions. Each point is the mean of 7 observations. The Km values are (mM): Control (×) 0.34; nifedipine 3×10^{-9} M (■) 1.2; 10^{-8} M (●) 3.0; BAY K8644 3×10^{-9} M (□) 0.12; 10^{-8} M (○) 0.05 and 3×10^{-8} (not shown) 0.06

latter study is shown in Fig. 4, and uses the sequential addition of increasing amounts of calcium to a depolarised vessels in calcium-free medium. The calcium is added extracellularly, and the contractions produced are almost certainly due to calcium acting intracellularly. The contractions produced then give a measure of calcium influx through the voltage-sensitive calcium channels activated by the high potassium depolarisation. (DHPs at the concentrations used do not affect calmodulin or intracellular events leading to contraction – see below.) The results of a representative experiment are shown in Fig. 4a, and indicate that whereas nifedipine *reduces* the calcium-induced contraction, BAY K8644 *increases* the calcium-induced contraction, i.e. BAY K8644 increases the calcium influx into the cell. Cumulated results of several such experiments with two concentrations of nifedipine and two of BAY K8644 are plotted in double reciprocal fashion in Fig. 4b. Firstly it can be seen that all the lines pass through the same point on the Y axis, showing again the competitive nature of the interactions of nifedipine and BAY K8644 with their binding site in the calcium channel. Secondly the "K_m" values can be calculated, and are 0.34 mM for the DMSO control, rise to 1.2 mM and 3.0 mM for nifedipine 3×10^{-9} M and 10^{-8} M respectively, and fall to 0.12 mM and 0.05 mM for BAY K8644 3×10^{-9} M and 10^{-8} M respectively.

The effect of BAY K8644 on calcium influx into potassium-stimulated aortic rings was also measured directly using the "lanthanum" method. Results with BAY K8644 and nifedipine are shown in Table 1. The inhibition of calcium up-

Table 1. Effects of potassium and nifedipine on the Ca-influx into aortic rings. From Schramm et al. [10]

Addition of (mol/l)	Ca-influx (µmol/g w. wt.)	n	Contraction (%)
Potassium			
0	253 ± 9	124	0
0.015	260 ± 13	55	2
0.080	391 ± 12	103	100
Nifedipine + 80 mmol/l K^+			
3×10^{-9}	374 ± 12	62	89
3×10^{-8}	318 ± 13	57	65
3×10^{-7}	298 ± 14	58	39
3×10^{-6}	300 ± 13	52	23
BAY K 8644 + 0 K^+			
3×10^{-6}	313 ± 16	35	0
BAY K 8644 + 15 mmol/l K^+			
3×10^{-9}	261 ± 11	32	7
3×10^{-8}	307 ± 11	54	53
3×10^{-7}	352 ± 12	63	69
3×10^{-6}	413 ± 11	56	63

Experiments with nifedipine were carried out in the presence of high potassium to depolarise and contract the rings; experiments with BAY K 8644 under partly-depolarising conditions to enable contractions to the agonist to be induced. "n" gives the number of rings in at least 7 experiments take produced by nifedipine correlated well with the relaxation of contraction of the rings, confirming similar results of Godfraind [33] in rat aorta. However the effects of BAY K8644 were more complex. Firstly it can be seen from Table 1 that the partial depolarisation with 15 mM K^+ did not affect the calcium influx, which is consistent with the lack of contraction. Increasing concentrations of BAY K8644 however show an increasing effect on calcium influx (see Fig. 5) which correlates well with the contraction up to 3×10^{-7} M.

As in other experiments (see Fig. 3), the BAY K8644-induced contraction peaks at around 3×10^{-7} M, and then diminishes slightly with higher concentrations. The BAY K8644-induced calcium influx, however, *increases* despite the diminished contraction. Thus we do not feel that BAY K8644 is calcium antagonistic at higher concentrations in this experimental model. The smooth muscle relaxant action of high calcium concentrations is well known (e.g. [33], or Fig. 4a, curve C) and there are other possible explanations. It has been shown that DHP's can stimulate calcium sequestration at high concentrations [34, 35], and it is not impossible that BAY K8644 also stimulates intracellular calcium uptake or calcium efflux. Thus the calcium *influx* would increase, as observed, but because the calcium *removal* from the cytoplasm also increases, the contraction would diminish slightly. Some evidence for such a mechanism is seen in Table 1, where the high concentration of BAY K8644 (3×10^{-6} M) *without* 15 mM K^+ depolarisa-

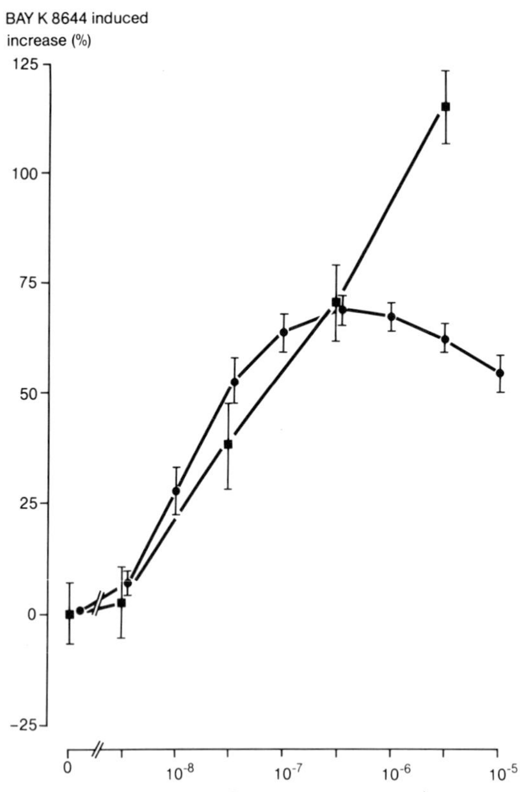

Fig. 5. Effects of BAY K8644 on contraction and Ca^{++}-influx of partly-depolarised (by addition of 15 mM K^+) rabbit aortic rings. The additional K^+ (addition of 15 mM K^+) has no effect on contraction (●) or Ca-influx (■). All values are normalised to the effects of 80 mM K^+, which are taken as 100%. The contraction values are means of at least four observations The Ca-influx values are taken from Table 1

tion markedly increases calcium influx but does *not* induce contraction, suggesting that this concentration of BAY K8644 also increases calcium removal from the cytoplasm.

Effects of BAY K8644 on "Skinned" Fibres

The major pharmacological locus of action of DHP calcium antagonists has convincingly been shown to be on the calcium channels located in the plasma membrane (for critical reviews see [36, 37]). Figure 6 shows the effect of BAY K8644 on the tension developed by Triton X-100-"skinned" aortic fibres. Note that in contrast to the effects of BAY K8644 on the calcium-tension relationship in intact muscle (Fig. 4a), the calcium-tension relationship in skinned muscle is unaffected by the calcium agonist. Thus the contractile effect of BAY K8644 is lost in triton-skinned tissue, which lacks a functioning membrane and sarcoplasmic reticulum. This too is compatible with the concept of BAY K8644 acting on membrane calcium channels. Several recent reports have shown that classical DHP calcium antagonists are without effect on skinned smooth muscle or cardiac fibres (e.g. [38, 39]) or do not (at pharmacologically relevant concentrations) affect calmodulin-dependent events involved in the intiation or maintenance of contraction (e.g.

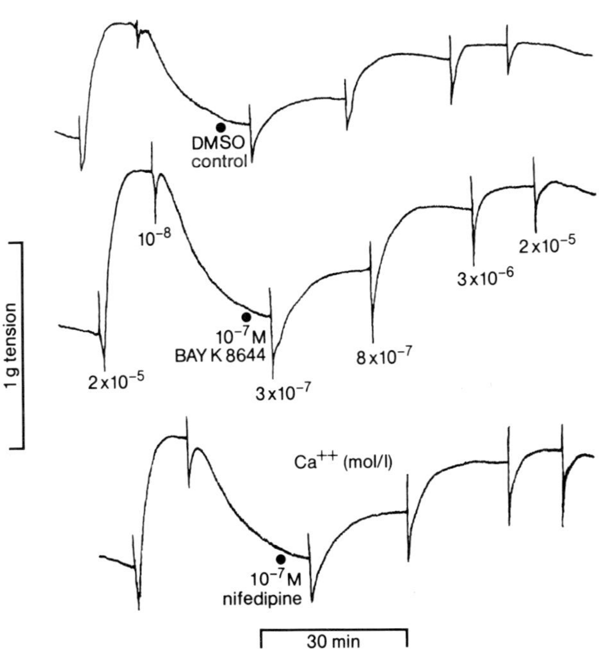

Fig. 6. Lack of effect of nifedipine or BAY K8644 on Ca^{++}-induced contraction of Triton X-100-skinned rabbit aortic rings. After an initial control conctraction using the "contracting solution" ($[Ca^{++}] = 2 \times 10^{-5}$ M) left, tissues were then relaxed using a "relaxing solution" ($[Ca^{++}] = 10^{-8}$ M). After administration of DMSO as a solvent control (*top*), BAY K8644 10^{-7} M (*middle*), or nifedipine 10^{-7} M (*bottom*), contractions were induced by immersion in increasing concentrations of Ca, obtained by appropriate mixtures of the "contracting" and "relaxing" solutions (see "Methods")

[40]). Recent results with saponin-skinned cardiac muscle also show loss of the BAY K8644 effect when the membrane is disrupted [41].

Recent results from Adelstein's group [42] also show that calmodulin-dependent myosin light chain kinase is unaffected by BAY K8644 in concentrations up to 10 μM, nearly two orders of magnitude greater than that required for maximal contractile effects.

Comparison of Effects of BAY K8644 on Cerebral and Peripheral Vessels

The effects of BAY K8644 on an isolated cerebral vessel, the rabbit basilar artery, and in a peripheral vessel, the saphenous artery, are shown in Fig. 7. Like the aorta, the saphenous artery was unresponsive to BAY K8644 (Fig. 7b) until par-

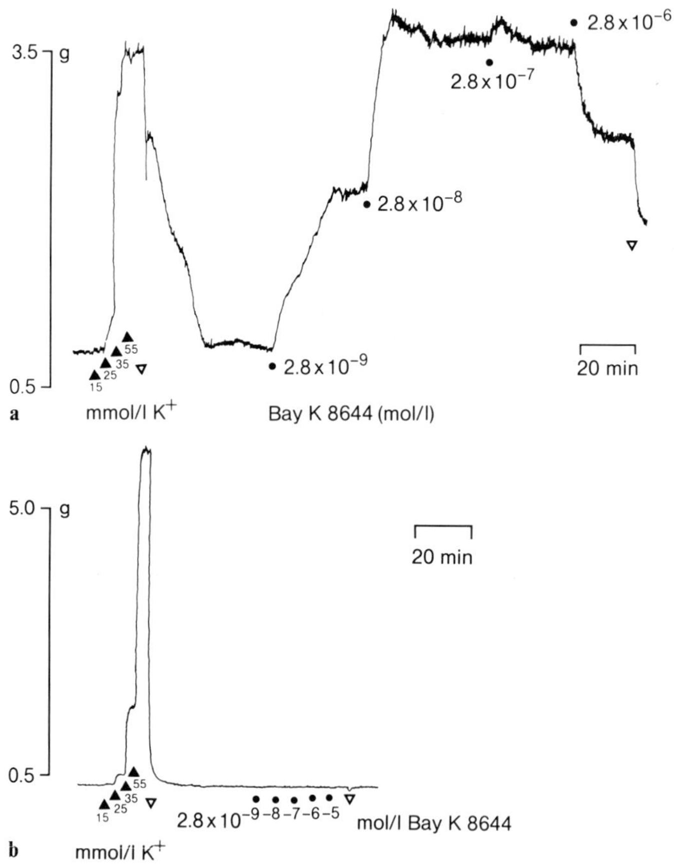

Fig. 7a–c. Effect of BAY K8644 on isolated cerebral and peripheral vascular rings. Rings of rabbit basilar (**a**) and saphenous artery (**b** and **c**) were contracted by addition of KCl (▲) as a positive control (*left*). Increasing concentrations of BAY K8644 (●) were then administered. Note that although the basilar artery (**a**) is contracted by BAY K8644 directly, the non-depolarised saphenous artery (**b**) is unaffected. A small depolarisation (addition of 20 mM K^+) is required to demonstrate the contractile affect of BAY K8644 on the saphenous artery (**c**). ▽ represents washing. Representative tracings are shown from many similar experiments

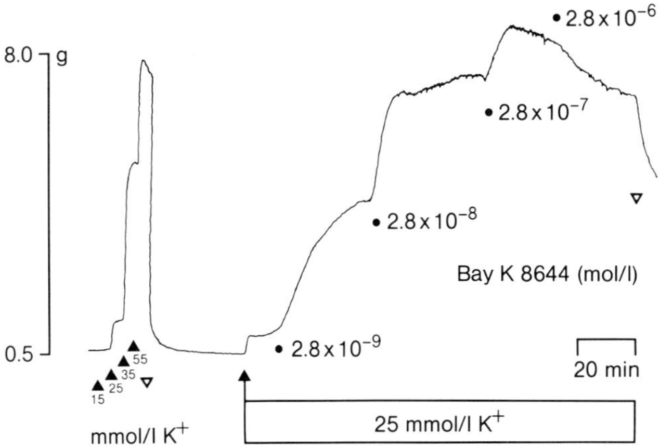

Fig. 7c

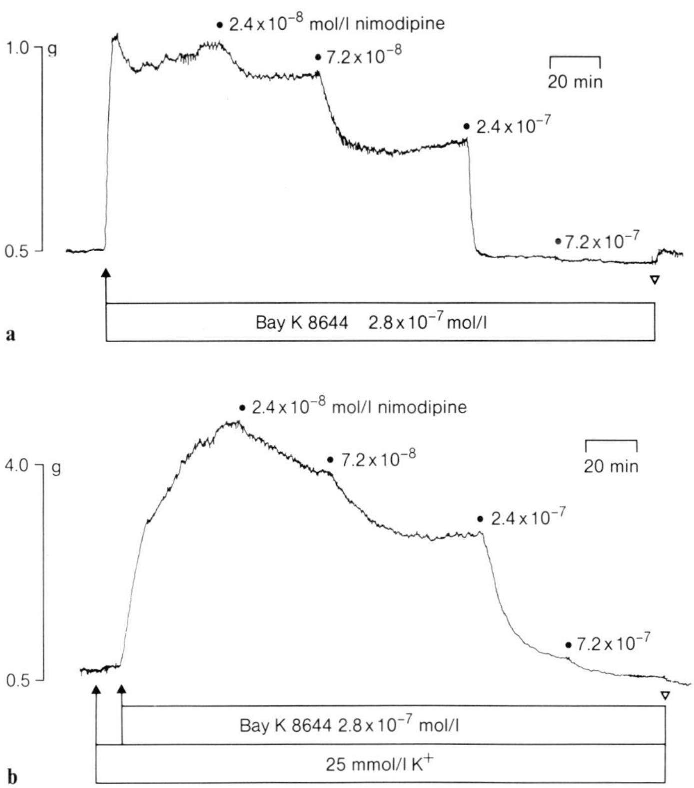

Fig. 8 a, b. Effects of the DHP calcium antagonist nimodipine on BAY K8644-induced contractions of the isolated basilar and saphenous arteries. Contractions were induced in basilar (**a**) and (partly depolarised) saphenous (**b**) artery rings using 2.8×10^{-7} M BAY K8644. Cumulative addition of nimodipine completely relaxed the basilar artery ($IC_{50} = 5.8 \times 10^{-8}$ M, 95% limits 5.3–6.5) and the saphenous artery ($IC_{50} = 8.2 \times 10^{-8}$ M, 95% limits 7.4–9.1)

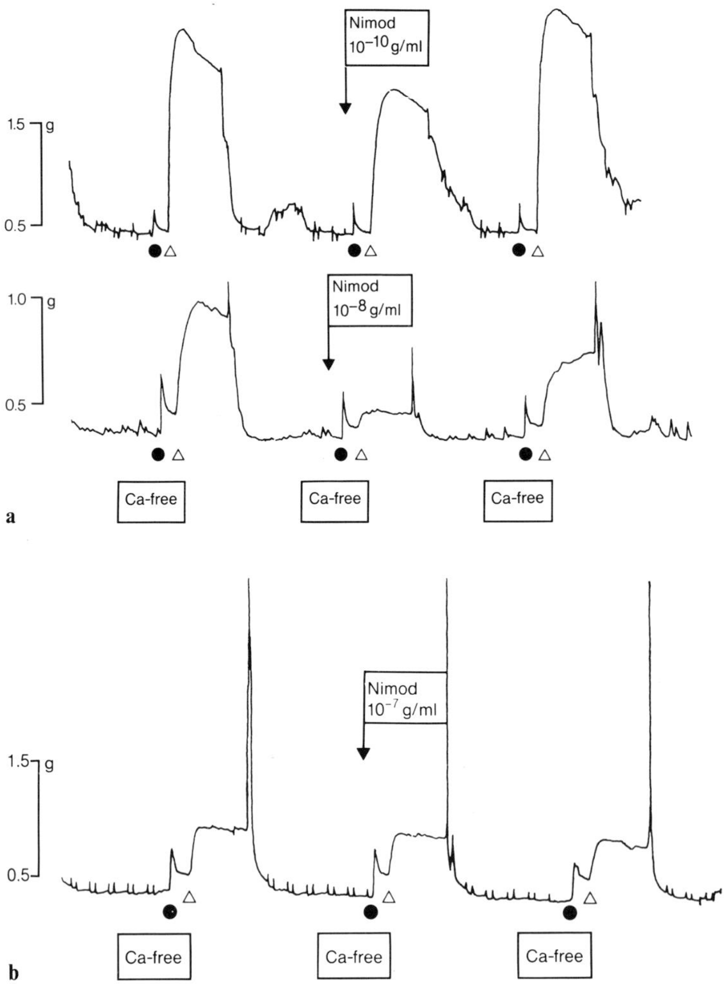

Fig. 9. Effect of nimodipine on agonist-stimulated calcium-influx contractions of isolated rabbit basilar artery (**a**) and saphenous artery (**b**). Addition of serotonin (2.5×10^{-7}mol/l) (●) after an 8 minute incubation in calcium-free solution produces a brief phasic contraction, probably due to intracellularly stored calcium. The readmission of calcium (△) 2.5 mmol/l then produces a sustained contraction which can be attributed to serotonin-stimulated calcium influx. Note that the contractions of the basilar artery are more potently inhibited by nimodipine than those of the saphenous artery. From Towart [13] by permission of the American Heart Association

tially depolarised by addition of K^+ (Fig. 7c). In contrast, the basilar artery was immediately responsive in the absence of further depolarisation (Fig. 7a). However this is probably another demonstration that BAY K8644 does not affect resting-state calcium channels in the (quiescent) saphenous artery, but does affect those in tissues which are spontaneously active. Vascular smooth muscle shows a wide range of electrophysiological behaviour (e.g. [43]), and the basilar artery under our conditions frequently exhibits spontaneous activity [44].

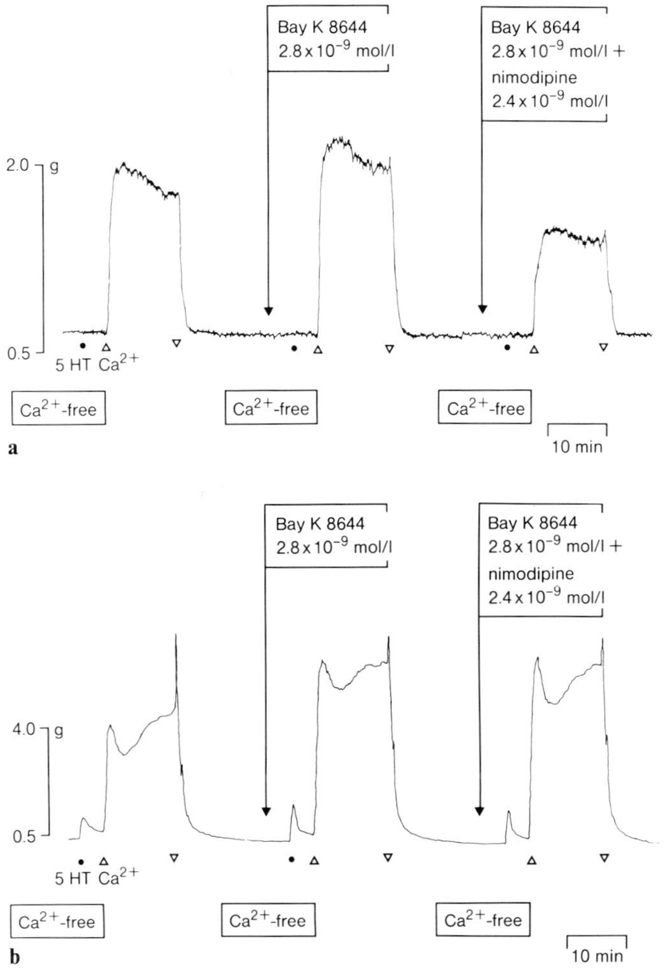

Fig. 10. Effect of BAY K8644 and nimodipine on agonist-stimulated calcium influx contractions of basilar (**a**) and saphenous arteries (**b**). Experimental protocol similar to that shown in Fig. 9. Note that both contractions are increased by BAY K8644, and that contractions of the basilar artery are more potently inhibited by nimodipine than those of the saphenous artery. Representative original tracings from experiments with several concentrations of nimodipine (see Fig. 11)

Figure 8 shows the effect of a classical DHP calcium antagonist on the contractions of the basiliar artery (above) and of the saphenous artery (below) induced by BAY K8644. As with the action of nimodipine on K^+-depolarisation-induced contractions (see [44]) the BAY K8644-induced contractions of the basilar artery are more rapidly inhibited by nimodipine. The effects of nimodipine on the cerebral vessel ($IC_{50} = 5.8 \times 10^{-8}$ M, 98% limits 5.3–6.5, n = 17) are slightly but significantly ($P < 0.05$) more potent than those on the saphenous artery ($IC_{50} = 8.2 \times 10^{-8}$ M, limits 7.4–9.1, n = 20).

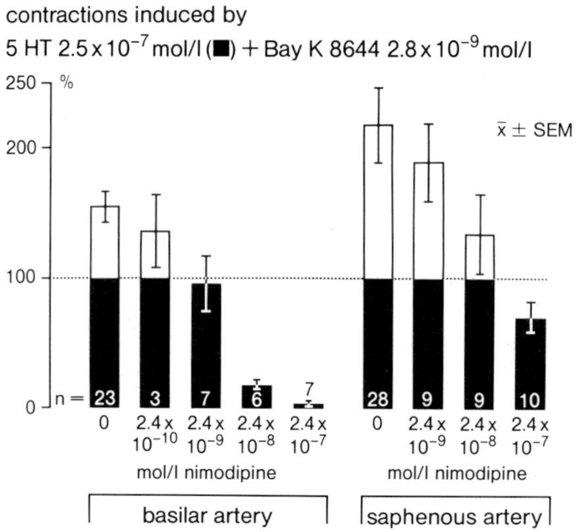

Fig. 11. Effect of nimodipine on the BAY K8644-induced potentiation of agonist-induced calcium influx contractions of the basilar artery (*left*) and the saphenous artery (*right*). Cumulated results of several experiments as shown in Fig. 10. The level of the serotonin-induced calcium-influx contraction in the absence of BAY K8644 is indicated by 100% (*solid columns*). The columns represent the mean ± s.e.m. of the combined effect of serotonin/BAY K8644 in the absence (0) and in the presence of increasing concentrations of nimodipine. "n" shows the total number of rings tested from several animals

Many authors have reported a much greater sensitivity of agonist-contracted cerebral vessels to calcium antagonists [e.g. (45, 46]). The close similarity (despite statistical significance) of the IC_{50} values of nimodipine on BAY K8644-contracted cerebral and peripheral vessels reinforces the view that BAY K8644 is effecting the contractions via an effect on the voltage-sensitive calcium channels.

In a previous study [13] we attempted to explain the differential effects of DHP calcium antagonists on agonist-induced contractions of cerebral vessels by proposing that the agonist-induced calcium influx into cerebral vessels was preferentially inhibited by DHPs such as nimodipine (see Fig. 9). We therefore performed similar experiments where the effects of BAY K8644 were compared on the agonist-induced calcium influx contraction of cerebral and peripheral vessels (see Fig. 10). Under these conditions the serotonin-induced calcium influx contraction (through Receptor Operated Calcium Channels?) was enhanced by BAY K8644, suggesting that in both basilar and saphenous arteries an additional, voltage sensitive channel activation was contributing to the enhanced contractions (see Fig. 11). A similar additive effect of agonist- and BAY K8644-induced calcium influx has recently been described in aortic strips [47]. We also examined the effect of various concentrations of the classical DHP calcium antagonist nimodipine on these contractions (Fig. 10, right). The concentration-effect relationships are illustrated in Fig. 11, and show that the effects of nimodipine on the agonist + BAY K8644 calcium influx contraction are some 30 × more potent on the cerebral vessel. In additon in the peripheral vessel the original agonist-induced calcium influx contraction (100% in Fig. 11) is much more resistant to nimodipine; the *additional* BAY K8644-induced contraction is reduced with an IC_{50} of around 10^{-8} M nimodipine, whereas in the basilar artery the whole agonist-BAY K8644 contraction is reduced with an IC_{50} of around 10^{-8} M nimodipine. This is consistent with the concept that the agonist-induced contraction of cerebral vessels involves a different, more DHP-sensitive calcium influx mechanism than that of peripheral vessels.

Conclusions

The novel DHP calcium channel agonist BAY K8644 has been used as a tool to investigate calcium movements across the vascular smooth muscle cell membrane. The pharmacological studies reported above have shown that it acts on the voltage-sensitive calcium channel, probably by interacting with the DHP receptor, to increase calcium influx. Its contractile effects may be competitively antagonised by classical DHP calcium antagonists. Cerebral vessels such as the isolated rabbit basilar artery are more sensitive to the effects of DHPs than peripheral vessels, suggesting basic differences in the calcium influx mechanisms, especially those mediated by receptor-operated channels.

Acknowledgment. The authors wish to thank Lynne Smith for typing this manuscript.

References

1. Fleckenstein A (1977) Specific pharmacology of calcium in myocardium, cardiac pacemakers, and vascular smooth muscle. Ann Rev Pharmacol Toxicol 17:49–66
2. Fleckenstein A (1983) Calcium antagonism in heart and smooth muscle. John Wiley & Sons, New York
3. Vater W, Kroneberg G, Hoffmeister F, Kaller H, Meng K, Oberdorf A, Puls W, Schloßmann K, Stoepel K (1972) Zur Pharmakologie von 4-(2-Nitrophenyl)-2,6-dimethyl-1,4-dihydropyridine-3,5-diacarbonsauredimethylester (Nifedipine, BAY a1040). Arzneim Forsch 22:1–14
4. Loev B, Goodman MM, Snoder KM, Tedeschi R, Macho E (1974) "Hantzch-Type" dihydropyridine hypotensive agents 3. J Med Chem 17:956–965
5. German Pat. Applic DOS 3130041 (1981)
6. Takenaka T, Maeno H (1982) A vasoconstrictive compound 1,4-dihydropyridine derivative. Proc. Jap. Parmacol. Soc., Abstract 213
7. Truog AG, Branner H, Criscione T, Falbert M, Kuhnis H, Meier M, Rogg H (1984) CGP 28392, a dihydropyridine Ca-entry stimulator. In: Rubin, RP, Weiss GB and Putney JW (eds) Calcium in biological systems. Plenum Press, New York
8. Groß R, Bechem M, Kayser M, Schramm M, Taniel R, Thomas G (1984) Effects of the Ca^{++}-agonistic dihydropyridine BAY K8644 on the heart. This volume
9. Schramm M, Thomas G, Towart R, Franckowiak G (1983 b) Activation of calcium channels by novel 1,4-dihydropyridines. Arzneim Forsch (Drug Res) 33:1268–1272
10. Schramm M, Towart R (1984) Modulation of calcium influx by the 1,4-dihydropyridines nifedipine and BAY K8644 (submitted for publication)
11. Ruegg JC, Meisheri K, Pfitzner G, Zeugner C (1983) Skinned coronary smooth muscle: calmodulin, calcium antagonists and cAMP influence contractility. Bas Res Cardiol 78:462–471
12. Towart R (1981). The selective inhibition of serotonin-induced contractions of rabbit cerebral vascular smooth muscle by calcium antagonistic dihydropyridines: An investigation of the mechanism of action of nimodipine. Circ Res 48:650–647
13. Towart R (1982) A new method for investigating the isometric contractile responses of small blood vessels. Brit J Pharmacol 75:150P
14. Schramm M, Towart R (1983) Modulation of calcium channel function with the 1,4-dihydropyridine structure. J Physiol 349:53P
15. Schramm M, Thomas G, Towart R, Franckowiak G (1983 a) Novel dihydropyridines with positive inotropic action through activation of Ca^{2+} channels. Nature 303:535–537
16. Schramm M, Towart R, Kazda S, Thomas G, Franckowiack G (1984) Calcium-agonism, a new mechanism for positive inotropy: haemodynamic effects and mode of action of BAY K8644. Adv Myocardiol 6:59–70

17. Massingham R (1973) A study of compounds which inhibit vascular smooth muscle contraction. Eur J Pharmacol 22:75–82
18. Schuemann HJ, Goerlitz BD, Wagner J (1975) Influence of papaverine, D600 and nifedipine on the effects of noradrenaline and calcium on the isolated aorta and mesenteric artery of the rabbit. Naunyn Schmiedebergs Arch Pharmacol 289:409–418
19. Towart R (1982) Effects of nitrendipine (BAY e5009), nifedipine, verapamil, phentolamine, papaverine, and minoxidil on contractions of isolated rabbit aortic smooth muscle. J Cardiovasc Pharmacol 4:895–902
20. Freedman SB, Miller RJ, Miller DM, Tindall DR (1984) Interactions of maitotoxin with voltage-sensitive calcium channels in cultured neuronal cells. Proc Natl Acad Sci USA 81:4582–4585
21. Garcia AG, Sala F, Reig JA, Viniegra S, Frias J, Fonteriz R, Gandia L (1984) Dihydropyridine BAY K8644 activates chromaffin cell calcium channels. Nature 309:69–71
22. Albus U, Habermann E, Ferry DR, Glossmann H (1984) Novel 1,4-dihydropyridine (BAY K8644) facilitates calcium-dependent (^{3}H)-noradrenaline release from PC12 cells. J. Neurochem. 42:1186–1189
23. Thomas G, Metzger G (1984) The effects of BAY K8644, a positive inotropic dihydropyridine, in the guinea-pig papillary muscle. IUPHAR 9th Int. Cong. Pharmacol. 1984, Abstract 23
24. Satoh K, Wada Y, Taira N (1984) Differential effects of BAY K8644 a presumed calcium channel activator, on sinoatrial nodel and ventricular automaticity of the dog heart. N-S Arch Pharmacol 326:190–192
25. Enyeart JJ, Hinkle PM (1984) The calcium agonist BAY K8644 stimulates secretion from a pituitary cell line. Biochem Biophys Res Comm 122:991–996
26. Lee KS, Tsien RW (1983) Mechanism of calcium channel blockade by verapamil, D600, diltiazem and nitrendipine in single dialysed heart cells. Nature 302:790–794
27. Kass RS (1982) Nisoldipine, a new more selective calcium current blocker in cardiac Purkinje fibres. J Pharmacol Exp Ther 223:446–456
28. Sangunetti MC, Kass RS (1984). Regulation of cardiac calcium current and contractile activity by the dihydropyridine BAY K8644 is voltage dependent. J Mol Cell Cardiol 16:667–671
29. Spedding M, Berg C (1984) Interaction between a "calcium agonist" BAY K8644 and calcium antagonists differentiate between calcium antagonist subgroups (to be published)
30. Glossmann H, Linn T, Rombusch M, Ferry DR (1983) Temperature dependent regulation of d-cis-(^{3}H)-diltiazem binding to Ca channels by 1,4-dihydropyridine channel agonists and antagonists. FEBS Let 160:226–232
31. Janis RS, Rampe D, Sarmiento JG, Triggle DJ (1984) Specific binding of a calcium channel activator, ^{3}(H)BAY K8644, to membranes from cardiac muscle and brain. Biochem Biophys Res Comm 121:317–323
32. Belleman P (1984) Binding properties of a novel calcium channel activating dihydropyridine in monolayer cultures of beating monocytes. FEBS Let 167:88–92
33. Godfraind T (1983) Actions of nifedipine on calcium fluxes and contraction in isolated rat arteries. J Pharmacol Exp Ther 224:433–450
34. Calvin RS, Pearson N, Messineo FC, Katz AM (1982) Effects of Ca channel blockers in Ca transport and Ca ATPase in skeletal and cardiac sarcoplasmic reticulum vesicles. J Cardiovasc Pharmacol 4:935–941
35. Pan M, Janis RA (1984). Effect of calcium antagonists on Na^+,K^+-AT Pase of smooth muscle. Biochem Pharmacol 33:787–791
36. Janis RA, Scriabine A (1983) Site of action of Ca channel inhibitors. Biochem Pharmacol 32:3499–3507
37. Schwartz A, Triggle DJ (1984) Cellular action of calcium channel blocking drugs. Ann Rev Med 35:325–339
38. Spedding M (1983) Direct inhibitory effects of some calcium antagonists and trifluoroparazine on the contractile proteins in smooth muscle. Brit J Pharmacol 79:225–231
39. Kanmura Y, Itoh T, Suzuki H, Ito Y, Kuriyama H (1983) Nifedipine actions on smooth muscle cells of pig and rabbit skinned and intact coronary arteries. In: Hashimoto K, Kawai C (eds) Asian Pacific Adalat-Symposium Tokyo, pp 3–30

40. Kreye VAW, Ruegg JC, Hoffman F (1983) Effects of calcium-antagonist and calmodulin-antagonist drugs in calmodulin-dependent contractions of chemically skinned vascular smooth muscle from rabbit renal arteries. N-S Arch Pharmacol 323:85–89
41. Thomas G, Gross R, Pfitzner G, Ruegg JC (1984) The positive inotropic dihydropyridine BAY K8644 does not affect calcium sensitivity or calcium release of skinned cardiac fibres. N-S Arch Pharmacol 328:378–381
42. Movesian MA, Adelstein RS (1984) Inhibition of turkey gizzard myosin light chain kinase activity by BAY K8644. Eur J Pharmacol 103:161–163
43. Harder DR (1983) Heterogeneity of membrane properties in vascular muscle from various beds. Fed Proc 42:253–256
44. Towart R, Wehinger E, Meyer H, Kazda S (1982) The effects of nimodipine, its optical isomers and metabolites on isolated vascular smooth muscle. Arzneim Forsch (Drug Res) 32:338–346
45. Allen GS, Banghart SB (1979) Cerebral arterial spasm. Part 9: in vitro effects of nifedipine on serotonin phenylephrine and potassium induced contractions of canine basilar and femoral arteries. Neurosurgery 4:37–41
46. Shimizu K, Ohta T, Toda N (1980) Evidence for greater susceptibility of isolated dog cerebral arteries to Ca antagonists than peripheral arteries. Stroke 11:261–266
47. Yamamoto H, Hwang O, van Breemen C (1984) BAY K8644 differentiates between potential and receptor operated Ca^{2+}-channels. Eur J Pharmacol 102:555–557

Discussion

(pp. 272–287)

Bühler: The interesting association between increased calcium influx and decreasing mechanical activity which you showed with BAY K 8644 could of course also be explained in terms of a differential effect on efflux. We recently looked at human platelets and found that the CIBA GEIGY agonist, CGP 28392 activates the calmodulin-stimulated calcium ATPase.

Towart: Experiments by Janis and by Katz and Schwartz have also shown this sort of effect with Ca^{2+}-antagonistic dihydropyridines. If BAY K8644 increases calcium efflux and sequestration then we could well have increased calcium influx, increased calcium efflux and a slight diminuition of the contraction. That could fit in quite nicely.

Fleckenstein: There is a possibility of a more simple explanation. If you would produce with high doses of the calcium agonists some sort of calcium overload, two things could happen: first the ATP-stores are exhausted and contractile activation would be depressed. Second intracellular acidosis could develop if the intracellular calcium concentration becomes very high. This accumulation of hydrogen ions would depress contractile force, too.

Towart: Certainly, I quite agree. We can't say anything about either the ATP or the pH inside the cells. But as you saw when we did the calcium dose-response curve, you see an increase in contraction up to about three to four millimolar calcium. Then you see the well-documented fall in contractility cause by high extracellular calcium concentrations.

Fleckenstein: You should use a TRIS buffer in order to test whether you can avoid this dissociation between calcium uptake and tension development.

Thomas: But then you shouldn't be able to overcome the depressant effect of high BAY K8644 concentrations by elevating the extracellular calcium concentration, as it is the case at least in the heart.

Fleckenstein: One should determine the intracellular high-energy phosphates in the myocardium under the influence of BAY K8644 in order to clear up the exact mechanism of its negative inotropic effects at high concentrations.

Taira: Intraarterial injections of the BAY K8644 into the saphenous arterial bed of the dog produced a tremendous increase in perfusion pressure. This means the saphenous vessels are still conducting vessels, because BAY K8644 caused constriction only in the presence of excess KCl.

Harper: These are very elegant results, especially the difference in response between the basilar and saphenous arteries. Could I add, however, one word of caution? As you know the vessels supplying the inflow tract of the brain do not necessarily have a blood brain barrier. They also have fibres which the intrinsic vessels in the brain do not have. As an illustration, e.g. 5-hydroxy-tryptamine (serotonin) will cause a very massive constriction of the internal carotid artery. It will not, however, affect the cerebral blood flow at all if infused into an internal carotid artery because it cannot cross the blood brain barrier. And therefore I wonder if you wouldn't consider using some of the techniques developed by Berne and his colleagues in Virginia of extracting one of the intraparenchymal resistence vessels which have, if they have a nerve supply at all, a connection with intrinsic fibre tracts. As it is in the intraparenchymal vessels that 65% of the cerebral vascular resistance lies, I wonder if you would consider expanding your studies to look at these very important vessels.

Towart: These are the perfused microvessels, are they not? The basilar artery was chosen purely because it was a very accessible vessel. You can do quite robust experimental procedures such as calcium withdrawal with these things.

Bayer-Symposium IX
Cardiovascular Effects of Dihydropyridine-Type
Calcium Antagonists and Agonists, 290–305

Effects of Ca^{++}-Agonistic and Ca^{++}-Antagonistic 1,4-Dihydropyridine Compounds on Tonic and Phasic Activation of Extramural Coronary Vasculature

G. FLECKENSTEIN-GRÜN, Y. MAKITA, Y.K. BYON, and A. FLECKENSTEIN

I. Introduction

The administration of calcium antagonists as antianginal, antiarrhythmic, antihypertensive or cardioprotective drugs, makes use of the different manifestations of one and the same elementary membrane action, i.e. inhibition of transmembrane Ca^{++} entry in myocardial fibres, nomotopic and ectopic cardiac pacemakers, as well as in various types of vascular smooth muscle cells [1] (Fig. 1). How-

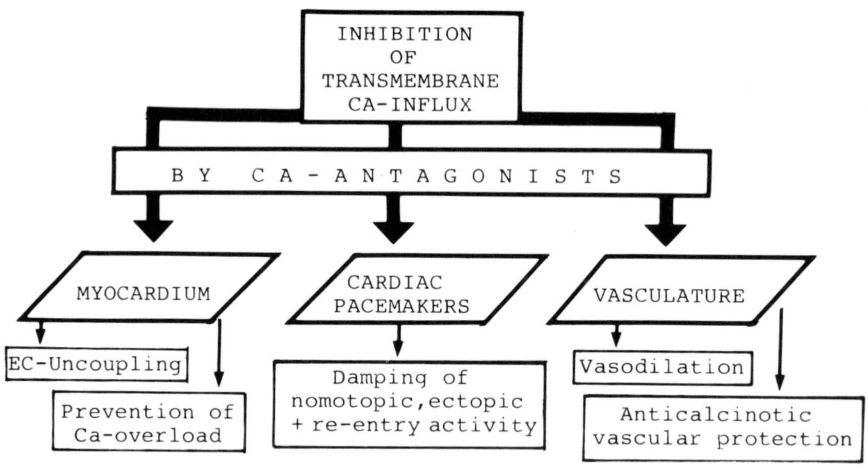

Fig. 1. Scope of Ca^{++}-antagonistic cardiovascular drug responses. From Fleckenstein-Grün et al. [17]

ever, it must be emphasized, that these particular effects are differently accentuated, depending on the individual calcium antagonist used. For instance, the classical calcium antagonists verapamil and D 600 (the generic name of D 600 is gal-

1 For details see Fleckenstein [1–4)

lopamil) exert their damping influence on myocardium, pacemakers, and arterial smooth muscle with comparable intensity. On the other hand, the BAYER compound nifedipine and further dihydropyridine calcium antagonists preferentially suppress Ca^{++}-dependent smooth muscle functions, whereas, at least in humans, the influence of such dihydropyridines on cardiac tension development and pacemaker activity in situ is rather modest. The fundamental Ca^{++}-antagonistic potency of the prototypical substance nifedipine on isolated myocardium and vascular smooth muscle has first been established by Fleckenstein and his group in the years 1969–1972 [5–11]. Since that time, a considerable number of further 1,4-dihydropyridine derivatives were synthesized in the BAYER laboratories and also elsewhere. All these compounds, listed in Table 1, share their preferential Ca^{++}-antagonistic action on the vascular system with the prototypical substance nifedipine. This is true of nimodipine, nisoldipine, nitrendipine, ryosidine, niludipine, felodipine, nicardipine and PY-108-068. However, with the recent discovery of other nifedipine-derivatives ("Calcium-Agonists") which promote transmembrane Ca^{++} entry (see Table 2), it became clear that 1,4-dihydropyridine compounds may exert a "Januslike" influence on passive transmembrane Ca^{++} transport.

Needless to say: Since 10 years scientific interest has concentrated on the outstanding ability of these dihydropyridine calcium antagonists to interfere with contractile activation of vascular smooth muscle in general. However, besides many observations on various types of systemic arteries and on systemic resistance vessels, the effects of these compounds on coronary vasculature, particularly of the large extramural coronary stem arteries, has remained the most important research topic. Thus it is the aim of the present paper to depict more recent results on the characteristic coronary actions of 1,4-dihydropyridine compounds with Ca^{++}-antagonistic *or* Ca^{++}-agonistic properties.

Table 1

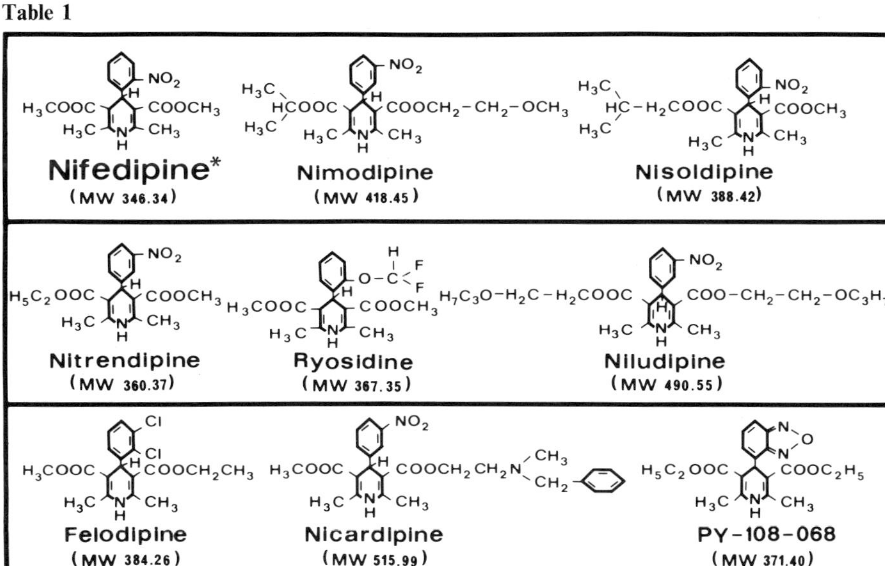

Table 2

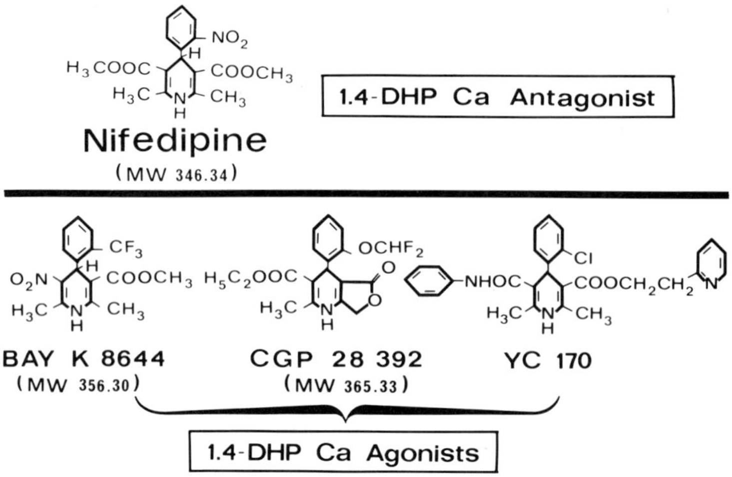

II. Outstanding Inhibitory Influence of Ca^{++} Antagonists on Ca^{++}-Dependent Excitation-Contraction Coupling of K^{+}-Depolarized Coronary (and Cerebral) Arterial Smooth Muscle

The most spectacular action of calcium antagonists on the coronary arterial vasculature, namely excitation-contraction uncoupling by blockade of voltage-dependent transmembrane Ca^{++} entry, can most clearly be demonstrated on K^{+}-depolarized preparations. For instance, Fig. 2a, b show the tremendous efficacy of nifedipine in relaxing two K^{+}-depolarized fully contracted vascular smooth muscle strips. One preparation originated from a rabbit coronary artery, the other preparation from a brain vessel (basilar artery of the same animal). However, with the help of successive small doses of nifedipine, full relaxation was finally obtained at a concentration as small as 3 μg nifedipine/l, i.e. at a concentration of 1×10^{-8} M.

The results of a comparative study carried out on pig coronary strips and on pig basilar artery strips with the use of different calcium antagonists, particularly of the dihydropyridine group, are represented in Figs. 3a, b. The ordinates indicate the percentages of excitation contraction uncoupling obtained on the K^{+}-depolarized strips. The abscissas show, on a logarithmic scale, the molar concentrations of the Ca^{++}-antagonistic compounds applied. As to the coronary vasculature, obviously all calcium antagonists tested in this series are more potent than papaverine. Verapamil and diltiazem are about 50–100 times, gallopamil 300 times, and nifedipine approximately 3,000 times stronger than papaverine. As it is evident from all our observations, the nifedipine derivatives nimodipine, nitrendipine, and ryosidine, exhibit at least the same outstanding coronary relaxing potency as the original compound nifedipine does. Only nisoldipine, nicardipine, and felodipine, are still stronger than nifedipine in this series. According to our data, nisoldipine exerts a coronary vasodilator action which surpasses that of pa-

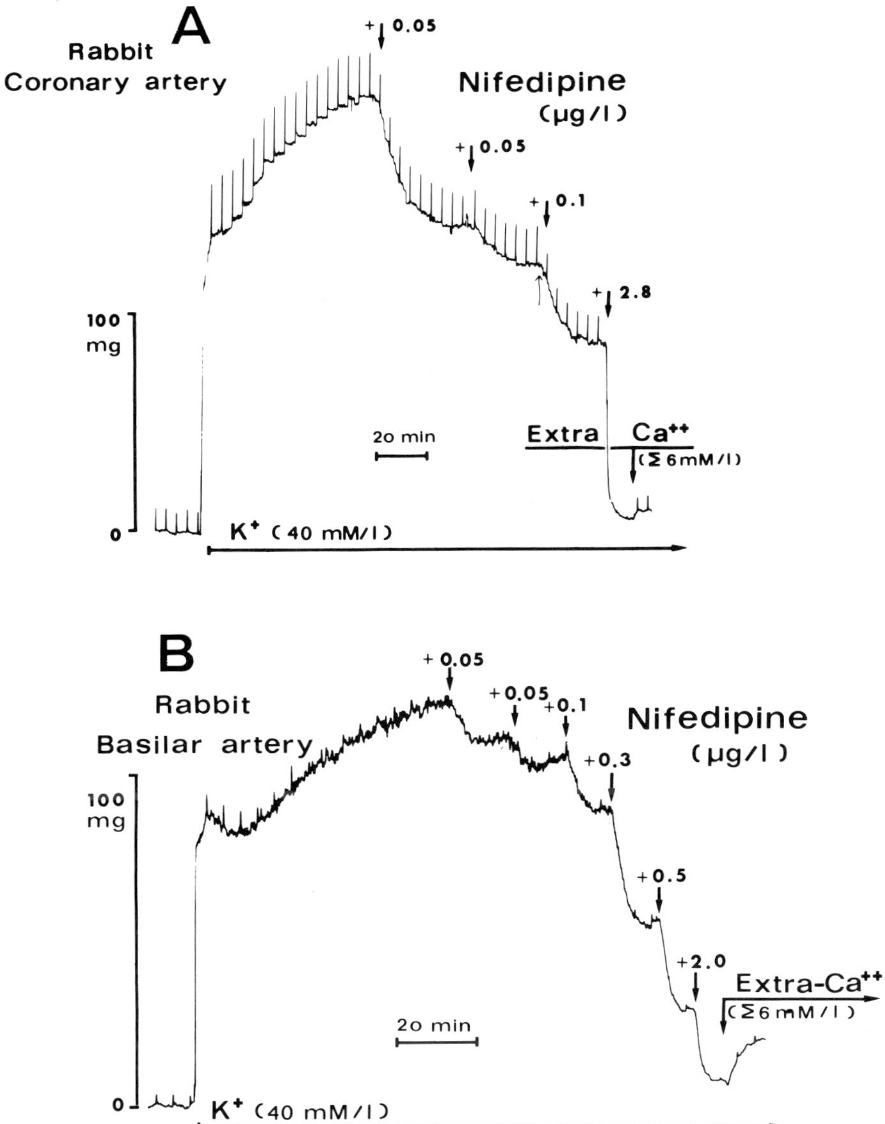

Fig. 2. Suppression by nifedipine of a spastic in vitro contraction of a rabbit coronary strip (**A**) and of a basilar strip (**B**) of the same animal. Depolarization with a high K^+ concentration (40 mM) in Tyrode solution. In addition to the high K^+ concentration, alternating electric square wave stimuli were applied to test excitability. Minute amounts of nifedipine, successively administered to the baths after the climax of shortening had been reached, produced gradual relaxation. With a total dose of 3 µg/l nifedipine (1×10^{-8} M) relaxation was completed and electric excitability abolished in both, coronary and basilar vasculature. From Fleckenstein-Grün and Fleckenstein [18]

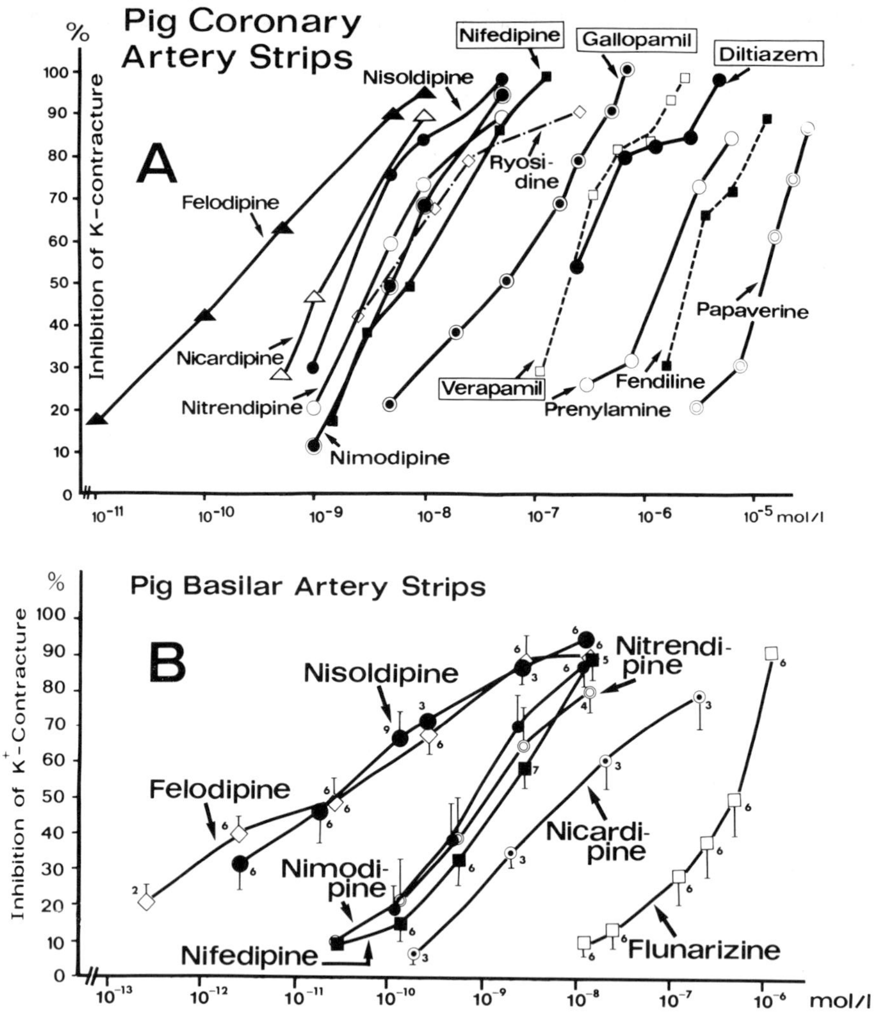

Fig. 3. A Suppression of K^+-induced contractures of pig coronary strips by Ca^{++}-antagonistic inhibitors of excitation-contraction coupling. The strips were depolarized with a K^+-rich Tyrode solution (43 mM KCl) for 40 min to produce full contractures. Then different concentrations of the Ca^{++}-antagonistic compounds were added, so that, depending on the dose applied, tension development was more or less inhibited. The degree of relaxation obtained is expressed as percent of peak tension just before addition of the Ca^{++}-antagonistic drugs. Each point represents the average relaxation calculated from at least 15 individual experiments for each concentration, S.E. not exceeding $\pm 2\%$. Before administration of the K^+-rich solution, the coronary strips (wet weight: 12–15 mg) were kept in a Tyrode solution with a normal K^+ content (concentrations in mM: NaCl 155; KCl 4; $NaHCO_3$ 11.9; $CaCl_2$ 1.0; NaH_2PO_4 0.48; glucose 5.6) for a period of 60 min under a load of 2.0 g. Throughout the experiment, a gas mixture of 97% O_2 and 3% CO_2 was used for oxygenation of the bath at a constant temperature of 35 °C and at a pH of 7.4. Isometric tension was continuously recorded with the use of a mechano-electronic transducer. Nifedipine was approximately 3,000, gallopamil 300, verapamil and diltiazem 50–100 times stronger than papaverine. Nisoldipine, a new 1,4-dihydropyridine calcium antagonist, turned out to be the most potent coronary dilator in this series. It surpasses papaverine by a factor of roughly 15,000. From Fleckenstein-Grün et al. [17]. **B** Suppression of K^+-induced contractures of pig basilar strips (wet weight: 2.8 ± 0.4 mg) by 1,4-dihydropyridine calcium antagonists in comparison with flunarizine. For experimental details see Fig. 3 A. In this series of experiments on brain vasculature, nisoldipine was about 10,000 times stronger than flunarizine

paverine by roughly 15,000 times. Using felodipine, a 50-percent blockade of excitation-contraction coupling was produced with a 10^{-10} molar concentration. Similarly, also on the pig cerebral vasculature obtained from basilar arteries, nisoldipine and felodipine were by far the most potent calcium antagonists (Fig. 3 b). If compared with flunarizine, which has been claimed to be a particularly efficient dilator of cerebral arteries, nisoldipine proved to be about 10,000 times stronger than flunarizine on the pig basilar artery.

III. Suppression by Calcium Antagonists of Acetylcholine-Induced Receptor-Mediated Coronary Smooth Muscle Activation

Another interesting type of spasm that we have studied on pig coronary strips in vitro is that produced with acetylcholine. This was for the following reasons:

1) It is well-known that in patients with spastic Prinzmetal's variant angina, coronary attacks preferentially occur under parasympathetic domination, that is to say at rest, after opulent meals, or during sleep.
2) Such coronary attacks can easily be provoked in Prinzmetal patients by injection of parasympathetic agonists, particularly methacholine.

As it is known from the work of Ginsburg et al. [12] and of Godfraind and Miller [13] on human coronary vasculature and from that of Taira et al. [14] on monkeys also in these cases, acetylcholine acts as a coronary vasoconstrictor, at least, of the big extramural coronary stem arteries. The same is true, according to our observations, of rabbit coronary strips. On the other hand in humans, calcium antagonists have proved to be particularly efficient against all spastic types of coronary disease. Thus it is an important fact that also in the pig's extramural coronary vasculature, acetylcholine and methacholine provoke spasms, and that

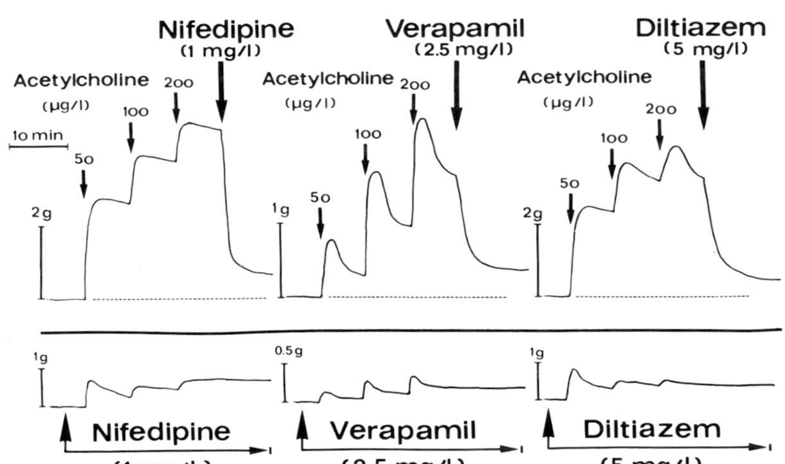

Fig. 4. Suppression of acetylcholine-induced spasms of pig coronary smooth muscle strips by different calcium antagonists, irrespective of whether they were added before or after acetylcholine. From Fleckenstein-Grün and Fleckenstein [18]

the calcium antagonists nifedipine, verapamil, and diltiazem readily suppress such acetylcholine-induced contractile responses also in vitro. In the upper panel of Fig. 4, the calcium antagonists produce an instantaneous relaxation at the climax of spasm which was previously elicited by administration of increasing doses of acetylcholine. In the lower panel, the calcium antagonists had been given beforehand, so that the acetylcholine-induced contractile responses remained very small.

IV. Ca^{++} Dependency of Receptor-Mediated Phasic and Tonic Coronary Constrictions, and Their Responsiveness to Calcium Antagonists

In the course of our studies with acetylcholine on pig coronary smooth muscle, it became obvious that the contractile responses to acetylcholine as well as to histamine and serotonin, are inhomogeneous. The situation resembles that of systemic arteries studied with norepinephrine by Godfraind and Kaba [15] and with norepinephrine, histamine, and serotonin by Bevan, Garstka, Su and Su [16]. Infact, these contractile responses consist of two parts: An initial phasic component A, which expires within 3 min, and a second long-lasting tonic part B, which is fully maintained at least during 20 min (see Fig. 5). According to current concepts derived from observations on rat aortae, phasic activation, that is to say part A, is usually attributed to a rapid Ca^{++} release from cellular stores. This type of phasic activation is considered rather resistant to calcium antagonists. On the other hand, tonic activation, that manifests itself as part B, is supposedly produced by voltage-dependent or receptor-operated transmembrane Ca^{++} influx which is highly susceptible to calcium antagonists. However, our results obtained on coronary smooth muscle clearly indicate that, in this type of vessels, no strict functional differentiation between tonic and phasic contractile activation – or in other words – between part A and part B exists.

In fact, as shown on pig coronary smooth muscle, calcium antagonists always counteract both the initial phasic part A and the long-lasting tonic part B of the acetylcholine-induced responses to nearly the same extent. The Figs. 6a, b show

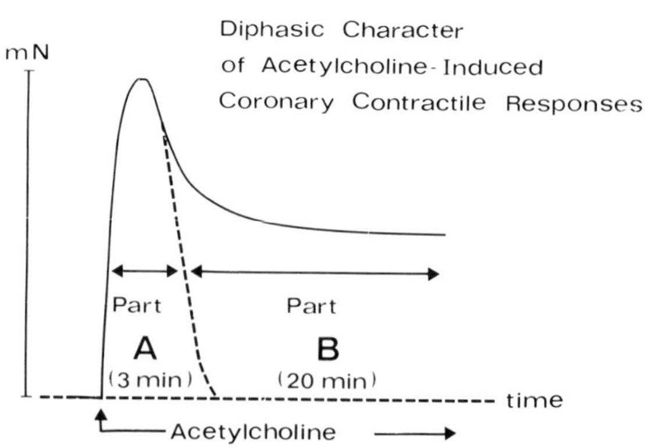

Fig. 5. Scheme of a mixed phasic/tonic contractile response of a pig coronary strip to acetylcholine. Also with histamine and serotonin similar inhomogeneous contractures were produced

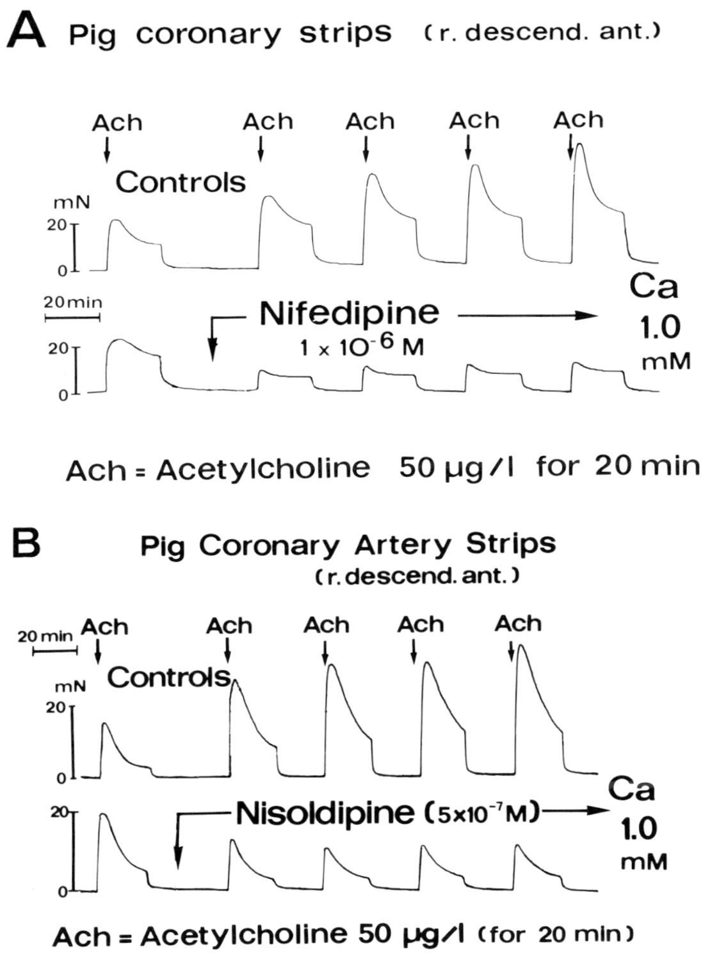

Fig. 6. Inhibition of acetylcholine-induced coronary contractures by nifedipine (1×10^{-6} M, **A**) or by nisoldipine (5×10^{-7} M, **B**). Acetylcholine, repeatedly administered in the low dose of 50 µg/l (2.8×10^{-7} M; incubation period 20 min each), produced constrictions with increasing phasic and tonic tension development ("positive staircase"). The 1,4-dihydropyridine calcium antagonists nifedipine and nisoldipine depressed both tonic and phasic coronary constrictions as well as the positive staircase phenomenon

the effects of nifedipine and nisoldipine. We conclude from these results, that not only the tonic part B, but also the phasic part A of the acetylcholine contractions require a transmembrane Ca^{++} supply which can be blocked by the calcium antagonists. Possibly, in coronary smooth muscle, Ca^{++} release from intracellular stores for phasic activation needs to be triggered by a small amount of Ca^{++} ions entering the cell via a Ca^{++} antagonist-sensitive transmembrane pathway.

Accordingly, the inhibitory actions of calcium antagonists such as verapamil and nifedipine on the phasic part A and on the tonic part B are always dramatically potentiated, if the availability of extracellular Ca^{++} is further reduced in a

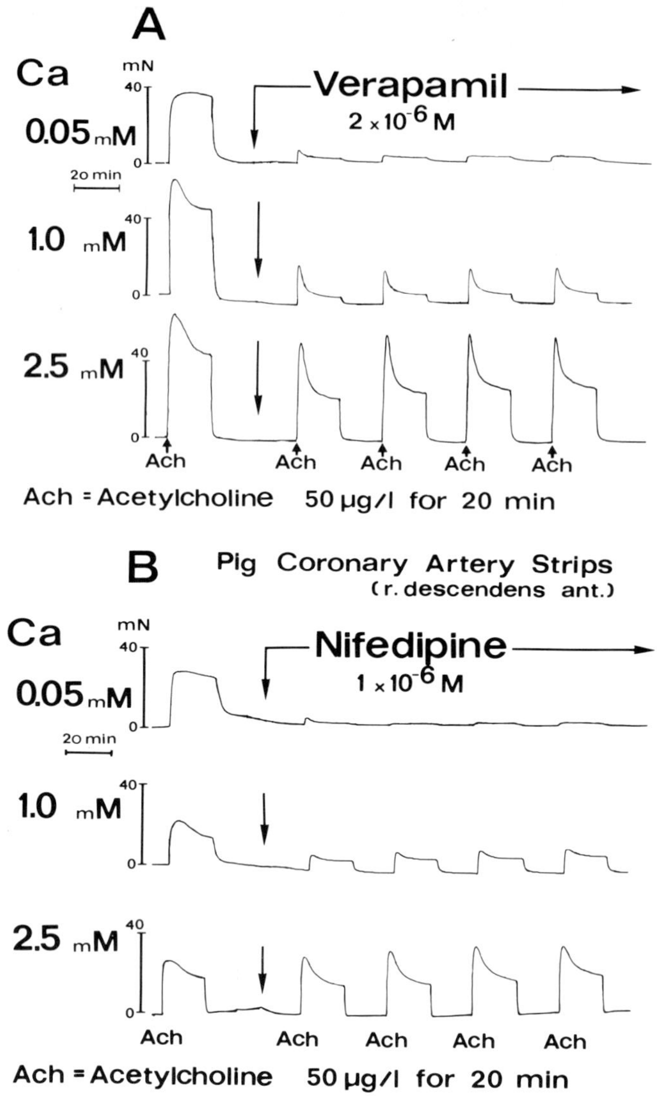

Fig. 7 A, B. Contractile responses of pig coronary strips to repeated 20 min exposures to a Tyrode solution with 50 µg/l (2.8×10^{-7} M) acetylcholine. Influence of extracellular Ca^{++} concentration on the degree of coronary relaxation produced by verapamil (**A**) and nifedipine (**B**). Whereas the effects of both calcium antagonists are potentiated by a low Ca^{++} concentration (0.05 mM), verapamil and nifedipine lose most of their relaxing potency in the presence of a high Ca^{++} concentration (2.5 mM). The tonic part of the acetylcholine-induced contractile responses is slightly more inhibited by the calcium antagonists than is the phasic part

solution with a low Ca^{++} content (0.05 mM). This is shown in the upper records of Fig. 7a, b. Conversely, calcium antagonists lose most of their inhibitory effects on part A and B if the transmembrane Ca^{++} supply is facilitated in a solution with an elevated Ca^{++} content (2.5 mM), as shown in the records on the bottom. In short, calcium antagonists exhibit a particularly broad scope of spasmolytic actions in the coronary vasculature, because, besides of lowering high coronary

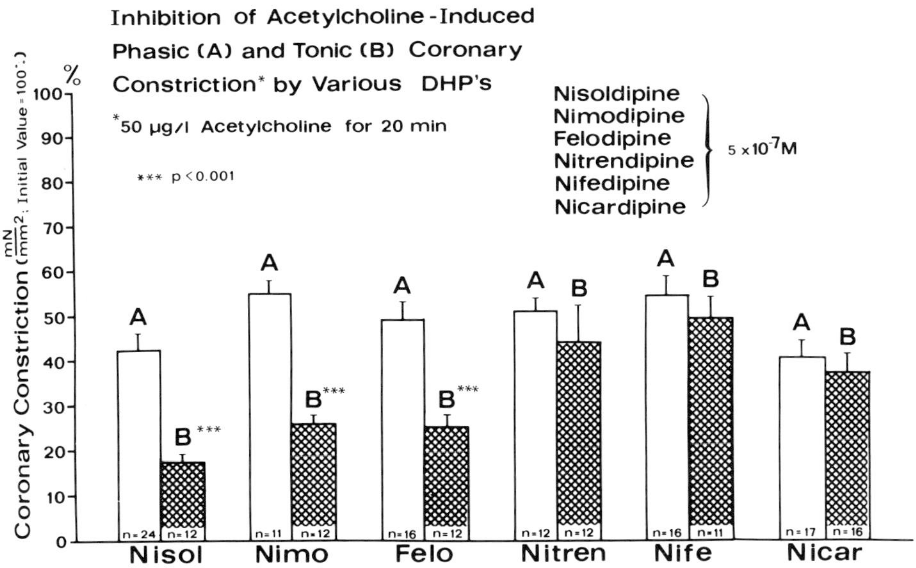

Fig. 8. Inhibition of acetylcholine-induced phasic (**A**) and tonic (**B**) coronary constriction by various DHP calcium antagonists. Experiments on isolated pig coronary artery strips (r. descendens anterior). Acetylcholine (2.8×10^{-7} M) was administered for 20 min (see Figs. 5 and 6) repeatedly. All DHP calcium antagonists used in this series depressed both tonic and phasic coronary contraction in a concentration of 5×10^{-7} M below the initial value (phasic contraction: 100% $= 31.9 \pm 2.4$ mN/mm^2; tonic contraction: 100% $= 14.8 \pm 2.1$ mN/mm^2). Only nisoldipine, nimodipine, and felodipine diminished tonic activation significantly stronger than the phasic responses

tone, these drugs also depress high contraction peaks of phasic character which also need a Ca^{++} supply through transmembrane pathways. As shown in Fig. 8, all dihydropyridine calcium antagonists, in a concentration of 5×10^{-7} M depress both phasic (P) and tonic (T) contractile tension development below the initial level which is taken as 100%. Only with nisoldipine, nimodipine, and felodipine, the decrease of tonic activation is significantly greater than that of the phasic responses.

V. Potentiation of Calcium Agonists of Voltage- or Receptor-Mediated Phasic and Tonic Coronary Contractile Responses

As already pointed out today by earlier speakers, the new calcium agonists, particularly Bay K 8644, facilitate voltage-dependent Ca^{++} uptake in vascular smooth muscle and thereby increase tonic vascular responses in a rather general way. Thus also in K^{+}-depolarized coronary smooth muscle strips, Bay K 8644 produces a dramatic rise in contractile tension. As shown in Fig. 9, successive addition of Bay K 8644 (in a concentration of 5×10^{-8} M or 5×10^{-7} M) potentiated tension development considerably. The columns in Fig. 10 represent quanti-

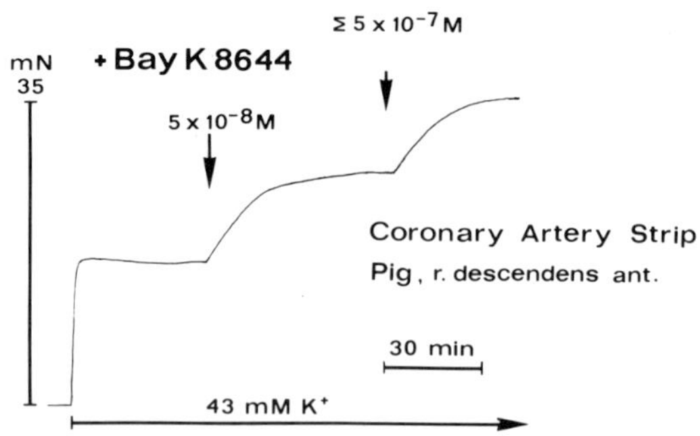

Fig. 9. Potentiation of a K^+-induced coronary contracture by the DHP calcium agonist Bay K 8644. Depolarization produced by elevation of the extracellular K^+ concentration up to 43 mM leads to a "voltage-dependent" Ca^{++} influx and activation of the coronary vasculature. Additional administration of Bay K 8644 (5×10^{-8} M and 5×10^{-7} M) increases tonic coronary tension development considerably

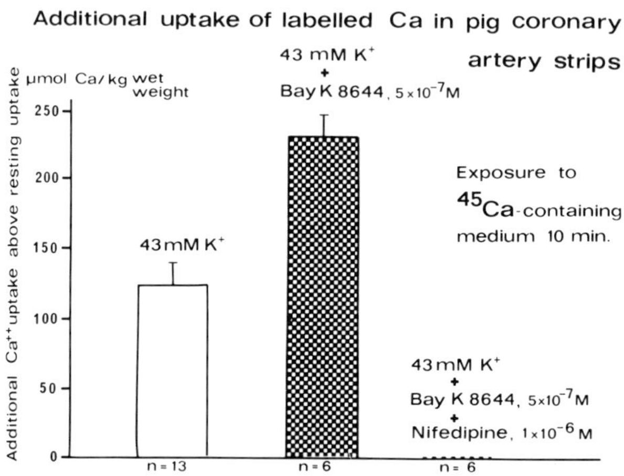

Fig. 10. Potentiation by Bay K 8644 (5×10^{-7} M) of net ^{45}Ca uptake into K^+-depolarized coronary vasculature. Reduction with nifedipine (1×10^{-6} M) of the net ^{45}Ca uptake in the K^+-depolarized, Bay K 8644-treated vasculature down to resting level. Experiments on isolated pig coronary artery strips (r. descendens anterior). Exposure to ^{45}Ca-containing medium each time for 10 min. ^{45}Ca influx measurements according to van Breemen et al. [19]

tative data (obtained with radioactive $^{45}Ca^{++}$) on the net transmembrane Ca^{++} uptake during a 10-min contracture in a depolarizing K^+-rich (43 mM) Tyrode solution, in the absence or presence of Bay K 8644. As can be easily seen from the hatched column, the net Ca^{++} uptake (underlying the contractile potentiation) is almost doubled in the presence of the calcium agonist Bay K 8644. If however, the coronary strips were forced to remain in a fully relaxed state by adding the calcium antagonist nifedipine to the K^+-rich Tyrode solution (still containing the calcium agonist Bay K 8644), the Ca^{++} uptake remained at resting level, i.e. at the baseline. All these results are in full agreement with the actual concepts about the reciprocal reactivity of voltage-dependent channels to calcium agonists and antagonists.

However, we emphasize that in coronary smooth muscle the promotion of transmembrane Ca^{++} influx by calcium agonists leads to both potentiation of voltage-dependent responses, and also to increases in receptor-dependent tonic and phasic contractility. Figures 11 and 12 exhibit (in the lower records) a series

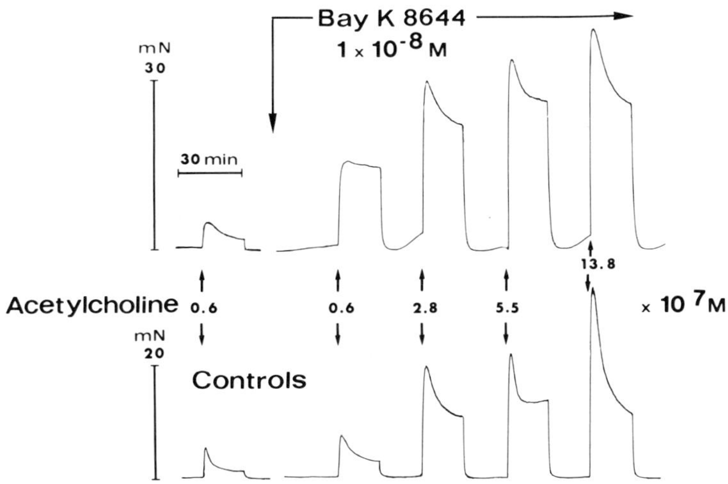

Fig. 11. Potentiation of acetylcholine-induced tonic and phasic coronary contractions by the DHP calcium agonist Bay K 8644 (1×10^{-8} M). Experiments on isolated pig coronary strips (r. descendens anterior). Acetylcholine was repeatedly administered in a concentration range of 0.6 to 13.8×10^{-7} M, each time for 20 min (followed by a washout period of 20 min) in the presence of Bay K 8644 (*upper part*) or in its absence (*lower part* of the figure)

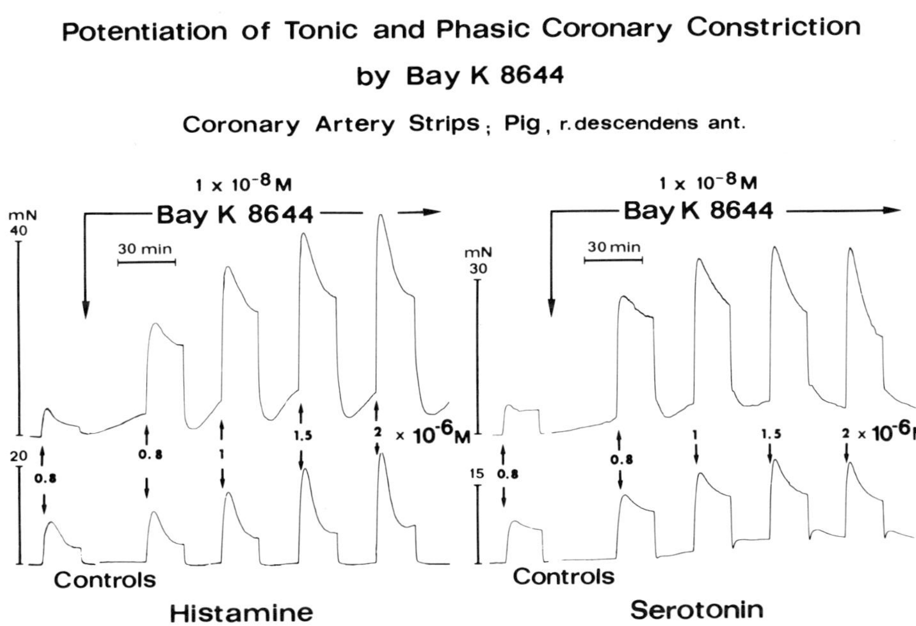

Fig. 12. Potentiation (upper records) of histamine- or serotonin-induced coronary contractile responses by the DHP calcium agonist Bay K 8644 (1×10^{-8} M). The control records without Bay K 8644 are shown on the bottom. Histamine and serotonin were administered in a concentration range of 0.8 to 2×10^{-6} M. Same experimental procedure as in Fig. 11

of coronary contractures which were produced by repeated administration of the 3 vasoconstrictor agonists acetylcholine, histamine, and serotonin, without addition of Bay K 8644. On the other hand, the upper series of contractures was carried out in the presence of the calcium agonist. In consequence, the initial phasic part A and the subsequent tonic part B were almost equally intensified by the calcium agonist. In other words: Also with respect to the influence on receptor-dependent phasic or tonic reactions of pig coronary smooth muscle, the calcium agonist Bay K 8644 acts oppositely to the calcium antagonist nifedipine.

VI. Similarities Between the Calcium Agonist Bay K 8644 and Cardiac Glycosides with Respect to Promotion of Ca^{++}-Dependent Coronary Constriction

In this context it is to be noted that there are many similarities between the enhancement of coronary spasms by the new calcium agonist Bay K 8644 and the sensitization to coronary vasoconstriction by cardiac glycosides. In fact, as we

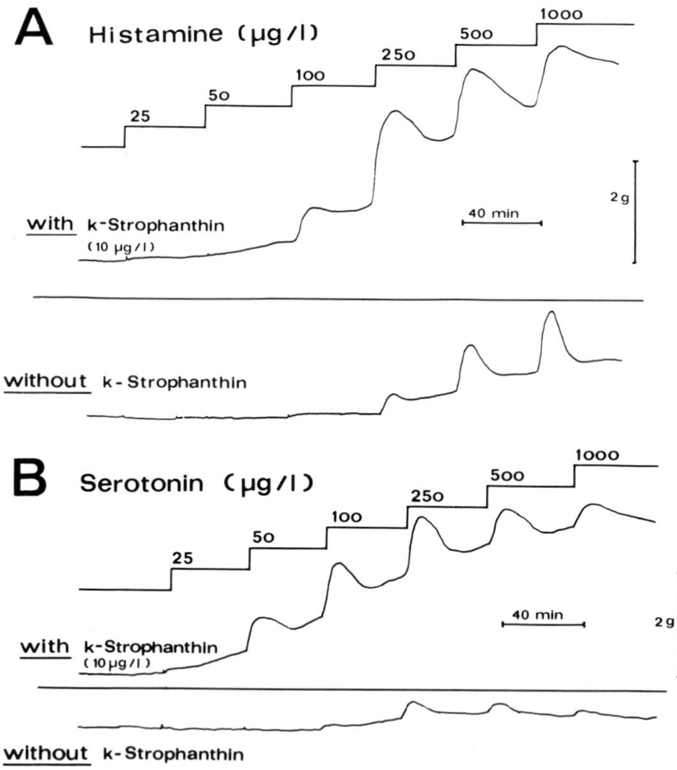

Fig. 13. Potentiation by k-strophanthin of phasic and tonic coronary contractile responses to histamine (**A**) or serotonin (**B**). Experiments on isolated pig coronary artery strips (r. descendens anterior). The vasoconstrictor agonists histamine and serotonin were administered at increasing concentrations (25 to 1,000 µg/l) in the presence or absence (=control series) of k-strophanthin. From Nakayama et al. [20]

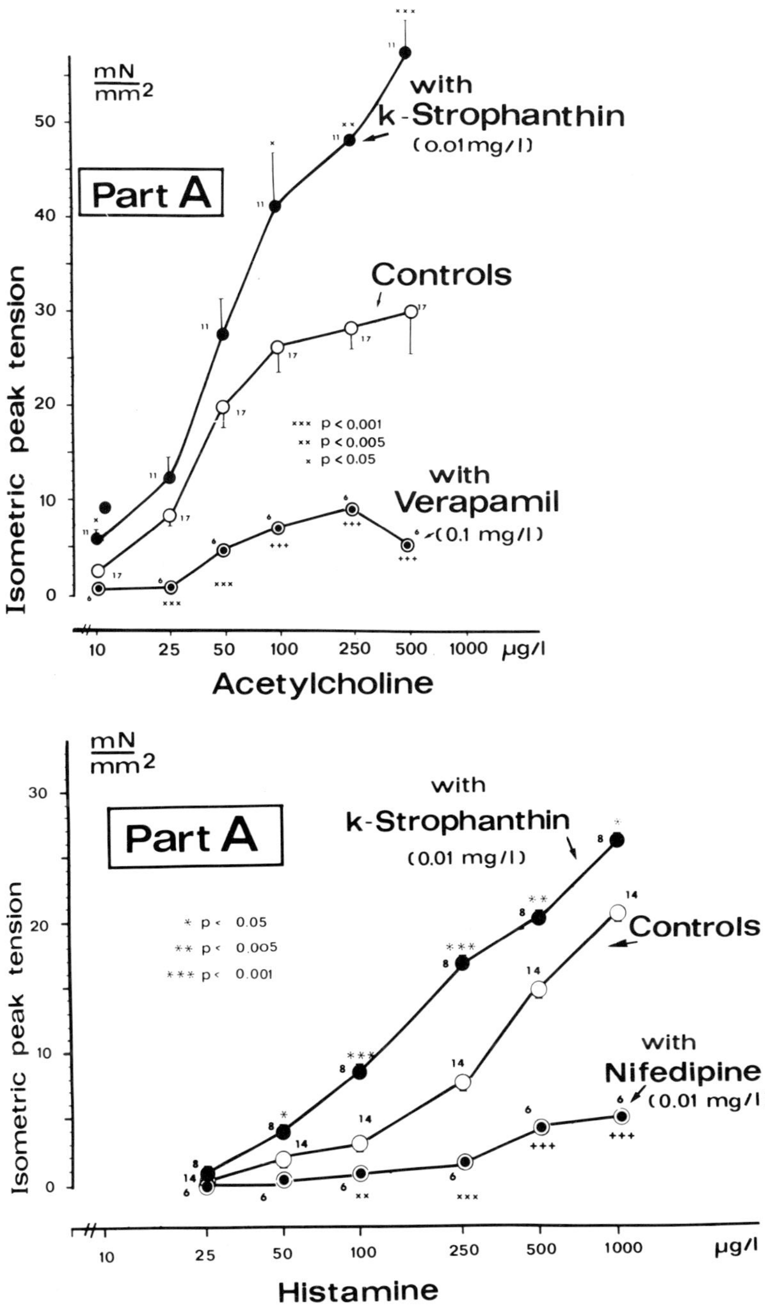

Fig. 14. Potentiation by k-strophanthin and suppression by calcium antagonists of the phasic parts (*A*) of the contractile responses of pig coronary strips to acetylcholine (*upper panel*) or to histamine (*lower panel*). Increasing doses of acetylcholine or histamine were successively added to Tyrode solutions containing k-strophanthin or the calcium antagonists verapamil or nifedipine. Isometric tension development is calculated as mN per square millimeter cross section, the coronary smooth muscle strips taken as cylindric. From Fleckenstein-Grün [21]

have found already 10 years ago, cardiac glycosides promote coronary vasoconstriction by facilitating calcium entry (for a detailed description and literature see Fleckenstein [4]). Accordingly, with k-strophanthin (Fig. 13a, b), the vasoconstrictor responses to acetylcholine, histamine, and serotonin, are as strongly potentiated as with Bay K 8644.

This fact becomes even more obvious from the summarizing graphs in Figs. 14a and 14b which reflect the transmembrane Ca^{++} entry promotion with strophanthin, and conversely, show the contractile depression produced by transmembrane Ca^{++} entry inhibition with the use of the calcium antagonists verapamil and nifedipine. In these two figures only the changes on the heights of the initial phasic part A of the acetylcholine-induced and histamine-induced coronary contractions are shown. The similarities between the effects of strophanthin and those of the calcium agonist Bay K 8644 (see Figs. 11 and 12) in potentiating the phasic part A of the acetylcholine or histamine contractures, is obvious. Thus the message of these observations is clear: In the coronary vasculature, not only the tonic part B, but also the phasic part A of receptor-mediated vasoconstriction requires a transmembrane Ca^{++} supply. Therefore, any change in Ca^{++} influx, i.e. inhibition by calcium antagonists, or conversely promotion by strophanthin and the new calcium agonists (particularly Bay K 8644) alter tonic *and* phasic contractile activation in parallel. Or in other words: In contrast with current concepts derived from observations on systemic arteries (mostly rat aortae), both tonic *and* phasic contractile activation of coronary smooth muscle exhibit fundamental similarities in their responsiveness to promoters and inhibitors of transmembrane Ca^{++} supply.

References

1. Fleckenstein A (1970/71 a) Specific inhibitors and promoters of calcium action in the excitation-contraction coupling of heart muscle and their role in the production of prevention of myocardial lesions. In: Harris P, Opie L (eds) Calcium and the heart. Proceed. of the Meeting of the Europ. Section of the Internat. Study Group for Research in Cardiac Metabolism, London, Sept. 1970. Academic Press, London New York, pp 135–188
2. Fleckenstein A (1977) Specific pharmacology of calcium in myocardium, cardiac pacemakers, and vascular smooth muscle. Ann Rev Pharmacol Toxicol 17:149–166
3. Fleckenstein A (1983) History of calcium antagonists. In: Schwartz A, Taira N (eds) Calcium channel-blocking drugs: A novel intervention for the treatment of cardiac disease. Monograph No. 95 of the American Heart Association, Circ. Research, Part II, vol 52, No. 2, pp 3–16
4. Fleckenstein A (1983) Calcium antagonism in heart and smooth muscle – Experimental facts and therapeutic prospects. Wiley, New York Chichester Brisbane Toronto Singapore
5. Grün G, Fleckenstein A, Tritthart H (1969) Excitation-contraction uncoupling on the rat's uterus by some "musculotropic" smooth muscle relaxants. Pflügers Arch Ges Physiol 264:239
6. Fleckenstein A (1970/71 b) Neuere Ergebnisse zur Physiologie, Pharmakologie und Pathologie der elektromechanischen Koppelungsprozesse im Warmblütermyokard. In: Vorträge der Erlanger Physiologentagung 1970. W. D. Keidel u. K. H. Plattig Hrsg., S 13–52, Springer, Berlin Heidelberg New York, 1971
7. Grün G, Fleckenstein A (1971) Ca-antagonism, a new principle of vasodilation. Naunyn-Schmiedeberg's Arch Exper Path Pharmakol 270 (Suppl), R 48

8. Grün G, Fleckenstein A, Byon YK (1971 a) Hemmung der Motilität isolierter Uterus-Streifen aus gravidem und nicht-gravidem menschlichem Myometrium durch Ca^{++}-Antagonisten und Sympathomimetica. Arzneimittelforsch (Drug Res) 21:1585–1590
9. Grün G, Fleckenstein A, Byon YK (1971 b) Ca antagonism, a new principle of vasodilation. In: Proceed. 25th Congress Internat. Union Physiol Sciences, Munich, 1971, vol 9, p 221
10. Fleckenstein A, Tritthart H, Fleckenstein B, Herbst A, Grün G (1969) A new group of competitive Ca antagonists (Iproveratril, D 600, Prenylamine) with highly potent inhibitory effects on excitation-contraction coupling in mammalian myocardium. Pflügers Arch Ges Physiol 307:R25
11. Grün G, Fleckenstein A (1972) Die elektro-mechanische Entkoppelung der glatten Gefäßmuskulatur als Grundprinzip der Coronardilatation durch 4-(2′-Nitrophenyl)-2,6-dimethyl-1,4-dihydropyridin-3,5-dicarbonsäure-dimethylester (Bay a 1040, Nifedipin). Arzneimittelforsch (Drug Res) 22:334–344
12. Ginsburg R, Briston MR, Harrison DC, Stinson EB (1980) Studies with isolated human coronary arteries. Chest 78 (Suppl) 180–186
13. Godfraind T, Miller RC (1983) Specificity of action of Ca entry blockers. A comparison of their actions in rat arteries and in human coronary arteries. In: Schwartz A, Taira N (eds) Calcium channel-blocking drugs: A novel intervention for the treatment of cardiac disease. Monograph No. 95 of the American Heart Association, Circ. Research, Part II, vol 52, No. 2, pp 81–91
14. Taira N, Satoh K, Maruyama M, Yamashita S (1983) Sustained coronary constriction and its antagonism by calcium-blocking agents in monkeys and baboons. In: Schwartz A, Taira N (eds) Calcium channel-blocking drugs: A novel intervention for the treatment of cardiac disease. Monograph No. 95 of the American Heart Association. Circ. Research, Part II, vol 52, No. 2, pp 40–46
15. Godfraind T, Kaba A (1969) Blockade or reversal of the contraction induced by calcium and adrenaline in depolarized arterial smooth muscle. Brit J Pharmacol 36:549–560
16. Bevan JA, Garstka W, Su C, Su MO (1973) The bimodal basis of the contractile response of the rabbit ear artery to norepinephrine and other agonists. Europ J Pharmacol 22:47–53
17. Fleckenstein-Grün G, Frey M, Fleckenstein A (1984) Calcium antagonists: mechanisms and therapeutic uses. In: Trends in pharmacological sciences, vol 5, No. 7. Elsevier Biomedical Press, Cambridge, pp 283–286
18. Fleckenstein-Grün G, Fleckenstein A (1978/80) Calcium-Antagonismus, ein Grundprinzip der Vasodilatation. In: Fleckenstein A, Roskamm H (eds) Calcium-Antagonismus, Proceed. eines Internat. Symp., Frankfurt, 1978. Springer, Berlin Heidelberg New York, pp 191–207
19. van Breemen C, Hwang OK, Meisheri KD (1981) The mechanism of inhibitory action of diltiazem on vascular smooth muscle contractility. J Pharmacol Exper Therapeutics 218, No. 2, pp 459–463
20. Nakayama K, Fleckenstein-Grün G, Byon YK, Fleckenstein A (1976) Opposite effects of cardiac glycosides and Ca-antagonistic compounds on vascular smooth muscle contractility under electrical, mechanical and pharmacological stimulation (Observations on helical strips from rabbit coronary and brain arteries). Pflügers Arch Ges Physiol Suppl to vol 365, R 7
21. Fleckenstein-Grün G (1985) Suppression of experimental coronary spasms by major calcium antagonists. In: Rubin RP, Weiss GB, Putney JW Jr (eds) Calcium in biological systems. FASEB-Meeting, Chicago, April 1983. Plenum, New York

Discussion

(pp. 290–305)

Hugenholtz: You mentioned the significance of the existing level of calcium in terms of the efficacy of the calcium antagonist. In the clinical situation we know that during nocturnal angina the free calcium content is higher, which has very bad connotation since there is a higher mortality. What variation (your range was from 0.05 to 2.5 mmol/l) is already enough to make a Ca^{2+}-antagonist less effective? The more so since we have seen in a number of patients that at night they break through their therapy.

Fleckenstein-Grün: I do not believe that in situ such degrees of an extracellular Ca^{2+} variation could occur which might change the sensitivity of vascular smooth muscle cells against Ca^{2+}-antagonists.

Kadowitz: I have a question about the intactness of the endothelium of the coronary vessels in your studies because in most coronary vessels the response to acetylcholine is endothelial dependent. We worked with bovine large and small coronary vessels. When the endothelium is intact, acetylcholine is a very potent vasodilator agent and it is true for some of the other vessels discussed.

Fleckenstein-Grün: Since many years we performed experiments with acetylcholine in pig coronary artery strips. In vascular strip preparations there is always a damage of the endothelium. We prefer these preparations because we are interested in the pathophysiological mechanism of coronary spasms and of the possibility to inhibit them by Ca^{2+}-antagonists. There might be a protective effect of an EDRF-released by an intact endothelium – against coronary artery spasms. Obviously there are extreme species differences: In coronary artery strips of pig, rabbit and men we can produce acetylcholine-, histamine-, and metacholine-induced spasms with very low concentrations; in dog coronary artery strips – treated under exactly the same conditions – we cannot. Therefore, dog coronary artery strips are poor preparations for studying coronary artery spasms and relaxing effects of Ca^{2+}-antagonists.

Hess: In many system including the neuro-muscular junction acetylcholine causes rapid desensitization. Could this be important in your system and could it explain why the contracture relaxes during maintained acetylcholine application?

Fleckenstein: This happens with high concentrations. We avoided such high concentrations of acetylcholine.

De Mey: The question rather is, whether there really is a part A and a part B with respect to excitation-contraction coupling.

Fleckenstein-Grün: No, I don't think so because of 2 reasons:

1. Under the influence of calcium antagonists the phasic part A is less influenced than the tonic part B.

2. In another series of experiments we added acetylcholine in a concentration of 50° µg/l for 3 min only followed by a washout period of several minutes and we repeated this procedure 10 to 12 times. In those experiments we never got any sign of the desensibilization of the receptors but we got a continuous increase of the acetylcholine induced answer and we interprete this as a positive stair-case phenomenon.

De Mey: It might be that part B is due to endogenous production of prostaglandins, since part B disappears in the presence of indomethacin.

Fleckenstein-Grün: In our experiments there was no influence of indomethacin on phasic or tonic acetylcholine-induced coronary constriction. Anyway, part A and part B must depend on the extracellular calcium concentration and a transmembrane Ca^{2+}-influx.

Van Breemen: We have found that during stimulation with an agonist the very initial influx is four times as high as the maintained influx of calcium. You only see that if you prelabel the tissue under non-stimulated conditions for about 3 to 4 min with $^{45}Ca^{2+}$. There appears to be a bound calcium fraction which has a half time of turnover of around 2 min which is released upon addition of an agonist. That given you a peak of influx and this may be responsible for the initial phasic portion. That, of course, is sensitive to calcium antagonists because it still has to cross the membrane.

Scriabine: What is the relative activity of various calcium antagonists on part A and B of the response to acetylcholine? Is it possible, that verapamil would inhibit both phases of acetylcholine-induced contractions at similar concentrations, but a drug like nisoldipine is relatively selective for the phase B?

Fleckenstein-Grün: We didn't carry out these comparative experiments with other calcium antagonists.

Cauvin: In the rabbit mesenteric resistance vessels, we also showed that the phasic contraction is sensitive to nisoldipine. All the other types of calcium antagonists also affect that phasic contraction because it is largely due to extracellular calcium entry. There does not seem to be any selectivity for various calcium antagonists with regard to inhibiting this phasic contraction.

Scriabine: Steinsland working in our laboratories found a great difference between verapamil and dihydropyridines on rabbit ear artery. Verapamil inhibits both the tonic and phasic contractions almost at the same concentrations, whereas nitrendipine was about 20 times or even more potent against the tonic than against phasic contractions caused by electrical stimulation.

Van Breemen: That may be due to the alpha blocking effect of verapamil.

Bayer-Symposium IX
Cardiovascular Effects of Dihydropyridine-Type
Calcium Antagonists and Agonists, 309–325

Effects of Dihydropyridines on Human and Animal Isolated Vessels

T. GODFRAIND, C. EGLEME, and M. WIBO

Introduction

In early studies on the role of calcium in the action of vasoconstrictors, Godfraind and Colleagues (Godfraind et al. 1968; Godfraind and Polster 1968; Godfraind and Kaba 1969) have reported that two pools of calcium are utilized by agonists, one being extracellular, the other intracellular. They also showed that potassium depolarization of vascular smooth muscle required the presence of calcium in the perfusion fluid to produce a contraction. The contraction evoked by calcium in depolarized smooth muscle is dose dependent and is specifically blocked by organic drugs such as cinnarizine, the first agent identified as an organic calcium antagonist (Godfraind and Polster 1968). From their experimental observations, Godfraind and Kaba (1969) have concluded that the inhibition by cinnarizine of the vasoconstriction evoked by catecholamines was due to blockade of calcium entry evoked by the alpha adrenergic agonist. The contraction resistant to cinnarizine blockade was similar to the one recorded in calcium free solution. This latter contraction was insensitive to cinnarizine. The concept of blockade of calcium entry as a main pharmacological action has been extended to several drugs of various chemical structures (see Cauvin et al. 1983; Fleckenstein 1983).

The purpose of this paper is to summarize the main experiments performed in our laboratory with the aim to examine how the concept of calcium entry blockade could be extended to the group of dihydropyridines which may be considered as the most important family of calcium antagonists. We will first consider the relation between inhibition of contraction and calcium movements in rat aorta. This tissue is an interesting model for in vitro studies on vascular smooth muscle, because its properties seem to be intermediate between those of large conducting and small resistant vessels. A special attention will be devoted to the interaction of dihydropyridines with adrenoceptors. Because endothelium has been shown to influence arterial contraction (Eglème et al. 1984; Godfraind et al 1984c), the role of this structure in Ca-antagonist action and in Ca-agonist effect will also be examined. We will also consider the interaction of dihydropyridines with K-depolarization and emphasize the problem of use-dependence. Because dihydropyridines are therapeutically important in cardiovascular diseases, we will examine their action in vessels obtained from hypertensive animals and in human isolated coronary arteries.

Methods

Twelve- to fifteen-week-old rats (Wistar, WKY, SHR), were killed by decapitation. Thoracic aorta and superior mesenteric artery were removed and cleaned. Rings of thoracic aorta (2 mm wide) were cut close to the aortic arch as reported elsewhere (Godfraind 1979). Some strips were left intact, other were stripped of their endothelial cells by mechanical rubbing. Selective removal of endothelium was deduced from the presence or absence of a relaxant response to acetylcholine (10^{-6} M) applied when the initial evoked contraction was stable.

Hearts were taken from patients within 5 h of sudden death (due to accident or non-cardiac-related vascular collapse). The terminal portions (about 2 cm) of the anterior descending branch of the left coronary artery and circumflex coronary artery were removed and cleaned of all loosely adherent tissue. Coronary and aortic arterials rings (2 mm wide) were suspended in 20- or 50-ml organ baths containing physiological solution.

The physiological solution employed in these experiments contained (millimolar): NaCl, 112; KCl, 5; $NaHCO_3$, 25; KH_2PO_4, 1; $MgSO_4$, 0.1; $CaCl_2$, 1.25; and glucose, 11.5. It was maintained at 37 °C and aerated with a gas mixture of 95% O_2–5% CO_2. For calcium flux studies, the physiological solution was prepared without phosphate in order to minimize Ca precipitation (Godfraind 1976). Therefore, parallel contraction experiments were also performed in this solution.

Rings of human coronary artery and of rat aorta and segments of superior mesenteric artery were suspended in organ chambers (50 ml) filled with physiological solution under a resting tension of 2 g. They were connected to an isometric lever with two strains gauges as part of a balanced bridge, the output of which was fed into a recorder. Experiments with dihydropyridines were conducted in a darkened room, using a Na lamp, in order to avoid drug degradation induced by daylight.

Drugs. The following drugs were used: norepinephrine bitartrate (Fluka AG, Buchs, Switzerland), clonidine-HCl (Boehringer), phentolamine mesylate (Ciba Pharmaceutical Company, Summit, NJ), prazosin hydrochloride (Pfizer, Inc., Groton, CT), and dihydropyridines (Bayer, Leverkusen, FRG), Norepinephrine and clonidine were dissolved in distilled water containing 7.9 mM Na_2SO_3 and 34 mM HCl. Dihydropyridines were dissolved in acetone (0.1–0.001 M) and diluted in physiological solution. The final acetone concentration was always lower than 0.01%.

Agonist Concentration-Response Curves. Contractions of arteries were evoked by cumulatively increasing the agonist concentration, until maximal contractions were achieved. After washout and relaxation, the vessels were incubated in physiological solution either containing or not containing a calcium antagonist. After 90 min, a second cumulative concentration-effect curve was obtained.

Inasmuch as Ca flux studies were done in a phosphate-free solution using 10^{-5} M norepinephrine, the action of Ca antagonists on the sustained contraction evoked by 10^{-5} M norepinephrine was also studied under the same conditions. In order to reduce sources of variation, these experiments were performed with rats selected at random from the same group of animals.

Depolarization-Evoked Contraction. The depolarizing solution used to evoke arterial contraction (Godfraind and Kaba 1969) comprised (millimolar): NaCl, 17; KCL, 100; $CaCl_2$, 1.25; $NaHOC_3$, 25; KH_2PO_4, 1; $MgSO_4$, 0.1, and glucose, 11.5).

Contraction was evoked by filling the organ chamber with this solution. For calcium flux studies, the solution was prepared without phosphate and appropriate controls for contraction were carried out as reported above for norepinephrine. In some experiments using higher calcium concentrations, $NaHCO_3$ concentration was reduced to 9 mM, so that the pH of the aerated physiological solution was not 7.4 but 7.2.

Calcium Concentration-Response Curves. The cumulative calcium contraction-response relationship was investigated in K depolarizing solutions containing either 100 mM KCl or 40 mM KCl. Arteries were preincubated for 10 min in Ca-free physiological solution containing 10^{-4} M ethylene glycol bis(β-aminoethyl ether)N,N'-tetraacetic acid, washed out with this solution (three times) and depolarized with K solution deprived of $CaCl_2$. The $CaCl_2$ additions were made cumulatively as soon as a plateau response had been obtained at the previous concentration. After the control curve, arteries were washed out with physiological solution until complete relaxation was obtained and then were incubated in physiological solution either containing or not containing nifedipine. Ninety minutes later, a second calcium concentration curve was obtained.

Measurement of ^{45}Ca Movements. Thoracic aorta was cut open longitudinally and segments weighing about 10 mg were used for the experiments. As previously reported, calcium influx and efflux were estimated by measuring changes in the specific activity of the calcium fraction resistant to displacement by lanthanum (Godfraind 1976). The norepinephrine-dependent ^{45}Ca influx was estimated after an equilibration period of 60 min in physiological solution and a preincubation of 90 min in the same solution with or without a dihydropyridine. The artery strips were incubated for 5 min in ^{45}Ca containing physiological solution (0.6 μCi of ^{45}Ca per ml) either containing or not containing a dihydropyridine, then for a further 2 min (unless otherwise stated) in the same solution also with or without norepinephrine 10^{-5} M. A similar procedure was followed with the ^{45}Ca depolarization solution. Thereafter, they were soaked for 5 min in La^{+++} solution (millimolal): NaCl, 122; KCl, 5.9; $MgCl_2$, 1.25; glucose, 11; $LaCl_3$, 50; and Tris-maleate, 15 (pH 6.8). The artery strips were then placed between two sheets of filter paper and pressed three times with a roller weighing 350 g. Each strip was weighed, and then dissolved in 0.1 ml of a solution composed of equal parts of perchloric acid (37% w/v) and H_2O_2 (30 volumes). This solution was heated for 15 min at 75 °C and, after cooling, 5 ml of Aqualuma (Lumac) was added. The radioactivity of the samples was counted as usual with appropriate controls in a liquid scintillation counter (Packard Tri-Carb 3375). The results of each determination have been converted to the apparent tissue content of ^{45}Ca (millimole per kilogram of wet (wt) =

$$\frac{\text{Dpm in muscle}}{\text{wet wt (kg)}} \times \frac{\text{nmol of Ca/l of medium}}{\text{Dpm/l of medium}}$$

Norepinephrine-dependent ^{45}Ca efflux was estimated in arteries preincubated for 120 min in ^{45}Ca containing physiological solution (3 μCi of ^{45}Ca/ml; a dihydropyridine being added or not during the last 90 min). The strips were then transferred to nonradioactive solution also with or without Ca antagonist and 5 min later to the same solution containing or not containing norepinephrine clonidine (10^{-5} M). The pieces of tissue were then treated as for influx experiments. In another series of efflux experiments arteries were loaded for 120 min in 100 ml of the ^{45}Ca physiological solution with or without nifedipine. Before the efflux experiment was started, the tissues were rinsed for 30 min (or less as otherwise stated) in a large volume of physiological solution. Thereafter they were transferred at 1- or 5-min intervals through a series of plastic scintillation vials containing the efflux medium. The tissues were allowed to move freely in 5 ml of physiological or K-depolarizing solution bubbled with gas mixture.

At the end of the efflux, experiment tissues were treated as in influx experiments and the radioactivity was counted as described above.

[^{3}H]-Nitrendipine Binding Assay. The light microsomal fraction from rat aorta was obtained as described by Godfraind and Wibo (1985) for ileal smooth muscle. The tissue fraction (30–50 μg protein) was incubated with [^{3}H]-nitrendipine (New England Nuclear) in a total volume of 0.55 ml at 30 °C for 45 min. The incubation medium contained (mM): NaCl, 106; KCl, 3.7; $MgCl_2$, 1; $CaCl_2$, 1; Tris 15 (pH 7.25) and sucrose, 100. Incubation was terminated by adding 3 ml of an ice-cold "stopping" solution (mM: NaCl, 145; KCl, 5; $MgCl_2$, 1.3; $CaCl_2$, 1.3; Tris, 20). the suspension was then filtered under vacuum through Whatman GF/F filters, and the filters were washed three times with 7 ml portions of ice-cold stopping solution. The filters were counted in a liquid scintillation counter. Nonspecific binding determined from samples incubated with 1 μM unlabeled nitrendipine, was subtracted from total binding to obtain specific binding. Unlabeled dihydropyridines were dissolved in ethanol to a concentration of 1 mM and further diluted with water. The final ethanol concentration was less than 0.5%.

Results and Discussion

1 Action on Contraction and Ca Movements

1.1 Contraction of Vascular Smooth Muscle, Role of Endothelium and Action of Dihydropyridines

The simplest experimental procedure to assess the relation between calcium entry and the development of contraction is to preincubate a smooth muscle in Ca-free physiological solution, to depolarize it with Ca-free KCl rich solution and gradually increase the calcium concentration in the bathing solution. This will result in an increase in tension dependent on Ca^{2+} concentration (Godfraind and Kaba 1969). When an agonist is used to stimulate the tissue, the calcium dependency of the response may also be examined. It must be pointed out that the response of a vessel to vasoconstrictors may depend upon the interaction of the agonist with its receptors but that it may be modulated by factors extrinsic to the muscle cell. Some of these factors may depend upon the endothelium. The essential role of endothelium as a mediator of relaxant responses induced in isolated vascular tissues by acetylcholine and other vasodilators is now well established (Furchgott 1984). We have examined the role of the endothelial tissue as a modulator of contractile effects of agonists on vascular smooth muscle. We first examined the influence of endothelium on the contractile response evoked by the adrenoceptor agonists noradrenaline and clonidine in rat isolated aorta (Eglème et al. 1984).

Noradrenaline concentration-effect curves obtained in the absence of endothelium were shifted to the left as compared to the concentration-effect curves obtained in the presence of endothelium. A similar shift was observed with other agonists, such as serotonin, $PGF_{2\alpha}$ and phenylephrine. On the other hand, removal of endothelium evoked a dramatic effect on the contractile responsiveness of rat aorta to clonidine. The maximum response increased by a factor of 9, and the EC_{50} value decreased. A similar observation has been made with other $alpha_2$ agonists such as UK 14-304-18 and oxymetazoline. It therefore appears that endothelium exerts specific inhibition for $alpha_2$ agonists and unspecific inhibition for other vasoconstrictors.

The action of dihydropyridines has been examined in depolarized aorta and in aorta stimulated by adrenoceptor agonists in the presence and the absence of endothelium.

In depolarized arteries different experimental protocols have been followed. Calcium dose-effect curves have been established in the presence of various concentrations of nifedipine or nimodipine (the racemic mixture and the two isomers) and in the presence of nifedipine. The results were similar except that the potency was different between these compounds. They produced a slight shift to the right and a progressive depression of the maximum response mainly noticeable at high doses. Such an effect is graphically similar to the interaction of some agonists with antagonists and justifies the use of the term "calcium antagonist" to characterize those dihydropyridines (Fig. 1).

Another protocol consisted in the analysis of the relaxing action of dihydropyridines on the contraction evoked by a K-depolarizing solution containing 100 mM KCl and 1.25 mM $CaCl_2$. In such experiments, it was observed that relaxation is dose-dependent (Godfraind and Miller 1983) and that the contraction can be completely abolished. In this respect, the princeps experiments performed with cinnarizine and lidoflazine (Godfraind and Polster 1968) were confirmed, since the relaxation is reduced by increasing the concentration of calcium in the perfusion fluid.

The third protocol is illustrated in Fig. 2 for three dihydropyridines. Contraction of rat aorta was evoked by K-depolarizing solution containing 100 mM KCl and 1.25 mM $CaCl_2$, then the preparations were incubated with various concen-

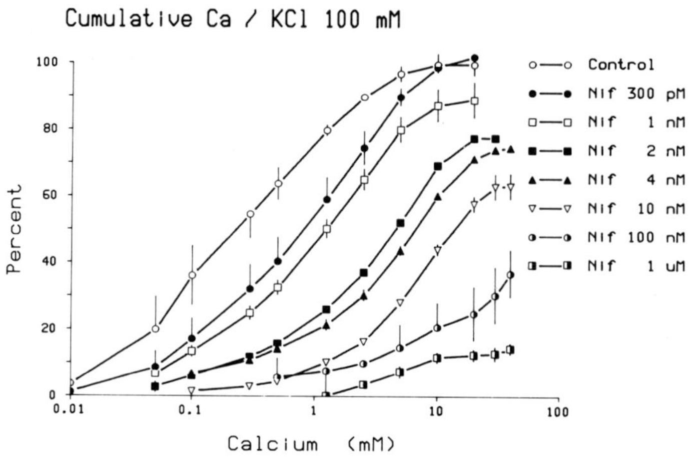

Fig. 1. Calcium dose-effect curve in depolarized rat aorta without and with pretreatment by various concentrations of nifedipine. Note apparent competition. From Godfraind (1983, modified)

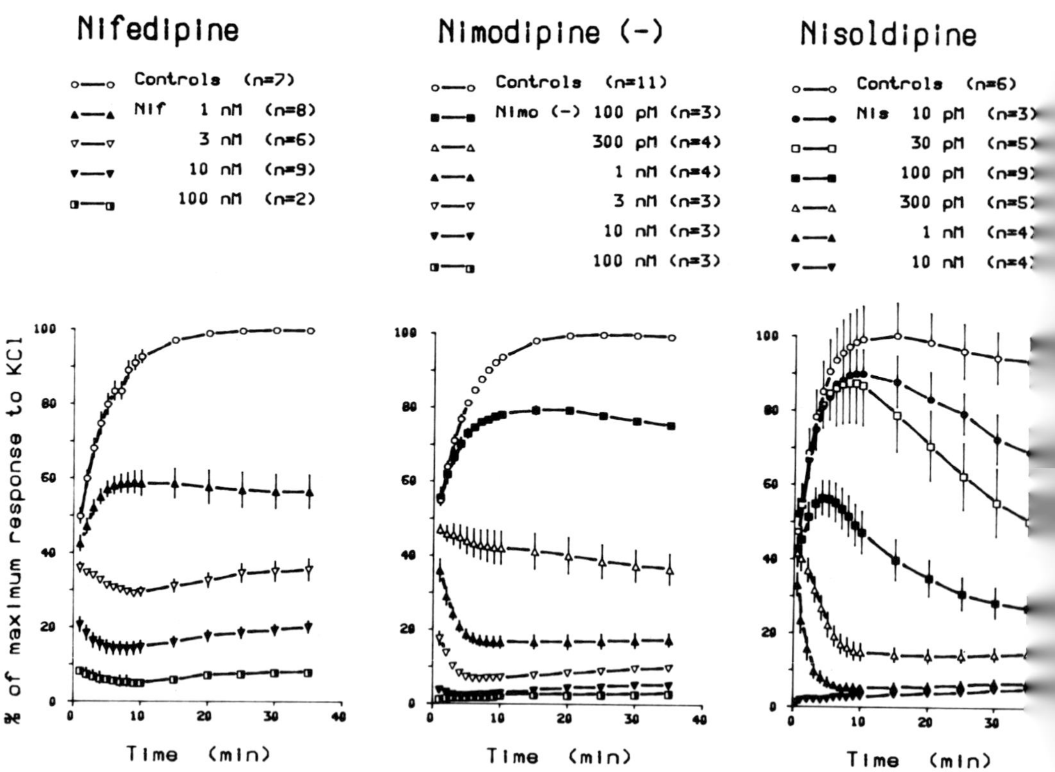

Fig. 2. Time course of the contraction of rat aorta evoked by K-depolarization before (control) and after 90 min preincubation with various concentrations of one of the dihydropyridines indicated on the graph. Note used-dependence mainly observable with nisoldipine

trations of nifedipine, nimodipine, and nisoldipine, as shown in Fig. 2. The time course of the contraction was different in controls and in treated preparations. For example, the contraction in the presence of nisoldipine 300 pM shows an initial phasic response followed by a secondary plateau; such a contractile pattern has been initially described by Godfraind and Dieu (1981) for flunarizine. These authors showed that it could be attributed to a use-dependent process: the inhibitory effect increasing with the duration of the depolarization. This increased inhibitory effect cannot be attributed to an insufficient preincubation time with the drug (it was equal to 90 min). Indeed, after washout of the K-solution by physiological solution containing nisoldipine, a second cycle of K-depolarization-evoked contraction shows the same pattern. As Fig. 3 illustrates, the decrease in IC_{50} resulting from this use-dependency is especially obvious with nisoldipine and less marked with nifedipine.

The action of the three dihydropyridines has been studied in rat aorta with and without endothelium, stimulated by $alpha_1$ and $alpha_2$ agonists. It has been previously shown by Godfraind et al. (1982) that the maximal inhibition of the response to $alpha_2$ agonists by calcium entry blockers was much greater than was the maximal inhibition of noradrenaline and phenylephrine responses. As Fig. 4 illustrates for noradrenaline and clonidine in the absence of endothelium, in the presence of the maximum effective concentration of nifedipine, the portion of the contraction resistant to the calcium entry blocker was much lower with clonidine than with noradrenaline. In addition, with noradrenaline, it has been reported by

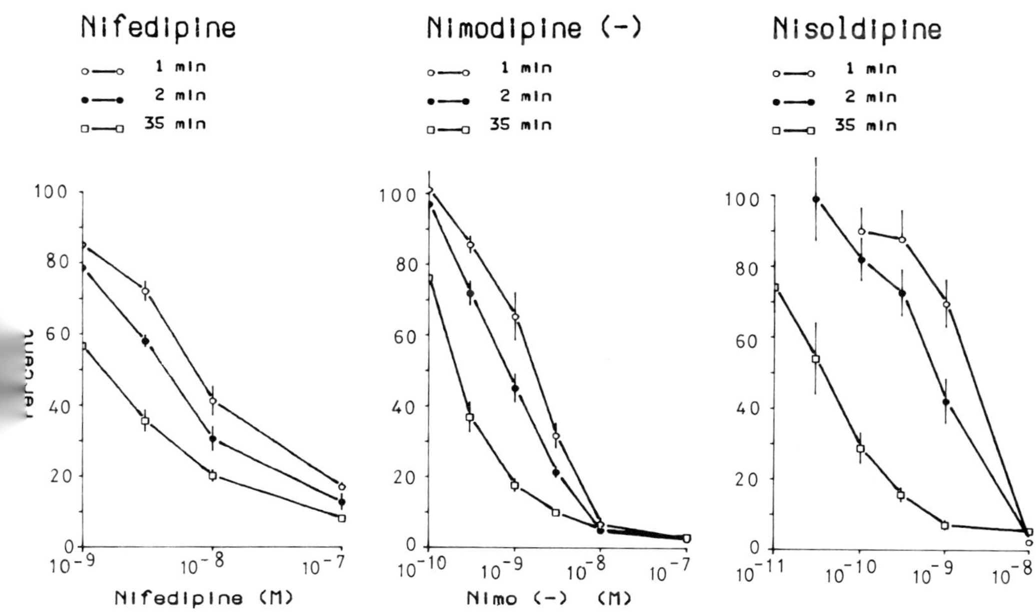

Fig. 3. Dose-inhibition curves of various dihydropyridines measured at various periods of the K-depolarization evoked contraction without or with a preincubation of 90 min. *Ordinate,* contraction in percent of control. *Abscissa,* concentration. Each point is a mean of at least 3 experiments

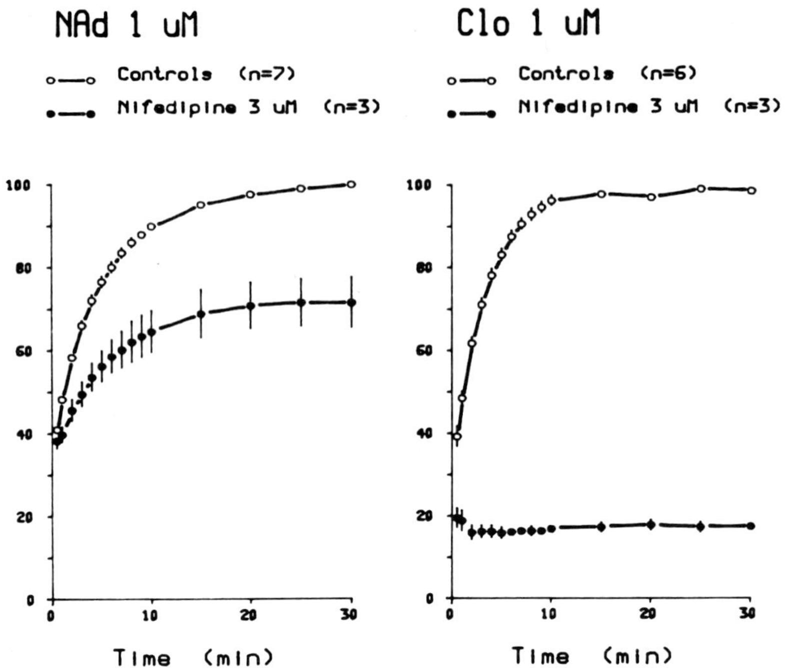

Fig. 4. Time course of the contraction evoked by noradrenaline and clonidine in rat aorta without endothelium, before and after treatment with a maximum effective concentration of nifedipine

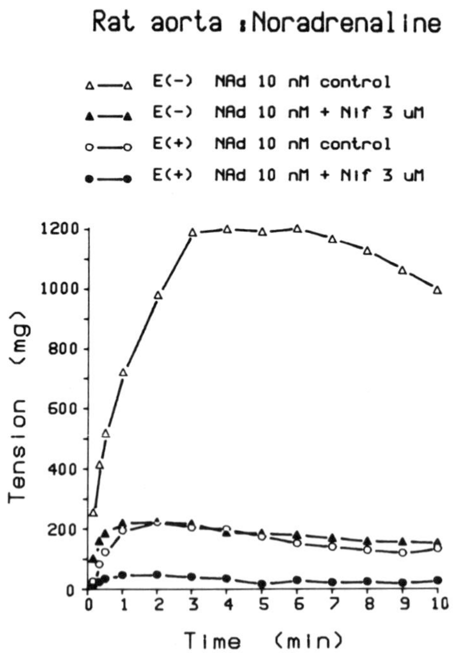

Fig. 5. Response of rat aorta to noradrenaline 10 nM, with (E+) and without (E−) endothelium; inhibition by nifedipine 3 uM

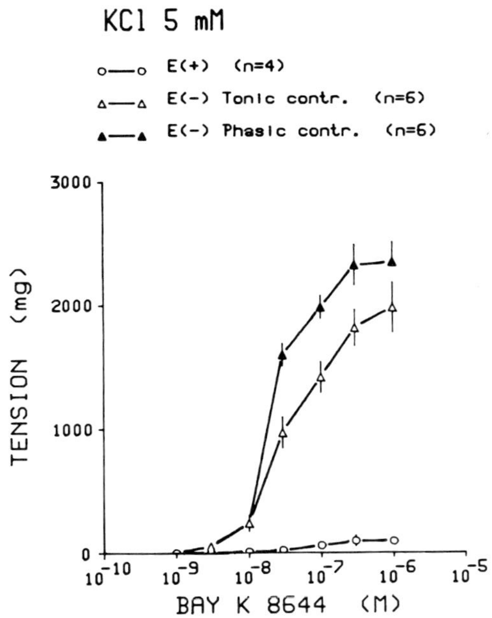

Fig. 6. Dose-effect curve of BAY K 8644 in rat aorta with (E+) and without (E−) endothelium in a solution containing only 5 mM KCl. In the absence of endothelium, the Ca agonist evoked a rhythmic activity abolished by the increase of KCl

Godfraind et al. (1984c) that the resistant response was larger in the absence than in the presence of endothelium and could account for most of the increased response evoked by a maximum dose of noradrenaline (3×10^{-6} M) after removal of endothelium. However with submaximum concentrations of noradrenaline, more close to those likely obtained after endogenous release, the response recorded in the absence of endothelium is highly sensitive to nifedipine (Fig. 5).

The calcium agonist BAY K 8644 evokes a vasoconstriction in vivo, as shown by Schramm et al. (1983) it can evoke the contraction of a vascular smooth muscle only when the K concentration of the medium is increased in order to slightly depolarize the preparation. Godfraind et al. (1984a) have shown in isolated taenia coli that the action of this dihydropyridine was to decrease the electrical threshold for opening of calcium channels. In the presence of 5 mM KCl, BAY K 8644 evokes barely no contraction of rat aorta with functional endothelium, but it can produce a marked contraction when the endothelium is removed (Fig. 6).

1.2 Ca Movements

The above observations show that several factors control or modulate the contractile responses of vessels. This emphazises the need for direct analysis of calcium fluxes and of calcium channels. Direct measurements of ^{45}Ca movements are not feasible in smooth muscle because they are not indicative of changes that could occur within the cell. Indeed, a large amount of calcium is bound on extracellular sites. Several attempts have been made to identify the biologically active calcium fraction and the most successful are based on the use of lanthanum. Lanthanum replaces Ca^{2+} on superficial binding sites and does not penetrate the cell.

Because lanthanum blocks transmembrane fluxes of calcium, it has been proposed that the calcium content of a muscle washed in a lanthanum solution could provide an estimate of cellular calcium. The ^{45}Ca fluxes across the smooth muscle cell membrane may be estimated in the rat aorta by measuring the ^{45}Ca turnover in the La^{3+}-resistant Ca fraction. This fraction corresponds to the amount of Ca that is not displaced when the tissue is soaked in 50 mM La^{3+} solution (Godfraind 1976). Noradrenaline increases the rate of uptake of ^{45}Ca into this calcium fraction. There is no net gain in tissue calcium and calcium efflux increases in a similar manner. The increase in the rate of ^{45}Ca uptake is dose-dependent. In the presence of the alpha-antagonist phentolamine, the dose-response curves for noradrenaline on ^{45}Ca uptake are displaced to the right in a manner suggesting a competitive antagonism, the pA_2 for phentolamine being equal to 7.8. Because of the resemblance of this pA_2 value to that obtained for the antagonistic effects of phentolamine on the contractile responses to norepinephrine, it appears that the activation of alpha-adrenoceptors is responsible for both the increased rate of Ca entry and the contraction. The observations suggest that alpha-adrenoceptor activation does open Ca pathways in the membrane, the actual accepted terminology is to consider that these pathways could consist of calcium channels closely associated with receptors, they have been termed ROC's (receptor-operated channels) (Bolton 1979). High K solutions also allow an increased influx of ^{45}Ca that presents some differences from the agonist-dependent influx, namely, as discussed below, its sensitivity to calcium antagonists. Those channels controlled by membrane potential have been termed POC's (potential-operated channels). In addition to ROC's and POC's, Bevan et al. (1982) have proposed the existence in some vessels, mainly in cerebral arteries, of channels sensitive to stretch (SOC's, strech-operated channels). The calcium electrochemical gradient is oriented inward, so that there is a powerful driving force that pushes calcium into the cell. The low intracytoplasmic concentration (below 10^{-7} M) may be attributed to the low permeability of the membrane of the resting cell to the cation and to its Ca pumps. The slow turnover of intracellular calcium at rest is likely to occur through Ca leak channels.

Most of the experimental observations accumulated over the last years indicate that inhibition of contraction by dihydropyridines is related to blockade of calcium entry through calcium channels operated by receptors and membrane potential. Experimental results show that blockade of stimuli-dependent calcium fluxes has similar concentration- and time-dependency as blockade of the contraction.

The lanthanum-resistant ^{45}Ca content of aortas was measured after various incubation periods in physiological solution containing ^{45}Ca and also after a preincubation of 5 min in ^{45}Ca-containing solution followed by further incubation in either the same solution containing noradrenaline (usually 10^{-5} M) or clonidine or in a ^{45}Ca-containing K-depolarizing solution. As shown by Godfraind (1976) and by Godfraind and Miller (1983), noradrenaline evoked an increased rate of ^{45}Ca influx, the maximum uptake being similar to that in control. In K-depolarizing solution both the initial rate of uptake and the maximum uptake of ^{45}Ca were increased; the increase of initial rate reached its peak after 2 min (Godfraind and Miller 1983).

Noradrenaline-dependent ^{45}Ca influx has been measured in aortas pretreated for 90 min with dihydropyridines. In agreement with previous observations (Godfraind and Dieu 1981; Godfraind and Miller 1983; Godfraind 1983), we found that the action of nifedipine and nisoldipine on the influx of ^{45}Ca was dose-dependent. The dose-effect curves for inhibition of contraction and Ca influx were superimposed, suggesting that reduction of noradrenaline effect on muscle tone was due to blockade of calcium entry.

In the absence of endothelium, clonidine enhanced ^{45}Ca influx. Clonidine-dependent ^{45}Ca influx was sensitive to nifedipine in a dose-dependent manner. However, at maximum effective nifedipine concentration, the clonidine-evoked ^{45}Ca influx remained equal to 15% of control influx as already reported with noradrenaline (Godfraind and Miller 1983). This observation confirms that calcium channels operated by adrenoceptors could not be completely blocked by dihydropyridines.

In previous reports, we have shown that the efflux of calcium evoked by noradrenaline was insensitive to nifedipine (Godfraind 1983). As Fig. 7 illustrates, this is also true for nisoldipine, both in physiological solution containing the normal concentration of calcium and in Ca-free solution. Figure 7 also shows that calcium efflux evoked by clonidine was absent in Ca-free solution. It was nevertheless still present although reduced in the presence of nifedipine 1 μM. This suggests that the calcium influx insensitive to nifedipine was able to activate calcium efflux from the cell. The experiments summarized above have also shown that calcium entry in a resting artery was only slightly affected by dihydropyrines, only when a maximum concentration was used.

K-dependent ^{45}Ca entry has also been examined in control aortas and in aortas pretreated during 90 min by various concentrations of dihydropyridines. When it was estimated after a stimulation of two minutes, allowing peak effect to be reached, I_{50} values were similar to IC_{50} values measured after the same period of time (Table 1). When the incubation time was prolonged, there was an ad-

Table 1. Concentration of dihydropyridines producing 50% of the maximum reduction of the contractile response (IC_{50}) or Ca influx in rat aorta (I_{50}), of maximum [^{3}H]-nitrendipine binding in rat aorta light microsomal fraction (K_i)

Ca antagonist		IC_{50} (nM)	I_{50} (nM)	K_I (nM)
Nifedipine	NAd	19	17	
	Clo	5.3	7.2	
	KCl 2 min	4.2		
	35 min	1.3	1.6	
	Binding			4.5
Nimodipine (−)	PGF_{2alpha}	0.73	0.9	
	KCl 2 min	0.8	1.1	
	35 min	0.2		
	Binding			1.2
Nisoldipine	NAd	0.82	0.62	
	KCl 2 min	0.41	0.74	
	35 min	0.03		
	Binding			0.93

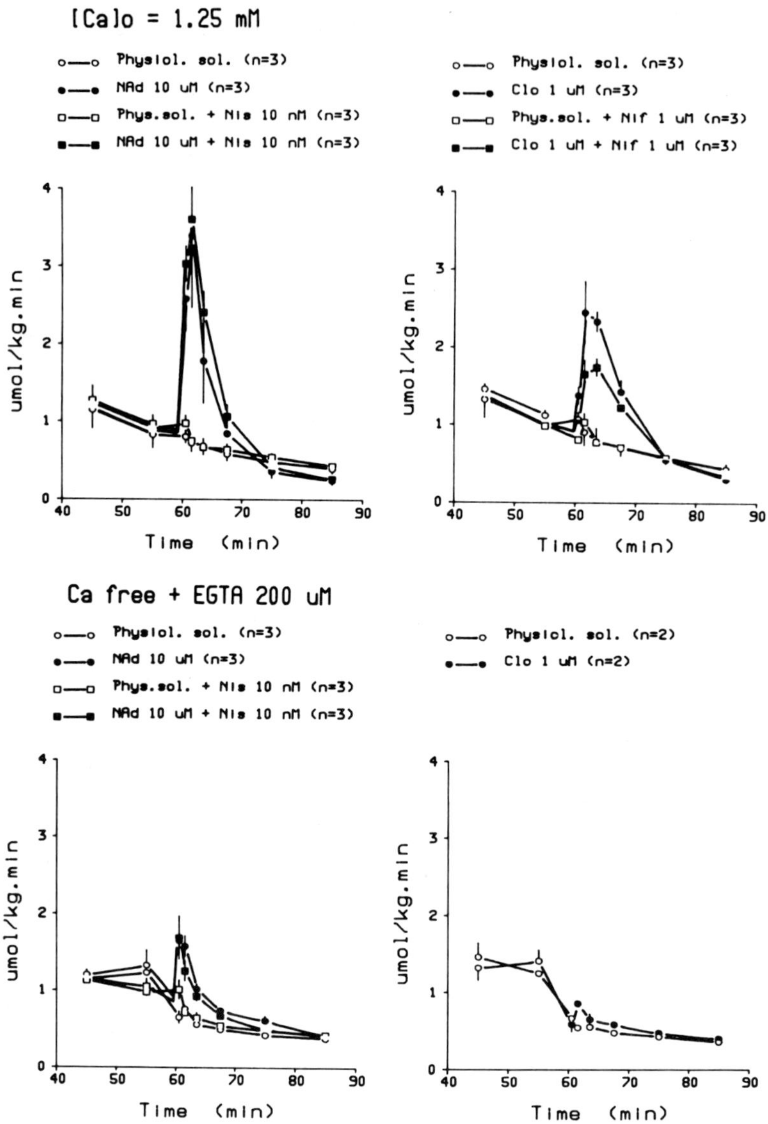

Fig. 7. Calcium efflux evoked in rat aorta by noradrenaline 10 uM and clonidine 1 uM (after removal of endothelium)

ditional inhibition of K-depolarization-dependent ^{45}Ca entry, consistent with the process of use-dependence already discussed (Fig. 1).

In Table 1 are compared estimates of the apparent dissociation constants of dihydropyridines in rat aorta measured by various approaches: contraction (IC_{50}), calcium entry (I_{50}), displacement of [H^3]-nitrendipine from its binding sites in rat aorta microsomes (K_i, calculated as described by Godfraind and Wibo 1985). Data reported on Table 1 indicate that the binding identified in microsomes could account for the action of dihydropyridines on ^{45}Ca influx during alpha agonists and K-solution stimulation. For each dihydropyridine so far examined, the three estimates are relatively close. There are however exceptions. One is the IC_{50} and I_{50} values for noradrenaline with nifedipine as an antagonist; these values are three time higher than those found with clonidine. Such a difference does not seem to exist with nisoldipine and needs further analysis. Another main difference is the IC_{50} ratios when K-depolarization was increased from 2 to 35 min. This ratio was equal to 3 with nifedipine, 4 with nimodipine and 11 with nisoldipine. This ratio is related to the potency of the dihydropyridines and to their lipophilicity. Because such a change in IC_{50} could reflect a change in binding affinity occurring during K-depolarization, some hypothesis may tentatively be proposed. If we except the results with noradrenaline-nifedipine and K-depolarization of 35 min, it is likely that dihydropyridines bind to one family of binding sites in a resting tissue. When Ca-channels are operated by change in membrane potential, the affinity of these binding sites could increase allowing a more efficient blockade of the channel (i.e. after 35 min K-depolarization). When Ca-channel is operated by receptors, this increase in affinity does not occur and the channel is incompletely blocked. Use-dependence observed during depolarization could therefore reflect this change in affinity. Another possibility to be examined is the existence of more than one family of POC's with different sensitivities to dihydropyridines.

2 Pathophysiological Models

2.1 Action of Dihydropyridines in Hypertensive Vessels

There are now several clinical reports showing the efficacy of dihydropyridines for the treatment of essential hypertension. Their hemodynamic mode of action is still controversial, since it had be attributed to the vasodilator effect of the compounds (for ref. see Kazda et al. 1982). It is therefore of interest to examine the characteristics of hypertensive vessels that could be related to calcium antagonists. We have compared the response to K-depolarization of aortas from hypertensive and normotensive rats in order to characterize the function of the potential operated calcium channels. The main observation was that relaxation following repolarization of the vessel occurred much more slowly in SHR than in WKY (Fig. 8), such an observation was also done with mesenteric arteries, an indication that this abnormality could be present in the whole arterial tree of the hypertensive rats. Such an effect might contribute to the increase in peripheral resistance observed in hypertensive animals. When arteries were pretreated with nisoldipine, the difference in the rate of relaxation was no longer apparent. Such an effect was observed with nisoldipine concentrations down to 10 pM. The latter concentration exerted similar effects on the contraction evoked by K-depolarization in SHR and WKY. This indicates that a specific action of nisoldipine in hypertensive vessels could be on the delayed relaxation after a contractile stimulus. This action might be involved in reduction of blood pressure observed after treatment of hypertensive rats with nisoldipine. It suggests that the hypertensive action of nisoldipine is not necessarily associated with its vasodilating properties.

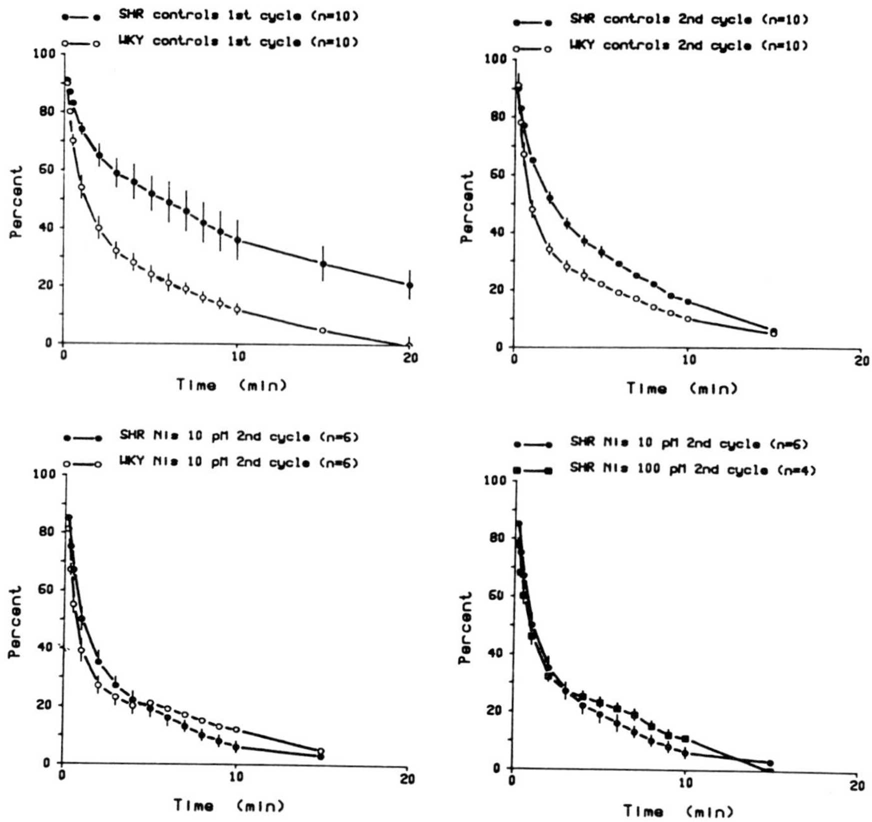

Fig. 8. Relaxation of rat aortas washed in physiological solution after contraction evoked by K-depolarization. Note that the delayed relaxation of SHR arteries is attenuated by pretreatment with nisoldipine (90 min preincubation)

2.2 Actions of Dihydropyridines in Human Isolated Coronary Arteries

In recent years, evidence has accumulated to suggest an important role of coronary vasospasm in the etiology of angina pectoris and myocardial infarction (see for example Maseri et al. 1978). Many spasmogens have been proposed as possible mediators of vasospasm but it may reasonably be assumed that whatever the initiating event or events are, the contractile response is dependent on a rise in the intracellular level of free calcium.

Human isolated coronary arteries display spontaneous activity (Godfraind and Miller 1983). The pattern of this activity varies according to the patient and to the segment examined. This activity is increased by several vasoactive agents including serotonin (the most potent), PGF2alpha (the most powerful), acetylcholine, histamine.

Nifedipine is a powerful inhibitor of both the spontaneous activity and the activity evoked by spasmogens (Godfraind et al. 1984b). The same is true for nisoldipine which appears to be the most potent inhibitor of the rhythmic contrac-

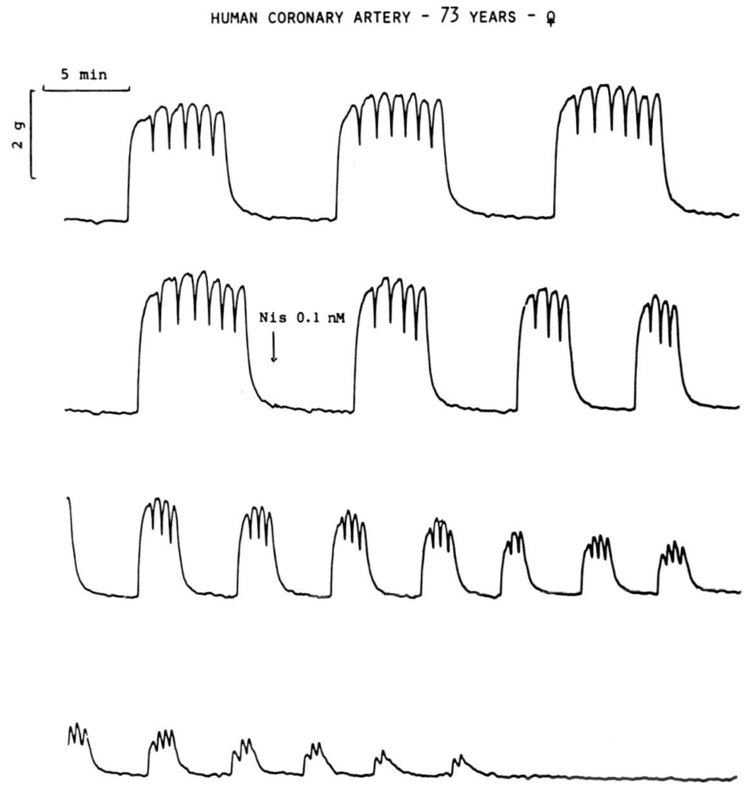

Fig. 9. Spontaneous contractile activity in human isolated coronary artery and its abolition by nisoldipine

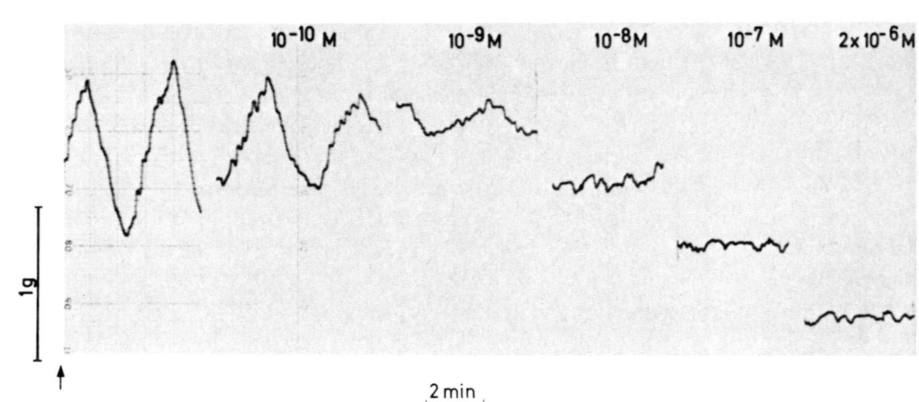

Fig. 10. Human isolated coronary artery stimulated by serotonin 10^{-5} M and treated by increasing concentrations of nifedipine (Godfraind et al. 1984, modified)

tions in human coronaries (Fig. 9). The action of nifedipine on coronary spasm is dose-dependent, this is illustrated by Fig. 10 for a human coronary artery that was contracted by serotonin. The abolition of the rhythmic activity was observed for concentrations (10^{-8} M) that were found in the blood after a therapeutic dose of nifedipine. Higher doses completely relaxed the artery. Studies of the sensitivity of the human myocardium to the depressant action of nifedipine have shown that depression of the coronary contraction was achieved without marked change in the contractility of trabecular muscle. This indicates that at therapeutic concentration the action of nifedipine is only on the coronary spasm.

Summary and Conclusions

In the present paper we have reported some of the experiments performed in order to analyse some mechanisms of the calcium antagonistic action of dihydropyridines. They were dealing with two main aspects: the analysis of the relation between Ca movements and contraction and the study of predictive pathophysiological models.

1. The relation between contraction and calcium movements has provided further evidence that the inhibition of contraction of smooth muscles by dihydropyridines may be attributed to blockade of calcium entry stimulated by depolarization or by receptors activation.

1.1. This has allowed to illustrate some of the characteristics of calcium channels in smooth muscle. Potential-operated channels are activated by changes in membrane potential, that can be evoked by K-rich solutions. They are completely blocked by calcium antagonistic dihydropyridines and the blockade shows use-dependence. They are open by calcium agonistic dihydropyridines. Receptor-operated channels are activated by the interaction of an agonist with its receptors; they are incompletely blocked by calcium antagonistic dihydropyridines and this blockade does not show use-dependence.

1.2. Endothelium appears to modulate the response of the adjacent smooth muscle to vasoconstrictors, mainly to alpha2 partial agonists. This might be, at least in part, attributed to a modulation by endothelium of calcium metabolism, both at the level of membrane channels and of intracellular stores. As a consequence, endothelium modulates the action of calcium antagonists.

2. We have analyzed two main pathophysiological models: isolated arteries obtained from hypertensive rats and human coronary arteries.

2.1. Isolated vessels from SHR show a delayed relaxation of the contractile response evoked by depolarization. This abnormality is attenuated by low doses of nisoldipine in such a way that hypertensive vessels behave like normotensive ones.

2.2. Human isolated coronary arteries are sensitive to nifedipine concentrations found in the blood of patients receiving therapeutic regimen. These concentrations do not alter the contractility of the isolated human myocardium.

The main conclusion that can be drawn from these experiments is that studies of isolated vascular smooth muscles allow to understand the mechanism of action of dihydropyridines and provide insight into their therapeutic properties.

References

Bevan JA, Bevan RD, Hwa JJ, Owen MP, Tayo FM, Winquist RJ (1982) Calcium, extrinsic and intrinsic (myogenic) vascular tone. In: Godfraind T, Albertini A, Paoletti R (eds) Calcium modulators. Elsevier North Holland Biomedical Press, Amsterdam New York Oxford, pp 125–132

Bolton TB (1979) Mechanism of action of transmitters and other substances on smooth muscle. Physiol Rev 59:606–718

Cauvin C, Loutzenhiser R, van Breemen C (1983) Mechanisms of calcium antagonists-induced vasodilation. Ann Rev Pharmacol Toxicol 23:373–396

Eglème C, Godfraind T, Miller RC (1984) Enhanced responsiveness of rat isolated aorta to clonidine after removal of the endothelial cells. Br J Pharmacol 81:16–18

Fleckenstein A (1983) Calcium antagonism in heart and smooth muscle. Wiley, New York

Furchgott RF (1984) The role of endothelium in the responses of vascular smooth muscle to drugs. Ann Rev Pharmacol Toxicol 24:175–197

Godfraind-De Becker A, Godfraind T (1980) Calcium transport system: a comparative study in different cells. Int Rev Cytol 67:141–170

Godfraind T (1976) Calcium exchange in vascular smooth muscle, action of noradrenaline and lanthanum. J Physiol (London) 260:21–35

Godfraind T (1979) Alternative mechanisms for the potentiation of the relaxation evoked by isoprenaline in aortae from young and aged rats. Eur J Pharmacol 53:273–279

Godfraind T (1983) Pharmacological importance of Ca movements in vascular tissue. In: van Zwieten PA, Schonbaum E (eds) Progress in pharmacology, vol 5/2. Gustav Fischer, Stuttgart New York, pp 11–22

Godfraind T, Dieu D (1981) The inhibition by flunarizine of the norepinephrine evoked contraction and calcium influx in rat aorta and mesenteric arteries. J Pharmacol Exp Ther 217:510–515

Godfraind T, Kaba A (1969) Blockade or reversal of the contraction induced by calcium and adrenaline in depolarized arterial smooth muscle. Br J Pharmacol 35:549–560

Godfraind T, Kaba A, Polster P (1968) Differences in sensitivity of arterial smooth muscles to inhibition of their contractile response to depolarization by potassium. Arch Int Pharmacodyn Ther 172:235–239

Godfraind T, Miller RC (1983) Specificity of action of Ca^{2+} entry blockers. A comparison of their actions in rat arteries and in human coronary arteries. Circ Res 52 (Suppl I) 81–91

Godfraind T, Miller RC, Socrates Lima J (1982) Selective $alpha_1$- and $alpha_2$-adrenoceptor agonist-induced contractions and ^{45}Ca fluxes in the rat isolated aorta. Br J Pharmacol 77:597–604

Godfraind T, Polster P (1968) Etude comparative de médicaments inhibant la réponse contractile de vaisseaux isolés d'origine humaine ou animale. Thérapie 23:1209–1230

Godfraind T, Hardy J-P, Morel N (1984a) Actions of the spasmogenic dihydropyridine BAY K 8644 on mechanical and electrical activities of guinea-pig taenia coli. J Physiol (London) 353:127P

Godfraind T, Finet M, Socrates Lima J, Miller RC (1984b) Contractile activity of human coronary arteries and human myocardium in vitro and their sensitivity to calcium entry blockade by nifedipine. J Pharmacol Exp Ther 230:514–518

Godfraind T, Egleme C, Al Osachie I (1985) Role of endothelium in the contractile response of rat aorta to α-adrenoceptor agonists. Clin Sci 68 (Suppl 10):65s–71s

Godfraind T, Wibo M (1985) Subcellular localization of [^{3}H]-nitrendipine binding sites in guinea-pig ileal smooth muscle. Br J Pharmacol 85:335–340

Kazda S, Garthoff B, Thomas G (1982) Antihypertensive effect of calcium antagonists in rats differs from that of vasodilators. Clin Sci 63:363s–365s

Maseri A, L'Abbate A, Baroldi G, Chierchia S, Marzilli M, Ballestra AM, Severi S, Parodi O, Biagini A, Distante A, Pesola A (1978) Coronary vasospasm as a possible cause of myocardial infarction. New Eng J Med 299:1271

Schramm M, Thomas G, Towart R, Franckowiak G (1983) Novel dihydropyridines with positive inotropic action through activation of Ca^{2+} channels. Nature (London) 303:535–537

Discussion

(pp. 309–325)

Cauvin: I have a question about your conclusion regarding the role of the endothelium in mediating a change in calcium-antagonist sensitivity of the norepinephrine activation. You said that the endothelial cells may regulate the size of the intercellular calcium pool. Have you measured contractions in Ca^{2+}-free solution in endothelial depleted tissues and with the endothelium present?

Godfraind: No. What I have done was to measure the exchangeable calcium fraction by isotope measurement and this is increased. But I have not yet done these crucial experiments you mentioned.

Fleckenstein: When the endothelium is removed you might not only remove endothelial cells but also damage to some extent the underlying smooth muscle. The concomitant depolarization would simply explain a lot of your observations, e.g. that the Ca^{2+}-agonist BAY K 8644 produces contractures in vessels in which you have removed the endothelium. A second possibility is that removing the endothelium causes artificial membrane leaks. If the membrane damage is great the possibility to inhibit this calcium influx by a calcium antagonist is diminished similar to the conditions of the "calcium-paradox" in the heart.

Godfraind: That is a very important question. Because of the possibility to damage the smooth muscle we also used methylene blue and haemoglobin, which interfere with the production or the disposition of the endothelial factor. Under these conditions we got the same results. You are right proposing that this also could be due to some depolarization of the smooth muscle. Regarding the sensitivity to Ca^{2+}-antagonists: We have been looking to the maximal stimulation which is able to release Ca^{2+} from the Ca^{2+} stores. But on the other hand when we look on the Ca^{2+} entry system, e.g. Ca^{2+} entry provoked by clonidine, this system is very sensitive. In conditions where we have no maximal activation of the adrenoceptor, then it could be that the Ca^{2+}-antagonists have the same effect without endothelium. The difference does only exist when we fully activate the preparation to release the intracellular Ca^{2+}.

Bayer-Symposium IX
Cardiovascular Effects of Dihydropyridine-Type
Calcium Antagonists and Agonists, 327–332

Endothelium-Dependent Vascular Relaxation*

J. G. De Mey

The responses of isolated large arteries to a number of vasodilators depend on the presence of endothelial cells (for a recent review see Furchgott 1983). The mechanism underlying this endothelium-dependent reactivity has been partly elucidated. The significance of the vasoactivity of the endothelium, depends on whether it applies to vessels and circumstances that participate in regulation of cardiovascular function and on whether it is altered in cardiovascular pathologies.

Large Arteries

Enzymatic or mechanical removal of the endothelium from isolated large arteries abolishes their relaxing responses to acetylcholine (Fig. 1). This was first described in the rabbit aorta by Furchgott and Zawadzki (1980), and was subsequently observed in large arteries from all mammalian species studed (Furchgott 1983). The arterial relaxing effect of a growing number of other substances also depends upon the presence of endothelial cells. Though not applicable to all types of arteries from all species these include: the inophore A23187, adenine nucleotides, arachidonic acid, bradykinin, histamine, serotonin and thrombin (Furchgott 1983; De Mey and Vanhoutte 1981; De Mey et al. 1982; Cherry et al. 1982; Van de Voorde and Leusen 1983; Singer and Peach 1982; Cocks and Angus 1983). Other agents such as adenosine, calcium antagonists, isoproterenol, nitroprusside, potassium and prostacyclin invariably relax arterial preparations with and without endothelium to the same extent (Furchgott 1983; De Mey and Vanhoutte 1981, 1982; De Mey et al. 1982).

Of the endothelium-dependent relaxing responses those to acetylcholine have been most thoroughly studied. They are antagonised by atropine. They are abo-

* Part of the authors research was performed at the Department of Human Physiology, University of California, Davis, USA and was supported by Fogarty International Research Fellowship TW03322-01

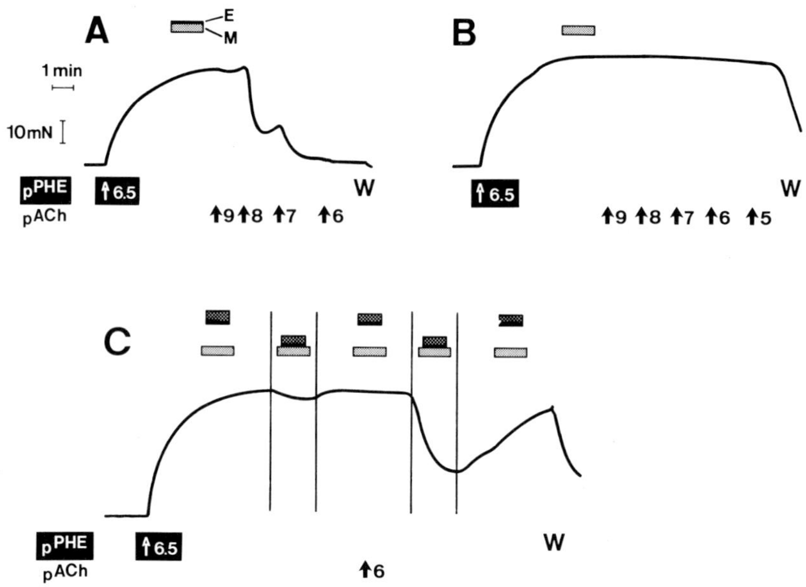

Fig. 1 A–C. Endothelium-dependency of relaxing responses to acetylcholine in cat thoracic aorta. Recording of isometric force versus time in a transverse strip at optimal length. During contraction induced by phenylephrine (*PHE*) the preparation was exposed to acetylcholine (*ACh*); concentrations shown as neg. log. molar; at *W* all agents were removed. **A** Preparation from which the lumenal surface was not intentionally damaged (partially intact endothelium, *E*). **B** Same preparation as in **A** following mechanical damage of the lumenal surface (removal of the endothelium). **C** Same preparation as in **B** now tested in the presence of a second aorta preparation that had not been damaged. This second preparation was separately mounted on a micromanipulator allowing spacing (10 mm) and contact between the lumenal and endothelial surface of the first assay preparation and the second "donor" preparation, respectively. Note the absence of relaxing responses to acetylcholine in the deendothelialised preparation (**B**) and its restoration in the close proximity of the endothelium of an other source.

lished by removal of the endothelium and restored when the endothelial layer of a donor preparation is placed in close proximity of the deendothelialised artery (Furchgott and Zawadzki 1980; Fig. 1). These experiments suggested stimulation by acetylocholine of the release of an endothelium derived relaxing factor (EDRF). This was confirmed by the observtion that the perfusate of isolated arteries, exposed to acetylcholine, relaxed deendothelialised arterial preparations (Griffith et al. 1984). The exact nature of EDRF remains to be established. Despite the key role of the endothelium in the vascular production of prostaglandins and lipoxygenase products (Moncada et al. 1977; MacIntyre et al. 1978; De Mey et al. 1982) EDRF is not a protaglandin and unlikely to be a lipoxygenase product. Indeed, endothelium-dependent reactivity is not affected by inhibitors of cyclooxygenase and inhibited by but some lipoxygenase inhibitors (Furchgott 1983; De Mey et al. 1982; Griffith et al. 1984). Endothelium-dependent responses to acetylcholine are abolished by inhibitors of guanyl cyclase. In addition, acetylcholine causes an increase in GMP in arterial preparations, provided that endothelial cells are present (Rapoport and Murad 1983; Furchgott 1983). Therefore

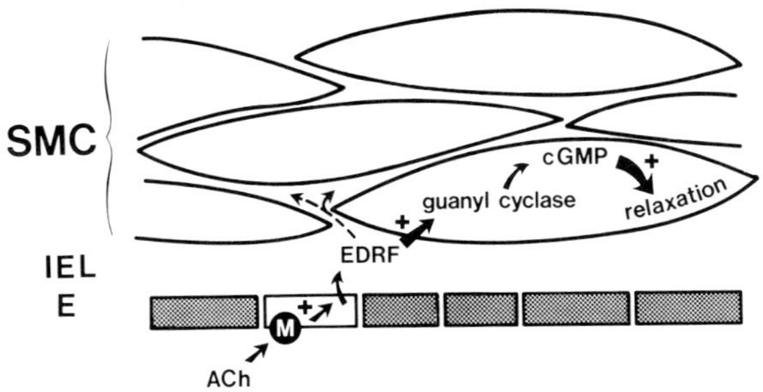

Fig. 2. Schematic representation of the mechanism underlying endothelium-dependent arterial relaxation in response to acetylcholine. Following interaction with muscarinic receptors (*M*) on the endothelium (*E*) acetylcholine (*ACh*) causes release of an endothelium derived relaxing factor (*EDRF*), which activates guanyl cyclase in the arterial smooth muscle cells (*SMC*). Whether EDRF reaches all smooth muscle cells by diffusion, or whether functional coupling between endothelial and smooth muscle cells is aided by conduction between smooth muscle cells, remains open. *IEL:* internal elastic lamina

endothelium-dependent responses to acetylcholine have been suggested to result from muscarinic stimulation of endothelial cells to release EDRF, which in turn activates arterial smooth muscle guanyl cyclase leading to increased levels of GMP which subsequently lead to relaxation (Fig. 2). It is at present unclear where in the above scheme a number of other properties of endothelium-dependent responses to acetylcholine fit. They are rapidly abolished by anoxia and by a variety of circumstances that inhibit electrogenic sodium transport (De Mey and Vanhoutte 1980, 1983; Furchgott 1983). Whether these refer to the release of EDRF or to the effects of EDRF on the smooth muscle is uncertain. Similarly the inhibitory effects of calcium removal and calcium antagonists (De Mey and Vanhoutte 1978, 1980; Singer and Peach 1982) are hard to situate. It is tempting though to interprete these as a representing calcium-dependent release of EDRF (Singer and Peach 1982).

Veins

In isolated veins, in contrast to arteries, acetylcholine causes but small endothelium-dependent relaxations, and at high concentrations contractions that do not depend upon the endothelium (De Mey and Vanhoutte 1982). Also for other agents quantitative and qualitative differences were observed between isolated canine arteries and veins. Endothelium-dependent relaxations to ATP are less pronounced in veins than in arteries, and partly masked by contractile effects that do not depend upon endothelium. Both arachidonic acid and thrombin cause endothelium-dependent contractions in veins and endothelium-dependent relaxations in isolated arteries form the dog (De Mey and Vanhoutte 1982). It is not clear at present whether these differences between arteries and veins reside in the endothelial or vascular smooth muscle cells.

Resistance Vessels

In isolated large blood vessels, endothelium-dependent reactivity is highly heterogeneous. It differs between types of blood vessels and animal species (Furchgott 1983). Consequently extrapolation from one set of circumstances to another is at least difficult. Whether endothelium-dependent responses are present in resistance vessels was therefore analysed directly. Small mesenteric arteries (optimal internal diameter $\simeq 200$ μm) were isolated from rats and mounted for recording of isometric force development (Mulvany and Halpern 1977). They maintained part of their endothelium in vitro. This could be selectively removed by short term exposure of the lumenal surface to detergent (Gospodarowsicz et al. 1980; De Mey and Gray 1984). Control and deendothelialised vessels contracted in response to norepinephrine. During such contractions acetylcholine, bradykinin and histamine caused relaxations in control but not in deendothelialised preparations. All preparations relaxed in response to nitroprusside and potassium (De May et al. 1984; De Mey and Gray 1984). Therefore, as in large arteries, the endothelium plays an obligatory role in some responses of vessels that are small enough to contribute to vascular resistance and its control. If anything, endothelium-dependent relaxing reactivity is more potent in small than large arteries (De Mey and Gray 1984). As in large arteries, the endothelium-dependent responses of resistance vessels to acetylcholine were abolished by methylene blue and ouabain.

Hypertension

From the above appears that arterial and resistance vessel endothelium is a possible source of an endogeneous vasodilator. Provided that endothelium-dependent vascular reactivity operates in vivo, defects in the release of EDRF or in the responsiveness of smooth muscle cells to EDRF can lead to increased peripheral resistance.

These considerations lead to the comparison of endothelium-dependent responses in resistance vessels from normotensive and genetically hypertensive animals. In mesenteric resistance vessels from adult (8 weeks and older), but not young (4 weeks and younger) spontaneously hypertensive rats significantly smaller endothelium-dependent relaxations were obtained in response to acetylcholine, bradykinin and histamine, than in those from age-matched Wistar-Kyoto rats (De Mey and Gray 1984). The relaxing responses to the endothelium-independent agents nitroprusside and potassium, were however comparable in both strains. A similar selective depression of endothelium-dependent relaxations was observed in mesenteric resistance vessels from Dahl sodium-sensitive rats on a high sodium diet (hypertensive) when compared to those from litter mates on a low sodium diet (normotensive).

Conclusion

The endothelium plays an obligatory role in responses of isolated arteries and resistance vessels to some relaxing agents. This endothelium-dependent reactivity is less apparent in veins and is decreased in resistance vessels from hypertensive animals.

Endothelium-dependent relaxations are mediated by an endothelium derived relaxing factor that activates vascular smooth muscle guanyl cyclase. More information on (1) the biology of endothelium, (2) the nature and properties of EDRF, (3) the mode of action of cyclic GMP, and on (4) the functional and structural organisation and interactions in the vascular wall, are needed for full understanding of the pharmacology and pathophysiology of functional myo-endothelial coupling.

References

Cherry PD, Furchgott RF, Zawadzki JV, Jothianandan D (1982) The role of endothelial cells in the relaxation of isolated arteries by bradykinin. Proc Natl Acad Sci USA 79:2106–2110

Cocks TM, Angus JA (1983) Endothelium-dependent relaxation of coronary arteries by noradrenaline and serotonine. Nature 305:627–630

De Mey JG, Gray SD (1984) Endothelium-dependent reactivity in resistance vessels. Prog Appl Microc

De Mey JG, Vanhoutte PM (1978) Calcium-dependency of the direct relaxant effect of acetylcholine on canine femoral artery. Arch Int Pharmacodyn Ther 236:296

De Mey JG, Vanhoutte PM (1980) Interaction between Na, K exchanges and the direct inhibitory effect of acetylcholine on canine femoral arteries. Circ Res 46:826–836

De Mey JG, Vanhoutte PM (1981) Role of the intima in cholinergic and purinergic relaxation of isolated canine femoral arteries. J Physiol (Lond) 316:437–455

De Mey JG, Vanhoutte PM (1982) Heterogeneous behavior of the canine arterial and venous wall. Circ Res 51:439–447

De Mey JG, Vanhoutte PM (1983) Anoxia and endothelium-dependent reactivity of the canine femoral artery. J Physiol (Lond) 335:65–74

De Mey JG, Claeys M, Vanhoutte PM (1982) Endothelium-dependent inhibitory effects of acetylcholine, adenosine triphosphate, thrombin and arachidonic acid in the canine femoral artery. J Pharmacol Exp Ther 222:166–173

De Mey JG, Gray SD, Mulvany MJ (1984) Effects of endothelial demage on reactivity of isolated 200 m arteries. Fed Proc 43:737

Furchgott RF (1983) Role of endothelium in responses of vascular smooth muscle. Circ Res 53:557–573

Furchgott RF, Zawadzki JV (1980) The obligatory role of endothelial cells in the relaxation of arterial smooth muscle by acetylcholine. Nature 288:373–376

Gospodarowicz D, Delgado D, Vlodavsky I (1980) Permissive effect of the extracellular matrix on cell proliferation in vitro. Proc Natl Acad Sci USA 77:4094–4098

Griffith TM, Eduards DH, Lewis MJ, Newby AC, Henderson AH (1984) The nature of endothelium-derived vascular relaxant factor. Nature 308:645–647

MacIntrye DE, Pearson JD, Gordon JL (1978) Localisation and stimulation of prostacyclin production in vascular cells. Nature 271:549–551

Moncada S, Herman AG, Higgs EA, Vane JR (1977) Differential formation of prostacyclin (PGX or PHI2) by layers of the arterial wall. An explanation for the anti-thrombotic properties of vascular endothelium. Throm Res 11:323–344

Mulvany MJ, Halpern W (1977) Contractile properties of small arterial resistance vessels in spontaneously hypertensive and normotensive rats. Circ Res 41:19–26

Rapoport RM, Murad F (1983) Agonist-induced endothelium-dependent relaxation in rat thoracic aorta may be mediated through cGMP. Circ Res 52:352–357

Singer HA, Peach MJ (1982) Calcium- and endothelial-mediated vascular smooth muscle relaxation in rabbit aorta. Hypertension 4 (suppl II): 19–25

Van de Voorde J, Leusen I (1983) Role of endothelium in the vasodilator response of rat thoracic aorta to histamine. Eur J Pharmacol 87:113–120

Discussion

(pp. 327–332)

Fleckenstein-Grün: We are very much interested in large coronary arteries, because in this region coronary spasms and stenoses occur in human pathophysiology and because Ca^{2+}-antagonists pocess distinct dilating effects in this particular part of the coronary bed. Did you ever remove the endothleium in large dog coronary arteries, and could you change the relaxing response to acetylcholine, methacholine or histamine into contractions in this type of vessels? If so, how did the contraction compare to potassium contractions?

De Mey: I have used LAD of the dog, following removal of the endothelium and that vassel contracts to 10^{-5} Mol/l acetylcholine. That is about 75% of the maximal response to potassium. The exact figures are in the July Volume 1984 of Circulation Research.

Bühler: This is an attractive concept but I have a conceptional problem with the endothelium-derived relaxant factor showing blunted responses in SHR and during aging. In both instances there was a smaller relaxation with isoproterenol and bradykinin, yet not difference with nitroprusside that couples to the guanyl cyclase, the effector system used for the EDRF. On the other hand, the isoproterenol is adenylate-cyclase-coupled. Is there a coupling defect behind the receptor both in rats and in man? How is this consistent with your argument?

De Mey: My data with isoproterenol and aging are compatible with what is know about aging and the adenylate-cyclase system. For the guanyl-cyclase system, I do not think there is any inconsistency. It does not seem to change with aging. The reason why I am reluctant to conclude that there would be a decreased release of EDRF in hypertension is that I am fully aware of the altered vascular morphology. As long as I do not know the exact morphological basis of this endothelium-dependent reactivity in quantitative terms, I cannot exclude that the morphological changes can result in the functional changes, I described.

Bühler: But why did you not find a morphological difference with the nitroprusside studies?

De Mey: Because nitroprusside is directly acting on smooth muscle cells. It does not need the endothelium to be there. The difference is that the endothelium-dependent agents first have to act upon the endothelium, then there is a release of EDRF, and subsequently EDRF interacts with the vascular smooth muscle cells. Nitroprusside and other direct activators of guanyl-cyclase on the orther hand act directly on the vascular smooth muscle cells.

Bevan: I want to add an exception to the generalisation you made in your summary slide concerning acetylcholine's action on the endothelium and the blood vessel. Dr. J. Brayden and I were interested in how in certain blood vessels which receive cholinergic nerves, the transmitter release from the nerves located at the endothelio-medial border causes dilation. Presumably it would have to diffuse across the media and release endothelium-derived relaxing factor. It turned out, however, that in these blood vessels, the acetylcholine receptors that lead to dilation are in the vascular smooth muscle cells. Removal of the intima makes little difference to the effect of the transmitter. There are always exceptions to every generalisation.

Cauvin: In line with the diffusion question, have you tried in some of the larger arteries to perfuse the inside and the outside of the vessels separately, so that you could determine whether the endothelial relaxing factor diffuses through the basement membrane or around the outside of the tissue?

De Mey: I have not done this kind of study. My approach has been to study endothelium-dependent reactivity in situations where vascular structure is altered. I have for instance compared endothelium-dependent reactivity throughout puberty and pregnancy in the uterine circulation. There endothelium-dependent reactivity is diminished when the thickness of the media increases. This is compatible with the diffusional model.

Fleckenstein: Under the influence of nitroglycerine and of sodium nitroprusside the cyclic GMP concentration tremendously increases according to some reports by a factor of 50. Does nitroglycerine, too, act directly on the vascular smooth muscle cell without mediation of the endothelium?

De Mey: In my experiments relaxation by nitroglycerine was endothelium-independent. One must, however, be very careful to generalise. This already appeared from what Dr. Bevan said, and also from my data illustrating that histamine is an endothelium-dependent relaxing agent in rat but not in dog resistance vessels. Endothelium-dependent reactivity is highly heterogeneous like the whole of vascular reactivity. One cannot extrapolate from one species to another and from one type of blood vessel to another.

Fleckenstein: Professor Taira had made the important observations that acetylcholine-injected into the coronary system of monkeys constricts the coronary arteries.

De Mey: I do not debate that large coronary arteries can be made to contract with acetylcholine. The same situation occurs in the coronary circulation with serotonin. It is a marvellous constrictor of the large coronary arteries and a dilator of the resistance vessels. A similar situation exists for noradrenaline.

Scriabine: I am not clear whether we can assume that the vasodilator effects of dihydropyridines are partially mediated by the release of endothelial factors or not. Dr. Godfraind demonstrated that the hypotensive effects of nifedipine were more pronounced in the presence of endothelium. Do you think that more work is needed in the area?

De Mey: I think there is more work needed on that. There is evidence that there is a basal release of EDRF in the intact blood vessel which is acting on the smooth muscle cells. If this agent is comparable to the EDRF which is released by acetylcholine, it will cause some stimulation of guanyl cyclase in vascular smooth muscle. There is already evidence for this as the levels of cyclic GMP are higher in an intact than in a deendothelialised artery. Since GMP affects excitation-contraction coupling, comparing a vascular smooth muscle cell in an intact arterial wall with a vascular smooth muscle cell in a de-dendothelialised arterial wall is problematic.

Glossmann: Behind your answer was there the idea that possibly 1,4-dihydropyridines increase the secretion of the relaxing factor?

De Mey: From my last picture I would expect the reverse, i.e. Ca^{2+}-antagonists could reduce the release of EDRF, and an agent like BAY K8644 could stimulate the release. It is hard to prodict what the overall effect will be on the whole vascular wall, since you would then have opposing effects.

Glossmann: But if one enantionmer would activate the release of EDRF and the other one would block the smooth muscle cell?

Chairman: The very fine talks that we heard from the smooth muscle experts prove – I think – that we are not really behind the myocardial officionados but that we simply have different and perhaps more problems.

Session V: Circulation

Chairman: A. Schwartz

Bayer-Symposium IX
Cardiovascular Effects of Dihydropyridine-Type
Calcium Antagonists and Agonists, 338–349

Coronary and Systemic Hemodynamic Effects of Dihydropyridines

D. C. Warltier and G. J. Gross

Introduction

The slow channel calcium blocking agents are a structurally diverse group of compounds which share a common property of interfering with excitation-contraction coupling in myocardium and vascular smooth muscle. Because these drugs have varying structures, their hemodynamic properties have been found to produce different cardiovascular actions. This is best documented for nifedipine, diltiazem and verapamil [1, 2]. Dihydropyridines form a subgroup within the general category of calcium antagonists. Many compounds with the basic dihydropyridine nucleus have been synthesized and whereas certain of these agents have been shown to possess calcium channel blocking activity in vitro and in vivo, more recently, others have been found to posses calcium agonist activity [3, 4]. The present investigation was undertaken to compare varying compounds with the dihydropyridine nucleus as to their systemic and coronary hemodynamic actions. The calcium antagonists, nifedipine, nisoldipine, nitrendipine, niludipine and FR 34235 and the calcium agonists, CGP 28392 and Bay k 8644 were studied in various doses. Because much of the previous work with these agents had been completed in anesthetized animals or in vitro, conscious dogs were used to avoid potential interactions with anesthetics and to maintain cardiovascular reflexes intact.

Methods

Adult mongrel dogs weighing 20–30 kg were anesthetized with sodium pentobarbital (30 mg/kg, i.v.), intubated with an endotracheal tube and respirated. Under sterile conditions, thoracotomy was performed at the fifth left intercostal space. Catheters were introduced into the internal mammary artery and vein and advanced to the aorta and superior vena cava for recording of arterial pressure and drug administration, respectively. A doppler flow probe was postioned on either the left anterior descending or left circumflex coronary artery for measurement of coronary blood flow velocity. A Koningsberg miniature micromanometer or fluid-filled catheter was inserted in the left ventricle through the apex for recording of left ventricular pressure and the maximum rate of rise of left ventricular pressure (peak +dP/dt), an index of global left ventricular contractility. In certain experiments, pairs of miniature ultrasonic segment length transducers were implanted in the subendocardium of the left ventricular free wall for measurement of regional myocardial contractility. Electrodes were also positioned on the internal thoracic wall for recording of the electrocardiogram. All catheters and leads were tunneled between the scapulae and exteriorized. The chest wall was closed and pneumothorax evacuated by a chest tube.

After surgery, each dog was allowed to recover for a period of 10 days. During this time each dog was trained to stand quietly in a sling and the animals were subsequently studied in the awake, unsedated state. End systolic segment length was determined at maximum negative dP/dt and end diastolic segment length was determined at the onset of left ventricular isovolumetric contraction. All hemodynamic data were recorded continuously on a polygraph and digitized on a microcomputer interfaced to an analog to digital converter.

Experimental Design

On the day of the study, each dog received multiple doses of a dihydropyridine calcium antagonist (nifedipine, nitrendipine, FR 34235, niludipine or nisoldipine) or agonist (CGP 28392 or Bay k 8644). Because all dihydropyrdines may be unstable in light, the intravenous line and syringe containing drug were protected from light by aluminium foil. In addition, all experiments were completed under light emitted from a sodium vapor lamp. Control hemodynamic data were obtained during intravenous infusion of drug vehicle (ethanol, polyethylene glycol, 0.9% saline).

In additional experimental groups, the effects of autonomic nervous system blockade (propranolol, phentolamine or methylatropine) on the hemodynamic effects of the calcium agonist, CGP 28392, were investigated. In other experimental groups, the influence of beta blockade and/or constant arterial pressure achieved with sodium nitroprusside infusion on the hemodynamic response to intravenous infusion of Bay k 8644 was studied.

Each experimental group consisted of 5 to 10 instrumented animals. Comparisons between doses of dihydropyridines and control data were completed with a one-way analysis of variance followed by Dunnett's modification of the t test. Comparisons between drugs at each dose was accomplished by use of a two-way analysis of variance for unbalanced data followed by Fisher's test of least significant difference. Correlations of hemodynamic changes produced by the various agents was completed by linear regression analysis.

Results

Systemic and Coronary Hemodynamic Effects of Dihydropyridine Calcium Antagonists

Each dog received 5 intravenous doses (1.0, 2.5, 5.0, 10.0 and 25.0 μg/kg/min for 5 min until a steady state was produced) of a dihydropyridine calcium antagonist. Hemodynamic changes were compared to the peripheral vasodilator, hydralazine (0.01, 0.025, 0.050, 0.10 and 0.25 mg/kg/min for 5 min). The drugs were administered on different days with or without pretreatment with propranolol (2 mg/kg, i.v.). Nifedipine, nitrendipine, FR 34235, niludipine, nisoldipine and hydralazine produced a dose-related reduction in mean arterial blood pressure. Whereas with the dihydropyridines a large change in diastolic pressure was observed, relatively smaller changes in systolic pressure occurred (Fig. 1). Significant changes in systolic arterial pressure were only noted with high doses of nifedipine. The dihydropyridines which caused the largest reduction in arterial pressure were nisoldipine

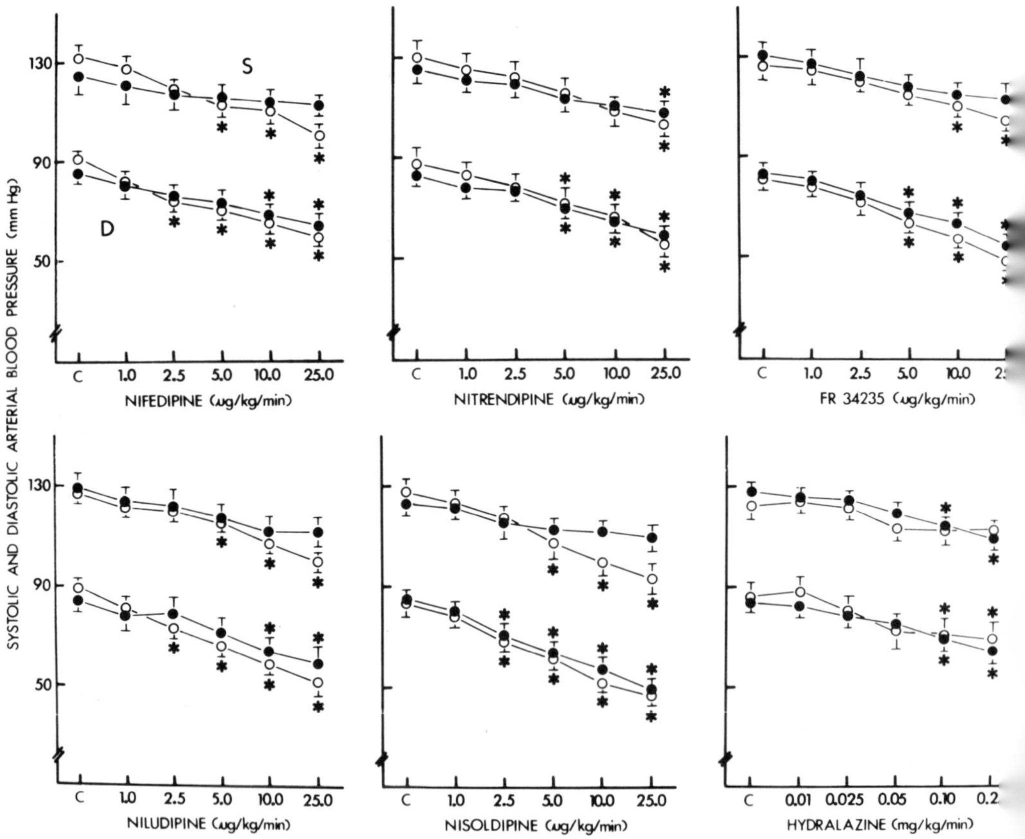

Fig. 1. Changes in systolic (*S*) and diastolic (*D*) blood pressure produced by intravenous infusion of calcium antagonists and hydralazine before (●) and after (○) beta blockade. *Significantly ($p < 0.05$) different from control (*C*)

Table 1. Efficacy of vasodilators on arterial pressure

Most effective:	Nitrendipine and nisoldipine
	FR 34235 and niludipine
Least effective:	Nifedipine and hydralazine

and nitrendipine. FR 34235 and niludipine were somewhat less effective and nifedipine and hydralazine least effective (Table 1). Although the dihydropyridines and hydralazine produced decreases in left ventricular systolic pressure, no changes in left ventricular end diastolic pressure were noted.

Concomitant with the vasodilator-induced reduction in arterial pressure was a dose-related increase in heart rate (Fig. 2). Changes in heart rate did not correlate solely with the degree of arterial pressure decrease produced by each agent (Fig. 3). Hydralazine at lower doses produced the largest reflex tachycardia. Of the dihydropyridines, nifedipine produced the greatest and niludipine the least re-

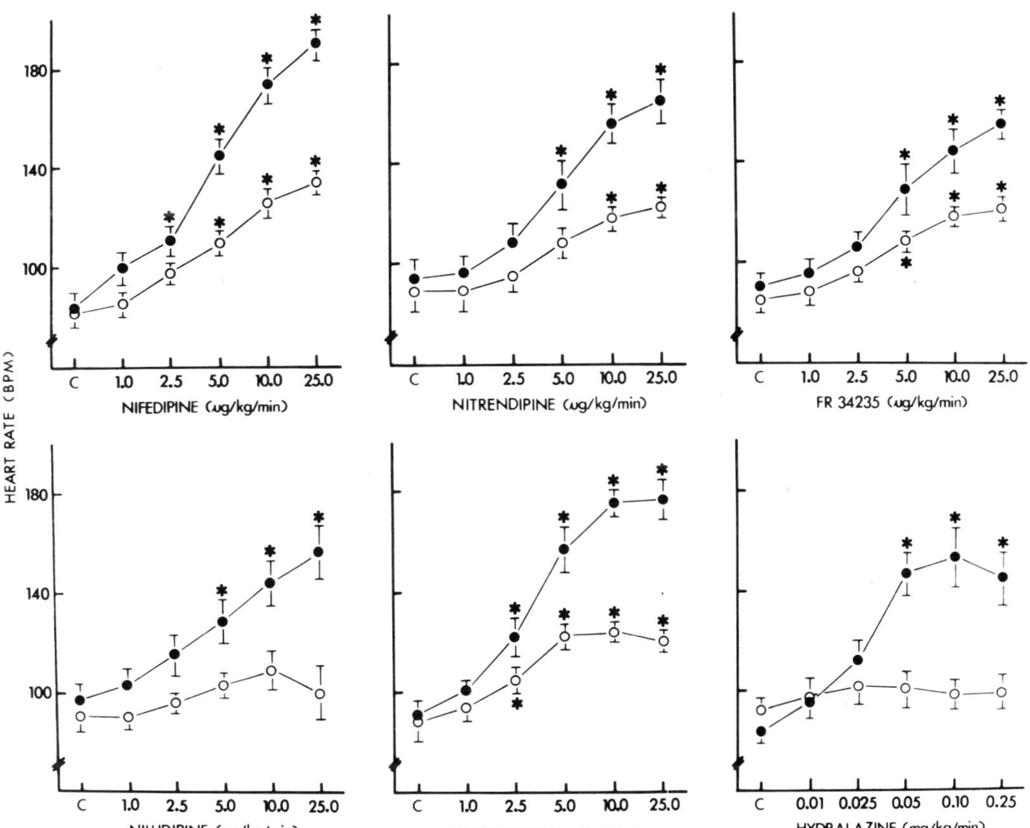

Fig. 2. Changes in heart rate produced by intravenous infusions of the calcium antagonists and hydralazine before and after beta blockade

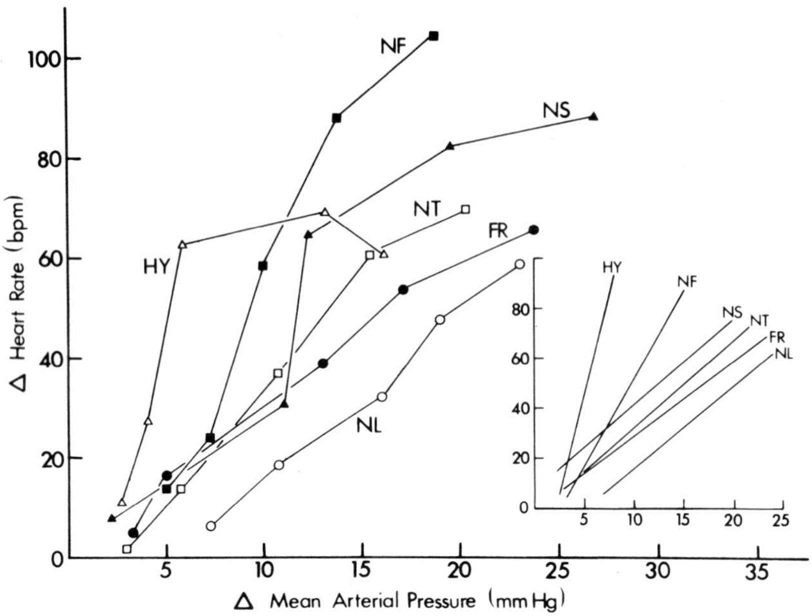

Fig. 3. Relationship between change of mean arterial pressure and heart rate after multiple doses of calcium antagonists or hydralazine. Insert at right represents all data points for each group analyzed by linear regression. *HY, NF, NS, NT, FR, NL* = hydralazine, nifedipine, nisoldipine, nitrendipine, FR 34235 and niludipine, respectively

flex tachycardia. The slopes of the regression lines generated by plotting changes in heart rate versus changes in mean arterial pressure for hydralazine and the dihydropyridine calcium antagonists are shown in Fig. 3.

Due to large changes in heart rate, the heart rate systolic pressure product, an index of myocardial oxygen consumption, was elevated by each of the drugs. Nifedipine and nisoldipine produced the largest changes in the rate-pressure product, while smaller changes were observed with nitrendipine, FR 34235, niludipine and hydralazine. Little change in global myocardial contractility (+dP/dt) was produced by the dihydropyridines, however a significant increase was observed with hydralazine (Fig. 4).

After beta blockade, the dihydropyridine calcium antagonists produced greater reductions in systolic arterial pressure and left ventricular systolic pressure (Fig. 1). No change in left ventricular end diastolic pressure was observed with combinations of high doses of calcium antagonists and propranolol. The reflex tachycardia observed prior to administration of propranolol was greatly attenuated (Fig. 2). Nevertheless, significant increases in heart rate still occurred with nifedipine, nitrendipine, FR 34235 and nisoldipine. No significant increase in heart rate was produced by niludipine and hydralazine after beta blockade. Because of the limitation of the reflex tachycardia and a significant fall in systolic arterial pressure, changes in the rate-pressure product after beta adrenergic blockade were minimal. Although small decreases in peak +dP/dt were observed with high doses of the calcium antagonists after propranolol, significant decreases only

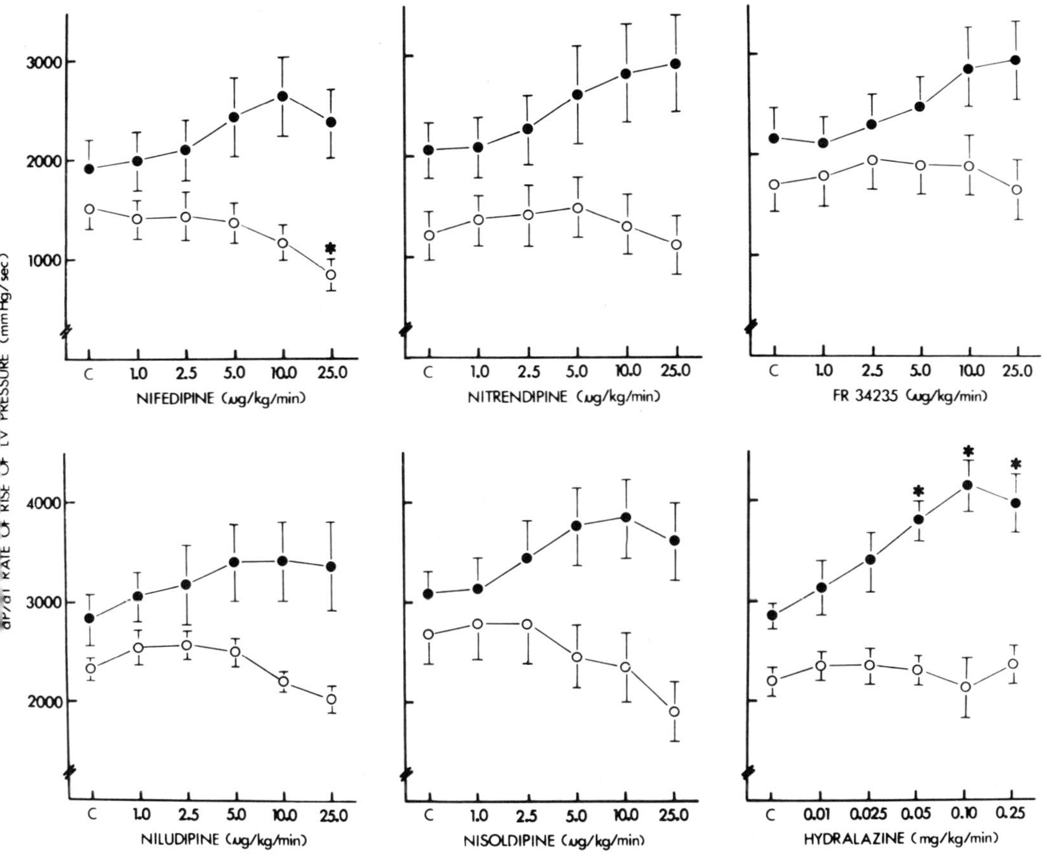

Fig. 4. Changes in left ventricular +dP/dt produced by intravenous infusions of calcium antagonists and hydralazine before and after beta blockade

occurred with the highest dose of nifedipine. Also, the reflex increase in contractility observed with hydralazine was blocked by propranolol (Fig. 4).

The effects of the dihydropyridine calcium antagonists and hydralazine on coronary blood flow before and after beta adrenergic blockade are summarized in Fig. 5. All drugs increased mean, diastolic and systolic coronary blood flow. Nisoldipine and FR 34235 produced the greatest increases in coronary perfusion while nitrendipine and hydralazine caused relatively smaller changes (Table 2). The increase in coronary perfusion observed with hydralazine was prevented by prior treatment with propranolol. Although the increase in flow following nifedipine was partially attenuated after beta adrenergic blockade, this was not observed with nitrendipine, FR 34235, niludipine and nisoldipine. The ratio of mean coronary blood flow to cardiac work (heart rate x systolic blood pressure) was significantly increased by nisoldipine, niludipine and FR 34235 but unchanged by hydralazine.

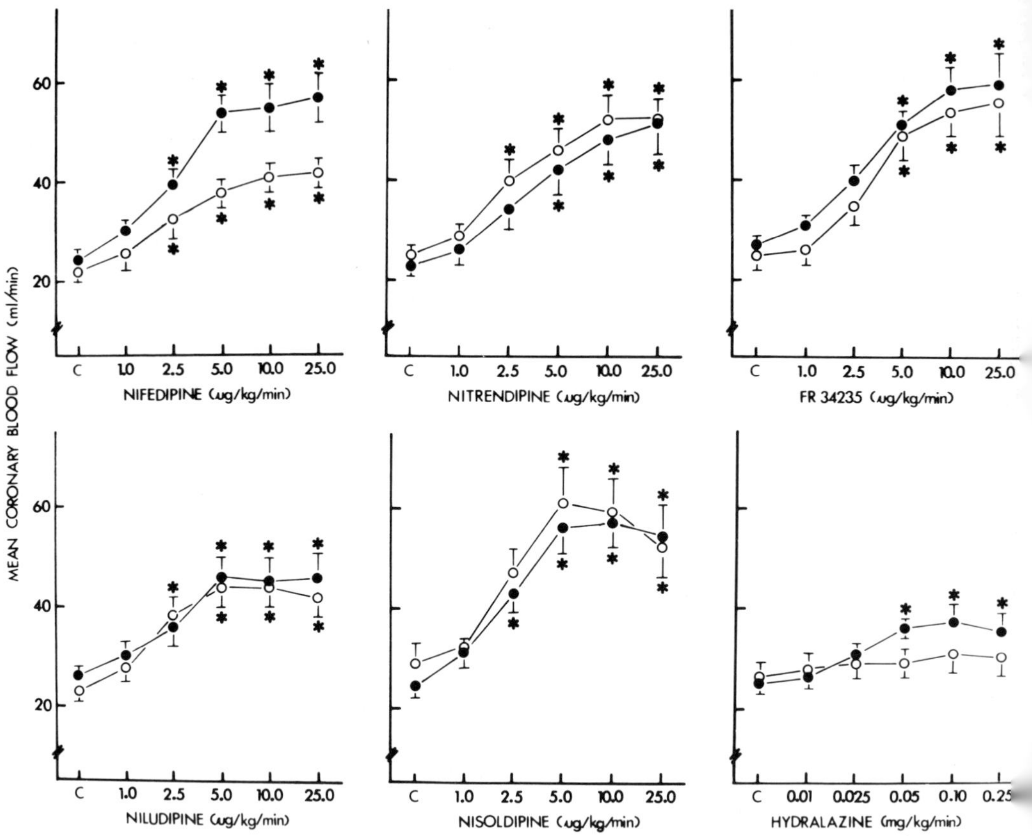

Fig. 5. Changes in mean coronary blood flow produced by calcium antagonists and hydralazine before and after beta blockade

Table 2. Efficacy of vasodilators on coronary blood flow

Most effective:	Nisoldipine and FR 34235
	Nifedipine and niludipine
Least effective:	Nitrendipine and hydralazine

Calcium Antagonist-Induced Change in Baroreflex Sensitivity

Baroreceptor reflex control of heart rate was assessed by the method of Smyth et al. [5]. Each dog received alternate intravenous injections of sodium nitroprusside (100 µg/kg) and phenylephrine (10 µg/kg) to reduce and elevate systolic arterial pressure, respectively. The cardiac interval was recorded from the electrocardiogram and plotted as a function of the preceding systolic pressure. On each day, three assessments of baroreflex sensitivity were made in each dog: control; following low doses of calcium antagonists (2.5 µg/kg/min) or hydralazine

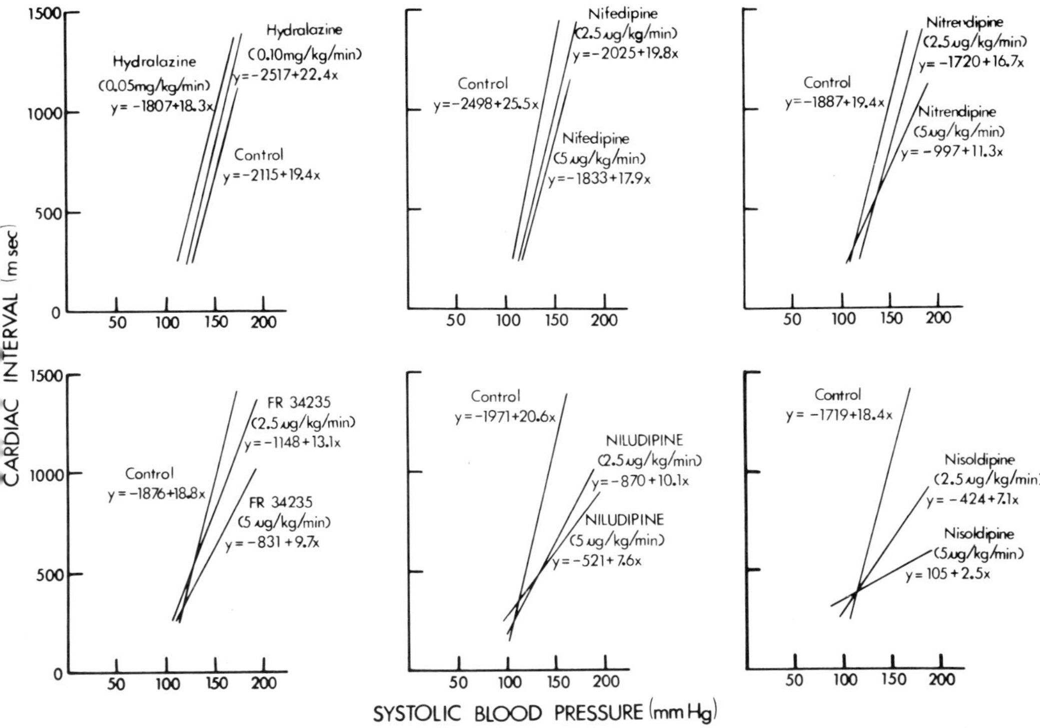

Fig. 6. Relationship between an increase in systolic arterial pressure and cardiac interval during control and after low and high doses of calcium antagonists or hydralazine. Straight lines generated by linear regression analysis

(0.05 mg/kg/min); following high doses of calcium antagonists (5.0 µg/kg/min) or hydralazine (0.10 mg/kg/min). Regression lines relating the reflex bradycardia associated with an increase in systolic arterial pressure in response to phenylephrine after administration of nifedipine, nitrendipine, FR 34235, niludipine, nisoldipine and hydralazine are shown in Fig. 6. No significant change in the sensitivity of the baroreflex was observed at low or high doses of hydralazine, nifedipine and nitrendipine. On the other hand, there was a significant dose-related decrease in sensitivity after administration of FR 34235, niludipine and nisoldipine. With the latter drugs, a smaller decrease in heart rate occurred with any given increase in arterial pressure than during control conditions. Only small changes in baroreflex sensitivity in response to a fall in arterial pressure were observed after any of the vasodilator drugs.

Systemic and Coronary Hemodynamic Effects of Dihydropyridine Calcium Agonists

Hemodynamic alterations elicited by the calcium agonist, CGP 28392 in conscious dogs are shown in Table 3. On the day of the study, each dog received

Table 3. Hemodynamic effects of CGP 28 392

	Control	CGP 28 392 (μg/kg)		
		50	100	150
HR	114± 10	87± 8	84± 10*	94± 11
BP	94± 4	111± 4*	118± 3*	129± 4*
+dP/dt	3,870±390	3,350±270	3,290±280	3,290±270
CBFV	63± 8	62± 11	61± 6	62± 9

4 doses (25, 50, 100 and 150 μg/kg) of CGP 28392 as an intravenous bolus. Hemodynamic effects were recorded with and without pretreatment with nifedipine (20 μg/kg/min). In other experimental groups, the contribution of the autonomic nervous system to drug actions was assessed by pretreatment with phentolamine (0.5 mg/kg), propranolol (1 mg/kg) or methyl atropine (1.5 mg/kg).

Intravenous administration of CGP 28392 resulted in a dose-related increase in systolic, diastolic and mean arterial blood pressure. There was also a significant elevation of left ventricular systolic pressure. Following bolus doses of 100 μg/kg, hemodynamics returned to the pre-drug state in approximately 2–4 min. During the peak effect of drug on arterial pressure, there was a corresponding reduction in heart rate. Also during the initial rise in arterial pressure following bolus administration of CGP 28392, there was a slight decrease in peak left ventricular +dP/dt. After the initial depression, a secondary transient rise in left ventricular +dP/dt commonly occurred. Small increases in both end diastolic and end systolic segment length following drug administration were observed, however no significant change in shortening of the myocardial segment occurred. The actions of CGP 28392 on coronary blood flow velocity were biphasic. Initially, CGP 28392 produced a small reduction in coronary blood flow velocity coincident with the peak effect of drug on arterial pressure. This was followed by a slight rise in coronary blood flow velocity coincident with a secondary increase in +dP/dt. Relative mean coronary vascular resistance was significantly increased by CGP 28392.

The influence of alpha and beta adrenergic blockade on the cardiovascular effects of CGP 28392 are summarized in Fig. 7. Alpha adrenergic receptor blockade produced by phentolamine had no effect on the increase in arterial blood pressure and coronary vascular resistance and decrease in heart rate produced by CGP 28392. Similarly, beta adrenergic blockade with propranolol had no effect on the increase in arterial pressure and coronary vascular resistance produced by CGP 28392. On the other hand, the reduction in heart rate was blunted presumably secondary to the relative bradycardia induced by beta adrenergic blockade. In one dog, there was no effect of methyl atropine on the increase in arterial pressure and coronary vascular resistance produced by CGP 28392, but the reduction in heart rate was attenuated, indicating the latter action of CGP 28392 to be a baroreceptor-mediated bradycardia. Following nifedipine, CGP 28392 had no effect on heart rate, arterial blood pressure, left ventricular systolic pressure or coronary blood flow velocity (Fig. 7).

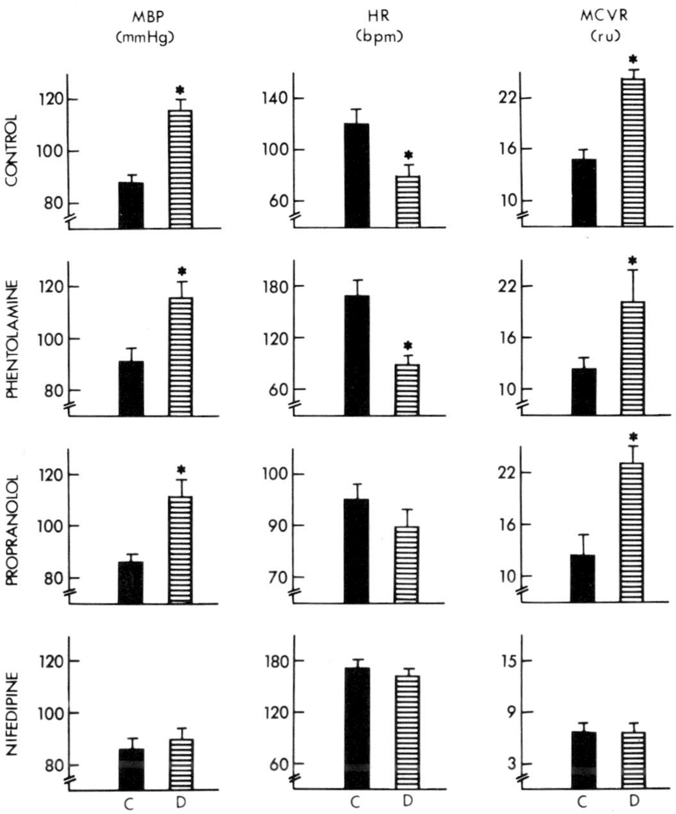

Fig. 7. Mean arterial blood pressure (*MBP*), heart rate (*HR*) and mean coronary vascular resistance (*MCVR*) during control (*C*) and following intravenous bolus administration of CGP 28392 (100 μg/kg; *D*) in control, phentolamine-, propranolol- and nifedipine-pretreated dogs

The hemodynamic actions of multiple intravenous infusions (2, 4, 8 and 20 μg/kg/min) of the calcium agonist, Bay k 8644 were assessed in conscious dogs before and after propranolol (1 mg/kg) and during a constant arterial pressure produced by simultaneous intravenous infusion of sodium nitroprusside. Bay k 8644 increased systolic, diastolic and mean arterial pressure and left ventricular systolic pressure. Heart rate remained unchanged. There was a dose-related positive inotropic effect as measured by peak +dP/dt and percent segment shortening. Coronary blood flow velocity increased at higher doses. At doses of 8 μg/kg/min dogs became excited and salivation and vomiting occurred. At higher doses self-limited grand mal type seizures developed in certain animals. Prior treatment with propranolol did not change any of the hemodynamic effects of Bay k 8644 (Figs. 8 and 9). Concomitant intravenous administration of sodium nitroprusside during infusions of Bay k 8644 in beta blocked animals prevented the increase in arterial pressure and resulted in enhanced segment shortening (Figs. 9 and 10).

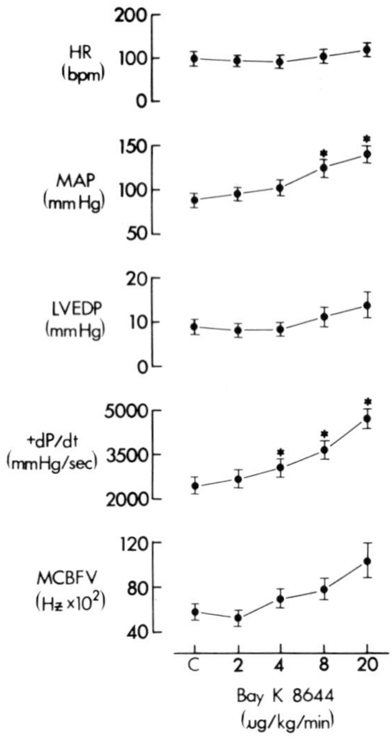

Fig. 8. Summarized hemodynamic actions of Bay k 8644 in conscious dogs pretreated with propranolol. *HR*, heart rate; *MAP*, mean arterial pressure; *LVEDP*, left ventricular end diastolic pressure; *MCBFV*, mean coronary blood flow velocity

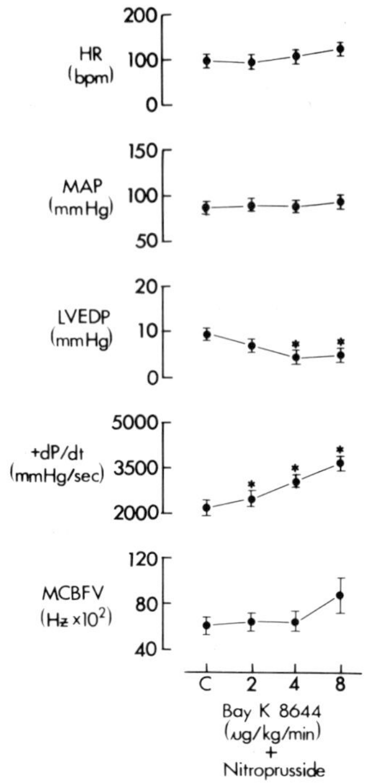

Fig. 10. Summarized hemodynamic actions of Bay k 8644 in conscious dogs pretreated with propranolol and intravenous infusion of nitroprusside used to control arterial pressure

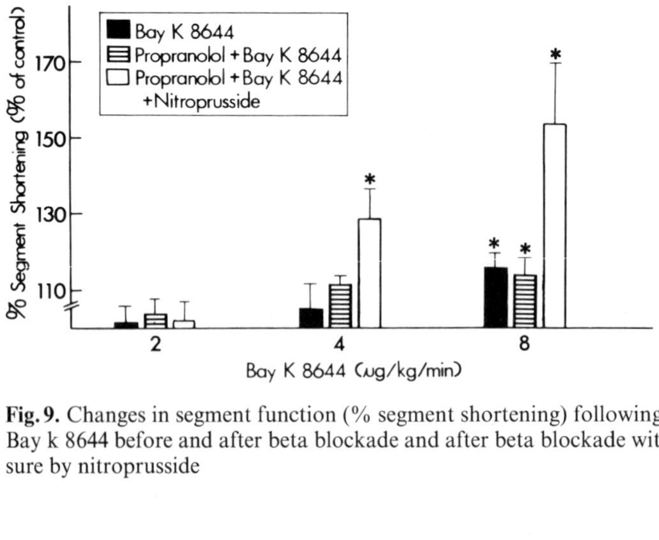

Fig. 9. Changes in segment function (% segment shortening) following intravenous infusions of Bay k 8644 before and after beta blockade and after beta blockade with control of arterial pressure by nitroprusside

Summary

Previous investigations have shown the structurally unrelated calcium antagonists, verapamil, diltiazem and nifedipine to have a variety of effects on systemic and coronary hemodynamics [1, 2]. The present results indicate that whereas the dihydropyridine calcium antagonists all produce a decrease in aterial pressure and an increase in coronary blood flow, the subtle structural modifications of the dihydropyridine nucleus have provided certain of the calcium antagonists with relative selectivities for peripheral versus coronary beds. Furthermore, certain of the dihydropyridine calcium antagonists produce more tachycardia than others. For example, dihydropyridines producing the greatest reduction of arterial pressure were nisoldipine and nitrendipine. Nifedipine was less effective. On the other hand, nifedipine produced the greatest and niludipine the least reflex tachycardia for any given change in arterial pressure. Nisoldipine and FR 34325 produced the largest increases in coronary conductance. Nitrendipine produced much smaller changes.

Other structural modifications of the dihydropyridine nucleus have produced agents with hemodynamic actions in direct opposition to those of the antagonists. Best recognized of these agents, the calcium agonists, are CGP 28392 and Bay k 8644 [3,4]. The calcium agonists produced elevations of arterial pressure and myocardial contractility. These hemodynamic effects were unchanged by alpha and beta adrenergic blockade but completely antagonized by nifedipine. The relative selectivities and specificities of the various dihydropyridine calcium antagonists and agonists may provide advantages for use of these agents in cardiovascular disease.

Acknowledgements. The authors extend their appreciation to Mr. Mark Zyvoloski for technical assistance and Ms. Lynn Binder for secretarial assistance. This work was supported by a grant from the American Heart Association with funds contributed in part by the AHA, Wisconsin Affiliate and Cardiovascular Research Training Grant No. 1 T32 HLO7546.

References

1. Henry PD (1980) Comparative pharmacology of calcium antagonists: nifedipine, verapamil and diltiazem. Am J Cardiol 46:1047–1058
2. Millard RW, Lathrop DA, Grupp G, Ashraf L, Grupp IL, Schwartz A (1982) Differential cardiovascular effects of calcium channel blocking agents: Potential mechanisms. Am J Cardiol 49:499–506
3. Schramm M, Thomas G, Towart R, Franckowiak G (1983) Activation of calcium channels by novel 1,4-dihydropyridines. Arzneim-Forsch 33:1268–1272
4. Preuss KC, Cheung NL, Brooks HL, Warltier DC (1984) Cardiovascular effects of the nifedipine analog, CGP 28392 in the conscious dog. J Cardiovasc Pharm 6:949–953
5. Smyth HS, Sleight P, Pickering GW (1969) Reflex regulation of arterial pressure during sleep in man. A quantative method of assessing baroreflex sensitivity. Circ Res 24:109–121

Discussion

(pp. 338–349)

Groß: Did you correlate the smaller increase in coronary blood flow under beta blockade to the lesser increase in heart rate? There is a very close correlation between change in heart rate and change in coronary flow.

Warltier: I think that is probably due to a reduction in oxygen consumption, secondary to a decrease in the rate-pressure product. I was somewhat surprised to see this, because nifedipine is a very effective coronary vasodilator. Apparently some of this vasodilation can be attributed to metabolic autoregulation. I might also add that in work previously published by Steven Vatner this was also found for nifedipine.

Hoffmeister: I would like shortly to comment on the cerebral actions of the agonist, BAY K 8644. We have shown that BAY K 8644 in intermediate doses has tranquilizing, "anxiolytic" effects in rodents as well as in rhesus monkeys.

In small rodents (mice and rats) very high doses of the substance lead to convulsions. These convulsions have a unique symptomatology and are not comparable to tonic or clonic seizures. In the EEG tracings there were no clear indications for seizures but they showed grapho-elements of cerebral activity.

Warltier: In the conscious dog these appeared as grand mal self limited seizures. Whether these are due to focal ischemia or activation of neurones within the CNS, we cannot be sure. We don't have electroencephalographic data on these animals. I have given a small amount of compound to a colleague who administered the drug intraventricularly in conscious rats. He saw no activity as far as seizures were concerned.

Fleckenstein: As to these experiments on rats concerning a central nervous stimulation by the BAYER agonist, I should like to say that the first sign of change in the central nervous system is that the rats become first of all highly aggressive.

Warltier: We have the same problem only it is with a very big dog. Although the seizures were usually selflimited at times we tried intravenous valium to interrupt them. In these cases the dogs did not develop a typical postictal depression, but became furious and had to be anesthetized.

Groß: Your finding is similar to what we found in conscious dogs, but it is different from what we saw in conscious rhesus monkeys and different from behavioural effects in rats; there are big species differences. Your dose-response curves of the CIBA-GEIGY agonist also did not reach a plateau. Did you see any central nervous effects with that drug?

Warltier: No, we didn't see any CNS effects with the CIBA-GEIGY compound but in the experiments with CGP 28392, the drug was administered as a bolus and the BAY K 8644 experiments were done by intravenous infusions. I think that could be a part of it.

Brown: An obvious signal to the problem with the Diazepam is: Did you try to prevent the seizures with nifedipine or one of the other antagonists?

Warltier: We really have not done that experiment in the way it should be done. We gave nifedipine on several occasions during the seizure and it abruptly decreased the arterial pressure in those animals but whether it stopped the seizure or whether the seizure had run its course, I really can't answer. Nimodipine might have been a better choice than nifedipine as it is a more lipophilic compound.

Hoffmeister: In mice we could not antagonize the convulsions with sedatives and antiepileptics, such as diazepam, diphenylhydantoin or phenobarbital although the doses used of those drugs completely inhibited electroconvulsive shock. In contrast, nifedipine blocked the BAY K 8644 seizures completely.

Scriabine: You used Ca^{2+}-antagonists together with propranolol. Did you see with this combination a negative dromotropic effect or effects on cardiac conduction? Did you do similar experiments with verapamil?

Warltier: No negative dromotropic effects were observed. We noted only effects on the SA node. I might also emphasize that this was a large dose of propranolol (2 mg/kg) and also a large dose of calcium antagonist (25 μg/kg/min). We did not notice any disturbances in conduction in these animals. We have not used verapamil in combination with propranolol.

Lichtlen: You found practically no change in the increase of coronary blood flow when you added propranolol. Flow increase was practically unchanged, although heart rate and DP/DT decreased. Thus, oxygen consumption clearly decreased.

Warltier: For most of the Ca^{2+} channel blockers this is ture. The only exception was nifedipine. With nifedipine we did see a significant fall in coronary perfusion after administration of propranolol. As far as the peripheral vasodilator, hydralazine, was concerned, its action to increase coronary flow was completely blocked by propranolol indicating it to be a very weak coronary vasodilator. Any increase in flow with hydralazine is probably secondary to an increase in myocardial oxygen consumption.

Lichtlen: How about nisoldipine and nitrendipine?

Warltier: In the case of these agents, no change in the increase in coronary flow was observed following pretreatment with propranolol.

Lichtlen: In a small series of patients we saw that despite nifedipine there is a significant decrease in blood flow after adding propranolol that would fit with your nifedipine group beside that heart rate was kept constant by pacing.

Warltier: If you keep heart rate constant by pacing, I would not expect this at all. I think in our consicious dogs oxygen consumption certainly would have increased following the administration of these drugs. This is in contrast to the condition present in the barbiturate anesthetized dog where there is already a very high spontaneous heart rate and arterial pressure due to the anesthesia. Under those conditions we have observed a significant decrease in oxygen consumption.

Nayler: Do you have any data on what is happening to the noradrenaline – turnover rate in these animals with the high dose of BAY K 8644?

Warltier: No, we don't have any data concerning norepinephrine levels, but we have used large doses of propranolol to block beta effects. Of course it is very difficult to block the endogenously released norepinephrine, but nevertheless we did use very large doses of beta blocker.

We did not measure norepinephrine in these experiments but based on our experiments with CGP 28392 where we pretreated with phentolamine, little of the action of the calcium agonist is due to alpha receptor stimulation.

Bayer-Symposium IX
Cardiovascular Effects of Dihydropyridine-Type
Calcium Antagonists and Agonists, 353–360

Effect of a Dihydropyridine-Type Calcium Antagonist on Cerebral Blood Flow and Metabolism

A. M. HARPER

Introduction

The calcium channel blocker, nimodipine, has been shown to have a preferential vasodilator action on the contraction of cerebrovascular smooth muscle induced by neurotransmitter and vasoconstrictor substances in vitro (Towart and Kazda 1982).

The present paper summarises some of the in vivo work undertaken in our laboratories over the past few years on the effect of nimodipine on cerebral blood flow and metabolism, both in "normal" animals and following occlusion of the middle cerebral artery (MCA).

Any study of cerebral blood flow (CBF) in animals must start with an awareness of certain anatomical and physiological principles. Firstly, the method used to measure CBF must take into account the widely varying cerebrovascular anatomy between species. For instance, the dog and the cat have many anastomoses between the intra- and extracranial circulations. They are therefore unsuitable for such methods as ^{133}Xenon clearance which depend on monitoring the clearance of the isotope from brain tissue alone.

Secondly, the interpretation of CBF measurements will depend on the recorded values for arterial blood pressure and the carbon dioxide tension in arterial blood. "Autoregulation" of CBF means the maintenance of a relatively constant flow in the face of changes in arterial blood pressure. When arterial blood pressure falls, the resistance vessels in the brain dilate and flow remains constant until a certain lower limit is reached. This is of importance when giving a vasodilator substance. If the drug lowers the blood pressure, then that in itself will cause a degree of cerebral vasodilatation, thus diminishing further vasodilation produced by the compound (for review, see Harper and McCulloch 1985).

As an illustration of this we can observe the changes in CBF with blood pressure when giving a powerful vasodilator, e.g., carbon dioxide. A reduction in arterial blood pressure when the vessels are already dilated with CO_2 causes the flow to fall with pressure, and impairs autoregulation – the vessels, being already dilated with CO_2, cannot further dilate to a sufficient extent to maintain a constant blood flow (Harper 1966). The reason for these introductory remarks will become clear when we consider the dose response effect of nimodipine on local CBF in the rat studies reported below.

Studies of Nimodipine on Regional CBF in Baboons

These experiments were performed on baboons anaesthetised with phencyclidine and nitrous oxide/oxygen on controlled respiration. The scalp and temporal muscles were removed to expose the calvarium. A bolus of ^{133}Xenon was injected into a branch of the carotid artery and the rate of clearance of the isotope detected from a collimated sodium iodide crystal mounted over the skull and connected to a ratemeter, scaler and recorder. Average flow through the area of the brain "seen" by the detector was calculated by the height/area method. Cerebral metabolic rate for oxygen ($CMRO_2$) was calculated from the flow multiplied by the cerebral arterio-venous oxygen difference – the cerebral venous blood being sampled from a catheter in the sagittal sinus.

Table 1 shows the effects of a continuous i.v. infusion of nimodipine at a dose of 2 μg kg^{-1} min^{-1}. After 50 min infusion there was an increase of approximately 25% in CBF, a decrease of 10% in mean arterial blood pressure, and no significant change in $CMRO_2$. The effects of continuous infusion of nimodipine into

Table 1. Effect of continuing intravenous infusion of nimodipine (2 μg kg^{-1} min^{-1}). (Harper et al. 1981)

Variable	Control	Nimodipine			Control	
		+10 min	+30	+50	10–15 after nimodipine min	30+ after nimodipine min
CBF						
Mean	62.6	67.2	74.8	79.8	71.2	61.2
Δ%	–	+ 7	+19	+27	+14	–
SE	3.6	4.7	6.3	3.7	5.1	5.8
p		ns	< 0.02	< 0.01	< 0.02	ns
$CMRO_2$						
Mean	4.38 (n=4)	4.14 (n=4)	4.75 (n=4)	4.08 (n=3)	4.91 (n=4)	4.49 (n=3)
Δ%		– 4	+ 8	– 7	+12	+ 3
SE	0.27	0.10	0.75		1.21	
P_{aCO_2}						
Mean	37.2	36.9	37.7	38.1	37.4	37.0
SE	1.1	1.6	1.0	1.1	1.2	1.2
		ns	ns	ns	ns	ns
MABP						
Mean	102	90	90	94	93	93
Δ%		–12	–12	– 8	– 9	– 9
SE	5	4	4	4	4	4
p		0.05	0.02	ns	ns	ns

Except otherwise indicated, n=5

Table 2. Effect of continuing intracarotid infusion of nimodipine (0.67 μg kg^{-1} min^{-1}) before and up to opening the blood-brain barrier with urea. From Harper et al. 1981

Variable	Control	Nimodipine		Nimodipine + urea		Post-infusion at 20 min
		+10 min	+30 min	+10 min	+30 min	
CBF						
Mean	61	89	96	114	87	65
Δ%		+46	+57	87	43	7
SE	4	6	7	6	17	14
p		< 0.05	< 0.05	< 0.01	ns	ns
P_{aCO_2}						
Mean	40	39	39	40	40	39
SE	1	1	1	1	1	1
p		ns	ns	ns	ns	ns
MABP						
Mean	96	88	84	94	91	92
Δ%		− 8	−12	− 2	− 5	− 4
SE	6	4	1	6	6	7
p		ns	ns	ns	ns	ns

Means for $n=4$ throughout

the internal carotid artery are shown in Table 2. At a dose of 0.67 μg kg^{-1} min^{-1} CBF increased by 45%. However, if the blood-brain barrier (BBB) was transiently disrupted by the infusion of hyperosmolar urea, the effect was more pronounced. CBF increased by over 80%. Twenty minutes later, when we would have expected the BBB to have closed again, the increase had returned to around 40%. This led us to speculate (Harper et al. 1982) that nimodipine might be especially effective in circumstances where there was pathological damage to the BBB.

Studies on Local Cerebral Blood Flow and Glucose Utilisation in Normal Rats

Methods. Local cerebral blood flow (lCBF) in 31 areas of the brain was measured in anaesthetised rats at constant body temperature and arterial PCO_2, using quantitative autoradiography with ^{14}C-iodoantipyrine as tracer (Sakurada et al. 1978). The method and experimental design have been described in detail (Mohammed et al. 1984). Local cerebral glucose utilisation (lCGU) was measured using the ^{14}C-2-deoxyglucose (2-DG) method of Sokoloff et al. (1977). The experimental design is described in detail elsewhere (Mohammed et al. 1985). In the blood flow experiments, i. v. infusion of either nimodipine or vehicle (a lutrol-glycerine-water mixture) was commenced 25 min before termination of the experiment and removal of the brain for autoradiography. In the 2-DG experiments, nimodipine or vehicle infusion was commenced 15 min before and continued for a further 45 min (during which time 2-DG was infused i.v.) before removal of the brain for autoradiography.

Results. Figure 1 demonstrates the lCBF responses of two strongly reacting areas (parietal cortex and medial geniculate) and two weakly reacting areas (globus pallidus and septal nucleus) to infusion of vehicle or nimodipine at doses of 1, 2 and 4 µg kg^{-1} min^{-1}. Neither globus pallidus nor septal nucleus showed significant changes. However, the parietal cortex and medial geniculate showed significant increases in flow of 107% and 63%, respectively. Increasing the dose of nimodipine from 1 to 2 and 4 µg kg^{-1} min^{-1} did not produce further increases in flow – in fact, the increase was less apparent. But it should be noted that the blood pressure fell markedly with higher doses. My remarks in the introduction now come into perspective. As the blood pressure is falling, that in itself will cause cerebral vasodilatation. Add a further vasodilatory stimulus such as nimodipine on to this – and it will not necessarily be more effective at a high dosage, than with 1 µg where there was a comparatively small drop in BP. With nimodipine *more* is not necessarily *better*.

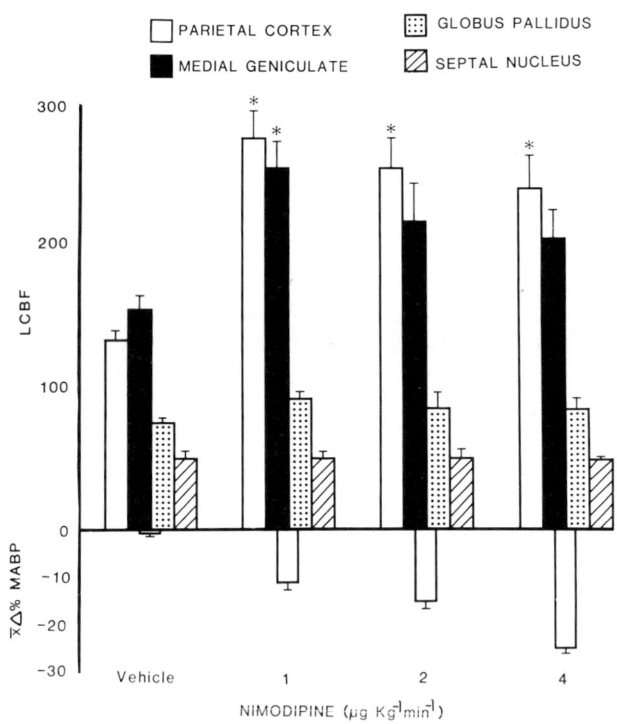

Fig. 1. Effect of vehicle and nimodipine at doses of 1, 2, and 4 µg kg^{-1} min^{-1} on local blood flow (*lCBF*) through parietal cortex, medial geniculate, globus pallidus and septal nucleus. LCBF is ml 100 g^{-1} min^{-1}. Δ% reductions in mean arterial blood pressure (*MABP*) are indicated by histograms below horizontal line. *Bars* indicate SEM. $* = p < 0.05$ using Student's t-test fro grouped data with Bonferroni correction. (Data from this figure and from Table 4 from A. A. Mohammed, O. Gotoh, D. I. Graham, K. A. Osborne, J. McCulloch, D. A. Mendelow, G. M. Teasdale, and A. M. Harper, 1984, unsubmitted observations)

Table 3. The effects of nimodipine (1 μg/kg/min, i. v.) upon local cerebral glucose utilisation and local cerebral blood flow

Region	Cerebral glucose utilisation		Cerebral blood flow	
	Vehicle n:6	Nimodipine n:7	Vehicle n:5	Nimodipine n:5
Caudate nucleus	91±4	82±2	136±12	183±16[a]
Genu of corpus callosum	30±1	28±1	46± 3	48± 1
Frontal cortex	91±3	90±2	179±17	249±12[b]
Sensory-motor cortex	96±4	94±4	165±16	248±13[b]
Parietal cortex	96±5	89±4	178±12	329±13[c]
Auditory cortex	127±8	115±4	188±14	309±22[b]
Visual cortex	98±5	92±3	140±15	186± 9[a]
Amygdala	48±1	50±3	95± 6	121± 3[b]
Nucleus accumbens	87±3	82±3	147±15	202±16[a]
Dentate gyrus	66±4	62±1	105± 5	131±15
Hippocampus	77±2	75±2	118± 9	161±12[a]
Thalamus (mediodorsal)	76±3	70±1	140±11	169± 3[a]
Substantia nigra (pars compacta)	59±2	55±1	117± 5	146± 4[b]
Lateral geniculate body	72±5	66±2	113± 6	182±15[b]
Medial geniculate body	94±5	87±3	160±11	243±20[b]

[a] $p<0.05$, [b] $p<0.01$ and [c] $p<0.001$, for the comparison between vehicle and nimodipine treatments
Data are presented as mean ±SE

Table 3 compares lCBF and $lCMR_{glu}$ values for vehicle and nimodipine infusion (1 μg kg^{-1} min^{-1}) from 15 selected areas of the brain. The full results are given in Mohammed et al. (1984, 1985), but the areas shown here were selected for presentation as being the areas which showed the most dramatic results in the next section of this paper. It can be seen that the most significant increases in flow were observed in cortical areas, hippocampus and thalamic nuclei. In no case was there any significant change in lCGU. This is important, as a cerebral vasodilator which also increased brain metabolism could be dangerous in the clinical situation – one would not wish to increase the metabolic requirements of the brain when its blood supply was already compromised.

Studies of lCBF in Rats with Middle Cerebral Artery Occlusion

Methods. In anaesthetised rats the middle cerebral artery (MCA) was occluded as described by Tamura et al. (1981). LCBF was measured as described previously. An infusion of nimodipine was commenced 30 min *before* MCA occlusion and continued for 30 min thereafter. At the end of this period the brain was removed for autoradiography.

Results. Figure 2 demonstrates the flow changes in parietal cortex and caudate nucleus. With nimodipine flow is more than doubled on the ipsilateral side compared with vehicle.

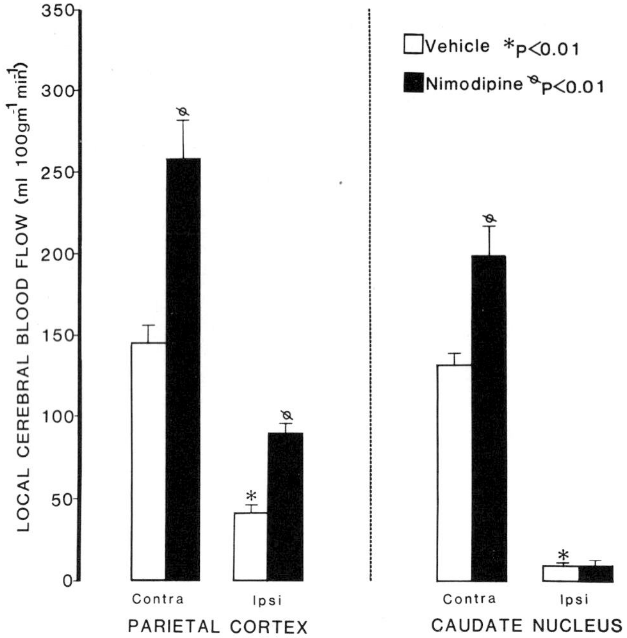

Fig. 2. Effect of nimodipine as compared to vehicle on lCBF following MCA occlusion in ipsilateral and contralateral parietal cortex. *Bars* indicate SEM

Table 4 shows the results from 15 areas of the brain, where the contralateral side is compared with the side ipsilateral to the lesion, using infusion of vehicle (as a control) and of nimodipine (1 $\mu g\ kg^{-1}\ min^{-1}$).

The administration of nimodipine modified the pattern of CBF disturbances in the contralateral and ipsilateral sides in most cortical and subcortical regions examined, compared with the corresponding sides during infusion of the vehicle. However, there was little change in areas in the centre of the ischaemic damage, such as the caudate nucleus.

On the ipsilateral side, the areas showing the greatest increases with nimodipine (as compared to control) were cortex, geniculate and thalamus. In effect, pretreatment and continuing treatment with the drug more than doubled cortical flow in the occluded side, but had no effect in the centre of the ischaemic lesion – namely, the caudate nucleus.

We examined 34 different brain structures in each animal in this series, and it is important to emphasise that in *no* case was any evidence of a "steal" phenomenon observed. In other words, there were no areas of the brain that had a *lower* flow with nimodipine than control.

Histopathological Studies. In a separate series of rats, infusion of nimodipine was commended 30 min before MCA occlusion and continued for 3 h. Thereafter perfusion fixation with FAM was performed; the head was fixed for 24 h at 4 °C. Coronal slices of the brain were embedded in wax and stained with haemotoxalyn eosin or cresyl violet/luxol fast blue. The areas of ischaemic damage were drawn on maps at 8 stereotactically determined coronal sections of the rat brain. By con-

Table 4. Effect of nimodipine on lCBF with middle cerebral artery occlusion

Structure	Vehicle n:5		Nimodipine n:5	
	Contralateral	Ipsilateral	Contralateral	Ipsilateral
Caudate nucleus	124± 7	9± 1^{C}	199±17^{b}	9± 3^{C}
Genu	32± 4	24± 2^{A}	40± 2	24± 3^{C}
Frontal cortex	126± 8	31± 3^{C}	243±23^{b}	61± 6^{bC}
Sensory-motor cortex	135±14	30± 3^{C}	246±20^{b}	61± 9^{bC}
Parietal cortex	147±10	43± 5^{C}	259±23^{b}	80± 6^{bC}
Auditory cortex	156±12	42± 5^{C}	289±14^{c}	96± 1^{cC}
Visual cortex	135± 2	53± 5^{C}	265±23^{c}	123±14^{bC}
Amygdala	99±12	78± 7^{A}	152±12^{a}	103±11^{C}
Nucleus accumbens	125±11	94±10^{B}	185±19^{a}	141±15^{aA}
Dentate gyrus	110± 4	88± 4^{C}	192±12^{c}	147±21^{aB}
Hippocampus	141±12	101± 3^{B}	225±13^{b}	182±18^{bC}
Thalamus (MD)	129± 3	89± 5^{C}	202±28^{a}	148±15^{aA}
Substantia nigra (compacta)	114± 7	87± 6^{C}	196±18^{c}	171±14^{cC}
Lateral geniculate	122±14	110± 6^{A}	220±24^{b}	181±20^{ac}
Medial geniculate	149± 9	128± 4^{A}	275±19^{c}	242±23^{bB}

Data are presented as mean ±SE. A, B, C significant difference between data on ipsilateral and contralateral sides within the same animals, $^{A}p<0.05$, $^{B}p<0.01$, $^{C}p<0.001$ (paired t-test). a, b, c significant difference between data for comparison between vehicle and nimodipine treated animals, $^{a}p<0.05$, $^{b}p<0.01$, $^{c}p<0.001$ (unpaired t-test)

ventional light microscopy, ischaemic areas were plotted on the maps. From the maps of the coronal section of the brain, the area of ischaemic damage was obtained from an image analyser function on a densitometer. Total volume of ischaemic damage was calculated by plotting areas of damage against 8 coronal levels and, knowing the distance between, the volume could be calculated from integration.

Results. There was necrosis of the neostriatum in all the animals with MCA occlusion. When the distribution of ischaemic damage at different stereotaxic levels was compared there was less extensive damage with nimodipine compared to control. The volume of hemispheric damage was reduced from 47 mm^3 ±7 with vehicle to 31±3 with nimodipine. The volume of cortical damage was reduced from 26 mm^3 ±6 to 16±3 with nimodipine. There was no significant change in the volume of the ischaemic lesion in the caudate nucleus (D. Graham 1984, unpublished observations).

Conclusion

There is clear evidence that nimodipine dilates cerebral vessels in vitro (Towart and Kazda 1979, 1982) and dilates pial vessels in vivo (Brandt et al. 1981). Over the past few years, our results in both baboons and rats have shown an unequivocal increase in CBF following the administration of nimodipine. We have also shown that doses of nimodipine higher than 1 to 2 μg kg^{-1} min^{-1} can be accompanied by unacceptably large decreases in arterial blood pressure which counteract the increase in CBF produced by the compound. Although not mentioned in the results, our studies (Mohammed et al. 1984) also showed that high doses of nimodipine were accompanied by a degree of hyperglycaemia which would be potentially dangerous in the clinical situation. Therefore, the dose of nimodipine, either clinically or experimentally, must be carefully controlled.

The observation that increases in flow are not accompanied by increases in cerebral metabolism will be comforting for the clinician.

It must be emphasis that the results following MCA occlusion presented here are with *pre-treatment* with nimodipine, and I do not think it appropriate in this paper to discuss the rather conflicting reports which have appeared when calcium channel blockers are given after an ischaemic or hypoxic insult. However, when nimodipine is administered before and during an ischaemic insult there are undoubted improvements in blood flow and the amount of histological damage in the periphery, but not the centre, of the lesion. Whether the improvement in pathological damage is due to better oxygen delivery due to increase in flow, or to more subtle biochemical changes involving prevention of Ca excretion from damaged neurophils, is a matter for further study.

References

1. Brandt L, Andersson K-E, Edvinsson L, Ljunggren B (1981) Effects of extracellular calcium and of calcium antagonists on the contractile responses of isolated human pial and mesenteric arteries. J Cereb Blood Flow &Metabol 1:339–347
2. Harper AM (1966) Autoregulation of cerebral blood flow: influence of the arterial blood pressure on the blood flow through the cerebral cortex. J Neurol Neurosurg Psychiat 29:398–403
3. Harper AM, Craigen L, Kazda S (1981) Effect of the calcium antagonist, nimodipine, on cerebral blood flow and metabolism in primates. J Cereb Blood Flow & Metabol 1:349–356
4. Harper AM, McCulloch J (1985) Cerebral blood flow and cerebrovascular disease. In: Kennard, Swash (eds) Scientific basis of neurology. Churchill Livingstone, pp 518–532
5. Mohammed AA, McCulloch J, Mendelow AD, Teasdale GM, Harper AM (1984) Effect of the calcium antagonist, nimodipine, on local cerebral blood flow: Relationship to arterial blood pressure. J Cereb Blood Flow & Metabol 4:206–211
6. Mohammed AA, Mendelow AD, Teasdale GM, Harper AM, McCulloch J (1985) Effect of the calcium antagonist, nimodipine, upon local cerebral blood flow and metabolic coupling. J Cereb Blood Flow & Metabol 5:26–33
7. Sakurada O, Kennedy C, Jehle J, Brown JD, Carbin GL, Sokoloff L (1978) Measurement of local cerebral blood flow with iodo [^{14}C] antipyrine. Am J Physiol 234:H59–H66
8. Sokoloff L, Reivich M, Kennedy C, Des Rosiers MH, Patlak CS, Pettigrew KD, Sakurada O, Shinohara M (1977) The [^{14}C]-deoxyglucose method for the measurement of local cerebral glucose utilization; theory, procedure and normal values in the conscious and anesthetized albino rat. J Neurochem 28:897–916
9. Tamura A, Graham DI, McCulloch J, Teasdale GM (1981) Focal cerebral ischaemia in the rat. 1. Description of technique and early neuropathological consequences following middle cerebral artery occlusion. J Cereb Blood Flow & Metabol 1:53–60
10. Towart R, Kazda S (1979) The cellular mechanism of action of nomodipine (Bay e 9736), a new calcium antagonist. Br J Pharmacol 67:409–410
11. Towart R, Kazda S (1982) Preferential vasodilator actions of the calcium antagonists nimodipine (Bay e 9736), nifedipine and verapamil on contraction of cerebral vascular smooth muscles induced by neurotransmitter and vasoconstrictor substances. In: Heistad DD, Marcus ML (eds) Cerebral blood flow: Effect of nerves and neurotransmitters. Elsevier-North Holland, New York, pp 29–38

Discussion

(pp. 353–360)

Steen: When looking at mid cerebral artery occlusion, Simon's group found edema formation much more with nimodipine than in the controls for the same cerebral blood flow level; can you give us any information from your own study, about edema formation or electrolytes.

Harper: I cannot give you any information on the electrolyte levels. Histopathologically we found no evidence of any edema, using this particular model, which is not quite the same as Simon's who used a complicated model.

Groß: Can you give an explanation why under maximal sympathetic stimulation the plateau of the autoregulation-curve in brain circulation is not depressed as seen in other autoregulating vascular regions, e.g. the kidney?

Harper: The cervical sympathetic only supplies the vessels, constituting the inflow tract to the brain and the pial vessels. There is a very poor cervical sympathetic nerve supply to the intraparenchymal vessels of the brain, where about 60–65% of the cerebral resistance lies. The function of the cervical sympathetic nerves is to protect against sudden episodes of hypertension. If your are running for a bus then you will presumably have an increased sympathetic tone, which will constrict the inflow vessels to your brain, therefore reducing the pressure distally and helping to prevent sudden increases in cerebral blood flow which might blow the top of your head! So what happens here is that with maximal sympathetic activity the inflow tract vessels are constricted and the whole autoregulatory curve is shifted to the right.

Bevan: How long after the occlusion did you make the flow-measurements; when did you kill the animal and studied the ischemic area? Did you follow the time course of the changes that occured?

Harper: We followed a time course very carefully: we had 2 different protocols. The neuropathologist insisted that we ran 3 h after occlusion. For the flow studies, the brain was removed 30 min after occlusion.

Bayer-Symposium IX
Cardiovascular Effects of Dihydropyridine-Type
Calcium Antagonists and Agonists, 362–367

Calcium, Dihydropyridines and Resistance Vessel Tone

J. A. BEVAN, J. J. HWA, I. LAHER, and M. P. OWEN

Until recently, technical limitations have precluded the study of small resistance vessels in vitro, and analysis of drug effects have been restricted to arteries of 300 μ O.D. and greater. The wire method of vessel mounting (Bevan and Osher 1972) and the development of an appropriate myograph (Mulvany and Halpern 1977) have allowed physiological and pharmacological analyses to be carried out on vessels as small as 70 μ O.D. As had been anticipated from findings with other less direct techniques, small arteries differ, sometimes quite remarkably, from their larger parent vessels not only in features related to their gross anatomy, but in a variety of other structural and particularly functional themes. The evidence is quite overwhelming that comparatively little can be infered concerning resistance vessels from the study of elastic or even the larger muscular arteries.

Since experimental results with these smaller vessels are relatively sparce, it is presently uncertain as to which of the changes that have been described to occur with diminution in arterial diameter are common to all vascular beds and which may be regionally specific. The available studies support the idea that as arteries in general get smaller, there is, 1) a diminution in cleft width (Rowan and Bevan 1983) with all the attendant changes in synaptic and transmitter economy, 2) an increase in relative size of myogenic or stretch-dependent tone (Bevan 1985), 3) an increase in the component of sympathetic vasoconstrictor control that is resistant to α-adrenoceptor blockade (Owen et al. 1983), and 4) in the dependence of agonist-induced responses on the continuous presence of calcium (Ca^{2+}) in the extracellular space (Cauvin et al. 1984 – also see below). In this chapter, we will examine briefly the role of Ca^{2+}, the Ca^{2+} activation or mobilization mechanisms, and the action of dihydropyridine Ca^{2+} channel blockers on some aspects of those phenomenon that seen to be particularly the province of the small resistance arteries.

Myogenic Tone

We have previously proposed that stretch-dependent tone, otherwise known as myogenic or intrinsic tone, may be dependent on Ca^{2+} activating mechanisms different from those involved with receptor-mediated or potential related tone (Bevan et al. 1982; Bevan and Hwa 1984). These conclusions were initially based upon the study of larger vessels, the rabbit basilar artery, and also the rabbit facial vein, a vessel that is probably unique and therefore not necessarily the most representative. The experimental evidence, although indirect, was dependent upon a variety of arguments involving different types of observations: 1) the stretch-induced mechanism is sometimes absent in vessels that develop both forms of tone, 2) relative sensitivity of the three modes of tone in the same blood vessel to vasodilators and to Ca^{2+} channel blocking agents, 3) differing relationships between external Ca^{2+} concentration and tone, and 4) differing susceptibility of the three types of tone to experimental damage.

The most important site of occurrence of myogenic tone is in the small resistance vessels, where it plays a major physiological role. Most smaller arteries develop this tone, although there are clearly quantitative regional differences. Myogenic tone makes a major contribution to resistance to blood flow in most regional vascular beds (Mellander and Johansson 1968). Experiments have been carried out in resistance vessels of the rabbit ear that demonstrate conclusively that the response to stretch is independent of the vessel nerve supply, the presence of the intimal endothelium, and do not involve known endogenous vasoconstrictor mechanisms nor established receptor pathways (Hwa and Bevan 1985). We have continued the pursuit of the evidence for the uniqueness of the Ca^{2+} mechanisms involved in the myogenic tone in these resistance vessels. Vessels from the rabbit ear were selected because of the large amount of background material that exists concerning this bed including some of its small blood vessels (Owen et al. 1983; Walmsley et al. 1983) and the absence of evidence that their myogenic response may be qualitatively different from that which occurs elsewhere in the circulation. In larger blood vessels the relative susceptibility of myogenic, potassium-induced and drug-initiated tone to organic and inorganic Ca^{2+} channel blockers is very different. In most instances myogenic tone is relatively resistant to blockade but not invariably so. This finding prompted us to consider the possibility that the mechanisms regulating Ca^{2+} movement, at least some aspects of the receptor-coupling-channel system involved in these modes of tone initiation, are different from each other. Some of this evidence will be presented.

Summarized in Table 1, are the ID_{50} values for a variety of inorganic and organic Ca^{2+} antagonists for stretch and high potassium-induced tone in resistance vessels of the rabbit ear. There are suggestions in the literature that at least in non-vascular smooth muscle, the intermediate step in the myogenic response is cell membrane depolarization. The sequence is similar in certain respects to the mechanism that couples the distortion of stretch or deformation sensory nerve terminals to afferent neuronal activity (see, for example, Loewenstein 1971). Thus, the main experimental burden in our study of resistance arteries was to distinguish between these two mechanisms. Although some agents, for example, diltiazem, block these two modes of tone in similar concentrations; others, such as nimodipine and magnesium, preferentially block one or the other of the two modes of tone development. ID_{50} values for these latter two substances – for stretch and potassium initiated tone – differ by more than two orders of magnitude.

There is additional evidence for the independence of the Ca^{2+} mechanisms. Barium will substitute for extracellular Ca^{2+} in both tone moieties in these small

Table 1. Rabbit ear resistance artery tone (ID_{50} M)

	Myogenic (Stretch)	K^+ (Phenoxybenzamine)
Nimodipine	$\gg 10^{-6}$	2×10^{-9}
Verapamil	5×10^{-8}	4×10^{-7}
Diltiazem	2×10^{-6}	6×10^{-7}
Mn^{++}	1×10^{-4}	2×10^{-3}
Mg^{++}	6×10^{-3}	$\gg 10^{-2}$

arteries, but to significantly different amounts. When Ba^{++} (1.6 mM) is substituted for Ca^{2+}, the myogenic tone that develops to a standard wall stress is approximately double control values; by contrast, potassium-induced tone is significantly reduced by this substitution. The effects of the dihydropyridine Ca^{2+} agonist. BAY K8644, can also be used to argue for the uniqueness of the two Ca^{2+} mechanisms. This agent will potentiate the response of the resistance vessels to stretch without changing the characteristics of the curve relating external Ca^{2+} concentration to tone development, i.e., without changing threshold, medium effective or peak Ca^{2+} concentrations. Potentiation of the high potassium response is not seen, in fact, there is evidence for its depression. The effects of this Ca^{2+} channel agonist have been used previously to argue for the separate identity of potential sensitive and receptor operated channels in rabbit aortic smooth muscle (Yamamoto et al. 1984). These several observations we have made support the hypothesis that originated in our study of larger vessels, namely that Ca^{2+} mechanisms responsible for stretch and potassium-induced tone have different identities. Such a conclusion implies that even if changes in membrane potential do occur in association with stretch, the electrical changes are probably not, or at least not necessarily, a causal intermediate step (see however, Harder 1984).

α-Adrenoceptor Resistant Sympathetic Tone

The second feature that appears – albeit on the basis of limited experiments – to occur when arteries get smaller is an α-adrenoceptor blocker resistant component of sympathetic vasoconstriction. This has been observed in electrophysiological studies, mainly on submucosal arterioles from the small intestine of the guinea-pig (Hirst and Neild 1981; Angus 1982) and also from in vitro observations of the contractions of blood vessels of the rabbit ear to field stimulation of their sympathetic nerve supply (Owen et al. 1983). The latter study showed that this resistance was greater the smaller the vessel – thus the more narrow the adrenergic synapse, and the higher the frequency of stimulation. In a vessel of approximately 70 μ O.D. at 8 Hz, it corresponded to about 15% of the total sympathetic response.

A number of explanations of these observations are possible. This resistant component could reflect the high concentration of norepinephrine that pertains within the synaptic cleft (Bevan et al. 1980), particularly when it is narrow as in small compared with the larger vessels and with higher stimulation frequencies when it might rise to the order of 10^{-4}–10^{-3} M. Reversible α-adrenoceptor antagonists cannot be used in sufficient concentration to influence these transmitter concentrations when restricted within the limits of their selectivity. Alternatively, the resistance to blockade could reflect the release of a non-adrenergic transmitter from the sympathetic nerve such as the polypeptide-neuropeptide Y (Lundberg et al. 1982). However, the low levels of this peptide present in ear artery vessels does not support this point of view (Edvinsson, personal communication). Finally, the phentolamine-resistant component could represent the action of the adrenergic transmitter on a receptor which is not an α-receptor and therefore possibly resistant to blockade. In the rabbit basilar artery where there is a paucity of α-adrenoceptors (Laher and Bevan 1985) and in other blood vessels after inactivation of a proportion of their α-adrenoceptor complement with phenoxybenzamine, a second population of sites can be demonstrated through which at high concentrations norepinephrine can cause contraction (Furchgott 1972; Duckles and Bevan 1976). Our experiments show that the contraction mediated through such a site, which has low discriminating requirements of chemical agonist activity, is Ca^{2+}-dependent. In the rabbit basilar artery at least, the contraction associated with this receptor has a similar susceptibility to nimodipine as that which occurs when norepinephrine acts through the α-adrenoceptor. This evidence, although preliminary, is consistent with the idea that both types of receptors are coupled to the same population of channels despite very marked differences in the affinity of norepinephrine for the two receptor types.

Calcium (Ca^{2+}) Dependence of Agonist-Induced Tone

In a preliminary paper, Cauvin et al. (1984) have compared Ca^{2+} related mechanisms in the aorta and a mesenteric vessel of the rabbit emphasizing the increased dependence of the small mesenteric vessels on external Ca^{2+}. This comparison, however, involves vessels that differ from each other in two important respects – between the aorta and its branches (Bevan and Yang 1982) (there is a vascular junction at the origin of the mesenteric artery from the aorta), and those changes involved with diminution in vascular diameter. In our own study, we have compared vessels of different diameter for the *same* regional bed – the rabbit ear – where the tissue supplied by the arterial system is reasonably homogeneous. Two types of experiments have been carried out. The first was designed to determine the time course of the fall-off in response to various agonists after Ca^{2+} had been removed from the tissue bath. Two parts of the response were identified – the initial phasic response that is generally considered to be associated with mobilization of Ca^{2+} from sequestered stores somewhere within the vascular smooth muscle cell, and the second, the equilibrium-component of contraction that is to a great extent in many vessels due to the entry of Ca^{2+} from the extracellular space into the cytoplasm. A number of trends of change in characteristics of agonist-induced response were distinguished that seemed independent of the agonist used. The rate of fall-off of both phases tended to be faster in the smaller compared with the larger vessels. After 30 min there was a clear cut residue in the central ear artery (300 μ O.D.) of both the phasic and the equilibrium part of the re-

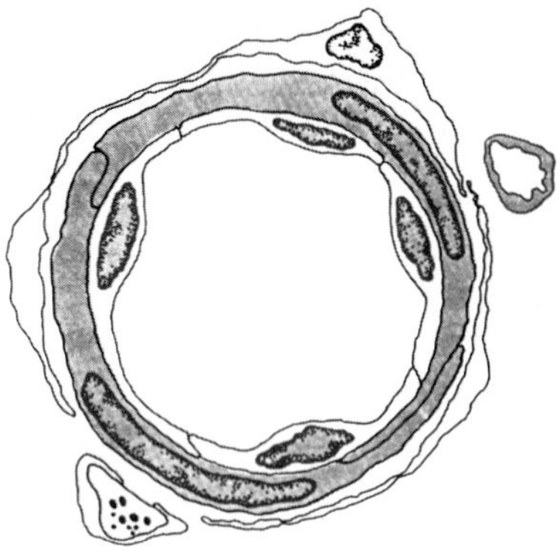

Fig. 1. Modes of resistance artery smooth muscle tone. (Drawn by J. Laher)

sponse. By contrast, in the smaller vessels the first part of the response had almost disappeared and the second completely by this time. These findings are consistent with the idea that phase I and a certain proportion of phase II in the central ear artery – of the order of 10% – is due to activator Ca^{2+} derived from stores resistant to depletion. In the resistance vessel on the other hand, Ca^{2+}, even that derived from "sequestered sites" is lost fairly rapidly to the extracellular space under such circumstances.

Complementing these experiments are others in which the relative effectiveness of nimodipine in reversing agonist-induced tone in three vessels of successively smaller size is measured. Unfortunately, nimodipine can only be used experimentally with a vehicle which we find itself markedly inhibits smooth muscle tone of the smaller vessels. Thus the effects of drug plus vehicle must be compared to those found with vehicle alone. The experimental evidence indicates an increased susceptibility of vessels smaller than the central ear artery to nimodipine with relatively little difference between vessels of 150 and 70 μ O.D. The nimodipine threshold is approximately three orders of magnitude lower in the smaller arteries compared with the central ear. It is clear that the changes in susceptibility of tone to this Ca^{2+} channel blocker do not parallel changes in dependence in external compared with sequestered Ca^{2+} amongst the three vessels.

Conclusion

Not only are there quantitative differences between vessels of different size from the same vascular bed, but new phenomena make their appearance as blood vessels get smaller. Ca^{2+} dependence and the susceptibility to dihydropyridine Ca^{2+} channel blockers of these new emergent features have been studied to a limited extent. Past experience shows the fallacy of trying to extrapolate to other vascular beds from the study of another. Our findings do, however, reveal increasing opportunities for selectivity of drug action on these different processes and provide the tantalizing opportunity for the subtle control of vascular tone with manipulations of the Ca^{2+} ion.

Acknowledgement. Research was supported by a grant from USPHS: HL32985.

References

Angus JA (1982) Sympathetic vasoconstriction – no role for α-adrenoceptors? Trends Pharmacol Sci 3:464–465

Bevan JA (1985) Myogenic or stretch-dependent tone. J Cardiovasc Pharmacol 7:5129–5136

Bevan JA, Bevan RD, Duckles SP (1980) Adrenergic regulation of vascular smooth muscle. In: Bohr DF, Somlyo AP, Sparks HV (eds) Handbook of physiology, sect 2, The cardiovascular system, vol 2, Vascular smooth muscle. American Physiological Society, Baltimore

Bevan JA, Bevan RD, Hwa JJ, Owen MP, Tayo FM, Winquist RJ (1982) Calcium, extrinsic and intrinsic (myogenic) vascular tone. In: Godfraind T, Albertini A, Paoletti R (eds) Calcium modulators. Elsevier, The Netherlands

Bevan JA, Hwa JJ (1984) Myogenic tone and cerebral vascular autoregulation: the role of a stretch-dependent mechanism. Fed Proc 43:449

Bevan JA, Osher JV (1972) A direct method for recording tension changes in the wall of small blood vessels in vitro. Agents and Actions 2:257–260

Bevan RD, Yang J (1982) Distinctive alpha-adrenergic properties of rabbit vascular smooth muscle cells define a central arterial compartment. Fed Proc Abstracts 41:4166

Cauvin C, Saida K, van Breemen C (1984) Extracellular Ca^{2+} dependence and diltiazem inhibition of contraction in rabbit conduit arteries and mesenteric resistance vessels. Blood Vessels 21:23–31

Duckles SP, Bevan JA (1976) Pharmacological characterization of adrenergic receptors of a rabbit cerebral artery in vitro. J Pharmacol Exp Ther 197:371–378

Furchgott RF (1972) The classification of adrenoceptors. In: Blashko H., Muscholl E (eds) Catecholamines. Springer, New York

Harder DR (1984) Pressure-dependent membrane depolarization in cat middle cerebral artery. Circ Res 55:197–202

Hirst GDS, Neild TO (1981) Localization of specialized noradrenaline receptors at neuromuscular junctions on arterioles of the guinea-pig. J Physiol 313:343–350

Hwa JJ, Bevan JA (1985) Stretch-dependent (myogenic) tone in rabbit ear resistance arteries. Am J Physiol (to be published)

Laher I, Bevan JA (1985) Alpha-adrenoceptor number limits response of some rabbit arteries to norepinephrine. J Pharmacol Exp Ther 233:290–297

Loewenstein WR (1971) Mechano-electric transduction in the Pacinian corpuscle: Initiation of sensory impulses in mechanoreceptors. In: Loewenstein WR (ed) Principles of receptor physiology. Springer, Berlin

Lundberg JM, Terenius L, Hokfelt T, Martling CR, Tatemoto K, Mutt V, Polak J, Bloom S, Goldstein M (1982) Neuropeptide Y(NPY)-like immunoreactivity in peripheral noradrenergic neurons and effects of NPY on sympathetic function. Acta Physiol Scand 116:477–480

Mellander S, Johansson B (1968) Control of resistance, exchange, and capacitance functions in the peripheral circulation. Pharmacol Rev 20:117–196

Mulvany MJ, Halpern W (1977) Contractile properties of small arterial resistance vessels in spontaneously hypertensive and normotensive rats. Circ Res 41:19–26

Owen MP, Quinn CL, Bevan JA (1983) Variation in phentolamine-resistant neurogenic vasoconstriction with artery diameter in the rabbit ear. Fed Proc Abstracts 42:620

Owen MP, Walmsley JG, Mason MF, Bevan RD, Bevan JA (1983) Adrenergic control in three artery segments of diminishing diameter in the rabbit ear. Am J Physiol 245:H320–H326

Rowan RA, Bevan JA (1983) Distribution of adrenergic synaptic cleft width in vascular and nonvascular smooth muscle. In: Bevan JA, Maxwell RA, Fujiwara M, Shibata S, Toda N, Mohri K (eds) Vascular neuroeffector mechanisms – IV. Raven Press, New York

Walmsley JG, Owen MP, Bevan JA (1983) Medial morphometry and mechanics of sequential rabbit ear arteries and myograph ring segments. Am J Physiol 245:H840–H848

Yamamoto H, Hwang O, van Breemen C (1984) BAY K8644 differentiates between potential and receptor operated Ca^{2+} channels. Eur J Pharmacol 102:555–557

Discussion

(pp. 362–367)

Schramm: To what an extent does myogenic tone contribute to total peripheral resistance. The reason for my question is the following: you showed that the most effective concentrations of BAY K 8644 and the Ciba-Geigy compound are the same. In all animal experiments, however, BAY K 8644 is 10 to 100 times more potent.

Bevan: I cannot explain the difference; I have only these observations in one blood vessel from one species. Regarding the importance of myogenic tone, I refer to the physiological Review by Johansson and Mallender in the late 1960s: On the basis of human and animal data, they estimated that at rest some 70 to 80% of peripheral resistance are due to myogenic tone.

Fleckenstein: We have studied that basal vascular tone, which is increased by stretch having pharmacologically excluded neurohormonal effects. This myogenic basal tone was highly dependent on calcium. Nifedipine as a representative of the 1,4-dihydropyridines and other Ca^{2+}-antagonists abolished this basal tone. These effects of the Ca^{2+}-antagonists could be overcome by excess Ca.

Bevan: Probably we should not generalise saying that myogenic tone is resistant or sensitive to a particular drug, I am sure that its sensitivity to drug action varies in different blood vessels. There is no evidence, however, for a differential sensitivity between myogenic tone and potassium-induced tone, in the rat portal vein, the rabbit mesenteric vein and portal vein, the rabbit facial vein, cerebral arteries of a number of species and in small arteries in the rabbit ear carried out by a number of investigators.

Fleckenstein: Our results are based on observations on rabbit ear vessels and on brain vessels.

Cauvin: Why is it that you don't want to call the other receptor mechanism activated by norepinephrine a gamma receptor? What is the difference in your interpretation of the phentolamine resistant contraction, as opposed to the interpretation of David Hirst?

Bevan: Calling this site a gamma-receptor implies that it is an adrenergic receptor. The selectivity of the receptor site has not been shown rather the contrary: The norepinephrine molecule can be changed in all sorts of ways and still there is a response via this receptor. It is not stereoselective. There is overwhelming evidence in the literature that one can block sympathetic influences on many blood vessels, with alpha adrenoceptor blocking agents. This is a mass of evidence against the universality of the hypothesis of Hirst and Neild.

Casteels: Can the effect of different concentrations of norepinephrine in the presence of phenoxybenzamine be partly explained by diffusion limitation to the same type of receptor?

Bevan: I do not think so, because in our experiments we wait for an equilibrium: we block alpha adrenceptors, block uptake 1 and uptake 2. Thus we presume that we are dealing with a tissue in which norepinephrine is not metabolised. We can show the same effect with a stable analogue of norepinephrine, too.

Casteels: Is there any analogy in other tissues for this type of "stretch induced Ca^{2+}-channel"? This assumption would actually make that we would have to consider in some vessels 3 types of Ca^{2+}-channels. Am I right in my interpretation?

Bevan: I use another word then channel for the entry pathway. Calcium gets in somehow, and I think the way it gets into the smooth muscle cell is different under the pressure of an agonist or high potassium.

Brown: Actually I think this relates exactly to the preceding question. There was a paper by Guharay, F. and Sachs, F. (1984, stretch-activated single ion channel current in tissue-cultured embryonic chick skeletal muscle. J Physiol Lond 352:685–701) on stretch-induced channels in skeletal muscle. These were relatively non-specific channels and they may be very similar in the smooth muscle: you might get a Ca^{2+} entry through a non-specific channel but that would not be a Ca^{2+}-channel in terms of antagonism by Ca^{2+}-antagonists. I suspect the stretch receptor is in fact an opening of non-specific channels through which Ca^{2+} can enter if present. Concerning the potassium stimulation I want to comment that raising extracellular potassium is not simply a depolarization according to the Nernst equation. The effect of barium on potassium stimulation says to me that there is more happening than that, because barium is a potassium channel blocker. Therefore, your membrane potential may be governed by a good deal more than by potassium, e.g. chloride might play a role.

Bevan: In previous publications we have listed a lot for considering stretch and receptor operated channels and SDC system to be different: e.g. the temperature dependence of the stretch-dependent mechanism is completely different from that for the other two sorts. In the facial vein, one cannot elicit a stretch response until the temperature is about 31° or 32 °C. It looks as if this is a critical temperature phenomenon.

Brown: Couldn't that be just temperature-dependence of the contractile mechanisms?

Bevan: It is not seen with the other agonists: it is something very specific for the stretch induced response.

Bayer-Symposium IX
Cardiovascular Effects of Dihydropyridine-Type
Calcium Antagonists and Agonists, 370–378

Differences Between Dihydropyridine and Non-Dihydropyridine Calcium Antagonists in Inotropic, Chronotropic, Dromotropic and Vascular Effects: Differences in Underlying Mechanism

N. TAIRA

It is generally accepted that nifedipine and nicardipine, dihydropyridine (DHP) calcium antagonists (Ca-antagonists), are less cardiodepressant that verapamil and diltiazem, non-dihydropyridine (non-DHP) Ca-antagonists, in therapeutic doses used in the treatment of angina pectoris and/or hypertension. Such a property of nifedipine is indeed one of its advantages over the two non-DHP Ca-antagonists. However, owing to this property nifedipine tends to produce reflex tachycardia which is thought to be one of its undesirable effects [1]. Among new DHP Ca-antagonists developed recently PY 108-068 [2] and PN 200-110 [3] have been claimed less likely to produce reflex tachycardia. Thus, the question arises whether some of DHP Ca-antagonists produced by some modifications of the chemical structure of nifedipine possess a low separation between the vasodilator and the cardiac effects as do verapamil and diltiazem. The present article first treats this question and afterwards discusses mechanisms underlying a high separation between the vasodilator and the cardiac effects in DHP Ca-antagonists. To settle the first question the article treats seven DHP Ca-antagonists, i.e., nifedipine, nicardipine, nimodipine [4, 5], nisoldipine [6], nitrendipine [7, 8], PY 108-068 [2] and PN 200-110 [3] and three non-DHP Ca-antagonists, i.e., verapamil, diltiazem and KB-944 [9, 10].

Coronary Vasodilator Activities

Nearly all of the Ca-antagonists discussed in the present article were initially developed or are going to be developed as antianginal drugs with coronary vasodilator activity. Thus, it appears reasonable to discuss their coronary vasodilator potencies. In Fig. 1 are shown dose-response curves for peak increase in blood flow through the anterior septal artery (ASA) determined with single bolus injections of Ca-antagonists into the ASA of isolated, blood-perfused papillary muscle preparations of dogs. These preparations were perfused through the ASA with arterial blood from donor dogs at constant pressure of about 100 mm Hg and the papillary muscles were stimulated at a rate of 120 stimuli/min as initially de-

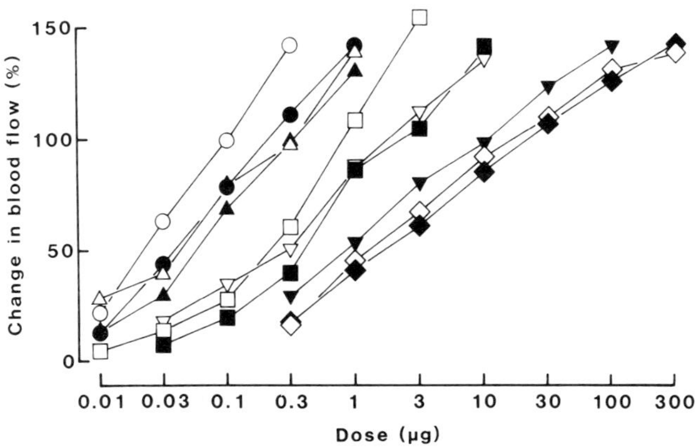

Fig. 1. Dose-response curves for peak increase in blood flow through the anterior septal artery produced by single bolus injections of Ca-antagonists into this artery in isolated, blood-perfused papillary muscle preparations of dogs. Data points are mean values of 5–8 preparations. Standard errors are not shown. Non-DHP Ca-antagonists: verapamil (▼) [12], diltiazem (◇) [12], KB-944 (◆) [13]. DHP Ca-antagonists: nifedipine (●) (Wada and Taira, unpublished), nicardipine (▽) [14], nimodipine (▲) [15], nisoldipine (□) [16], nitrendipine (■) [17], PY 108-068 (○) [18], PN 200-110 (△) [19]. All the curves are reproduced from the referenced articles with permission of the authors and publishers

Table 1. Doses of Ca-antagonists which produced a 100% increase in blood flow through the anterior septal artery (ASAFED 100%) determined in isolated, blood-perfused papillary muscle preparations of dogs

Drug	ASAFED 100% in µg	Reference
PY 108–068	0.10[a] (0.04–0.24)[b]	18
Nifedipine	0.21 (0.13–0.39)	Wada and Taira, unpublished
PN 200–110	0.25 (0.06–0.60)	19
Nimodipine	0.62 ± 0.23[c]	15
Nisoldipine	0.78 (0.49–1.15)	16
Nitrendipine	1.9 ± 0.6	17
Nicardipine	4.3 ± 0.9	14 (partly)
Verapamil	9.4 ± 3.6	12
Diltiazem	20.8 ± 6.2	12
KB–944	43.5 ± 13.5	13

[a] Determined from dose-response curves fitted by linear regressions
[b] Confidence limits for 0.95 probability
[c] Mean ± S. E.

scribed [11]. Under these conditions ASA flow was 5–7 ml/min and the papillary muscle was preloaded so as to develop maximum tension. In these preparations the ASA supplies nearly exclusively working heart muscle, i.e., the papillary muscle and the ventricular septum to which the former is attached, and the ASA bed well maintains vascular tone but is free from the central nervous system and intraventricular pressure. Thus, it appears reasonable for the drug effect on ASA flow to represent that on coronary circulation.

As clearly seen in Fig. 1, all the Ca-antagonists increased ASA flow up to about 150% of the baseline value with increasing doses. The doses which doubled ASA flow (ASAFED 100%) are tabulated in Table 1. Generally speaking the DHP Ca-antagonists were more potent than any of the non-DHP Ca-antagonists on a weight basis. However, such differences in coronary vasodilator potencies among Ca-antagonists are not so important, because similar efficacies are obtainable by dose matching.

Coronary Vasodilator Effect Versus Negative Inotropic, Chronotropic and Dromotropic Effects

All Ca-antagonists are capable of producing negative inotropic, chronotropic and dromotropic effects in addition to vasodilatation. Therefore, the clinically important thing is whether a Ca-antagonist is selective for vasculature compared with cardiac tissues. As briefly discussed in the introduction, a highly vasoselective Ca-antagonist has its own advantage and disadvantage over a non-vasoselective Ca-antagonist. The same would be true for non-vasoselective Ca-antagonists. For example, a non-vasoselective Ca-antagonist capable of producing a negative dromotropic effect in coronary vasodilator doses should be cautiously prescribed to patients with atrioventricular (AV) conduction disturbances. In contrast such a Ca-antagonist can be used in the treatment of paroxysmal supraventricular tachyarrhythmias.

The selectivity of a Ca-antagonist for coronary blood flow versus sinoatrial (SA) nodal automaticity, AV nodal conduction, intraventricular conduction, ventricular automaticity and myocardial contraction was determined by use of isolated, blood-perfused SA node, AV node and papillary muscle preparations of dogs as shown in Table 2. In the paced papillary muscle preparation the dose doubling ASA flow (ASAFED 100%) and the dose reducing developed tension of the papillary muscle by half the baseline value (DTID 50%) were determined. Unless stimulated the papillary muscle beats spontaneously at a rate of about 40 beats/min [20]. This ventricular automaticity is thought to originate in Purkinje fibres within the ventricular septum [20]. In these preparations the dose reducing the rate of ventricular automaticity by 15% of its baseline value (VRID 15%) was tried to be determined.

Isolated, blood-perfused SA node preparations beat spontaneously at a rate of about 100 beats/min [21]. When injected into the right coronary artery most Ca-antagonists reduce sinus rate down to about 70 beats/min but rarely below this value. Atrial standstill ensues from further increasing doses. By use of these preparations the dose reducing sinus rate by 15% of the bascline value (the dose producing a half maximum decrease in sinus rate) (SRID 15%) was determined.

Isolated, blood-perfused AV node preparations consist essentially of the right atrium and the ventricular septum. The preparations were perfused through the right coronary artery, the posterior septal artery (PSA) and the ASA with arterial blood from donor dogs at constant pressure of about 120 mm Hg as described

Table 2. Items investigated, preparations used and variables measured

Item	Preparation	Measured variable
Coronary vasodilatation	Isolated, blood-perfused papillary muscle preparation of the dog (P)	Dose doubling ASA flow (ASAFED 100%)
Suppression of SA nodal automaticity	Isolated, blood-perfused SA node preparation of the dog	Dose reducing sinus rate by 15% of the baseline rate (SRID 15%)
Suppression of AV nodal conduction	Isolated, blood-perfused AV node preparation of the dog (AV)	Dose prolonging AV conduction time by 15% of the baseline value when injected into the PSA [AVCTID 15% (in ASA)]. Dose doubling PSA flow (PSAFED 100%)
Suppression of intraventricular conduction	AV	Dose prolonging AV conduction time by 15% of the baseline value when injected into the ASA [AVCTID 15% (in ASA)]
Suppression of ventricular automaticity	P	Dose reducing rate of automaticity by 15% of the baseline rate (VRID 15%)
Suppression of cardiac muscle contraction	P	Dose reducing developed tension by half the baseline value (DTID 50%)

previously [22]. When the right atrium is paced at a rate of 150 stimuli/min AV conduction time is about 130 msec. The PSA mainly supplies the AV node, whereas the ASA mainly supplies the more distal conduction system, i.e., the His-Purkinje-ventricular system. Therefore, changes in AV conduction time produced by injection of a drug into the PSA reflect those in AV nodal conduction. In contrast, changes in AV conduction time produced by intra-ASA injection of a drug is attributable to those in intraventricular conduction. In these preparations the intra-PSA dose doubling PSA flow (PSAFED 100%) and the intra-PSA dose increasing AV conduction time by 15% of the baseline value [AVCTID 15% (in PSA)] were determined. With a Ca-antagonist injected into the PSA AV conduction time increases continuously up to about 130% of the baseline value but scarcely beyond this value. Further increasing doses results in the second- or third-degree AV block. Therefore, the dose producing a 15% increase in AV conduction time is the one which produces a half maximum increase in AV conduction time. Such doses were determined. Similarly the intra-ASA dose producing a 15% increase in AV conduction time [AVCTID 15% (in ASA)] was tried to be determined.

From these values the selectivity of a Ca-antagonist for coronary blood flow versus cardiac activities was calculated as defined in Fig. 2. Selectivity spectra of the three non-dihydropyridine Ca-antagonists are depicted in Fig. 3. Although there appear to be minor differences in selectivity spectra, in these three drugs the doses doubling coronary blood flow are very close to those producing a 15% re-

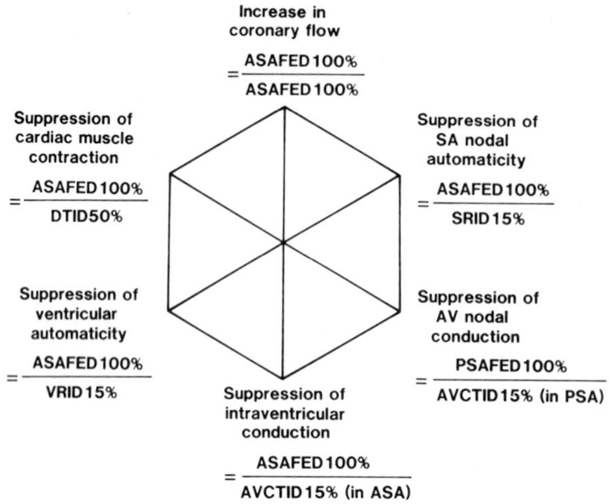

Fig. 2. Definition of the selectivity of a Ca-antagonist for coronary blood flow versus cardiac variables and its plot on a hexagonal plan

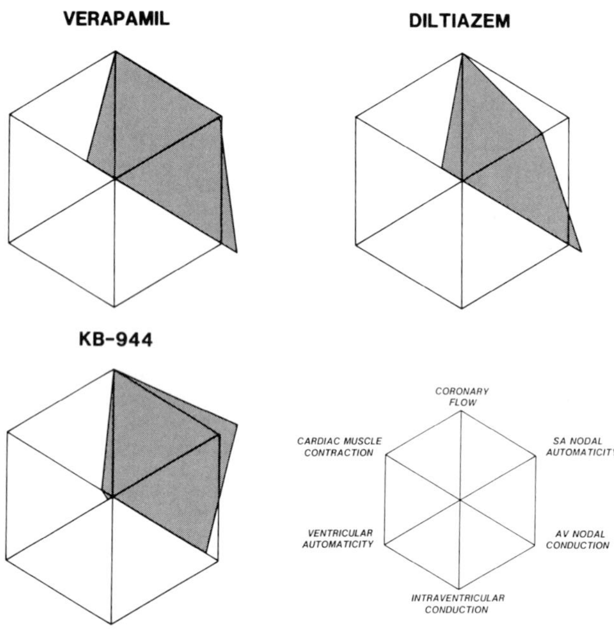

Fig. 3. Selectivity spectra of verapamil, diltiazem and KB-944. Data for verapamil are adopted from the articles [12, 23–25] and those for diltiazem are from the articles [12, 23, 24, 26]. The spectrum of KB-944 is reproduced from the article [13] with permission of the authors and publisher

duction of sinus rate and a 15% prolongation of AV conduction time. Thus, they can be characterized as Ca-antagonists producing a half maximum decrease in sinus rate and a half maximum prolongation of AV conduction time (the first-degree AV block) in doses doubling coronary blood flow. Needless to say, these negative chronotropic and dromotropic effects can be lessened by sympathetic re-

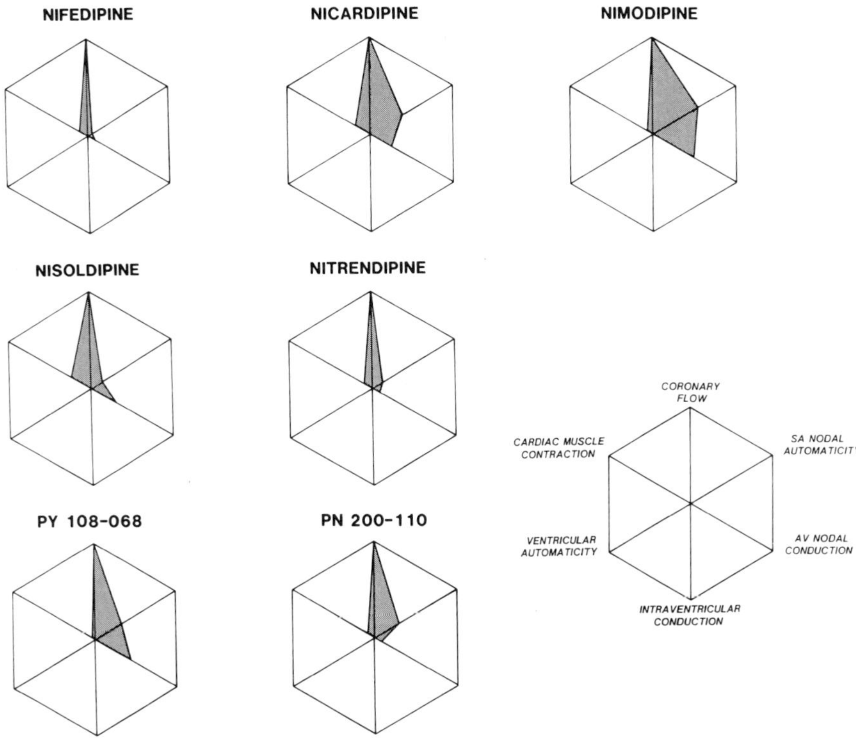

Fig. 4. Selectivity spectra of nifedipine, nicardipine, nimodipine, nisoldipine, nitrendipine, PY 108-068 and PN 200-110. Data for nicardipine are adopted partly from the article [14]. The spectra of nimodipine [15], nisoldipine [16], nitrendipine [17], PY 108–068 [18] and PN 200-110 [19] are reproduced from the referenced articles with permission of the authors and publishers. Data for nifedipine are unpublished (Wada and Taira)

flex triggered by a fall of systemic arterial pressure when these Ca-antagonists are given systemically. Nevertheless, such tendency can be retained, and indeed it is true.

In Fig. 4 are shown selectivity spectra of DHP Ca-antagonists. Although minor, there are differences in selectivity spectra among them. Nifedipine and nitrendipine are the most selective for coronary blood flow compared with any of cardiac variables. For example there are about a 10-fold difference between the dose doubling coronary blood flow and the dose producing a half maximum reduction of sinus rate. The selectivity for coronary blood flow versus cardiac activities diminished in the following order: Nifedipine ≒ nitrendepine > PN 200-110 > PY 108-068 > nisoldipine > nicardipine ≒ nimodipine. Although the selectivity of the latter two Ca-antagonists is lower than that of nifedipine and nitrendipine, it is still higher than that of non-DHP Ca-antagonists. All the ten Ca-antagonists are virtually ineffective on intraventricular conduction suggesting the virtual lack of the effect on the fast sodium channel. All the Ca-antagonists except KB-944 are virtually ineffective on ventricular automaticity originating in Purkinje fibres.

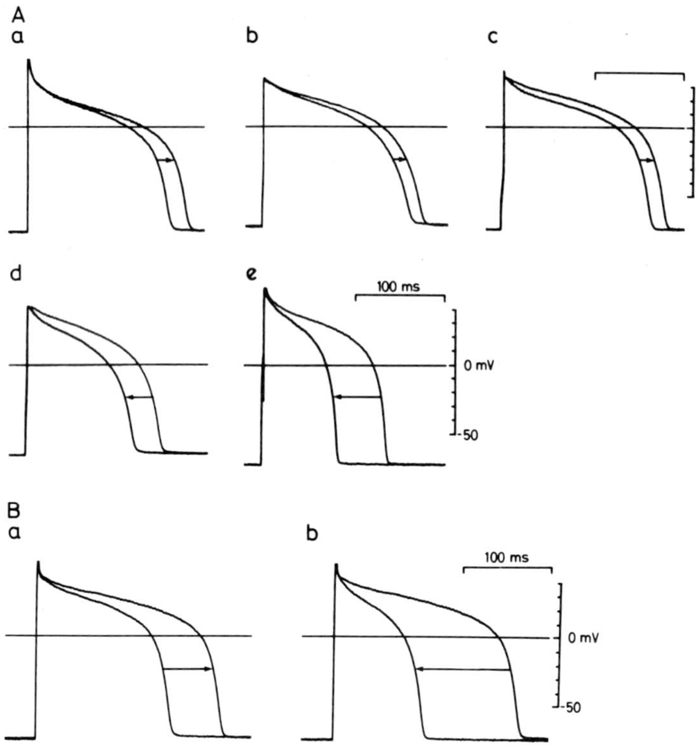

Fig. 5. A Effect of intracellularly applied nifedipine, nicardipine, isobutylmethylxanthine (IBMX), D600 and diltiazem on action potentials recorded from single guinea-pig ventricular cells by the "whole cell recording" technique. In panels a–e an action potential just after rupture of the patch membrane (control) and that 2–3 min after the rupture (the effect of a drug inside the cell attained a maximum) are superimposed. **a** 1 μM nifedipine; **b** 10 μM nicardipine; **c** 30 μM IBMX; **d** 1 μM D600; **e** 100 μM diltiazem. **B** Similar recordings obtained from one and the same single cell with 1 μM nifedipine inside the cell (**a**) and successive superfusion of the cell with 1 μM nifedipine (**b**). Directions of changes in action potential are shown by arrows. Reproduced with permission of the authors and publisher from the article [27]

Differences in Underlying Mechanism

Several pieces of evidence showing that DHP Ca-antagonists and non-DHP Ca-antagonists have different sites of action on putative Ca-channels and different electrophysiological modes of action on the Ca-channels in sarcolemma have been presented. However, none of these appears to give a satisfactory explanation to major differences in cardiovascular profile between DHP Ca-antagonists and non-DHP Ca-antagonists. Recently we found that when applied intracellularly to single guinea-pig ventricular cells by use of patch clamp microelectrodes nifedipine (1 μM) and nicardipine (10 μM) augmented the action potentials, whereas D600 (1 μM) and diltiazem (100 μM) only abbreviated them via the same route of application (Fig. 5) [27]. Needless to say, when these Ca-antagonists were

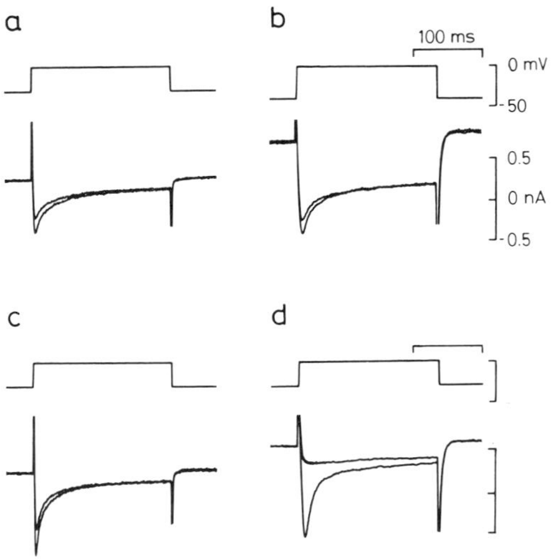

Fig. 6. Effects of intracellularly applied nifedipine, nicardipine and IBMX, and of extracellularly applied nifedipine on the slow inward current of single guinea-pig ventricular cells. Membrane potentials were clamped at −30 (**a, c** and **d**) or −40 (**b**) mV and 200 msec depolarizing clamp pulses to 0 mV were applied. Upper and lower recordings show the clamp potentials and the membrane currents, respectively. In each panel clamp potentials and the membrane currents obtained just after rupture of the patch membrane and those during maximum drug effects are superimposed. In **a** 1 μM nifedipine, in **b** 10 μM nicardipine and in **c** 30 μM IBMX were applied intracellularly, and in **d** 1 μM nifedipine was applied extracellularly. Reproduced with permission of the authors and publisher from the article [27]

applied extracellularly the action potentials were abbreviated. The action potentials augmented by intracellular nifedipine (1 μM) were abbreviated when the cells were superfused with Tyrode solution containing nifedipine (1 μM) (Fig. 5) [27]. In keeping with the results on the action potentials nifedipine (1 μM) and nicardipine (10 μM) when applied intracellularly increased the peak slow inward current scarcely affecting the holding potential (Fig. 6) [27]. In contrast nifedipine (1 μM) applied extracellularly abolished the slow inward current [27].

The effects of intracellularly applied nifedipine and nicardipine were mimicked by isobutylmethylxanthine (IBMX) (30 μM) (Figs. 5 and 6) [27]. IBMX is a potent inhibitor of cyclic AMP phosphodiesterase (hereafter simply called PDE). Nicardipine was first described as a vasodilator with a potent inhibitory action on PDE [28]. Afterwards nicardipine was shown to increase intracellular cyclic AMP in rat uterine smooth muscle in association with relaxation [29]. Recently nifedipine has been also shown to inhibit selectively peak I PDE activity, whereas D600 and diltiazem lack virtually such an activity [30]. Our electrophysiological data taken together with biochemical ones suggest that the increase in the slow inward current produced by the two dihydropyridines applied intracellularly can be ascribed to their inhibition on PDE and the resultant increase in intracellular cyclic AMP. This mechanism would counteract their blocking action on the Ca-channel in cardiac cells and leads to the less cardiopressant action. The Ca entry blockade and PDE inhibition both leads to vasodilatation. Unlike

DHP Ca-antagonists, the non-DHP Ca-antagonists, D600 and diltiazem only inhibited the slow inward current whether they were applied intracellularly and extracellularly. This leads only to cardiodepression. The dual mechanism of action of DHP Ca-antagonists would underlie their less cardiodepressant action compared with their vasodilator action.

References

1. Ebner F (1975) In: Lochner W, Braasch W, Kroneberg G (eds) 2nd International Adalat Symposium. New therapy of ischemic heart disease. Springer, Berlin Heidelberg New York, p 348
2. Hof RP, Hof A, Neumann P (1982) J Cardiovasc Pharmacol 4:352
3. Hof RP, Hof A, Scholtysik G, Menninger K (1984) J Cardiovasc Pharmacol 6:407
4. Kazda S, Hoffmeister F (1979) Naunyn-Schmiedeberg's Arch Pharmacol 307:R43
5. Kazda S, Garthoff B, Krause HP, Schloßmann K (1982) Arzneim-Forsch 32:331
6. Kazda S, Garthoff H, Meyer H, Schloßmann K, Stoepel K, Towart R, Vater W, Wehinger E (1980) Arzneim-Forsch 30:2144
7. Meyer H, Bossert F, Wehinger E, Stoepel K, Vater W (1981) Arzneim-Forsch 31:407
8. Knorr A, Stoepel K (1981) Arzneim-Forsch 31:2062
9. Morita T, Yoshino K, Kanazawa T, Ito K, Nose T (1982) Arzneim-Forsch 32:1037
10. Morita T, Kanazawa T, Ito K, Nose T (1982) Arzneim-Forsch 32:1043
11. Endoh M, Hashimoto K (1970) Am J Physiol 218:1459
12. Himori N, Ono H, Taira N (1976) Jpn J Pharmacol 26:427
13. Taira N, Kawada M, Satoh K (1983) J Cardiovasc Pharmacol 5:349
14. Satoh K, Yanagisawa T, Taira N (1981) Clin Exp Pharmacol Physiol 7:249
15. Satoh K, Kawada M, Wada Y, Taira N (1984) Arzneim-Forsch 34:563
16. Takahashi K, Taira N (to be published) Arzneim-Forsch
17. Satoh K, Wada Y, Taira N (1986) Arzneim-Forsch
18. Wada Y, Satoh K, Taira N (1984) J Cardiovasc Pharmacol 6:881
19. Wada Y, Satoh K, Taira N (1985) J Cardiovasc Pharmacol 7:190
20. Endoh M, Kimura T, Hashimoto H (1974) Jpn J Pharmacol 24:771
21. Kubota K, Hashimoto K (1973) Naunyn-Schmiedeberg's Arch Pharmacol 278:135
22. Hashimoto K, Iijima T, Hashimoto K, Taira N (1972) Tohoku J Exp Med 107:263
23. Ono H, Himori N, Taira N (1977) Tohoku J Exp Med 121:383
24. Narimatsu A, Taira N (1976) Naunyn-Schmiedeberg's Arch Pharmacol 294:169
25. Endoh M, Yanagisawa T, Taira N (1978) Naunyn-Schmiedeberg's Arch Pharmacol 302:235
26. Taira N (1979) In: Bing RJ (ed) New drug therapy with a calcium antagonist. Diltiazem Hakone Symposium 1978. Excerpta Medica, Amsterdam Princeton, p 91
27. Iijima T, Yanagisawa T, Taira N (1984) J Moll Cell Cardiol 16:1173
28. Sakamoto N, Terai M, Takenaka T, Maeno H (1978) Biochem Pharmacol 27:1269
29. Nishikori K, Takenaka T, Maeno H (1981) Jpn J Pharmacol 31:701
30. Norman JA, Ansell J, Phillips MA (1983) Eur J Pharmacol 93:107

Discussion

(pp. 370–378)

Kazda: Years ago in Essen we found in cooperation with Prof. Schümann and Dr. Brodde that nimodipine inhibited the phosphodiesterase from brain homogenates much more than papaverine did whereas nifedipine did not. Afterwards we spent a lot of time and work looking for the possible equivalents in vivo. We treated rats with nimodipine and didn't find any changes in the cyclic AMP, neither in the brain homogenates nor in the heart muscle.

Taira: CIBA-GEIGY people have shown that dihydropyridine Ca^{2+}-antagonists inhibit cyclic AMP phosphodiesterase from bovine hearts with IC 50 values of the order of 10^{-6} M. In the present experiments we haven't measured cyclic AMP. But I suggested one of possibilities.

Hess: As you said most of these substances are very lipophilic. Why then it should make a lot of difference whether you apply them from the inside or from the outside of the cell? In our patch clamp studies we are adding dihydropyridines to the outside of the cell. In order to act on the patch it has to go inside the cell probably through the lipid phase of the membrane. So I do not understand why you don't see a block when you apply it to the inside.

Taira: I believe the dihydropyridine applied within the cell has a greater chance to act from the inside of the membrane than from the outside. We saw a block only with high concentrations of dihydropyridine Ca^{2+}-antagonists applied within the cell.

Fleckenstein: As to the site of action of 1,4-dihydropyridine-Ca^{2+}-antagonists, we found – using the electron microscopic potassium pyroantimonate technique – that the accumulation of calcium on the outer surface of the sarcolemma membrane of heart muscle under the influence of high doses of isoproterenol we could remove this calcium from the surface if we added enough nifedipine. The action of nifedipine in these particular experiments is from outside by displacing Ca^{2+}.

Taira: Of course, I cannot deny such a mechanism of action of dihydropyridines.

Kass: Compounds that are at physiological pH predominantly in a charged form such as verapamil and D 600, require that the Ca^{2+} channel first opens before the drugs can act. Dihydropyridines, such as nisoldipine and nitrendipine, that are predominantly in the neutral form at physiological pH, channel opening is not a prerequisite for drug activity. Nicardipine's pK is on the order of 7 and thus it is partially in the charged form and partially in the neutral form at physiological pH. Its requirements for channel opening lie somewhere intermediate to verapamil and to the other dihydropyridines, suggesting that channels must first open before nicardipine can exert its full effect. It the site of action of this compound were on the outside of the membrane, it doesn't make sense that the channels must first open before the drug can act.

Taira: At a pH of 7.4 66% of the molecules of nicardipine are in the non-ionised form. I believe these non-ionised nicardipine molecules can permeate into the cell and act like nifedipine molecules.

Bayer-Symposium IX
Cardiovascular Effects of Dihydropyridine-Type
Calcium Antagonists and Agonists, 381–407

Effects of Calcium Antagonists on Fixed and Dynamic Obstructions in Patients with Severe Coronary Artery Disease

P. R. LICHTLEN and W. RAFFLENBEUL

Ischemia and angina pectoris due to an increase in vasomotor tone of large epicardial coronary arteries resulting in a critical reduction in lumen size have long been thought to be a distinct clinical entity. As long ago as 1772 Heberden [1], in his first description of angina pectoris, mentioned "spasmodic" alterations as a primary cause of the disease. The possibility of a functional component (spasm) in coronary artery disease leading to angina pectoris („funktionelle Störungen an den Koronararterien in Form von vasomotorischen Krampfzuständen") was again discussed at a special meeting on angina pectoris held in Vienna in 1924 [2]. Furthermore, in 1947, Blumgart [3], in a famous editorial in the American Journal of Medicine on "The Question of Spasm of the Coronary Arteries," analysed clinical events which in his opinion were provoked by spasm and enumerated several factors leading to increased vasomotor tone; he referred to a typical case of angina at rest accompanied by transient ST elevations, which had been published by Wilson and Johnston in 1941 [4]. A similar case was published in 1942 by Duchosal and Henny [5], who reported angina at rest with ST elevation in a patient suffering from hyperthyroidism. The breakthrough in the clinical characterization of "vasospastic angina" and its pathophysiology was brought about by observations of transient ST elevations recorded both in patients with angina at rest and in animals with ischemia, which were published by Prinzmetal et al. in 1959 [6, 7]; the authors concluded that these phenomena were definitely due to a "hypertonus of an atherosclerotic artery." Nevertheless, for approximately another 15 years the notion of "coronary spasm" as a distinct cause of angina pectoris at rest, and in specific cases also during exercise, was not widely accepted among cardiologists, although there were a few anecdotal reports supporting the idea [8, 9, 24]. Acceptance had to wait until Maseri et al. [10–12], through systematic analysis of such patients, were able to present precise data on the incidence and clinical appearance of variant (spastic) angina as well as on its pathophysiology. This knowledge was finally extended by the concept of dynamic and fixed obstructions, with evidence based both on animal studies [13] and on observations recorded in patients [14]. These clinical terms were finally supported by the anatomic characterization of coronary artery stenoses of large epicardial arteries with and without persisting normal smooth muscle tissue [15–17] depending on the degree of involvement of the atherosclerotic process.

Pathophysiology of Increased Vasomotor Tone – "Fixed" Versus "Dynamic" Obstructions

Dynamics obstructions [13, 14] are considered to be present when the degree of luminal narrowing varies with changes in smooth muscle tone of the residual normal wall segment caused either by contraction leading to a further reduction in lumen size or by relaxation resulting in widening of the obstructed section.

Fixed obstructions are defined as narrowings where no spontaneous changes in lumen size and tone induced by pharmacological agents are observed. This is usually due to complete destruction of the normal smooth muscle cells, i.e., circumferential atherosclerotic involvement of the coronary artery, or occurs when smooth muscle cells are still present, but their contraction is inhibited in the presence of extensive atherosclerosis, the artery forming a rigid tube at this point (Fig. 1). Postmortem studies, including coronary angiography and extensive histological analysis, performed by us on 384 stenotic coronary segments of extramural epicardial arteries revealed a high incidence of obstructions within the residual normal wall segment [17] (Fig. 1). Of the obstructions analysed in each heart 35% proved to have a residual normal wall segment comprising at least 25% of the entire circumference of the arterial wall, and 75% of all obstructions had a normal area comprising at least 10% of the circumference (Fig. 2). Furthermore, the incidence of a normal wall segment within a high-grade obstruction was highest in the proximal left anterior descending branch (41%) and lowest in the left main coronary artery (8%). Similar findings were reported by Vlodaver and Edwards [15] and Hort et al. [16]. In view of these anatomic findings it seemed preferable to characterize these obstructions as eccentric and concentric, as their morphology does not allow any assessment of their functionality. It should, however, be mentioned at this point that pharmacological interventions allow a clear separation of eccentric from dynamic stenoses.

The distinction between eccentric and concentric stenoses can also be made during life by means of coronary angiography. There are marked angiographic differences which can be assessed very easily by morphometric analysis of these obstructions viewed from different angles at least 90° apart (see below). Furthermore, as mentioned above and discussed below, concentric obstructions usually do not respond to pharmacological agents that relax smooth muscle tone, in contrast to eccentric ones.

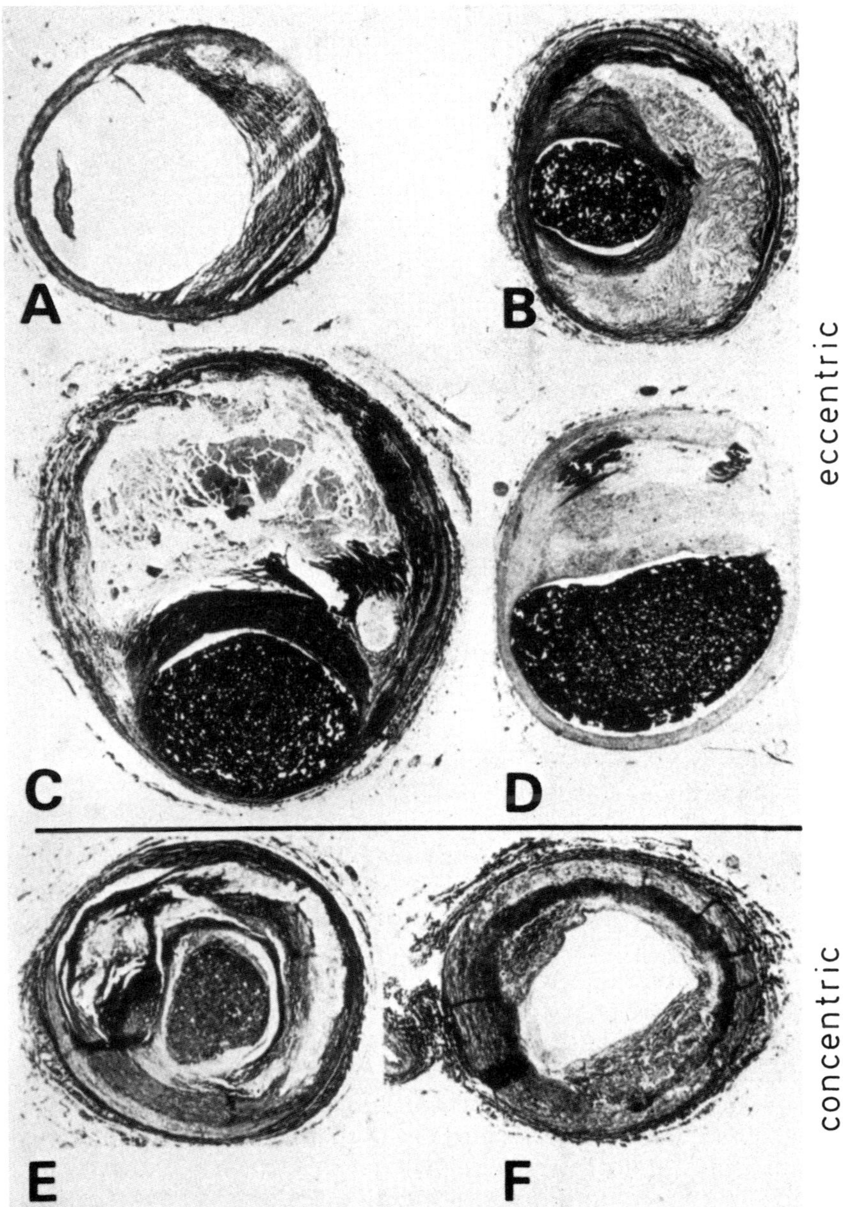

Fig. 1. Histological cross sections of eccentric and concentric stenoses. Eccentric stenoses (A, B, C, D) still have normal wall segments of various lengths, the residual lumen (in some of them filled with contrast material after postmortem coronary angiography) varying in diameter. Note that the atherosclerotic plaque is half-moon shaped, which suggests a circular lumen. In concentric stenoses (E, F) the entire arterial wall is involved in the atherosclerotic process, so that there are no wall segments with normal smooth muscle [17]

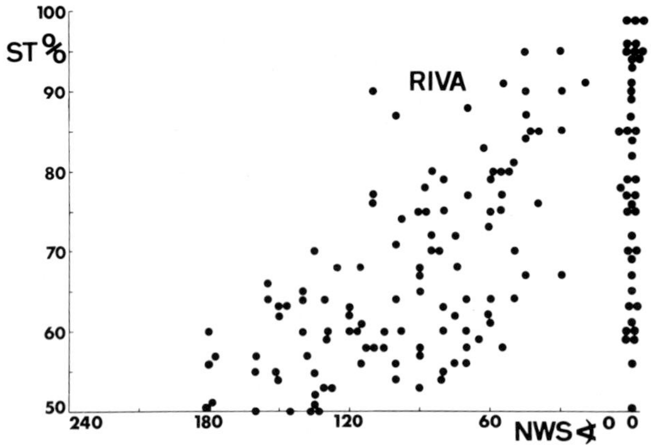

Fig. 2. Relation between the extent of stenosis (ST%) (*ordinate*) determined from the histological cross section and the extent of normal wall segment (*NWS*) (*abscissa*) observed in 156 LAD obstructions; the angle (*abscissa*) relates to the total arterial circumference, i.e., the entire cross section. The concentric obstructions (angle = 0) are entered on the *right*. The correlation between extent of the NWS and ST% is a loose one; however, it should be noted that even in 80% stenoses the NWS is still in the range of 60% ($^1/_6$th of the circumference = 17%), leaving enough normal smooth muscle to contract and cause a further increase in the degree of obstruction. From [17]

Clinical Aspects

The clinical implications of these observations become evident when the relation between coronary flow and the degree of obstruction, i.e., the most stenotic diameter in high-grade obstructions, is analysed more closely. Animal studies [18] and careful investigations in human subjects [19–21] have revealed that in high-grade obstructions (degree of stenosis more than 80%, luminal diameter at point of worst stenosis smaller than 1.0 mm) this relation is not a linear but an exponential one, the decrease in flow exceeding the corresponding decrease in lumen size. It follows that in this range of obstruction even minimal changes in the stenotic diameter lead to relatively large changes in flow (Fig. 3); hence, drugs relaxing smooth muscle tone can be quite effective in these circumstances.

In view of the above-mentioned recent anatomic findings regarding the presence of eccentric and concentric obstructions, it seemed to be of the utmost importance to demonstrate their clinical relevance. The analysis immediately showed that the evidence for the presence of so-called dynamic obstructions is mainly indirect (Tables 1–3). Nevertheless, there are distinct clinical equivalents indicating that changes in vasomotor tone can, indeed, lead to ischemia. Several features are suggestive for *angina at rest:*

1. Myocardial oxygen consumption is usually not increased and coronary sinus oxygen saturation starts to decrease before ST segment changes (ST elevation in transmural and ST depression in endocardial ischemia) occur [22]; this is an indirect sign of a primary decrease in flow leading to ischemia. Hence, ischemic ECG signs and abnormal hemodynamics typical for ischemia (abnormal increase

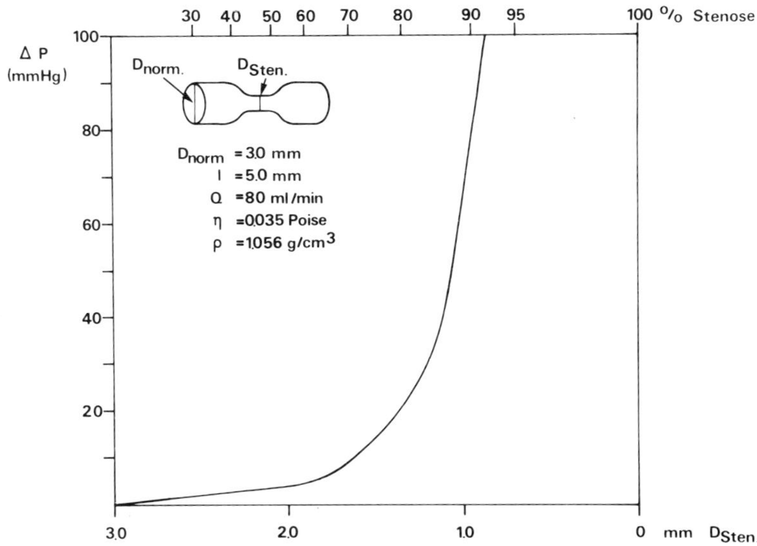

$$\Delta P = \Delta P_S + \Delta P_C + \Delta P_E$$

$$\Delta P = \frac{8\eta l}{\left[\frac{D_{norm}}{2}\right]^4} Q \left(\frac{A_1}{A_2}\right)^2 + \frac{4.8\eta}{\left[\frac{D_{norm}}{2}\right]^3} Q \left(\frac{A_1}{A_2}\right)^{3/2} + \frac{\rho}{\left[\frac{D_{norm}}{2}\right]^2} Q \left(\frac{A_1}{A_2}\right)^2$$

Fig. 3. Relation between pressure drop ($\triangle P$, *ordinate*) and degree of obstruction (% stenosis), i.e., the most stenotic diameter (D_{Sten}) (*abscissa*) in severe obstructions. Calculations are based on animal experiments and an experience in humans, assuming a constant flow of 80 ml/min; the assumptions are indicated at upper left: D_{norm}, prestenotic diameter; l, length of stenosis; Q, coronary flow; v, blood viscosity; p density. The *formula* for $\triangle$P is given below the graph: $\triangle P_s$, total pressure drop across the stenotic segment: $\triangle P_c$, pressure drop at entrance to (contraction of blood), $\triangle P_e$ pressure drop at exit from the obstruction (expansion); the calculation is indicated below (A = prestenotic and stenotic area). Note that the total pressure drop does not follow a linear but an exponential relation [14]

in left ventricular end-diastolic pressure, decrease in positive dp/dt_{max}) without a rise in CK values, i.e., without signs of myocardial necrosis, follow the decrease in flow, i.e., oxygen delivery. It should be stressed that in this situation ST segment changes are often present without angina, especially if the ischemic episode is short, usually of less than 3 min duration [23].

2. There is *angiographic proof* of increased vasomotor tone and spasm during spontaneous attacks of angina, especially in patients with an increased incidence of anginal attacks at rest [8, 24, 25], i.e., unstable angina pectoris; in addition, in these patients a high incidence of eccentric obstructions or even normal coronary arteries is found [26].

3. Thallium scintigrams, performed at rest during attacks of variant angina have revealed a transient reversible perfusion defect in the corresponding myocardial area, also indicating the presence of ischemia [27].

4. Finally, a high incidence of positive *ergonovine tests* (up to 20%) was found in patients with spontaneous attacks of angina at rest [28]. The excellent response

Table 1. Evidence for increased coronary vasomotor tone (spasm) as a cause of angina at rest (variant angina)

During angina, MVO_2 is not increased, coronary sinus O_2 decreases before ECG changes occur, ischemic ECG changes (ST elevation or ST depression) and abnormal hemodynamics as in ischemia are always present; however, no increase in CK values
Angiographic proof during spontaneous attacks of angina; coronary angiogram with a high incidence of eccentric obstructions or normal aspects (Prinzmetal)
^{201}Tl-scintigraphy at rest during attacks with areas of decreased activity, typical for ischemia
High incidence of positive ergonovine tests (ECG, angiograms) (15%–20%)
Excellent response to drugs leading to relaxation of coronary vasomotor tone (Ca antagonists, nitrates)

Table 2. Evidence for increased coronary vasomotor tone (spasm) as a cause of angina at effort

Variable exercise tolerance (time to ST depression, total exercise time, amount of exercise)
"Walk-through" phenomenon unexplained by collaterals
Events of transient ST elevation during exercise in patients with eccentric obstructions
Increased vasomotor tone (spasm) at angiography during various types of exercise (handgrip, bicycle)
Good response to Ca antagonists, sometimes poor response to beta blockers (deterioration)
Positive ergonovine test in approx. 5% of these patients
Angina at effort and at rest

Table 3. Evidence for increased coronary vasomotor tone (spasm) as a cause of acute myocardial infarction

Altered sensitivity for increased vasomotor tone in acute and subacute myocardial infarction, high incidence of positive ergonovine tests (20%) in weeks immediately after MI
Ergonovine-induced spasm can lead to MI
Angiography revealing complete occlusion leading to MI, released by NTG, in the presence of high-grade obstructions, but no platelet thrombus (Oliva)
Development of MI in coronary regions where previously spasm was observed (Marzilli, Maseri)
Residual high-grade obstructions after thrombolysis can dilate further under influence of NTG and Ca antagonists

to treatment with drugs leading to relaxation of coronary vasomotor tone (nitrates, calcium antagonists) in these patients represents additional indirect proof [29, 30].

In *stress-induced* angina it is more difficult to find evidence for dynamic obstructions as a primary cause of ischemia; nevertheless, various observations suggest their involvement:

1. It is well-known that in many patients with effort angina the *daily exercise tolerance* varies considerably; this applies both to the duration of the test and to the degree of ST depression and is often not explained by a so-called walk-through phenomenon based on opening of collaterals; it must rather be attributed to dynamic obstructions, especially when not only ST depressions but also *transient ST elevations* are observed during exercise (Fig. 4). This is further substantiated by the observation of increased vasomotor tone recorded by angiography performed during various types of exercise, e.g., bicycle ergometry [31–35] and handgrip [36, 37]. Yasue [35] was able to demonstrate that the induction of ischemia by spasm during exercise could be prevented by the administration of calcium antagonists, whereas administration of beta blockers to the same patients exacerbated their ischemia.

2. In patients with variant angina and positive exercise tests the number of positive ergonovine tests was found to be higher than in the population with stable angina pectoris [28].

3. Many of these patients exhibit angina both at effort and at rest [24] and belong to the large group of patients with both fixed and dynamic obstructions.

Finally, spasm was also suggested as a primary cause of *acute myocardial infarction*. The evidence, however, is still controversial although it is suggested by several observations:

1. The majority of acute myocardial infarctions occurs at rest, often at night, at a time of "low coronary blood flow"; it is therefore not surprising that an increase in myocardial oxygen consumption and an insufficient response in flow – as in exercise-induced angina – is usually not the precipitating factor. In contrast, as a rule, myocardial infarction is due to a primary decrease in flow, usually in the presence of high-grade obstructions with rupture of the plaque followed by thrombus formation and total occlusion of a vessel.

2. In contrast, patients with variant angina can develop myocardial infarction even when their coronary angiograms are normal, and in these cases spasm cannot be ruled out as a primary cause [10, 24, 38].

3. Myocardial infarction sometimes occurs in the same perfusion area, i.e., in the coronary region where spasm has been seen in previous angiograms [39].

4. Coronary angiograms performed very soon (less than 1 h) after the onset of myocardial infarction sometimes reveal that the affected coronary artery is patent even though a high degree of obstruction is present [40, 41].

5. A high proportion of positive ergonovine tests (approximately 20%) was found in the first 6 weeks after myocardial infarction [28].

Nevertheless, all these observations appear to constitute rather weak suggestive evidence, and the whole problem of spasm in myocardial infarction needs further investigation.

a

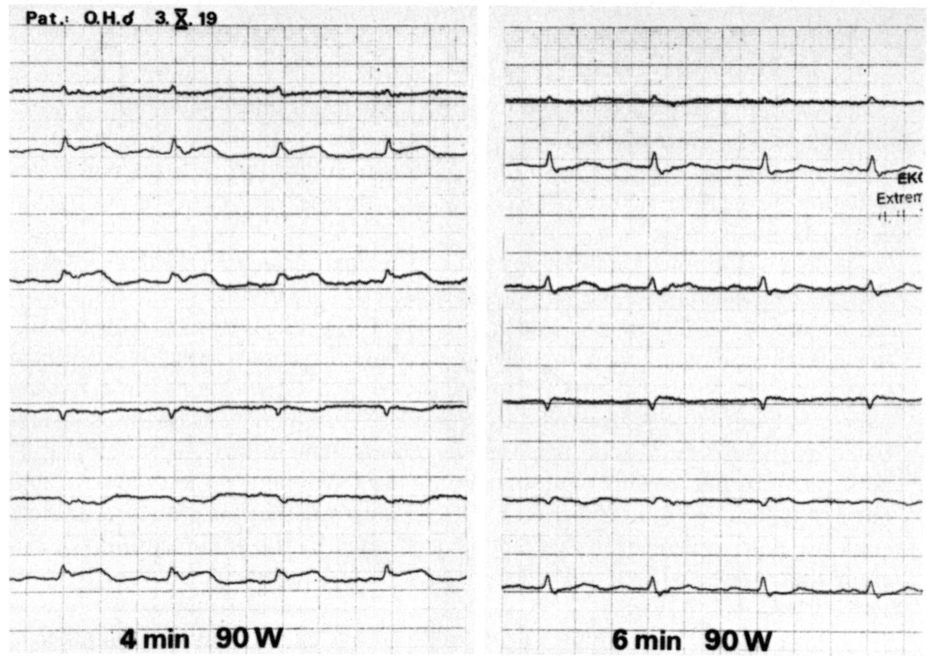

b

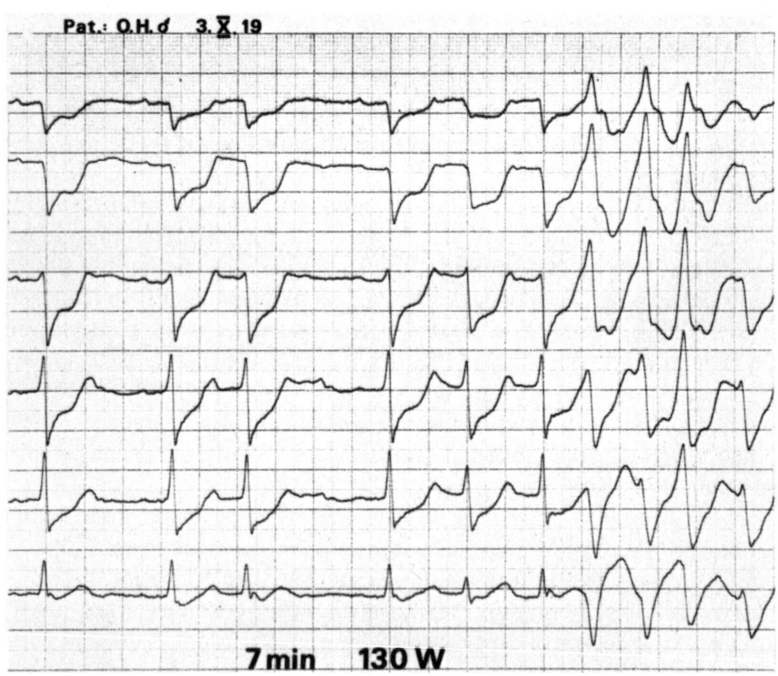

Fig. 4 a–d. Spasm of the right coronary artery during exercise in a patient with typical unstable angina pectoris, i.e., anginal pain both at rest and during exercise. **a** ECG during exercise at 4 min, last min at 90 W (bicycle ergometry), showing typical ST elevations in leads II, III, and aVF (*top* to *bottom*: leads I, II, III, aVR, aVL, and aVF); at 6 min, last 3 min at 90 W, ST segments have normalized. **b** At 7 min, last min at 130 W, severe anginal pain, ST depression in leads V_1–V_6, and ST elevations in leads II, III, and aVF (not shown), followed by a short run

c
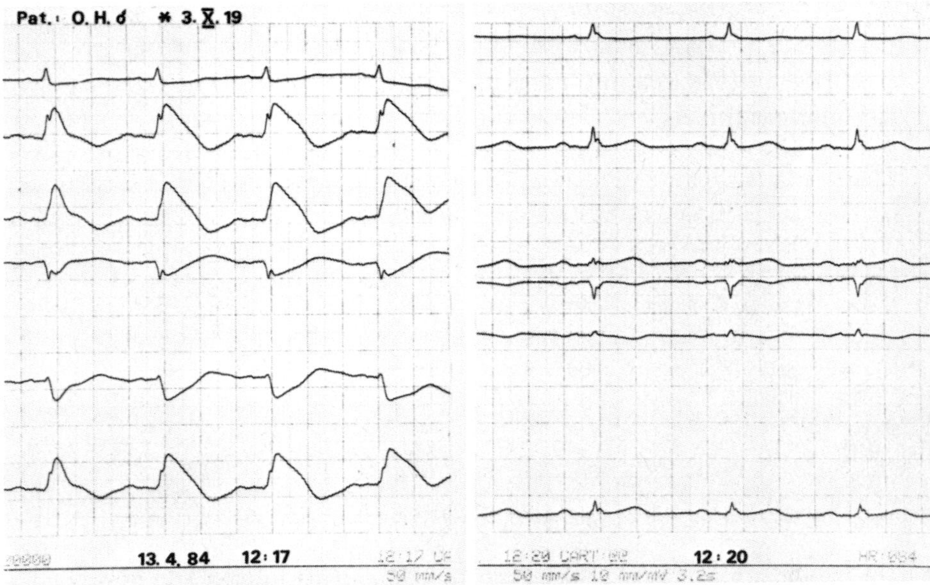

d
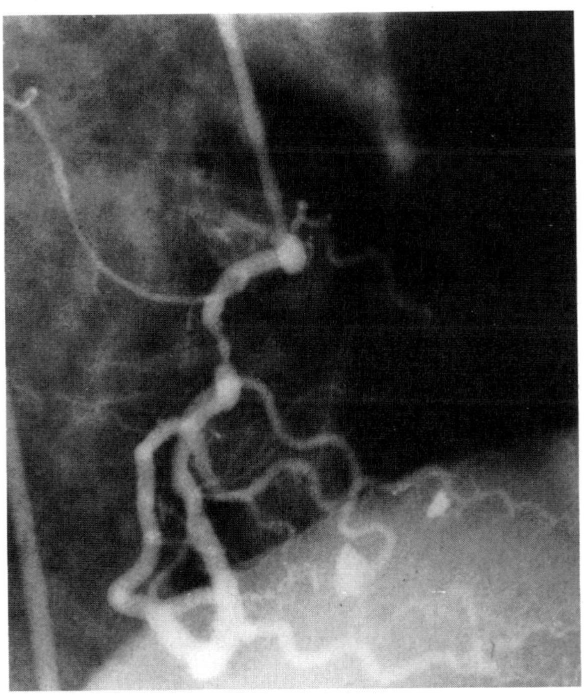

of ventricular tachycardia. **c** ECG 1 h after the exercise test during an attack of angina at rest, accompanied by ST elevations in leads II, III, and aVF lasting for about 3 min, successfully stopped by sublingual nifedipine (20 mg). **d** The coronary angiogram performed 3 days later showed eccentric obstructions in both the proximal RCA and the LAD (not shown). The patient underwent successful bypass grafting to the RCA and LAD and has since remained free of pain

Evaluation of Vasomotor Tone in Coronary Arteries in Human Subjects

Changes in vasomotor tone (VMT) leading to a substantial though transitory constriction or relaxation of large epicardial arteries, both in normal segments and in obstructions, can readily be observed in man during coronary angiography. In contrast, at the arteriolar level, changes in vasomotor tone can only be assessed indirectly by measuring coronary blood flow and resistance, as the resolution of the present angiographic equipment is not sufficiently sensitive to visualize vessels of this size (500 μm and less).

Morphometric Analysis of Coronary Arteries by Angiography

The first quantifications of the lumen size od coronary arteries and obstructions observed at angiography were performed in our laboratory in the early 1970s (Rafflenbeul 1975, 1976, 1981) [42–44]. These measurements were done with the aid of a vernier caliper with an accuracy of 0.05 mm, projecting the angiogram on a Tage-Arno projector. Calibration was performed by measuring the tip of the catheter (Sones or Judkins catheter, the tip of both catheters being approximately 1.8 mm across). Later, a tabletop computer was added for automatic calculation of the most stenotic diameter and the degree of stenosis (percent diameter stenosis, area stenosis). Today, in addition, a fully automatic computerized system (CAAS system, Rotterdam) is in use, since extensive tests demonstrated a high correlation between computerized measurements and those performed by the vernier caliper system [44]. The accuracy of these systems was further checked by analysing both the intraobserver and the computer variability; variabilities ranged around 10% for the caliper measurements and around 2% for computer assessments. Hence, changes in coronary diameters below 10% are not regarded as biologically valid in our laboratory, even if they are statistically significant. Finally, extensive comparisons were made between the angiographic aspects of coronary obstructions during life and at autopsy in approximately 60 patients for further assessment of the accuracy of quantification [45].

Measurements of the diameters of obstructions are always performed in at least four projections, two of them being at least 90° apart. The smallest stenotic area is assessed by averaging the measurements in the four projections; if the term "diameter-stenosis" is applied to characterize the obstruction, the most stenotic diameter is selected from the various projections: for instance, in 80% to 90% obstruction the most stenotic diameter of the proximal left anterior descending branch is usually less than 1.0 mm.

The stenotic diameters in various planes are also applied to characterize *eccentric and concentric obstructions.*

A typical example for an eccentric obstruction in the proximal left anterior descending branch is shown in Fig. 5. In one plane, the most stenotic diameter averaged 1.31 mm (average of 5 measurements), while in another plane at an

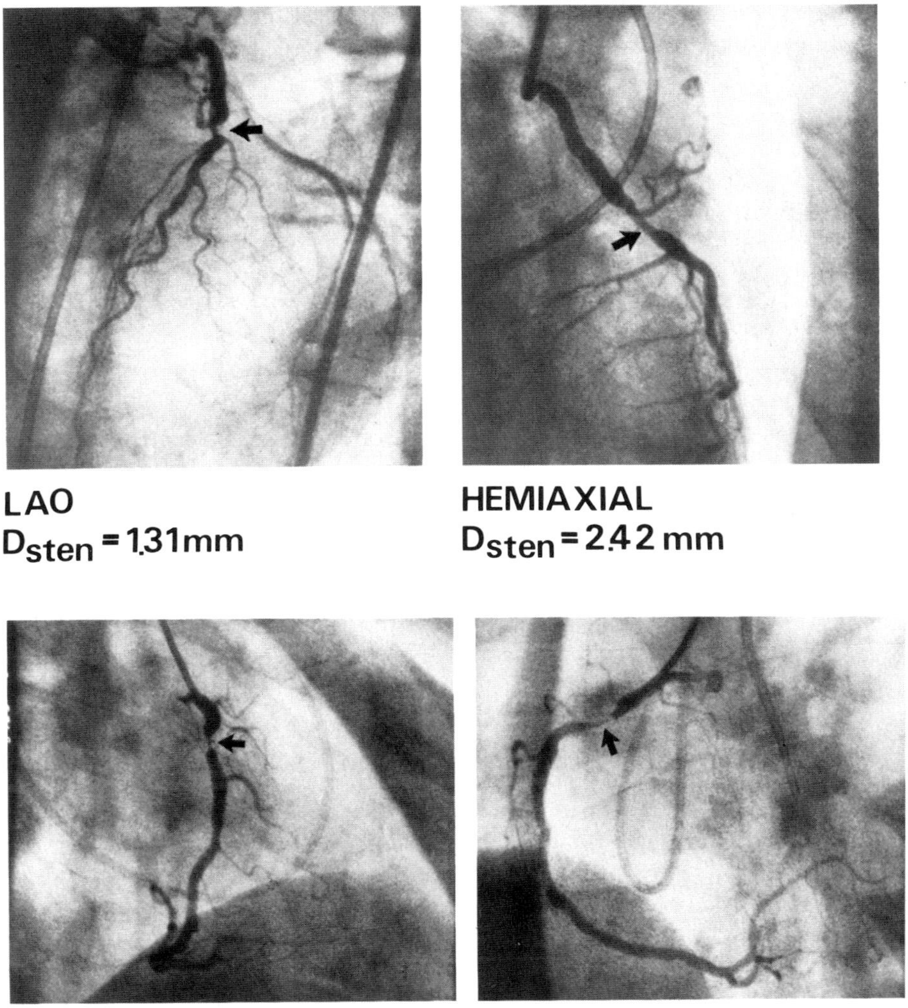

Fig. 5. Eccentric (**a**) and concentric (**b**) obstructions found at angiography. Angiograms were taken in two projections at least 90° apart. Measurements of the luminal diameter at the point of the most stenotic diameter were done with the aid of a vernier caliper (accuracy 0.05 mm); for calibration the tip of the catheter was measured (approximately 1.8 mm in diameter). (For details see text)

angle of approximately 90° to the first, it averaged 2.42 mm, the difference in length between the two diameters amounting to 84.7%. Based on pharmacological studies (see below), a 25% difference in length between two diameters of a stenosis measured in projections at least 90° apart was accepted as the lower limit for the characterization of eccentric obstructions. Hence, the obstruction of the proximal right coronary artery demonstrated in Fig. 5 is by definition a concentric one, the diameter in the two planes being almost identical with averages of 1.68 and 1.64 mm (difference 2.4%).

Pharmacological Effects on Epicardial Arteries, Especially on Obstructions

Several drugs decrease vasomotor tone in large epicardial arteries.

Nitroglycerin, Nitrates

The coronary dilatory effect of sublingual nitroglycerin and isosorbide dinitrate is well-known. Several morphometric studies have been published on this subject during the last decade [20, 36, 46–49, 52, 53]. Large epicardial coronary arteries and smaller side branches with an angiographically normal aspect show a dilatation by more than 20% of the most stenotic diameter and of the normal lumen, both in the area of the LAD and LCX and of the RCA 5–10 min after sublingual administration of 5 mg ISDN (isosorbide dinitrate) or 0.8 mg nitroglycerin. With regard to the dilatation of obstructions, two types of reaction were observed (Fig. 6): Some obstructions showed only biologically insignificant changes or none at all of the most stenotic diameter (an increase of less than 10%), while in others the dilatation at this point reached an average of 28% and in some instances up to 40%; by this they reached a diameter of 2 mm and more and a luminal size outside the clinically critical range.

As mentioned above, the vasomotor tone of the *arteriolar system* has to be assessed indirectly, i.e., by recording regional myocardial blood flow, both in the normal and poststenotic region. This can be achieved by applying precordial

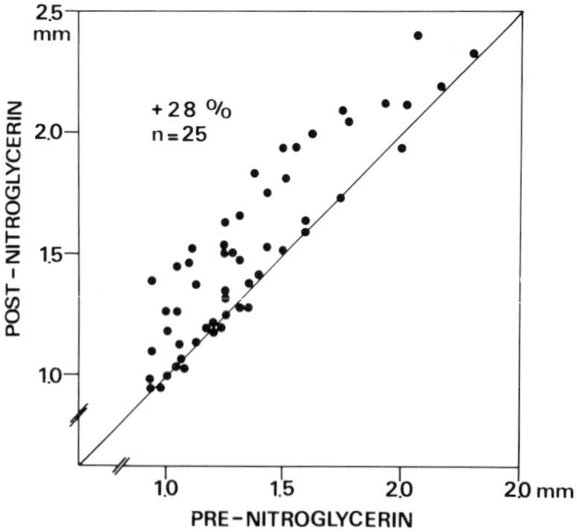

Fig. 6. Dilatation of 54 severe obstructions after administration of 0.8 mg nitroglycerin sublingually. Most stenotic diameter before administration of nitroglycerin (*abscissa*) and 10 min after drug intake (*ordinate*). (For details see text)

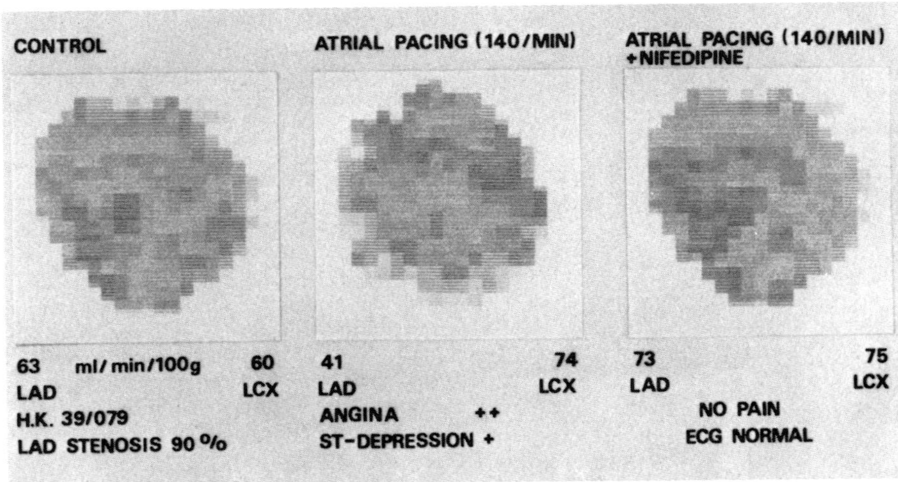

Fig. 7. Typcial example of the changes in regional myocardial blood flow in the normal and the poststenotic area (90% stenosis of the proximal LAD). Panels indicate flow images taken in an LAO projection of 60°, the *left* part of each panel corresponding to the area perfused by the LAD and the *right* part, to the area of the LCX. The panels demonstrate matrix points of the gamma camera (approx. 400 for the entire heart); matrix points in red correspond to the highest flow values, flow decreasing in 6% steps from red to orange, green, and blue. At rest (*left hand panel*) flow was with 63 and 60 ml/min per 100 g tissue about equal in the poststenotic and normal area. During control pacing with 140 beats/min up to severe angina and ST depressions >0.2 mV (*middle panel*) flow decreased in the poststenotic region to 41 ml/min per 100 g tissue and increased in the normal area to 74 ml/min per 100 g tissue. This indicates that during ischemia flow in the endocardial region was very low or even stopped, resulting in a marked drop in transmural flow. 15 min after 20 mg nifedipine sublingually pacing was repeated for the same duration and at identical heart rates (*right hand panel*); flow increased in the poststenotic area to 73 ml/min per 100 g tissue, i.e, to the level achieved in the normal area even before nifedipine; the patient was free of pain and the ECG normalized. (For details see text)

Xenon-clearance technique, the only one allowing a clear separation of transmural flow in the myocardial areas perfused by the LAD, the LCX, and the distal RCA (for details see: Lichtlen [21, 54]). Xenon-133 10–20 mCi is injected into the left main coronary artery, and the speed of washout of Xenon-133, i.e., the decrease in the precordial radioactivity, which correlates closely to coronary flow, is recorded by a Pho gamma 3 camera connected to a computer system (CDC 1100, 16 k). Flow is expressed both in millimeters per minute per 100 g myocardium and in an analogous way as a so-called flow image (a typical example is shown in Fig. 7). Studies were performed at rest and after atrial pacing up to the development of angina and/or ischemia, i.e., ST segment depression of at least 0.1 mV in leads V5 and V6 before and after administration of antianginal drugs, the heart rate being the same in the second period of pacing, which was also of identical duration.

Under *nitroglycerin* both at rest and during atrial pacing up to a heart rate of 147 beats/min (Fig. 8), flow decreased significantly both in the normal and poststenotic areas, which in these studies generally means the region perfused by the left anterior descending branch [55, 56]; this small decrease in flow after a nitrate

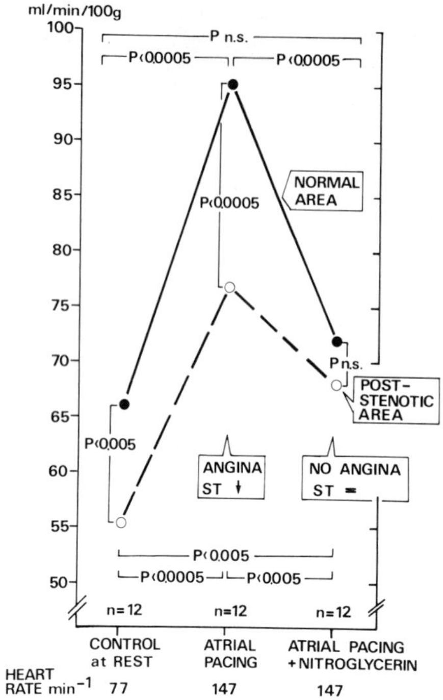

Fig. 8. Behavior of transmural regional myocardial blood flow at rest (*left*) and during control atrial pacing (*middle*), and pacing after 0.8 mg nitroglycerin sublingually (*right*) in 12 patients with isolated severe (>75%) obstructions of the LAD or LCX. *Solid points* and *lines*, flow in the normal area (mainly the LCX); *open circles* and *broken lines*, flow in the poststenotic region, mainly of the LAD. Even at rest, average flow was lower in the poststenotic than in the normal area and remained lower during pacing-induced ischemia. After nitroglycerin, flow during pacing of identical duration and with the same heart rate decreased mainly in the normal area following the decrease in myocardial oxygen consumption, i.e., in the rate-pressure product, from 180 to 151 $mmHg \times min^{-1} \times 10^2$ so that flow became homogeneous throughout the heart, although at a lower level than was recorded before nitroglycerin; this led to an equalization of oxygen demand and delivery in the poststenotic and normal areas

occurred despite improvement or even complete abolition of angina and ischemia; it must therefore be interpreted as an autoregulatory decline in flow following the decrease in oxygen consumption. Hence, under the effect of nitroglycerin a different behavior is observed at the arteriolar level from that in epicardial arteries with regard to vascular smooth muscle tone; in the latter nitroglycerin leads to relaxation of vascular smooth muscle tone, whereas in the arterioles smooth muscle tone remains unaffected, at least in the doses administered sublingually and leading to a significant reduction in venous return; this is further supported by the lack of changes in total coronary resistance, especially in patients with fixed obstructions. Only when nitroglycerin is administered directly into a coronary artery does flow increase by approximately 50%, as was demonstrated both by videodensitometry [57] and by the precordial Xenon washout technique for recording coronary flow [58, 59]; this is of short duration, however (approximately 5 min), and is obviously the result of a transient but complete saturation of all receptors, at the levels of both large epicardial arteries and arterioles. With sublingual or IV administration of nitroglycerin, however, such a pronounced arteriolar dilatation was never observed.

Calcium Antagonists

Sublingual administration of 20 mg nifedipine leads to a strong dilatation both of normal segments of epicardial arteries and of eccentric coronary obstructions (Figs. 9 and 10). In 42 obstructions, most of them in the proximal left anterior

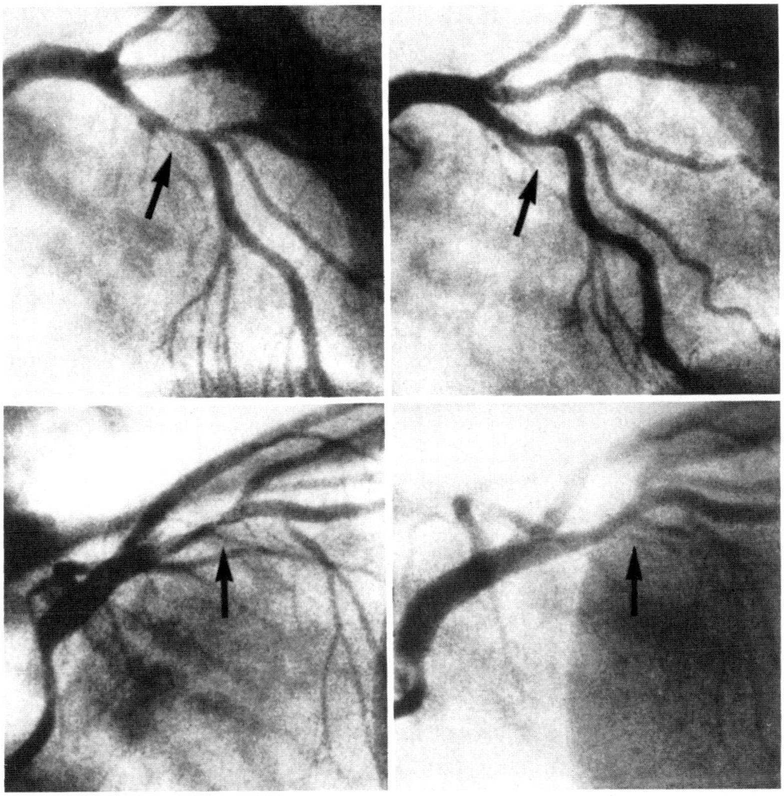

Fig. 9. Angiogram of the LCA in a left and right half-axial projection before (*left*) and 15 min after (*right*) 20 mg nifedipine sublingually. Note that the concentric "obstruction" of the proximal LAD (*arrow*), probably representing mild spasm, was completely relieved by nifedipine. The average increase in diameter of the normal sections amounted to 36%. Cine films were taken in absolutely identical projections and at the same magnification

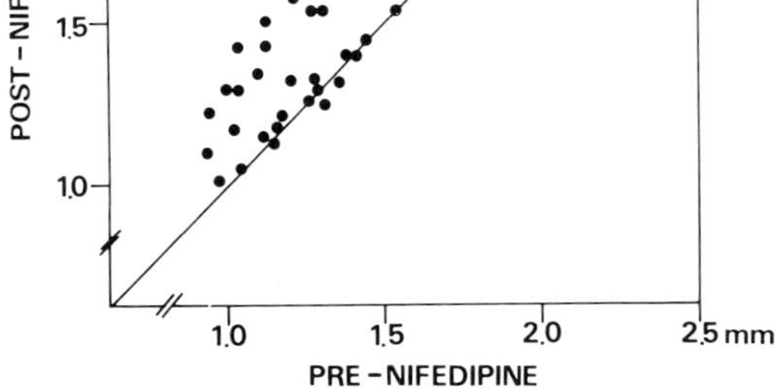

Fig. 10. Effect of 20 mg nifedipine sublingually. Luminal diameter at the point of most severe stenosis in 42 high-grade obstructions (>75%), mainly of the proximal LAD, before (*abscissa*) and 10 min after (*ordinate*) administration of the drug. Note that only half the cases had an increase in lumen size. (For details see text)

descending branch, an average dilatation of 31% was observed in 28 stenoses dilated by more than 10% [20, 29]. However, under the influence of nifedipine, too, some obstructions were dilated by 40% or more, achieving an increase of the most stenotic diameter up to 2 mm or more, which is well outside the clinically critical range. The question arises as to whether higher doses would have led to an even more pronounced dilatation. Observations recorded during repeated administration of sublingual capsules of nifedipine during angioplasty suggested to us, however, that this is very unlikely; repeated administration of nifedipine within less than 30 min was not followed by further dilatation. This was also substantiated by the observations of other groups combining sublingual and intracoronary administration of nifedipine [50, 51, 60]. We have also observed similar degrees of dilatation of epicardial arteries with other calcium antagonists, especially after 10 mg diltiazem IV, when the most stenotic diameter increased by 17% in 8 cases [61, 62]. In contrast to these observations, Feldman et al. [53] reported an insignificant increase in size both of the normal lumen and of coronary obstructions after nifedipine, averaging merely approximately 4%. Only when these authors added nitroglycerin did they find an increase of up to 20% in the diameter of large epicardial arteries. These striking differences from our own observation need further explanation.

Feldman et al. [53] excluded all patients who were symptomatic or had typical ischemic ECG changes at the time of the study. Furthermore, nine patients who were receiving constant treatment with betablocking agents during the study were included, seven of whom were receiving propranolol (up to 320 mg/day) and two, nadolol (up to 120 mg/day). In contrast, in our own study, beta blockers were stopped 3–5 days before the investigation, together with all other antianginal drugs except for nitroglycerin capsules, which were allowed up to 6 h before catheterization. In addition, in ten of Feldman et al.'s patients, only 10 mg nifedipine was administered, whereas all our patients received 20 mg sublingually. Finally, in Feldman's study nitroglycerin was administered directly into the left main coronary artery (200 μg), whereas our patients received a sublingual dose of 0.8 mg (Fig. 8). Hence, substantial dissimilarities in the methods applied, the greated being the simultaneous administration of beta blockers, might explain the different outcome of these studies.

The behavior of the arteriolar resistance under nifedipine has been described extensively in earlier publications [21, 56, 63] (Fig. 11 and Tables 4 and 5) and is well-known. Nifedipine leads to a considerable increase in coronary flow both in the normal and poststenotic area. At rest, flow in the poststenotic region increased more than in the normal area (19% vs 11%). During atrial pacing up to heart rates leading to angina and ischemia a further increase in flow was observed only in the poststenotic region while in the normal area flow remained unchanged or decreased mildly (Fig. 11). A similar effect on coronary blood flow was observed with nisoldipine (0.15 μg/kg) (Tables 4 and 5); regional blood flow increased by approximately 30% at rest in this case and showed a small but insignificant decrease in both the stenotic and the normal areas during pacing. Furthermore, similar changes, although of different duration, were observed with verapamil and diltiazem (Table 4) at rest and during atrial pacing. Hence, calcium antagonists lead to an increase in flow in the normal and poststenotic region at rest as well as dur-

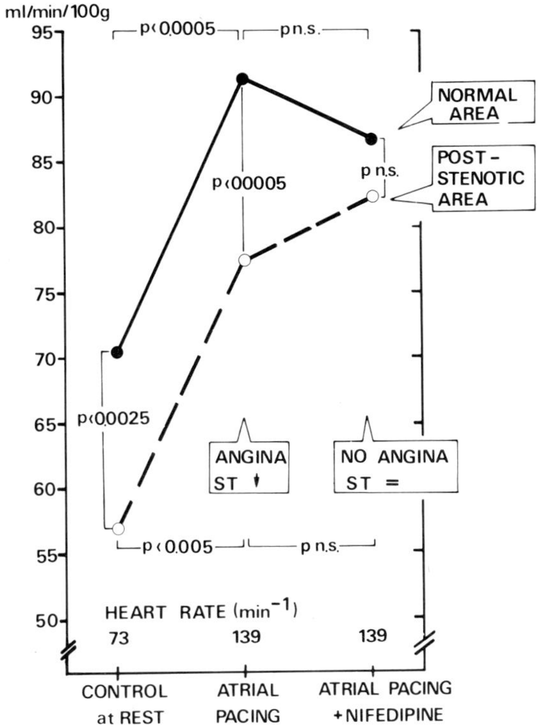

Fig. 11. Behavior of regional myocardial blood flow in 11 patients with isolated high-grade coronary obstructions (>75%), mainly of the LAD, at rest (*left*) and during control atrial pacing (*middle*) and pacing 15 min after administration of 20 mg nifedipine sublingually (*right*). Note that nifedipine was followed by a further, although not significant increase of flow in the poststenotic area, reaching the level of flow in the normal region and again rendering flow homogeneous throughout the heart; in contrast to nitroglycerin (Fig. 8), however, this was on a higher flow level, in spite of a significant decrease in oxygen demand, i.e., of the rate-pressure product from 182 to 142 mmHg × $\text{min}^{-1} \times 10^2$. (For details see text)

Table 4. Changes in regional myocardial blood flow at rest following nifedipine, verapamil, and diltiazem, during control pacing, and during pacing after drug intake

	n	MBF (ml/min per 100 g)			RPP (mmHg min^{-1} O^2)
		PA	NA	HR	
1. Resting control	10	58.8±13.0	70.8±19.9	79	104.0
2. Resting nifedipine		69.6±15.6*	78.7±14.4*	88****	100.3
3. Pacing to ischemia	11	77.6±20.7	91.2±18.5	139	181.7
4. Pacing with nifedipine		82.8±14.8	86.8±11.8	139	142.0***
1. Resting control	7/2[a]	57.2±15.9	61.7±15.7	75	107.7
2. Resting with verapamil		66.3±18.9*	73.7±18.2**	80*	111.9
3. Pacing to ischemia	5	72.6±18.9	90.2±15.1	124	182.7
4. Pacing with verapamil		76.3±10.9	84.6± 9.3	122	166.9
1. Resting control	13/6[a]	56.1±11.1	58.4±11.9	70	89.0
2. Resting with diltiazem		67.5±13.8**	75.3±17.1****	75**	82.1**
3. Pacing to ischemia	6	71.5±13.9	85.3±13.8	130	165.6
4. Pacing with diltiazem		79.3±15.0	92.3±19.4	130	149.8**

PA, area beyond stenosis; NA, normal area; RPP, rate-pressure product

[a] Coronary patients/normal subjects

*$P<0.05$; **$P<0.005$; ***$P<0.01$; ****$P<0.001$

Table 5. Regional myocardial blood flow at rest following nisoldipine 0.15 µg/kg, during control pacing, and during pacing after drug intake

	Regional myocardial blood flow		Blood pressure		Rate-pressure product (mmHg × min^{-1} × 10^{-2})	Heart rate (min^{-1})
	NA (11) (ml/min per 100 g)	PA (5)	Systolic (mmHg)	Diastolic		
Control, resting	54.9 ± 9.4	55.0 ± 8.2	132.3	74.6	92.7	70.1 ± 10
Control, pacing	76.3 ± 18.3	86.2 ± 9.8	110.9	79.9	154.1	139.0 ± 17
Nisoldipine, resting	72.2 ± 17.2	76.6 ± 4.7	112.0	67.8	88.6	79.1 ± 9
Nisoldipine, pacing	76.7 ± 15.2	80.4 ± 12.5	106.1	74.1	149.1	140.5 ± 21
% Difference						
Drug/Control Resting	+ 31.5%	+ 39.2%	− 15.3%	− 9.1%	− 4.3%	+ 12.8%
Drug/Control Pacing	+ 0.5%	− 6.7%	− 4.3%	− 7.3%	− 3.3%	+ 1.1%
Control: Resulting pacing	+ 38.9%	+ 56.7%	− 16.2%	+ 7.1%	+ 61.1%	+ 98.3%
Nisoldipine Resting pacing	+ 6.2%	+ 4.9%	− 5.3%	+ 9.3%	+ 68.3%	+ 77.6%

NA, normal area; PA, area beyond stenosis

ing atrial pacing leading to ischemia; they maintain coronary blood flow despite a significant drop in oxygen demand due to a decrease in afterload, and by this means they are able to release or prevent angina in almost all instances. It is note worthy that the intracoronary administration of nifedipine also leads to an increase in flow, as one might expect, but that at the same time a marked and significant reduction in all hemodynamic parameters (left ventricular systolic pressure, aortic pressure, and positive and negative dp/dt_{max}) is observed, while end-diastolic pressure considerably increases [64]; this negative inotropic effect is shortlasting (approximately 3 min), however, and is more short-lived than the effect on coronary flow, which under these circumstances remains increased up to approximately 10 min. This underlines the differing action of the drug on cardiac and vascular smooth muscle.

There are many reasons for the *improvement of regional myocardial blood flow* in the ischemic areas after administration of dihydropyridines, especially nifedipine. First, there is further and persistent relaxation of smooth muscle tone both in the epicardial arteries and in the intramurally located arterioles; this decrease in vascular smooth muscle tone most likely also takes place in the ischemic zone, i.e., in the endocardial layers, where probably not all arterioles are maximally dilated during ischemia. Indeed, there is strong evidence from animal studies and from observations recorded in humans that during ischemia arteriolar dilatation is not complete.

Second, the decrease in afterload leads to a drop of the elevated end-diastolic pressure during stress-induced ischemia [65], and by this results in a "decompression" of the endocardial region. Third, nifedipine was found to lead to a decrease in wall stiffness, which leads also to a decline in myocardial resistance during diastole [64, 66]. All these events favor the increase in flow, especially as autoregulation is attenuated although not completely abolished. The latter is demonstrated by the fact that, although resting flow increases after nifedipine, coronary blood flow is still capable of increasing further during exercise, i.e., during a further rise in oxygen demand [67]. This is in contrast, for instance, to the effects of dipyridamole, where maximum flow is achieved even at rest and no further increase is seen during exercise [67]. Fourth, in some patients, in addition to the decrease in arteriolar resistance, a decrease in the degree of proximal obstructions, the proximal resistance, can be observed; this might contribute further to the improvement of flow during increased oxygen demand. Nevertheless, it should be mentioned that, so far, it is difficult to make a separate assessment in humans of the contribution to the flow increase brought about by the two resistance areas (proximal and distal).

Combination of Nitroglycerin and Nifedipine

The most marked dilatation of epicardial arteries and obstructions can be observed after combined administration of nitroglycerin and nifedipine. Obstructions that dilated significantly, i.e., by more than 10%, averaged an increase of 49% of the most stenotic diameter (Fig. 12). Furthermore, this intervention led to a distinct separation between so-called dynamic and fixed obstructions. Hence,

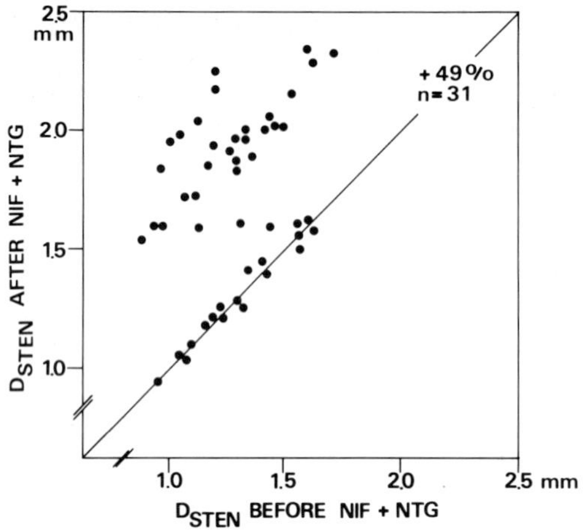

Fig. 12. Effects of the combined administration of 20 mg nifedipine and 0.8 mg nitroglycerin sublingually on the most stenotic diameter in 50 high-grade coronary obstructions (>75%) (same format as Figs. 6, 8, and 11). Note the clear separation between dilating and nondilating stenoses; furthermore, the degree of dilatation achieved far exceeds the one observed when the drugs were given alone. (For details see text)

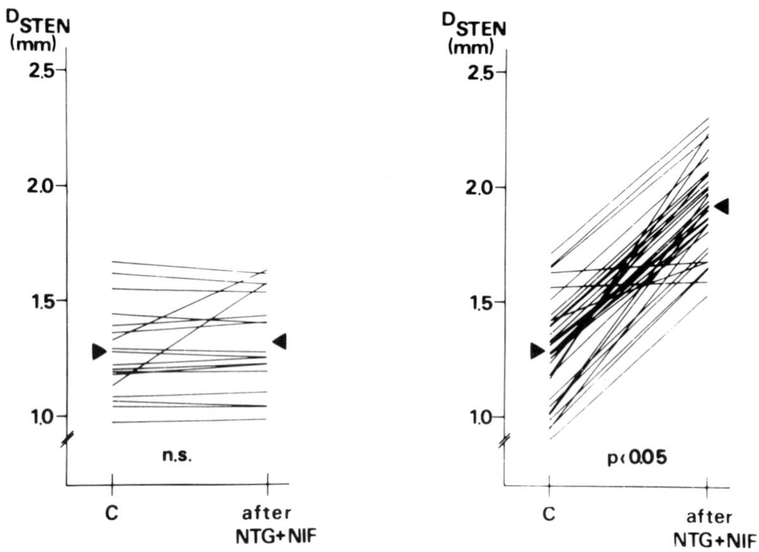

Fig. 13. Comparison of the pharmacological effect of the combined administration of nifedipine and nitroglycerin sublingually on 50 high-grade obstructions, i.e., the most stenotic diameter (*ordinate*) with the angiographic definition of concentric and eccentric obstructions. Concentric obstructions (*left*, $n = 18$) were defined as those where the difference between the most stenotic diameter differed by less than 25% in two projections 90° apart; and eccentric ones (*right*, $n = 32$) as those in which these diameters differed by more than 25%. A good correlation between the functional and anatomic definitions was found. (For details see text)

the assumption that dynamic obstructions were the eccentric ones was confirmed by successful reclassification by an independent observer. By dividing the obstructions according to the above-mentioned angiographic criteria into eccentric and concentric ones and comparing them with the reaction to this pharmacological intervention, i.e., the combined administration of sublingual nifedipine and nitroglycerin, this observer correctly reclassified 16 of 18 angiographic concentric obstructions (98%) and 29 of 32 angiographic eccentric obstructions (90%) (Fig. 13). This indicates that the previous assumption that the dynamic obstructions are usually the eccentric ones is valid and of considerable clinical importance.

Duration of Changes in Vascular Smooth Muscle Tone

So far, no studies are available on the long-term behavior of vascular smooth muscle tone in severe obstructions. Hence, it is not surprising that the duration of relaxation of smooth muscle tone in large epicardial arteries and the influence of nifedipine on any development of tolerance are rarely known. The behavior of smooth muscle tone in large epicardial arteries was therefore studied in our laboratory in 36 patients undergoing angiography on two occasions 23 days apart, the second study being performed in connection with balloon dilatation. The reaction of vascular smooth muscle tone to the second intervention was found to be unaltered, although in the meantime these patients had received large doses of nifedipine (up to three or four doses of 20 mg/day); at the first angiogram the average dilatation of the most stenotic diameter amounted to 48%, while on the second occasion, approximately 12 h after the last drug intake, to 38% (Fig. 14). It is of interest to note that these obstructions were not in a dilated stage before

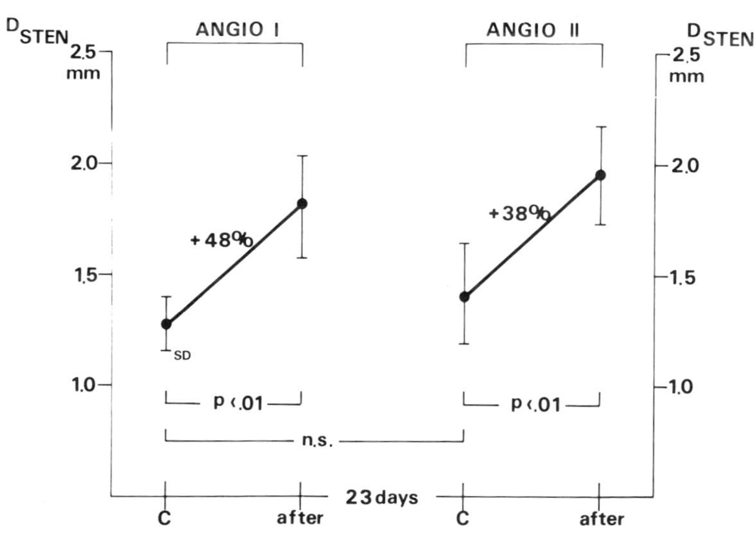

Fig. 14. Long-term course of residual vascular tone in 36 isolated obstructions of the proximal LAD, analysed from angiograms performed at an average of 23 days apart in the same projections. Note that the second pharmacological intervention achieved the same degree of dilatation, indicating absence of tolerance, although these patients received high doses of oral nifedipine (up to 60 or 80 mg/day) and oral nitroglycerin (up to 3 × 40 mg/day) during the interval. The second study was performed approximately 6–8 h after the last drug intake. (For details see text)

administration of the drug, although all these patients suffered from severe exercise-induced ischemia, as demonstrated by the presence of typical ST depressions greater than 0.1 mV and of angina pectoris; in addition, approximately one-third of these patients also suffered from attacks of angina at rest; in all cases a high degree of obstruction, mainly of the proximal left anterior descending artery, was present at angiography, so that patients were considered for angioplasty. This observation also suggests that there is no feedback mechanism between the ischemic area and the perfusing epicardial artery, where the increased vasomotor tone within the obstruction may persist despite ischemia and maintain this vicious circle. Finally, this level of vasomotor tone in the stenotic area prevailed in spite of daily pharmacological dilatation with 3 × 20 mg nifedipine and often, in addition, 3 × 20 mg ISDN over 3 weeks, vasomotor tone increasing again as soon as the drug effect disappeared.

Discussion

In recent years it has been shown that changes in coronary vasomotor tone play a major role in the understanding and treatment of coronary artery disease. Two major vascular areas are involved, the epicardial arteries, where physiologically only small changes in diameters and resistance take place, and the arteriolar bed, where the main changes in resistance occur by way of alterations in arteriolar tone, mediated through neurogenic, humoral, or metabolic factors. Hence, a massive increase in vasomotor tone in epicardial arteries, especially when leading to ischemia, has to be regarded as pathologic, especially spasm, i.e., transient occlusion of a major coronary branch due to increased vasomotor tone. Whether spasm occurs in entirely normal coronary arteries or only when abnormalities of the vessel wall, especially of atherosclerotic origin, are present is still a matter of debate and needs further investigation. Furthermore, chronically increased vasomotor tone in a normal segment of a high-grade eccentric stenosis has to be regarded as "unphysiologic," as it contributes considerably to the elevated total vascular resistance and the abnormal decrease in regional flow in that epicardial branch. Obviously, the abnormally increased vasomotor tone in epicardial arteries, especially in eccentric obstructions, is a phenomenon that occurs independently of changes in tone at the arteriolar level. This is shown by the fact that ischemia does not lead to reflex relaxation of vasomotor tone in the epicardial artery even when dilatation is present in the arterioles.

Relaxation of vascular smooth muscle tone can be achieved by various drugs influencing calcium metabolism in smooth muscle cells, especially by nitrates and calcium antagonists. All these drugs relax both large epicardial arteries and arterioles, although to different degrees. Nitrates and calcium antagonists in particular exhibit a strong dilating effect on large epicardial arteries, and because of this on eccentric obstructions. Due to their different mode of action, calcium antagonists reducing the transmembrane calcium flux by acting at the cell membrane [68] while nitrates act within the cell, removing calcium from the contractile apparatus by stimulating cycling GMP [69], these drugs exhibit a strong synergistic action in relaxing the vasomotor tone of epicardial coronary arteries. In contrast, they act differently at the arteriolar level; nitrates given systemically do not influence arteriolar resistance, which means that autoregulatory changes in regional coronary flow following a decrease in myocardial oxygen consumption are fully preserved both at rest and during exercise; calcium antagonists, in contrast, mildly inhibit autoregulation and lead to an increase in flow at rest distal to the stenosis, even in the presence of a decrease in myocardial oxygen consumption. However, this partial inhibition of autoregulation observed under calcium antagonists is different from the effect seen following administration of dipyridamole, a powerful phosphodiesterase inhibitor, which leads to a complete blockade of autoregulation resulting in maximum arteriolar relaxation and maximum increase in coronary flow up to coronary reserve even at rest; with dipyridamole no further increase in flow is therefore observed during exercise, in contrast to calcium antagonists [67]. This explains the frequent occurrence of a steal phenomenon with dipyridamole [55, 70, 71] and its absence under calcium antagonists where – after doses given clinically – arteriolar relaxation is incomplete and during exercise flow increases further up to coronary reserve. A similar behavior of smooth muscle tone after administration of vasodilating drugs including adenosine was also observed by Berne et al. [72] when recording action potentials in smooth muscles of epicardial arteries and arterioles in dogs. They found that adenosine, the most powerful natural dilator of small coronary arteries, blocked the calcium-dependent action potential in arterioles but not in epicardial arteries; in contrast, nitroglycerin had an effect only in the epicardial arteries, whereas nifedipine – in doses equivalent to those used under clinical conditions – blocked the calcium-dependent action potential in both epicardial and small coronary arteries.

The different actions of these drugs have to be taken into account in the treatment of patients with angina pectoris. Both nitrates and calcium antagonists decrease blood pressure; nitrates, however, have only a mild effect and act predominantly through a decrease in cardiac output and not in resistance, so that afterload is usually unaffected by nitrates. In contrast, calcium antagonists act mainly through a decrease in peripheral resistance, i.e., in afterload, and cardiac output – as venous return is unaffected – is often increased due to mild secondary betastimulation. Nitrates have their most marked effect on preload, i.e., relaxation of venous tone, whereas calcium antagonists, as already mentioned, affect venous tone only indirectly. It should therefore be stressed that the action of the two drugs is only identical with regard to the dilatation of large epicardial arteries. Nevertheless, their combination leads to vasodilatation both of the peripheral venous and of the arteriolar system, and especially of the epicardial coronary smooth muscle vasculature, an observation of considerable clinical importance. When both drugs are given simultaneously perfusion is greatly improved both in unstable and stable angina pectoris. Hence, this combination is a favorable one and should be used more often in vasospastic angina.

References

1. Heberden W (1772) Some account of a disorder of the breast. Med Trans Col Physician (London) 2:59–67
2. Wenckebach KF (ed) (1924) Angina pectoris. Verhandlungen der Gesellschaft für Innere Medizin und Kinderheilkunde. Moritz-Perles, Wien
3. Blumgart HL (1947) The question of "spasm" of the coronary arteries. Am J Med 2:129
4. Wilson FN, Johnston FD (1941) The occurrence in angina pectoris of electrocardiographic changes similar in magnitude and in kind to those produced by myocardial infarction. Am Heart J 22:64
5. Duchosal PW, Henny G (1942) Angine de poitrine et hyperthyroidisme. Cardiologia 5:372
6. Prinzmetal M, Kennamer R, Merliss R, Wada T, Bor N (1959) Angina pectoris. I. A variant form of angina pectoris. Am J Med 27:375
7. Prinzmetal M, Ekmekci A, Toyoshima H, Kwoczynski JK (1959) Angina pectoris. III. Demonstration of a chemical origin of ST elevation in chronic angina pectoris, its variant form, early myocardial infarction, and some non-cardiac conditions. Am J Cardiol 3:276–293
8. Lichtlen PR, Schönbeck M (1974) Ischämischer Koronarspasmus bei Angiographie. Z Kardiol 63:311–319
9. Lichtlen PR (1981) Introductory remarks – some thoughts about unstable angina pectoris. In: Rafflenbeul W, Lichtlen PR, Balcon R (eds) Unstable angina pectoris. Thieme, Stuttgart, pp 1–7
10. Maseri A, L'Abbate A, Pesola A, Ballestra AM, Marzilli M, Severi S, Maltini G, DeNes M, Parodi O, Biaggini A (1977) Coronary vasospasm in angina pectoris. Lancet 1:713–717
11. Maseri A, Severi S, DeNes M, L'Abbate A, Chierchia S, Marzilli M, Ballestra AM, Parodi O, Biaggini A, Distante A (1978) Variant angina: one aspect of a continuous spectrum of vasospastic myocardial ischemia. Pathogenetic mechanisms, estimated incidence and clinical and coronary arteriographic findings in 138 patients. Am J Cardiol 42:1019
12. Maseri A, L'Abbate A, Chierchia S, Parodi O, Severi S, Biaggini A, Distante A, Marzilli M, Ballestra AM (1979) Significance of spasm in the pathogenesis of ischemic heart disease. Am J Cardiol 44:788–792
13. Gould KL (1980) Dynamic coronary stenosis. Am J Cardiol 45:286
14. Rafflenbeul W, Lichtlen PR (1982) Zum Konzept der dynamischen Koronarstenose. Z Kardiol 71:439–444
15. Vlodaver Z, Edwards JE (1971) Pathology of coronary atherosclerosis. Prog Cardiovasc Dis 14:256–274
16. Hort W, Moosdorf R, Kalbfleisch H, Köhler F, Milzner-Schwarz U, Frenzel H (1977) Postmortale Untersuchungen über Lokalisation und Form der stärksten Stenosen in den Koronararterien und ihre Beziehung zu den Risikofaktoren. Z Kardiol 66:333–340
17. Freudenberg H, Lichtlen PR (1981) The normal wall segment in coronary stenoses – A postmortal study. Z Kardiol 70:863–869
18. Gould KL, Lipscomb K (1974) Effect of coronary stenoses on coronary flow reserve and resistance. Am J Cardiol 34:48
19. Engel HJ, Lichtlen PR, Hundeshagen H (1982) Relations between coronary obstructions, left ventricular wall motion and regional myocardial blood flow in single vessel coronary artery disease. Z Kardiol 71:326–333
20. Rafflenbeul W, Lichtlen PR (1983) Quantitative coronary angiography: Evidence of a sustained increase in vascular smooth muscle tone in coronary artery stenosis. Z Kardiol 72 (Suppl 3):87–91
21. Lichtlen P, Engel HJ, Hundeshagen H (1985) Assessment of regional myocardial blood flow using invasive techniques, especially the precordial Xenon clearance technique. In: Diethelm L, Heuck F, Olsson O, Vieten H, Zuppinger A, Hundeshagen H (eds) Nuklearmedizin. Springer, Berlin Heidelberg New York, pp 65–111 (Handbuch der medizinischen Radiologie, vol 15)
22. Chierchia S, Maseri A, Simonetti I, Bondelli C (1977) Oxygen myocardial extraction in angina at rest. Evidence of a primary reduction of blood supply. Circulation 55/56 (Suppl 3):37

23. Selwyn A (1985) Values of continuous ECG in detecting ST depression and arrhythmias. In: Controversies in the treatment of angina pectoris. Eur Heart J (in press)
24. Lichtlen PR (1980) Klinik, Diagnostik und Therapie der unstabilen Angina pectoris. Internist 21:636–645
25. Lichtlen PR (1983) Unstabile Angina pectoris und Präinfarkt-Syndrom. Internist 24:372–382
26. Lichtlen P (1984) Coronary heart disease, clinical aspects and drug therapy. Deutscher Ärzte-Verlag, Köln
27. Maseri A, Parodi O, Severi S, Pesola A (1976) Transient transmural reduction of myocardial blood flow, demonstrated by 201-Thallium Scintigraphy as a cause of variant angina. Circulation 54:280
28. Bertrand ME, Lablanche JM, Tilmant PY, Thieuleux FP (1981) Provoked coronary arterial spasm. In: Delius W, Gerlach E, Grobecker K, Kübler W (eds) Catecholamines and the heart. Springer, Berlin Heidelberg New York, pp 257–267
29. Rafflenbeul W, Lichtlen PR (1983) Release of residual vascular tone in coronary artery stenoses with nifedipine and glyceryltrinitrate. In: Kaltenbach M, Neufeld HN (eds) 5th international adalat symposium. Excerpta Medica, Amsterdam, pp 300–308
30. Lichtlen PR, Engel HJ, Rafflenbeul W (1984) Calcium entry blockers, especially nifedipine, in angina of effort. Possible mechanisms and clinical implications. In: Opie LH (ed) Calcium antagonists and cardiovascular disease. Raven, New York, pp 221–236
31. Yasue H, Omote S, Takizawa A, Nagao M, Miwa K, Tanaka S (1979) Exertional angina pectoris caused by coronary arterial spasm: effect of various drugs. Am J Cardiol 43:647–652
32. Yasue H, Omote S, Takizawa A, Nagao M, Miwa K, Tanaka S (1979) Circadian variation of exercise capacity in patients with Prinzmetal's variant angina: role of exercise-induced coronary arterial spasm. Circulation 59:938–948
33. Yasue H, Omote S, Takizawa A, Masao N, Hyon H, Nishida S, Horie M (1981) Comparison of coronary arteriographic findings during angina pectoris associated with ST elevation or depression. Am J Cardiol 47:539–546
34. Matsuda Y, Ogawa H, Moritanika K, Fujii T, Yoshino F, Katayama K, Miura T, Toma Y, Matsuda M, Kusukawa R (1984) Coronary angiography during exercise-induced angina with ECG changes. Am Heart J 108:959–966
35. Yasue H (1984) Coronary artery spasm and calcium ions. In: Opie LH (ed) Calcium antagonists and cardiovascular disease. Raven, New York, pp 117–128
36. Brown BG (1983) Dilation of coronary artery stenosis: A major mechanism of the effect of nitrates. Z Kardiol 72 (Suppl 3):77–81
37. Lee AB, Brown BG, Bolsen EL, Dodge HT (1982) Coronary stenosis constriction as a major factor in ischemic left ventricular dysfunction induced by isometric handgrip. Circulation 66 (Suppl 2):249
38. Oliva PB, Breckinridge JC (1977) Arteriographic evidence of coronary arterial spasm in acute myocardial infarction. Circulation 56:366
39. Marzilli M, Goldstein S, Trivella MG, Palumbo C, Maseri A (1980) Some clinical considerations regarding the relation of coronary vasospasm to coronary atherosclerosis: a hypothetical pathogenesis. Am J Cardiol 45:882–886
40. Lichtlen PR (1979) Die Koronarographie beim akuten Infarkt. Z Kardiol 68:237
41. Rentrop P, Blanke H, Karsch KR, Kaiser H, Köstering H, Leitz K (1981) Selective intracoronary thrombolysis in acute myocardial infarction and unstable angina pectoris. Circulation 63:307–317
42. Rafflenbeul W, Dzuiba M, Henkel B, Lichtlen P (1975) Morphometric analysis of coronary obstructions during life. Circulation 51/52 (Suppl 2):27
43. Rafflenbeul W, Heim R, Dzuiba M, Henkel B, Lichtlen P (1976) Morphometric analysis of coronary arteries. In: Lichtlen PR (ed) Coronary angiography and angina pectoris. Thieme, Stuttgart, pp 255–265
44. Rafflenbeul W, Reiber JHC, Bouman F, Freudenberg H, Lichtlen PR (1981) Zuverlässigkeit verschiedener Methoden zur Graduierung von Stenosen im Koronarangiogramm. Z Kardiol 70:302

45. Freudenberg H, Lichtlen P (1979) Postmortale Koronarangiographie. In: Lichtlen PR (ed) Koronarangiographie. Straube, Erlangen, pp 341–357
46. Rafflenbeul W, Amende I, Simon R, Engel HJ, Lichtlen P (1976) Qualitative and quantitative angiography before and after nitroglycerin. In: Roskamm H, Hahn CH (eds) Ventricular function at rest and during exercise. Springer, Berlin Heidelberg New York, p 53
47. Rafflenbeul W, Urthaler F, Russell RO, Lichtlen P, James TN (1979) Dilatation of coronary artery stenosis after isosorbiddinitrate in man. Br Heart J 43:546
48. Brown BG, Bolson E, Petersen RB, Pierce CD, Dodge HT (1981) The mechanism of nitroglycerin action: stenoses vasodilation as a major component of the drug response. Circulation 64:1089
49. Schulz W, Wendt P, Klepzig H, Kober G (1982) Der Einfluß von intrakoronarem SIN 1 und Nitroglycerin auf koronar-venöse Sauerstoffsättigung und Weite von Koronargefäßen und Stenosen. In: Molsidomin – Symposium, Januar 1982, Rottach-Egern
50. Schulz W, Wendt P, Kaltenbach M, Kober G (1983) Active and passive changes in coronary artery diameters after vasodilation. In: Kaltenbach M, Neufeld HN (eds) 5th International adalat symposium. Excerpta Medica, Amsterdam, pp 309–317
51. Schulz W, Anderten W, Reiber JHC, Bernauer R, Kaltenbach M, Kober G (1983) Active and passive coronary vasodilation after intracoronary and sublingual nitroglycerin. Z Kardiol 72 (Suppl 3):82–86
52. Conti CR, Hill JA, Feldman RL, Conti JB, Pepine CJ (1984) Comparison of nifedipine and nitrates: clinical and angiographic studies. In: Opie LH (ed) Calcium antagonists and cardiovascular disease. Raven, New York, pp 269–275
53. Feldman RL, Hill JA, Conti JB, Conti CR, Pepine CJ (1983) Analysis of coronary responses to nifedipine alone, and in combination with intracoronary nitroglycerin in patients with coronary artery disease. Am Heart J 105:651–658
54. Lichtlen PR, Engel HJ (1979) Assessment of regional myocardial blood flow using the inert gas washout technique. Cardiovasc Radiol 2:203–216
55. Lichtlen P, Engel HJ, Amende I, Rafflenbeul W, Simon R (1976) Mechanisms of various antianginal drugs. Relationship between regional flow behaviour and contractility. In: Jatene AD, Lichtlen PR (eds) 3rd International adalat symposium. Excerpta Medica, Amsterdam, pp 14–29
56. Engel HJ, Lichtlen PR (1981) Beneficial enhancement of coronary blood flow by nifedipine; comparison with nitroglycerin and beta-blocking agents. Am J Med 71:658–666
57. Simon R, Amende I, Lichtlen PR (1982) Differential effects of nifedipine and nitroglycerin on hemodynamics in single coronary arteries in man. Circulation 66:II–119
58. Bernstein L, Friesinger GC, Lichtlen PR, Ross RS (1966) The effect of nitroglycerin on the systemic and coronary circulation in man and dogs. Myocardial blood flow measured with Xenon-133. Circulation 33:107–116
59. Lichtlen P, Halter J, Gattiker K (1974) The effect of isosorbiddinitrate on coronary flow, coronary resistance and left ventricular dynamics under exercise in patients with coronary artery disease. Basic Res Cardiol 69:402–421
60. Schulz W, Kraus G, Kaltenbach M, Kober G (1981) Einfluß von intrakoronarem und intravenösem Nifedipin auf die allgemeine und lokale Gefäßweite von epikardialen Koronararterien bei stabiler Angina pectoris – ein antianginöser Wirkaspekt? Z Kardiol 70:809
61. Rafflenbeul W (1983) Dilatation of coronary artery stenoses with diltiazem i.v. In: Fleckenstein A, Hashimoto K, Herrmann M, Schwartz A, Seipel L (eds) New Ca-antagonists – recent developments and concepts. Fischer, Stuttgart, p 181
62. Bonzell T, Wollschlager H, Lölgen H, Müzel T, Wehrle B, Just H (1984) Effect of intravenous diltiazem on coronary artery diameter in patients with coronary artery disease. J Am Coll Cardiol 3:578
63. Malacoff RF, Lorell BH, Mudge GH, Holman BL, Idoine J, Bifolck L, Cohn PF (1982) Beneficial effects of nifedipine on regional myocardial blood flow in patients with coronary artery disease. Circulation 65 (Suppl 1):32–37
64. Amende I, Simon R, Hood WP, Hetzer R, Lichtlen PR (1983) Intracoronary nifedipine in human beings: magnitude and time course of changes in left ventricular contraction/relaxation and coronary sinus blood flow. J Am Coll Cardiol 2:1141–1145

65. Lichtlen P (1975) The influence of nifedipine on left ventricular and coronary dynamics at rest and during exercise in patients with coronary artery disease. In: Hashimoto K, Kimura E, Kobayashi T (eds) 1st International nifedipine (adalat) – symposium. Tokyo Press, Tokyo, pp 114–120
66. Amende I, Simon R, Hood WP, Daniel W, Lichtlen PR (1981) Differential effects of intracoronary nitroglycerin and nifedipine on coronary flow and myocardial function in man. Circulation 64:293
67. Lichtlen P (1975) Coronary and left ventricular dynamics under nifedipine in comparison to nitrates, betablocking agents and dipyridamole. In: Lochner W, Braasch W, Kroneberg G (eds) 2nd International adalat – symposium. Springer, Berlin Heidelberg New York, pp 212–224
68. Fleckenstein-Grün G, Fleckenstein A (1980) Calcium-Antagonismus – ein Grundprinzip der Vasodilatation. In: Fleckenstein A, Roskamm H (eds) Calcium-Antagonismus. Springer, Berlin Heidelberg New York, pp 191–206
69. Kukowetz WR, Holzmann S (1983) Mechanism of nitrate-induced vasodilation and tolerance. Z Kardiol 72 (Suppl 3):14–19
70. Tauchert M, Behrenbeck DW, Hützel J, Hilger HH (1976) Ein neuer pharmakologischer Test zur Diagnose der Koronarinsuffizienz. Dtsch Med Wochenschr 101:35
71. Tauchert MA, Osterspey J, Hützel J, Hilger HH (1976) Medikamentöse Induktion einer Angina pectoris als neuer Test in der Vorfelddiagnostik der koronaren Herzkrankheit. Verh Dtsch Ges Inn Med 1982:1153
72. Berne RM, Belardinelli L, Harder DR, Speralakis N, Rubio R (1980) Response of large and small coronary arteries to adenosine, nitroglycerin, cardiac glycosides, and calcium antagonists. In: Fleckenstein A, Roskamm H (eds) Calcium-Antagonismus. Springer, Berlin Heidelberg New York, pp 208–220

Discussion

(pp. 381–407)

Groß: There might be the possibility of compressing epicardial arteries mechanically by the epicardium under ischemic conditions. Did you ever see a further reduction of cardiac diameter due to the preload reduction of nitroglycerin which may explain the additive effect of nitroglycerin and nifedipine?

Lichtlen: That's a good question. We have measured geometry after nitroglycerin, mainly during diastole, but also during systole. Although geometry changes a lot, the heart gets smaller, the enddiastolic volume decreases, and the left ventricle becomes elongated. We have, however, not seen a compression of epicardial arteries (Amende et al: Circulation 1978).

Bühler: In the spastic type of angina with the use of betablockers alone there is unopposed alpha$_1$- and possible alphy$_2$-adrenoceptor-mediated vasoconstriction and both could be eliminated with the Ca^2-antagonist. There is therefore no reason to incriminate the betablocker for the lack of dilator effect you referred to.

Lichtlen: I agree, up to now the evidence we have is small but from what we have seen in flow studies there is some evidence. I am not sure, whether this is the explanation for Conti's results differing from ours. 4 years ago Holman at the American Heart Meeting showed no increase of coronary blood flow in his patients after nifedipine. In the discussion it came out that all these patients were under propranolol. About 2 years later, he showed new results in patients who had no propranolol and they had a typical increase of flow. Finally we saw some patients with typical Prinzmetal-angina who did very well under a Ca^{2+}-antagonist. However, when the family doctor added a betablocker, these patients immediately had again their attack of angina, although they were still under the Ca-Antagonist. Finally, Dr. Fleckenstein showed an increase in tone when he added noradrenaline after betablockade.

Fleckenstein: Yasue, too, in Japan injected noradrenaline after betablockade and increased coronary tone in patients considerably. We did it in animals and it was the same. May I comment on spasm? For me it is always a mystery why for about 40 years all these ancient papers were completely forgotten. Everybody who used the term "coronary spasm" was really bombarded by the cardiologists. We suffered from such bombardments when we propagated their ability of Ca^{2+}-antagonists to relax coronary artery spasm.

Lichtlen: Maseri rediscovered and reintroduced it actually.

Hugenholtz: One can even go back to Heberden's original description: it really sounds very much as if it was such a case. Concerning the interaction between betablockers and Ca^{2+}-antagonists, the positions are not all that far apart, if you take the dose more into account. In open chest pig studies we studied the coronary flow and the dimension of the vessels at varying doses and at varying combinations. When you have a dominant effect of the betablocker, clearly flow will go down as one has to expect, but if you give enough of the calcium antagonist, you can completely undo that "damage" and get your dilatation. It is a matter of the dose in the human situation: when it works fine we leave it, if it is not enough you will not see antyhing, and we say the drug is no good. I would not fear anymore the combination therapy provided the patient with betablocker is given enough Ca^{2+}-antagonist in addition.

Lichtlen: That is a good point, because Conti used 10 mg nifedipine and some patients had more than 300 mg propranolol. That might really explain it.

Session VI: Hypertension

Chairman: F. R. Bühler

Bayer-Symposium IX
Cardiovascular Effects of Dihydropyridine-Type
Calcium Antagonists and Agonists, 412–420

Effects of Calcium Antagonistic and Agonistic Dihydropyridines on Experimental Hypertension and Vascular Damage

S. Kazda, B. Garthoff and G. Luckhaus

Summary

Due to their specific effect on the gated calcium entry into the vascular smooth muscle cell, the antagonistic and agonistic 1,4 dihydropyridines can be used as a tool for assessing the role of calcium ions in different forms of experimental hypertension. Chronic treatment with nifedipine prevents the genetically determined hypertension, cardiac hypertrophy and renal ischemia in spontaneously hypertensive rats for more than the half of their life span. However, this treatment does not abolish the primary genetical defect since discontinuation of therapy results in a very rapid increase of blood pressure even in an advanced age of these rats.

Calcium antagonisms by nifedipine prevented salt-induced hypertension, vascular damage and mortality in sensitive Dahl rats. Chronic treatment with the calcium agonist BAY K 8644 accelerated the development of the salt induced hypertension in sensitive rats, but did not affect blood pressure in salt loaded resistant rats. In some sensitive rats on low salt diet BAY K 8644 induced renovascular damage without sustained hypertension. Calcium modulating dihydropyridines do not change the different genetical predisposition to hypertension.

In the salt loaded stroke-prone spontaneously hypertensive rats (SP-SHR) the calcium antagonist nimodipine largely prevented tissue damage and mortality but did not decrease the extremly high blood pressure. Similar protective effect without substantial influence on high blood pressure in salt loaded SP-SHR was achieved by bilateral surgical parathyreoidectomy.

Hypertension associated vascular damage must not necessarily be dependent on the systemic intravascular pressure. It is suggested, that in malignant hypertension the deleterious calcium overload can be activated or inhibited independently of the regulation of arterial blood pressure. In this sense, the protective effect of calcium antagonistic dihydropyridines mimics that of parathyreoidectomy.

Nifedipine as a protagonist of the calcium antagonistic dihydropyridine derivatives has been accepted in the antihypertensive armamentary mainly because of its vasodilating effect, resulting in the reduction of the elevated peripheral vascular resistance.

However, careful observation of hypertensive patients and further experimental research revealed effects clearly distinguishing calcium antagonistic compounds from the other known vasodilators. In addition to peripheral vasodilation the calcium antagonistic DHP's improve renal excretion of sodium and have a complex effect on the renin-angiotensin-aldosterone system. Altogether they seem to affect the most important events involved in the pathogenesis of essential hypertension.

Do the Calcium Antagonists Represent a Causal Therapy of Spontaneous Hypertension?

Spontaneously hypertensive rats (SHR) remain normotensive when the chronic treatment is started in the early, prehypertensive age. In Fleckenstein's experiment [1] SHR were followed for 24 weeks. In our experiments we investigated the effect of the long term therapy for 60 weeks, which represents roughly $^2/_3$ of the life span of these rats. Whereas the untreated controls developed sustained hypertension within the first four months of life, rats treated chronically with nifedipine remained normotensive.

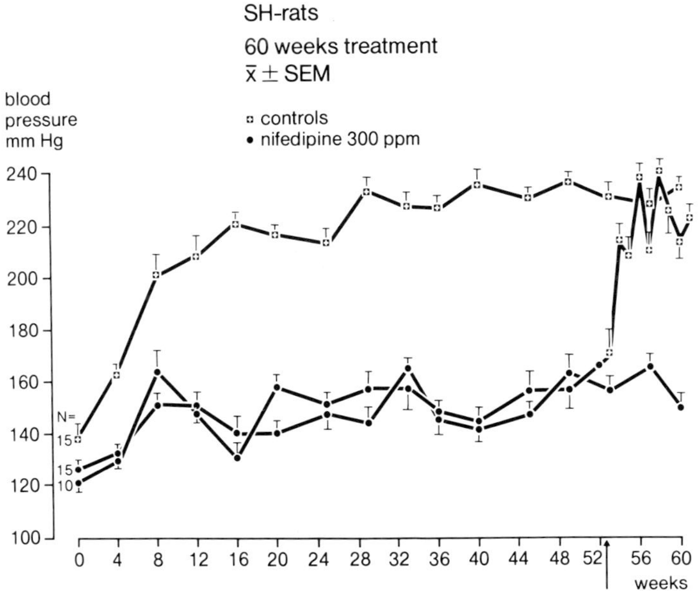

Fig. 1. Development of hypertension in male spontaneously hypertensive rats from the age of 8 weeks (=0). Chronic treatment with nifedipine for 60 weeks prevented hypertension. After discontinuation of therapy at week 52 blood pressure increased to the hypertensive values of non-treated controls within 4 weeks

In our experiment the hypertensive cardiac hypertrophy has been almost totally prevented by nifedipine. Also increase in the plasma renin activity and plasma aldosterone concentration were reduced after 60 weeks treatment with nifedipine [2]. With the progression of the hypertensive disease in SHR obviously the progredient renal ischemia resulted in an increasing stimulation of renin secretion, which can be inhibited by a long term treatment with nifedipine.

Do these results indicate that the primary genetical defect in spontaneously hypertensive rats resides in the increased transmembrane availability of calcium ions for vascular contraction – in the peripheral or in the renal vessels – which can be abolished by the early treatment with nifedipine?

Probably not. In one group of our SHR the nifedipine treatment was stopped at the advanced age of 52 weeks. In these rats the blood pressure rapidly increased to the level of their untreated controls within 4 weeks. At this age the rats needed much less time for development of high blood pressure as needed by the untreated animals in the prepubertal age (Fig. 1).

This finding demonstrates that some superior regulating mechanisms are involved in the realization of genetic predisposition for hypertension whose efficacy is only therapeutically suppressed by chronic administration of nifedipine. Whenever this pharmacological suppression is discontinued the primary defect can be realized by the very rapid increase of blood pressure independently of the age of the animals.

Apart from its theoretical importance this finding has also therapeutic consequences. Even using calcium antagonists as a possible "pathogenetic principle", the treatment should not be interrupted. Only a consequent life long treatment can prevent the scondary hypertension-bound pathology and related mortality.

Calcium Overload as a Cause of Hypertensive Vascular Damage?

The role of the kidney in the development of hypertension and the presumably specific renovascular action of calcium antagonists can be evaluated using the salt sensitive (S) and salt resistant (R) Dahl-rats. When loaded with high salt diet the S rats develop malignant hypertension within few weeks, whereas the R-strain remains normotensive and survives for a long period of time [3].

In the S-rats the high salt diet resulted in vascular damage usually described as hypertensive vasculopathy. Especially in the renal vessels a subendothelial fibrin deposition, medial hypertrophy and periarteritis were observed. Fibrinoid necrosis of the vasa afferentia led to progressive glomerular changes including collapse and hyalinization (Fig. 2) [4].

When treated with nifedipine simultaneously to the high salt diet the S rats do not develop hypertension and resemble in this sense the rats of R strain (Fig. 3). The R rats did not experience any change in blood pressure under high salt diet with or without nifedipine and also their kidneys and other organs remained morphologically intact. It would appear that nifedipine changed the sensitive strain to a resistant one as the S rats tolerate the high salt diet without increasing blood pressure and without developing any morphological changes in the kidney when protected by permanent treatment with nifedipine [5, 4].

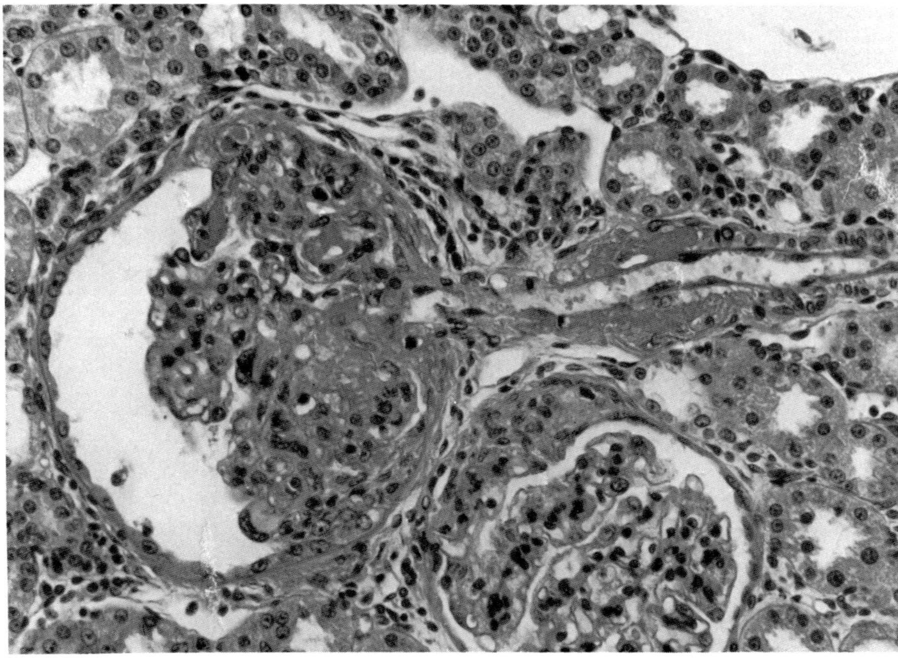

Fig. 2. Subendothelial fibrin deposition causing a luminal stenosis of the vas afferens and secondary glomerular collapse in the hypertensive S-Dahl rat

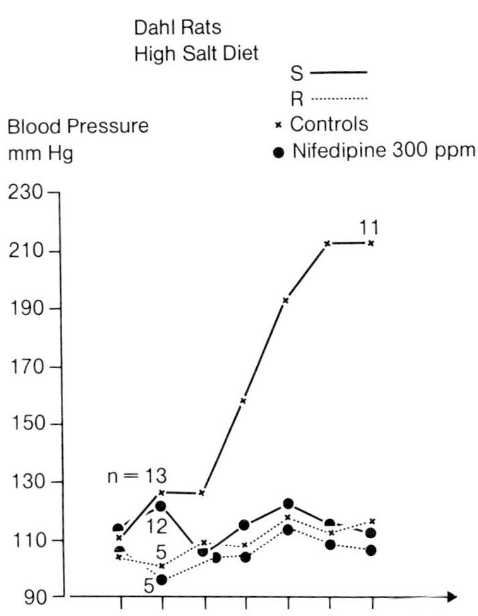

Fig. 3. Development of salt-induced hypertension in S-Dahl rats. Nifedipine prevented hypertension in S-rats but had no effect on blood pressure in salt loaded R-rats

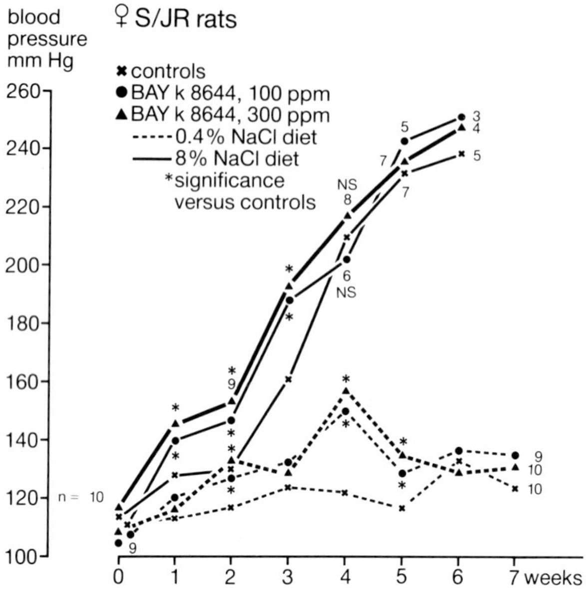

Fig. 4. Effect of the calcium agonist BAY K 8644 on blood pressure and survival rate (numbers over the curves) in sensitive (*S*) Dahl rats of John Rapp colony (*JR*) on high and low sodium diet

Does this mean that in the R rats some endogenous "calcium antagonist" is blocking the vascular calcium channels and thus preventing the increase of blood pressure and vascular damage in answer to the hypertensinogenic sodium challenge? If it is so, would it be possible to overcome this hypothetical block in the R rat by treating it with the *calcium agonist* in addition to the high salt diet? In other words, would it be possible to change the R rat to S rat by chronic treatment with BAY K 8644?

The answer is: Probably not. Feeding the R rats with high concentrations of BAY K 8644 in the diet in addition to the high concentration of NaCl did not result in any increase in blood pressure and in any morphological damage of the kidney.

In the S rat a chronic treatment with BAY K 8644 accelerated the development of salt induced hypertension, especially in the first four weeks of administration (Fig. 4). The difference between the agonist treated and non-treated animals does not seem to be very high. In fact the difference is probably much more important than it can be demonstrated in this diagram of blood pressure.

BAY K 8644 has many attractive pharmacological properties but unfortunately it does not taste very good. In the first week the food consumption of the animals was reduced – as shown also by the initial retardation of the growth curve (Fig. 5). Therefore the animals consumed a very limited amount of BAY K 8644 and, what is extremely important, they consumed very limited amount of NaCl which is also mixed to the food. The hypertensive effect of sodium chloride in Dahl rats is "dose dependent". Consequently, these two groups – medicated and

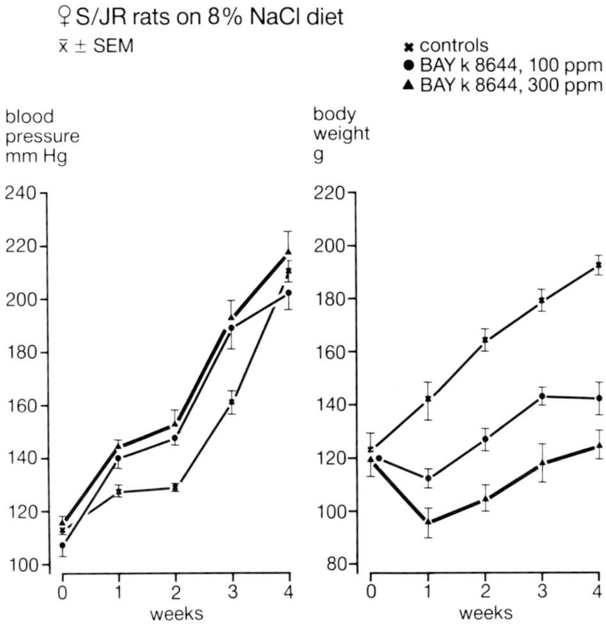

Fig. 5. BAY K 8644 accelerates the development of salt induced hypertension in the sensitive rats of John Rapp colony (*left pannel*). The retardation of the growth curve (*right pannel*) reflects the dose dependent reduction of food consumption by the compound

not medicated – are not quite comparable with regard to their sodium intake. Despite this BAY K 8644 produced a fulminant increase in blood pressure and resulted in early vascular damage of the kidney and in early death.

Curiously in S rats on low salt diet, who normally do not develop hypertension BAY K 8644 produced some temporary increase in blood pressure. At the end of the experiment some of these agonist treated low salt rats had a high serum urea concentration and high plasma renin acitvity. These 4 animals treated with BAY K 8644 actually developed slight to moderate vascular changes in the kidney which never develops on a low salt diet. Such vasculopathy is normally observed only in severely hypertensive S rats on a high salt diet. In the agonist treated animals vasculopathy developed without permanent increase in blood pressure.

Prevention of Calcium Overload Protects the Tissue from Damage Without Affecting High Blood Pressure?

These findings substantiate the conclusion that the vascular damage in sensitive rats must not necessarily be dependent on the systemic intravascular pressure. It is possible that in malignant hypertension different calcium regulating systems are activated. The systems responsible for vascular tone and for cellular viabilitiy do

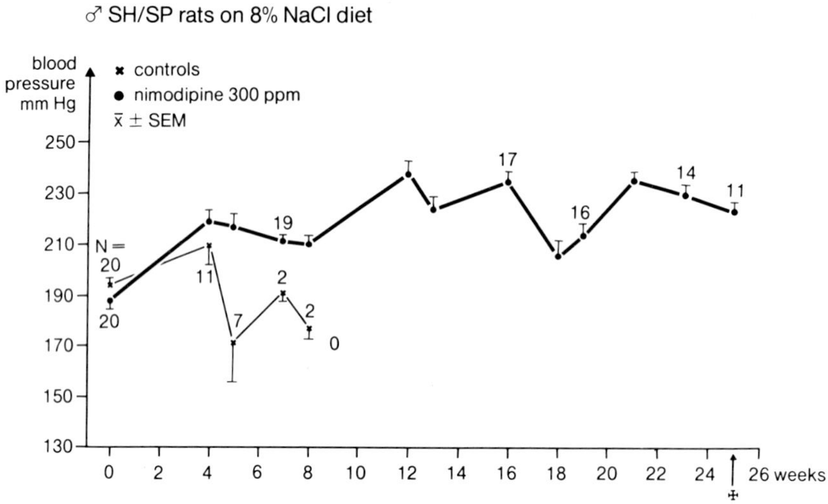

Fig. 6. Chronic treatment with nimodipine increases the survival rate (numbers over the curves) in salt loaded stroke-prone spontaneously hypertensive rats without decreasing the high blood pressure. (With kind permission of Elsevier Biomedical Press)

not have to be identical. We found arguments in favour of this hypothesis in experiments with another strain of hypertensive rats. In the stroke-prone substrain of spontaneously hypertensive rats cerebral apoplexy and renal lesions with high mortality were induced by a high salt diet.

Simultaneous treatment with nitrendipine produced a small but significant decrease of the high blood pressure. 11 out of 20 controls died within 9 weeks and all had lesions in various organs. All the nitrendipine treated rats survived and the incidence and degree of lesions were reduced. A dramatic reduction in mortality and vascular lesions was achieved by nimodipine. In this experiment all the more sensitive young stroke-prone SHR died within 9 weeks as a result of high salt diet. However, more than half of the treated animals survived 25 weeks. Nimodipine is a calcium antagonistic compound having very weak peripheral vascular effect. In this experiment the high blood pressure was not reduces by nimodipine. In contrast, in the very ill controls the blood pressure dropped ante finem; on average it was lower than that of the nimodipine treated animals (Fig. 6). These findings support our hypothesis that the vascular damage in hypertensive or hypertension-prone animals is not entirely dependent on high blood pressure [6].

Presumably other factors in addition to the high blood pressure are also involved in vascular damage induced by calcium overload. There are some clinical and experimental observations indicating that the avitivity of the parathyroid gland is involved in malignant hypertension.

Stimulated by these findings in a pilot experiment we performed bilateral parathyroidectomy (PTX) in young stroke-prone SHR and loaded them with high salt diet. All operated animals developed tetania on the first postoperative day. This however, disappeared after few days on calcium treatment. Other than

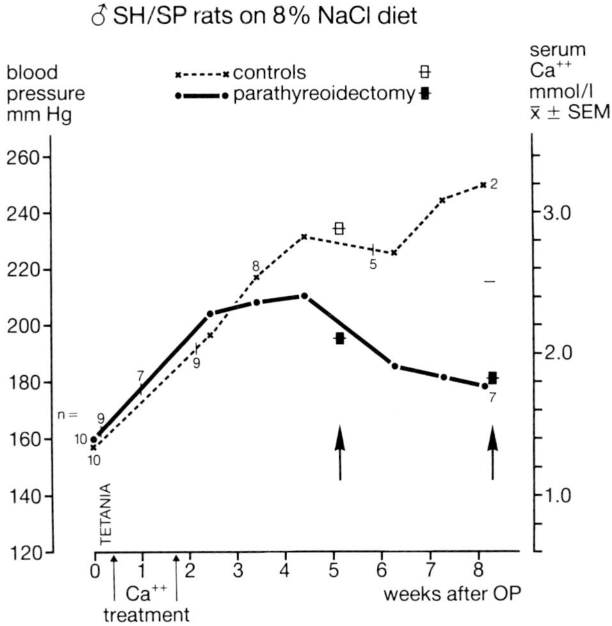

Fig. 7. Effect of bilateral parathyreoidectomy on blood pressure, survival rate (numbers over the curves) and total serum calcium concentration in young, salt-loaded stroke-prone spontaneously hypertensive rats. All operated animals developed tetania and 3 out of 10 died within the first week after parathyreoidectomy

that and initial loss of body weight the animals developed very well. The control animals on a high salt diet became heavily ill, they lost weight and successively died. In contrast the PTX animals tolerated the high salt diet without any problem.

The increase in blood pressure was not influenced by PTX over 3 weeks on high salt diet. Later, the blood pressure slightly decreased in the PTX animals whereas in the two surviving controls it continued to increase. The serum calcium concentration in the PTX rats was reduced by approximately of 30% (Fig. 7).

Histologically all the intercurrently died control animals revealed severe angiopathy in the brain, heart and kidneys. In the two surviving animals, sacrificed at week 9, morphological changes have been found in the kidneys. In contrast, in none of the PTX-animals morphological changes have been found in any organs.

Parathyroidectomy seems to mimic the protective effect of dihydropyridine calcium antagonists in preventing the malignization of the hypertensive disease. It can be speculated that the parathyroid gland is activated in malignant hypertension. Whether the tissue protective effect of calcium antagonistic dihydropyridines is mediated by their effect on parathyriod gland still has to be investigated.

References

1. Von Witzleben H, Frey M, Keidel A, Fleckenstein A (1980) Normalization of blood pressure in spontaneously hypertensive rats by long term treatment with verapamil and nifedipine. Pflugers Arch Ges Physiol (Suppl 384) R 9
2. Kazda S, Garthoff G, Luckhaus G (1983) Calcium antagonists in hypertensive disease: experimental evidence for a new therapeutic concept. Postgrad Med J 59 (Suppl 2) 78–83
3. Dahl LK, Heine M, Tassinari L (1962) Role of genetic factors in susceptibility to experimental hypertension due to chronic salt ingestion. Nature (London) 194:480–482
4. Luckhaus G, Garthoff B, Kazda S (1982) Prevention of hypertensive vasculopathy by nifedipine in salt-loaded Dahl rats. Arzneim Forsch/Drug Res 32:1421–1425
5. Kazda S, Garthoff B, Dycka J, Iwai J (1982) Prevention of malignant hypertension in salt loaded "S" Dahl rats with the calcium antagonist nifedipine. Clin Exp Hypertension A4:1231–1241
6. Kazda S, Garthoff B, Luckhaus G (1983) Calcium antagonists prevent brain damage in stroke-prone spontaneously hypertensive rats (SHR-SP) independent of their effect on blood pressure. J Cerebral Blood Flow Metab 3 (Suppl 1):526–527

Discussion

(pp. 412–420)

Casteels: Could one conclude from your results that the high concentration of ionised Ca^{2+} in plasma is somehow responsible for damage of the blood vessels in brain? Do you have any idea why this damage is mainly localised at the brain vessels?

Kazda: I am not so sure, that the plasma Ca^{2+} per se could be decisive. The responsible factor is something which enhances or inhibits the transmembrane entry of Ca^{2+}.

Bühler: Your parathyroidectomized animals nevertheless increase blood pressure. In other words although the parthyroid hormone may be involved in vascular toxicity, it doesn't seem to be involved in cellular Ca^{2+}-overload. Is that correct?

Kazda: I don't know. This preliminary experiment does not permit us this conclusion. In this experiment we have taken for certain reasons very young animals. In the other experiments with Ca^{2+}-antagonists, I showed, we have used animals with already established hypertension. So I cannot compare these two experimental groups.

Towart: In the work of John Laragh there is some indication that in essential hypertension there is a very mild form of hyperparathyroidism. If that is true and it would go with your data, then in fact this mild form of hyperparathyroidism would not contribute to hypertension, but it may contribute to the vascular toxic aspects of hypertension.

Kazda: That is what I am speculating.

Lichtlen: Together with our endocrinologist we studied a large group of patients with severe coronary artery disease and by and large these had a significantly higher parathyroid hormone level than the normal patients or patients with normal coronary arteries or with valve failure.

Fleckenstein: In normal rats one week after parathyroidectomy we have measured about 50% of the normal plasma-Ca^{2+}-level. To what extent was Ca^{2+}-level decreased in your parathyroidectomized rats?

Kazda: The reduction was roughly 30% of the total serum Ca^{2+} concentration in comparison to the controls. Rats have obviously some accessory parathyroid tissue which allows them to survive the removal of the two main glands even without calcium supplementation.

Hall: I am constantly surprised that so many people add salt to the diet. If you want to get excess salt into the animal you don't add it to the diet, you add it to the water, because all you have to do if you add it to the diet is drink more water and that tends to wash it out. If you add it to the water, there is no way it can do that.

Kazda: Dietary salt addition is much more effective in stimulating hypertension. The rats have free access to water and can easily dilute the ingested salt. The possibility to increase salt intake by giving it to the water is limited. Even 2% NaCl are toxic. In our experiments we need high amounts of NaCl.

Van Breemen: What is the nifedipine or nimodipine doing when it prevents vascular damages without reducing the blood pressure? Can you also get a situation where you have no increase in blood pressure, but still have vascular damage which is preventable by Ca^{2+}-antagonists?

Kazda: In some of the sensitive rats without salt, the agonist BAY K 8644 produced damage in vessels without inducing hypertension.

Van Breemen: How do you imagine now where does that Ca^{2+} got to cause the damage? If it goes into the cell it should give you the contraction and the high blood pressure. So there seems to be another place it can go where it can cause vascular damage other than the cytoplasm.

Garthoff: It is certainly possible that you can cause vascular damage without elevating blood pressure. Another classical model would be the infusion of angiotensin II which has been done in the rabbit. Microinfarctions have been produced with subpressor doses of angiotensin II.

Knorr: Louis Tobian from Minneapolis has very similar results in Dahl-rats in which high potassium diet also prevented widely the lesions without changing the high blood pressure.

Cauvin: In human hypertensives spasms are often seen particularly at bifurcations in arteries. So it is possible that the Ca^{2+}-antagonist may be more effective in reducing spasms than overall blood pressure and that the spasms may produce the strokes and the renal infarctions.

Kazda: It is possible, that the high sodium diet exaggerated the vasoconstrictory autoregulation which may produce the extreme spasm and damage in organs, without changing systemic blood pressure. It is very apparent that these necroses occur mainly in organs with marked autoregulation in kidney and brain.

Bayer-Symposium IX
Cardiovascular Effects of Dihydropyridine-Type
Calcium Antagonists and Agonists, 423–434

On the Antihypertensive Properties of Nitrendipine, with Observations of Its Effects on Electrolyte Excretion

C. E. HALL and S. HUNGERFORD

Summary

The weekly implantation of 25 mg nitrendipine pellets effectively prevented spontaneous and DOC-salt hypertension and were well tolerated. In the latter model steroid-induced "diabetes insipidus-like" syndrome was also prevented.

Nitrendipine acted differently in rats with spontaneous hypothalamic diabetes insipidus than it did in normal Long-Evans rats. When 0.7% NaCl was used as the loading solution, the latter responded with polyuria, lowered urine osmolality, natriuresis and kaliuresis, none of which occurred in DI rats. When the loading solution consisted of 0.45% NaCl + 0.25% KCl, nitrendipine caused polyuria in normal rats, without any effect on electrolyte excretion, and decreased electrolyte excretion without affecting urine volume in DI rats.

When loading solutions of 0.9% NaCl, 0.9% KCl and 5.1% glucose were used, the response to nitrendipine was again different. In the first instance the drug caused polyuria, hypernatremia and hyperkalemia without affecting urine osmolality: in the second it had no effect, and in the third it caused hyponatremia. When dual solute solutions of NaCl + glucose, NaCl + KCl, or KCl + glucose were used, there were still different responses. With the first, nitrendipine reduced urinary Na^+ and K^+, with the second it also reduced urine volume, and with the third it increased urine output while diminishing urine osmolality and K^+ excretion.

Introduction

Experimental [1–4] and clinical [5–8] studies indicate calcium-entry blocking drugs have antihypertensive effects, presumably inhibiting the calcium entry into smooth muscle cells of resistance vessels (arterioles) which precedes and initiates contraction.

The following studies examined the antihypertensive properties of the calcium-entry blocker, nitrendipine (NIT), in spontaneous, and deoxycorticosterone

– salt hypertension. Also to be reported are its influence on renal electrolyte excretion, since NIT [9] and its congeners such as felodipine [10] and diltiazem [11] have natriuretic properties, a significant finding in view of the known interrelationship between Na^+ and hypertension. In the cardiovascular studies, NIT was compressed into 25 mg pellets, which were subcutaneously implanted.

In the urinary studies, the effect of NIT was first compared in normal Long-Evans (LE) rats and in Brattleboro (DI) rats with hypothalamic diabetes insipidus, and then on the urine composition of Sprague-Dawley (SD) rats given loading solutions of differing chemical composition.

Materials and Methods

Experiment 1

Eighteen five week old male SHR were divided into two equal groups. Into one of these, a 25 mg NIT pellet was implanted on day 0 and on day 7, 14, 21, 30, 41, 63, and 70. The others served as controls. They are individually caged in an environmentally-controlled, windowless room lighted 8 AM–8 PM, and given Purina Laboratory Chow and tap water ad lib.

Conscious systolic blood pressure were measured initially, and then at approximately weekly intervals, on the tails of warmed, restrained rats. The equipment consisted of a Mark IV Physiograph integrated with a PE 300 Programmed Electrosphygmomanometer (Narco Biosystems, Houston, TX). Repetitive measurements were made until three consecutive values agreed to within 10 mm Hg, which were then averaged to obtain the value recorded. Values above 150 mm Hg were regarded as hypertensive. Pellet implantations were always made immediately following blood pressure determinations.

Experiment 2

Twenty-two female SD rats weighing 95–130 g were divided into three groups and mononephrectomized under ether anesthesia. They were housed and treated as in experiment 1, but received 1% NaCl solution to drink. Animals of groups 1 and 2 (n = 8) received 5 mg deoxycorticosterone pivalate (DOCP) initially and at weekly intervals in a commercial suspending medium (Ciba-Geigy), of which controls (n = 6) received the same volume. Animals of group 2 also received a 25 mg NIT pellet initially and on days 7, 14, 21, 43, and 50, and a single subcutaneous injection of 30 mg/kg (in propylene glycol) on the 64th day. On the 64th day, animals of the other two groups were injected with propylene glycol. Conscious systolic blood pressures were measured and evaluated as in experiment 1, initially and at approximately weekly intervals.

On the 51st day, and on the 64th day (one hour after a 30 mg/kg injection of NIT), the urinary excretion pattern was evaluated by a modification of methods described elsewhere [12, 13]. Each rat received 3 ml/100 g body weight of an 0.45% NaCl + 0.25% KCl solution intraperitoneally, and then placed in a metabolism cage for a 5 h urine collection. Bladders were voided manually initially, (the sample discarded) and terminally, this sample being added to the voided volume. Urine Na^+ and K^+ were measured by flame photometry, and on the 64th day urine osmolality was also determined (Wescor Vapor Pressure Osmometer, Model 5100 C).

On the 65th day cardiac blood was drawn for serum Na^+ and K^+, and the animals were killed.

Experiment 3A

Two groups of 6 five-week old female Brattleboro (DI) rats, homozygous for the responsible gene (di/di) and age-matched groups of Long-Evans (LE) rats were used. They had free access to Purina Laboratory Chow and tap water until one hour before the studies, when both were withdrawn.

Six of each strain received 30 mg/kg NIT in polyethylene glycol subcutaneously and the remainder received vehicle. Thirty minutes later they all received 30 mg/kg of a 0.45% NaCl and 0.25% KCl solution intraperitoneally. The procedure outlined in experiment 2 was followed thereafter.

Experiment 3B

The foregoing experiment was repeated, except that urine was collected for 6 hours.

Experiment 4A

In this experiment the respective groups were constituted and treated as in the foregoing, but the rats were given 30 ml/kg of an 0.7% NaCl solution. Groups 1 and 2 consisted of DI rats and 3 and 4 of age-matched LE. Each rat received an 0.2 ml injection of polyethylene glycol subcutaneously which, in groups 1 and 3, contained 15 mg/ml of NIT. Electrolyte solution was given i.p.

Experiment 4B

This was a repetition of the preceding experiment, excepting that the fluid volume administered was increased to 40 ml/kg.

Experiment 5A

Groups of 16 female SD rats weighing 150–175 g were used for each of the loading solutions employed in these studies. Eight received 30 mg/kg of NIT subcutaneously, the other the same volume of vehicle, and the solutions were given intraperitoneally immediately thereafter. A one hour period of food and water deprivation preceded the experiment. The first group of 16 received 30 mg/kg of an 0.9% NaCl solution, the second, one of 0.9% KCl, and the third, a 5.1% glucose solution. Urine was collected over a 6 hour period.

Experiment 5 B

The protocol and procedures were identical to those of the previous experiment except that a double-solute solution was used in each case. The first consisted of 0.45% NaCl and 2.55% glucose, the second of 0.45% NaCl and 0.45% KCl and the third of 0.45% KCl and 2.55% glucose.

In all of the foregoing studies "Student's" double-tailed "t" test for unpaired samples was used for statistical analysis.

Results

Experiment 1

The blood pressures of NIT-treated and control SHR were identical prior to pellet implantation. Thereafter until the 30th day of the experiment, when they might be considered as growth dependent, they rose in parallel in the two groups, albeit a few mm Hg lower in the implanted groups. By the 30th day, however, pressures in the two groups differed significantly. Although they continued to increase in untreated SHR, the treated group levelled off and remained normotensive. Between days 41 and 60 there were no pellet implantations, and although pressures

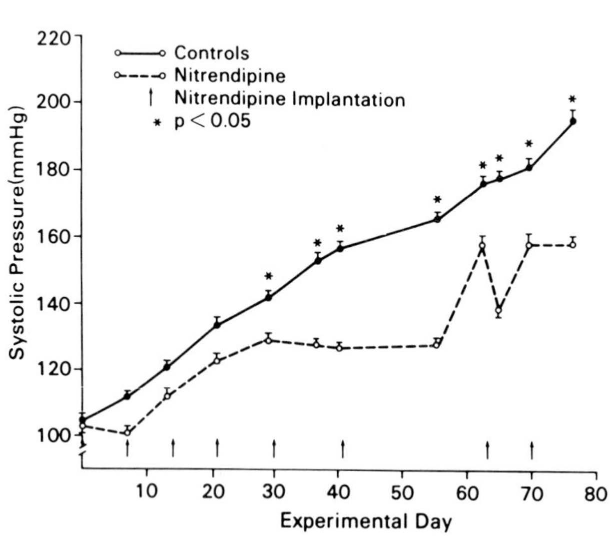

Fig. 1. Effect of nitrendipine pellet implantation on the development of hypertension in SHR. The *asterisks* indicate significant differences from control values ($P < 0.05$)

were still normal through day 56, they had risen sharply by day 62. Pellet implantation on this day caused a prompt fall in blood pressure, however, by day 70 pressures had again risen to the levels of day 62. Implantation of another pellet prevented a further rise, although it did not produce a further fall (Fig. 1). All of the pellets were recovered at autopsy.

Experiment 2

The systolic pressure of unprotected animals given DOCP+NaCl was significantly above that of NIT-treated or control rats, which were alike by the second week. Despite the fact no pellets had been implanted after the 21st day, the two had almost identical pressures on day 30. From that day onward the pressures diverged, and on day 42 they had risen considerably in the NIT-treated group. An implanatation on day 43 produced a distinctive decline within a day (Fig. 2). By day 48 they were again rising, and another pellet induced a slight drop. The pressures in NIT-treated rats exceeded that of untreated controls only on days 42 and 48, but never entered the hypertensive range.

Urinary studies on day 51 and 64 gave similar results. DOCP alone produced polyuria, excessive Na^+ excretion, an elevated Na^+/K^+, and urinary dilution. All of these were abolished by NIT. On the 61st day, but not on the 51st day, steroid-treated rats exhibited kaliuria, which was not modified by NIT. NIT had no effect on the hypernatremic and hypokalemic effect of steroid treatment (Table 1). All pellets were recovered at autopsy.

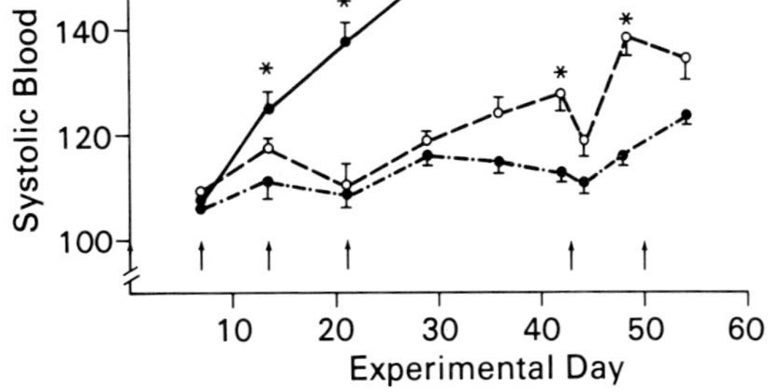

Fig. 2. Influence of implanted nitrendipine pellets on the course of DOC-salt hypertension. Significant differences from control values (P<0.05) are indicated by *asterisks*

Table 1. Effect of nitrendipine on urine volume and electrolyte excretion and serum Na^+ and K^+ of DOC-treated rats

Data	DOCP (N=7)	DOCP + Nitrendipine (N=7)	Controls (N=6)
	Day 51		
Urine, ml/kg/5 h	33.6 ± 8.9*[a]	16.2 ± 5.3	15.2 ± 5.6
Total Na^+	5.68 ± 0.90[a]	3.53 ± 0.40	2.82 ± 0.40
Total K^+ μmol/kg/5 h	1.93 ± 0.18	1.72 ± 0.08	1.60 ± 0.22
Na^+/K^+	3.00 ± 0.43[a]	2.02 ± 0.18	1.81 ± 0.20
	Day 61		
Urine, ml/kg/5 h	36.4 ± 4.8[a]	17.6 ± 4.2	15.4 ± 3.9
Osmolality, mosmol/kg	753 ± 57[a]	1,392 ± 158	1,391 ± 266
Total Na^+	8.41 ± 0.70[a]	4.72 ± 0.87	4.02 ± 0.74
Total K^+ μmol/kg/5 h	1.69 ± 0.19[a]	1.71 ± 0.06[b]	1.28 ± 0.19
Na^+/K^+	5.25 ± 0.59[a]	2.74 ± 0.45	3.18 ± 0.40
	Day 64		
Serum Na^+ mEq/L	145.4 ± 1.5[a]	143.5 ± 1.6[b]	139.2 ± 0.7
Serum K^+ mEq/L	3.3 ± 0.2[a]	3.1 ± 0.1[b]	4.6 ± 0.3
Na^+/K^+	44.1 ± 3.3[a]	46.3 ± 3.1[b]	30.3 ± 4.6

*Mean ± SEM
[a] Significantly different from controls ($P<0.05$)
[b] Significantly different from controls ($P<0.025$)

Experiment 3 A

NIT significantly increased urinary volume, but had no effect on the excretion of Na^+ or K^+, or on urine osmolality in LE rats. Control DI rats excreted much larger urine volumes than LE, and this was slightly but not significantly reduced by NIT treatment. The drug reduced Na^+ excretion considerably, and K^+ excretion less, reducing urinary Na^+/K^+. Urine osmolality was slightly, but not significantly, increased (Table 2 A).

Experiment 3 B

This experiment yielded the same results as the foregoing. In LE rats urine volume was increased by NIT, which had no significant effect on excretion of Na^+ or K^+ or on urine osmolatily. Control DI rats exhibited polyuria. NIT slightly decreased urine volume and Na^+ excretion. Na^+/K^+ fell, and urine osmolality rose (Table 2 B).

Table 2. Effect of nitrendipine on urinary volume, electrolyte excretion and osmolality in sodium and potassium loaded DI and LE rats

Data	DI Rats		LE Rats	
	Nitrendipine	Controls	Nitrendipine	Controls
A. Injectate = 30 ml/kg 0.45% NaCl + 0.25% KCl				
N	6	6	6	6
Urine, ml/kg/5 h	79.1 ± 7.1*	89.5 ± 7.5	23.4 ± 0.9[b]	15.8 ± 2.6
% injected vol.	265 ± 36	298 ± 24	78 ± 3[a]	52 ± 8
Na^+	2,248 ± 371[c]	4,256 ± 264	2,079 ± 302	1,855 ± 214
K^+ μMol/kg/5 h	3,611 ± 148[b]	4,618 ± 339	3,415 ± 347	3,280 ± 240
Na^+/K^+	0.67 ± 0.08[b]	0.93 ± 0.04	0.65 ± 0.14	0.56 ± 0.03
mMol/kg	370 ± 13[a]	303 ± 24	930 ± 42	1,138 ± 169
B. Injectate = 30 ml/kg 0.45% NaCl + 0.25% KCl				
N	6	6	6	6
Urine, ml/kg/6 h	73.3 ± 9.8	90.6 ± 8.3	36.2 ± 2.4[c]	17.8 ± 2.4
% injected vol.	228 ± 29	278 ± 27	104 ± 12[b]	61 ± 8
Na^+	3,551 ± 197[d]	5,699 ± 221	3,494 ± 197	2,829 ± 358
K^+ μMol/kg/6 h	4,992 ± 464	5,156 ± 288	4,500 ± 290	4,889 ± 221
Na^+/K^+	0.73 ± 0.17[d]	1.11 ± 0.05	0.70 ± 0.04	0.56 ± 0.06
mMol/kg	444 ± 18[c]	376 ± 10	1,251 ± 268	1,257 ± 160

* Mean ± SEM
[a] Significantly different from corresponding controls ($P<0.05$)
[b] Significantly different from corresponding controls ($P<0.025$)
[c] Significantly different from corresponding controls ($P<0.01$)
[d] Significantly different from corresponding controls ($P<0.001$)

Experiment 4 A

NIT increased urine volume and the total excretion of both Na^+ and K^+ in LE rats without affecting the Na^+/K^+. Urine osmolality was reduced. In DI rats urine volume was increased by NIT, but excretion of Na^+ and K^+ was not affected (Table 3 A).

Experiment 4 B

The effect of NIT in LE rats ws the same as in the previous experiment. Urine volume was increased and osmolality decreased. The excretion of Na^+ and K^+ was augmented, but Na^+/K^+ was not affected. In DI rats, NIT had no effect on electrolyte excretion, urine volume or osmolality (Table 3 B).

Experiment 5 A

When an 0.9% NaCl solution was given, NIT significantly increased urine volume, natriuresis and kaliuresis, and Na^+/K^+. Urine osmolality was not affected (Table 4).

Table 3. Effect of nitrendipine on urinary volume, electrolyte excretion and osmolality in sodium loaded DI and LE rats

Data	DI Rats		LE Rats	
	Nitrendipine	Controls	Nitrendipine	Controls
A. Injectate = 30 ml/kg 0.70% NaCl solution				
N	6	6	6	6
Urine, ml/kg/6 h	78.7 ± 2.8*[a]	64.3 ± 5.9	17.0 ± 1.4[d]	8.4 ± 1.2
% injected vol.	263 ± 11[a]	216 ± 20	57 ± 5[d]	28 ± 4
Na^+	4,635 ±405	3,805 ±346	2,102 ± 30[d]	1,335 ± 43
K^+ μMol/6 h	3,824 ±360	3,689 ±446	2,331 ± 39[d]	1,539 ± 62
Na^+/K^+	1.24 ± 0.15	1.06 ± 0.10	0.90 ± 0.01	0.87 ± 0.03
mMol/kg	320 ± 5[c]	367 ± 12	1,255 ± 74[d]	2,112 ± 41
B. Injectate = 40 ml/kg 0.70% NaCl solution				
N	6	6	6	6
Urine, ml/kg/6 h	81.4 ± 5.8	86.1 ± 4.0	34.8 ± 4.4[b]	16.0 ± 5.6
% injected vol.	203 ± 14	214 ± 10	87 ± 11[b]	40 ± 14
Na^+	4,560 ±522	6,517 ±430	4,902 ±559[d]	2,269 ±463
K^+ μMol/6 h	3,577 ±303	4,066 ±228	3,334 ±198[d]	2,210 ± 74
Na^+/K^+	1.28 ± 0.11	1.60 ± 0.14	1.46 ± 0.19	0.95 ± 0.16
mMol/kg	342 ± 17	335 ± 6	546 ± 57[d]	1,600 ±319

* Mean ± SEM
[a] Significantly different from corresponding controls ($P<0.05$)
[b] Significantly different from corresponding controls ($P<0.025$)
[c] Significantly different from corresponding controls ($P<0.01$)
[d] Significantly different from corresponding controls ($P<0.001$)

The 0.9% KCl solution markedly reduced Na^+ and increased K^+ excretion of controls as compared with those given the 0.9% NaCl solution, reducing Na^+/K^+. NIT had no effect on urine volume, electrolyte excretion or osmolality. Both osmolality and Na^+/K^+ were much lower in both groups than when 0.9% NaCl was given (Table 4).

A 5.1% glucose solution led to greater urine volume in controls than was found with either of the two previous solutions, but NIT had no effect on urine volume or osmolality. The latter was low and comparable to that seen when 0.9% KCl was given. Urinary Na^+ was reduced and urinary K^+ unchanged, but Na^+/K^+ fell (Table 4).

Experiment 5B

When NaCl + glucose solution was given, urine volume was intermediate between what it had been when either was given alone in a solution of the same osmolality. Nitrendipine reduced both Na^+ and K^+ excretion. Neither urinary Na^+/K^+ nor osmolality were affected (Table 5).

With the 0.45% NaCl and 0.45% KCl solution, NIT reduced urine volume and the excretion of both Na^+ and K^+. Urine osmolality was slightly but not sig-

Table 4. Effect of nitrendipine on urine composition of rats given single-solute solutions

Data	Nitrendipine-treated	Controls
Injectate: 30 ml/kg of 0.9% NaCl		
N	8	8
Urine vol. ml/kg/6 h	24.4 ± 2.2[c]*	16.8 ± 1.0
As % of injected vol.	82 ± 7[b]	56 ± 3
Osmolality (mMol/kg)	1,128 ±111	1,388 ± 71
Na^+	3,355 ±248[c]	2,126 ±197
K^+ μMols/kg/6 h	3,655 ±156[a]	3,151 ±171
Na^+/K^+	0.92± 0.05[b]	0.66± 0.07
Injectate: 30 ml/kg of 0.9% KCl		
N	8	8
Urine vol. ml/kg/6 h	28.0 ± 2.5	26.2± 1.1
As % of injected vol.	93 ± 8	87 ± 4
Osmolality (mMol/kg)	695 ± 45	738 ± 32
Na^+	564 ±186	441 ±187
K^+ μMols/kg/6 h	4,352 ±313	4,775 ±200
Na^+/K^+	0.12± 0.04	0.07± 0.03
Injectate: 30 ml/kg of 5.1% glucose		
N	8	8
Urine vol. ml/kg/6 h	44.9 ± 8.0	41.3 ± 5.5
As % of injected vol.	149 ± 27	139 ± 2.1
Osmolality (mMol/kg)	534 ± 33	618 ± 53
Na^+	1,227 ±311[a]	2,072 ±289
K^+ μMols/kg/6 h	2,451 ±283	2,489 ±244
Na^+/K^+	0.49± 0.09[b]	0.97± 0.13

* Mean ± SEM
[a] Significantly different from controls ($P<0.05$)
[b] Significantly different from controls ($P<0.025$)
[c] Significantly different from controls ($P<0.005$)

nificantly reduced, and since Na^+ excretion was depressed more than that of K^+, Na^+/K^+ fell (Table 5).

NIT increased urine volume, decreased osmolality and K^+ excretion when the 0.45% KCl+2.55% glucose solution was given. The Na^+ excretion of controls was lowest in this instance than had been seen with either of the other solutions, but was not affected by NIT. Decreased K^+ excretion led to increased Na^+/K^+ (Table 5).

A summary of NIT effects in experiments 5 and 6 is given in Fig. 3.

Discussion

Both spontaneous and DOC-salt hypertension in rats were effectively prevented by subcutaneous implantation of NIT pellets, and in the latter model development of the "diabetes insipidus-like" syndrome was also obviated, but not ste-

Table 5. Effect of nitrendipine on urine composition of rats given double-solute solutions

Data	Nitrendipine-treated	Controls
Injectate: 30 ml/kg 0.45% NaCl+2.55% glucose		
N	8	8
Urine vol. ml/kg/6 h	36.0 ± 4.5*	33.8 ± 2.4
As of injected vol.	119 ± 15	113 ± 8
Osmolality (mMol/kg)	758 ± 93	816 ± 56
Na^+	2,069 ±357[c]	3,407 ±206
K^+ µMols/kg/6 h	3,319 ±210[a]	4,071 ±521
Na^+/K^+	0.72 ± 0.12	0.90 ± 0.06
Injectate: 30 ml/kg 0.45% NaCl+0.45% KCl		
N	8	8
Urine vol. ml/kg/6 h	24.3 ± 2.0[c]	39.6 ± 4.2
As % injected vol.	81 ± 7[c]	132 ± 14
Osmolality (mMol/kg)	983 ± 91	796 ± 49
Na^+	1,293 ±245[c]	3,874 ±521
K^+ µMols/kg/6 h	4,490 ±133[c]	6,074 ±277
Na^+/K^+	0.30 ± 0.04[c]	0.63 ± 0.07
Injectate: 30 ml/kg 0.45% KCl+2.55% glucose		
N	8	8
Urine vol. ml/kg/6 h	33.2 ± 2.3[a]	25.5 ± 2.4
As % injected vol.	110 ± 7[a]	85 ± 8
Osmolality (mMol/kg)	558 ± 38[b]	847 ± 94
Na^+	291 ± 95	299 ±124
K^+ µMols/kg/6 h	2,922 ±253[b]	3,889 ±290
Na^+/K^+	0.11 ± 0.03	0.06 ± 0.02

* Mean ± SEM
[a] Significantly different from controls ($P<0.05$)
[b] Significantly different from controls ($P<0.025$)
[c] Significantly different from controls ($P<0.01$)

Fluid Administered	U_V	U_{Na}	U_K	$U_{Na/K}$	U_{OSM}
0.9 % NaCl	↑	↑	↑	↑	↔
0.9 % KCl	↔	↔	↔	↔	↔
5.1 % Glucose	↔	↓	↔	↓	↔
0.45% NaCl + 0.45% KCl	↓	↓	↓	↓	↔
0.45% NaCl + 2.55% Glucose	↔	↓	↓	↔	↔
0.45% KCl + 2.55% Glucose	↑	↔	↓	↔	↓

Fig. 3. Influence of nitrendipine on urine characteristics as affected by chemical composition of the fluid load administered

roid-induced hypernatremia and hypokalemia. This suggests a renal site of action. Such pellets were well tolerated, causing no detectable local injury.

A natriuretic action of NIT was confirmed for two strains of rat when 0.9% or 0.7% NaCl solution constituted the volume overload, but did not occur in normal rats when either 0.45% NaCl+0.25% KCl, 0.9% KCl or 5.1% glucose was used instead. The solutions containing only NaCl also caused polyuria in normal rats and usually lowered urine osmolality. In DI rats NIT caused antinatriuresis when 0.45% NaCl+0.25% KCl was used, and urine osmolality was slightly increased, but had no effect on Na^+ excretion when 0.7% NaCl was infused. When 0.9% KCl was the loading solution, the drug had no effect on urine composition of normal rats and when 5.1% glucose was employed antinatriuresis resulted, even though urine volume did not change. In rats given 0.45% KCl+0.45% NaCl or 0.45% KCl+2.55% glucose, NIT reduced the excretion of urine, Na^+ and K^+ in the first instance, and had the same effect on electrolyte excretion without modifying urine volume in the second.

Since NIT had an antinatriuretic effect in DOC-salt hypertensive rats; in DI rats loaded with 0.45% NaCl and 0.25% KCl; and in normal rats loaded with 5.1% glucose, NaCl+glucose or NaCl+KCl, it can not be considered as natriuretic in the same sense as sodium diuretic drugs. Positive effects were limited to conditions where only NaCl loading was employed, and were accompanied by increased urine volume. These are separable, since polyuria resulted when KCl+glucose was used without concurrent natriuresis.

Acknowledgements. These studies were supported by grants from Miles Laboratories, Inc. and the National Institutes of Health (HL09911). The authors are indebted to Dr. Alexander Scriabine of Miles Laboratories, Inc. for generous supplies of nitrendipine.

References

1. Hiwatani M, Taira N (1979) Antihypertensive effect of niludipine (Bay a 7168) on conscious renal hypertensive dogs. Arzneim Forsch 29:1373–1376
2. Kazda S, Garthoff B, Dycka J, Iwai J (1982) Prevention of malignant hypertension in salt-loaded "S" Dahl rats with the calcium antagonist nifedipine. Clin Exper Hyper 44:1231–1241
3. Fleckenstein A, Fleckenstein-Grün G (1980) Cardiovascular protection by Ca antagonists. Eur Heart J 1(Suppl B):15–21
4. Hall CE, Hungerford S (1983) Prevention of spontaneous and glucocorticoid hypertension in rats by nisoldipine. Physiol Behav 30:899–903
5. Hansson L, Andrén L, Orö L, Rymen T (1983) Pharmacokinetic and pharmacodynamic parameters in patients treated with nitrendipine. Hypertension 5(Part 2):25–28
6. Guazzi M, Olivari MT, Polese A, Fiorentini C, Magrini F, Moruzzi P (1979) Nifedipine, a new antihypertensive with rapid action. Clin Pharmacol Ther 22:528–532
7. Lewis GRJ, Morley KD, Lewis BM, Bones PJ (1978) The treatment of hypertension with verapamil. N Z Med J 87:351–354
8. Leary WP, Asmal AC (1979) Treatment of hypertension with verpamil. Curr Ther Res 25:747–752
9. Garthoff B, Kazda S, Knorr A (1982) Nitrendipine increases sodium excretion in acutely saline loaded rats. Biochem Pharmacol 31:3015–3016
10. DiBona GF, Sawin LL (1984) Renal tubular site of action of felodipine. J Pharmacol Exp Ther 228:420–424

11. Morita H, Nasao T, Yabana H, Yamaguchi I (1983) Hypertensive and diuretic action of diltiazem in spontaneously hypertensive and Wistar-Kyoto rats. J Pharmacol Exp Ther 227:472–477
12. Gomez-Sanchez CE, Holland OB, Higgins JR, Mathieu R, Gruber M, Kaplan NM (1976) Mineralocorticoid activity of 16 β hydroxy-dehydroepiandrosterone and related steroids. J Lab Clin Med 88:571–577
13. Hall CE, Gomez-Sanchez CE, Hungerford S, Gomez-Sanches EP (1981) Mineralocorticoid and hypertensive properties of 19-nor progesterone. Endocrinology 109:1168–1175
14. Hall CE, Hungerford S (1982) Inhibition of DOC-salt and adrenal-regeneration hypertension with the calcium blocker nifedipine. Clin Exper Hypertension 4:1217–1230

Discussion

(pp. 423–434)

Garthoff: I am a little bit confused about your results in the Brattleboro rat strain of Long-Evans rats. Is there any possibility to get an idea of whether nitrendipine is anti-natriuretic or anti-diuretic in these rats like diuretics in diabetes insipidus?

Hall: All I can say is that we got variable responses depending on the solution that was administered, antidiuresis in some cases, diuresis in others, but we don't have a detailed analysis, we cannot predict the effect. When sodium is given as a sole cation, even when it is given in hypotonic solution as with the 0.7% NaCl-solution everything goes up, increased urine volume, increased sodium, increased potassium. When you give the other solutions, the result is not predictable.

Bühler: The addition of glucose, increases sodium reabsorption in the proximal tubule and this has been shown by Early a number of years ago.

Hall: But why should nitrendipine increase this? When you give glucose you probably get glucosuria, we did not test for that, but it is very probable. If you do, you undoubtedly would get a much increased urine volume and you might get a sodium washout effect in controls, too.

Scriabine: Did you test any of the thiazide diuretics under similar conditions? Is the nitrendipine effect similar to that of thiazide diuretics in rats with diabetes insipidus?

Hall: Thiazide diuretics do not do much in the Brattleboro rat, for they have such a severe polyuria anyway. But we have not tested thiazide diuretic against any of the dihydropyridines for urinary effects.

Steen: Isn't it hard to say much from these experiments when you don't know what the glomerular filtration rate is? We have published studies that show that Ca^{2+} is a very effective blocker of sodium reuptake in the distal tubule, as you block sodium-potassium ATPase.

Hall: I admit one would like to have all of that data. Everyone agrees that dihydropyridines cause vasodilation in the reno-vascular circulation. Whatever you get increased or decreased renal blood flow depends on how much vasodilation you get in other vascular beds. If you get enough vasodilation elsewhere you will impair the renal vascular system and reduce renal blood flow, whereas if the other vascular beds are not comparably reduced then you get increased renal blood flow. And what will finally determine the electrolyte effects will be the renal blood flow, the glomerular filtration rate on the one hand the tubular reabsorption capacity in the other, and that means that in each you have to study the renal blood flow, which we have not done.

Bayer-Symposium IX
Cardiovascular Effects of Dihydropyridine-Type
Calcium Antagonists and Agonists, 437–442

The Use of Calcium Antagonists in the Treatment of Arterial Hypertension

G. Leonetti, L. Sampieri, C. Cuspidi, M. Fruscio, R. Gradnik, L. Terzoli, L. Rupoli, and A. Zanchetti

It is well known that an increase of total peripheral resistances is responsible of the blood pressure elevation in the majority of hypertensive patients [1–3]; for this reason vasodilating drugs should theoretically be preferred to other antihypertensive drugs with different mechanisms of action. Despite this pathophysiological consideration, the use of the vasodilating drugs has been very limited in antihypertensive treatment in the past due to the occurrence of two side effects interfering with their efficacy and reducing the patient's compliance. These side effects are sodium and water retention and reflex activation of the sympathetic nervous system [4, 5].

Under these aspects, the new class of vasodilating agents, represented by calcium antagonists, seems to differ from previous vasodilators such as hydralazine, minoxidil, guancydine and diazoxide [6], and in this paper we shall evaluate the clinical usefulness of these drugs by considering their antihypertensive efficacy, their effect on sodium and water balance and the degree of reflex activation of the sympathetic nervous system they may induce.

Acute Study. In 14 patients with moderate essential hypertension we have compared the acute antihypertensive effects, the sodium and water excretion and the degree of sympathetic nervous system activation after the oral administration of a single dose of nifedipine (10 mg) and verapamil (160 mg) [7]. The data are summarized in Fig. 1.

Both nifedipine and verapamil significantly reduced supine systolic and diastolic blood pressure, when compared to the blood pressure levels of the placebo period. Although the blood pressure reductions were of similar degree, the blood pressure lowering was more prompt after nifedipine (peak effect after 30–60 min) than after verapamil (peak effect reached at the 4th h).

30 and 60 min after nifedipine administration there was a short-lasting increase of heart rate, while after verapamil there was a trend toward a heart rate decrease: if we consider the heart rate changes as an indirect sign of reflex activation of the sympathetic nervous system we should admit that only nifedipine caused some activation of the sympathetic nervous system.

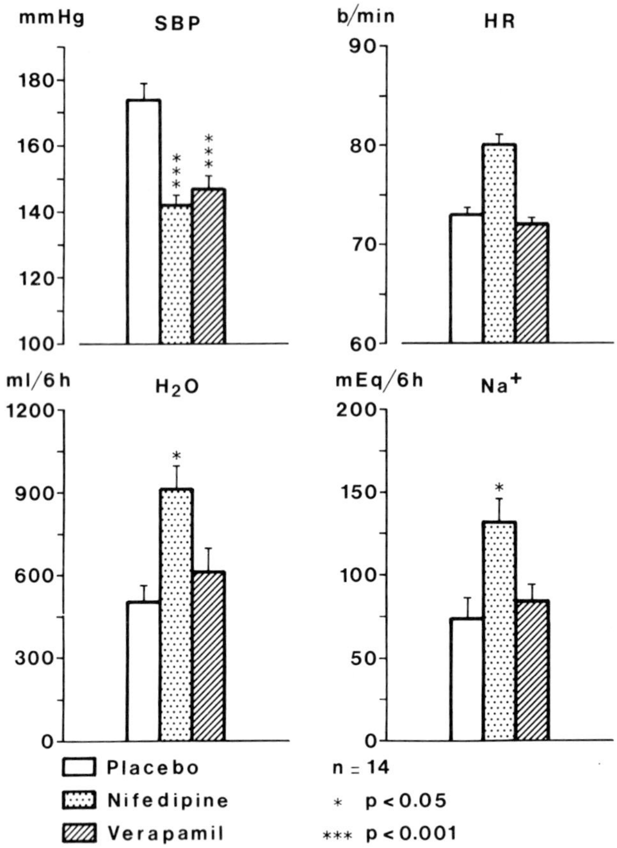

Fig. 1. Supine systolic blood pressure and heart rate values and 6-h urine and sodium excretion in 14 essential hypertensive patients during placebo, nifedipine or verapamil administration (means ± SE)

The measurement of plasma catecholamines confirms that only after oral administration of nifedipine there was a transient and significant increase in plasma noradrenaline (pretreatment 216 ± 14 pg/ml, treatment 302 ± 20 pg/ml, $p < 0.05$) which was coincident with the peak rise of heart rate. No change of plasma noradrenaline was observed after verapamil administration.

During the 6 h following administration of both calcium antagonists there was an increase in urine volume and sodium excretion, which was however statistically significant only after nifedipine administration. There was no change of creatinine clearance after verapamil and nifedipine administration and this suggests that also in man calcium antagonists may increase sodium excretion through a direct tubular action, as it has been shown in animal experiments [8–11].

Our study, in agreement with other publications [12, 13], indicate that both verapamil and nifedipine acutely decrease blood pressure in hypertensive patients and this blood pressure reduction does not cause sodium retention, while the reflex activation of the sympathetic nervous system is mild or absent.

Short-Term Study. In 3 different short-term studies in hospitalized patients we have evaluated the antihypertensive and renal effects of 3 different calcium antagonists: verapamil, nifedipine and felodipine.

1) After a placebo run-in period, verapamil [14] was orally administered to 12 patients with essential hypertension of moderate degree at a dose of 80 mg tid for 5 days; thereafter the dose was increased to 160 mg tid for another 5 day period, if diastolic blood pressure was still above 95 mm Hg, or otherwise it remained unmodified. The lower dose of verapamil significantly reduced supine and upright blood pressure (Fig. 2) and a further blood pressure reduction was observed when the dose of verapamil was increased. Despite the blood pressure reduction, there was no concomitant change of supine and upright heart rate.

As far as, sodium balance is concerned (expressed as average of 5-day sodium excretion), we have found a slight increase of sodium output during the first 5-day period (baseline 107 ± 15 mmol/24 h; 1st period 113 ± 15 mmol/24 h) which was however back to control value during the second 5 days period. No significant changes of potassium and urine volume were found.

2) Olivari et al. [5] in another short term study with Nifedipine 10 mg q.i.d. have shown that the antihypertensive effect observed acutely, during the 1st and 2nd day of treatment, was still present or slightly augmented after 20 days of therapy. An increase of the heart rate was found only the first hour following Nifedipine administration: the average daily heart rate was however unchanged.

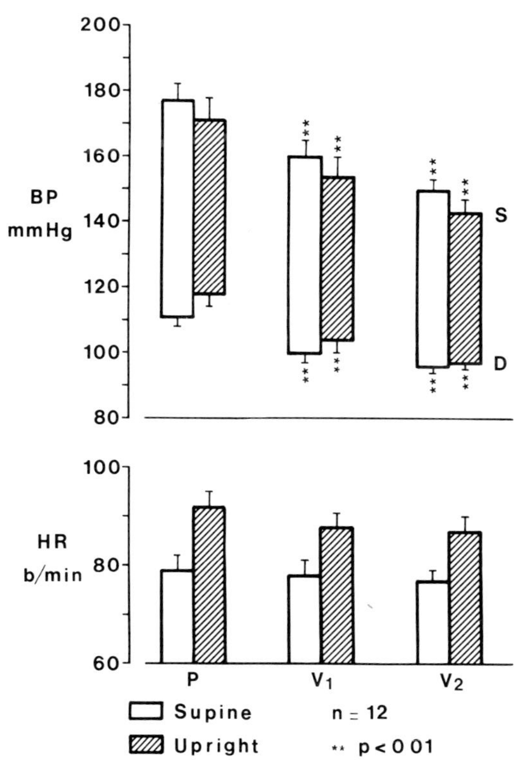

Fig. 2. Supine and upright blood pressure and heart rate in 12 essential hypertensive patients during placebo and after 5 (V1) and 10 (V2) days of verapamil treatment (means ± SE)

There was an increase of urine volume during the 1st day of Nifedipine administration which was back to control value in the remaining part of the study.

3) Recently we have investigated in 9 patients with mild or moderate essential hypertension, the antihypertensive efficacy and the water and sodium effect of a new dihydropyridine derivative, felodipine, administered as tablet of 10 mg bid. Supine and upright blood pressures were already significantly reduced during the first day of oral treatment and the blood pressure reduction was slightly increased in the 1st day of felodipine and to a minor extent thereafter. The sodium output was increased during the 1st and 2nd day of felodipine administration and the negative sodium balance was maintained in the following days. After the withdrawal of felodipine there was a slow progressive rise of blood pressure toward the pretreatment values which were reached after 5 days.

From these studies it appears that the antihypertensive effects of the calcium antagonists found during the first day of therapy is still present or slightly increased in the following days and that reflex activation of the sympathetic nervous system and sodium and water retention do not represent relevant side effects of this class of drugs. For some of the previously available vasodilators, such as minoxidil, guancydine and diazoxide there were already signs of sodium retention after 5–7 days of therapy.

Chronic Studies. There are many aspects of the clinical response to a new antihypertensive drug that can be considered for assessing its therapeutic role: the blood pressure reduction and the incidence and importance of side effects are among the most important aspects to be considered especially in comparison to other antihypertensive drugs.

For this purpose in a chronic out-patient study we have investigated [16, 17] the clinical usefulness of verapamil, by comparing its antihypertensive efficacy and adverse reactions with those of a well established beta-adrenergic blocker, propranolol. In 31 patients with mild or moderate hypertension, verapamil and propranolol, at the doses we have investigated, were equipotent in reducing supine and upright systolic and diastolic blood pressure (Fig. 3). On the contrary, heart rate was significantly reduced during propranolol therapy, while no change was found during verapamil administration (Fig. 3).

Monotherapy with diuretics, beta-blockers and converting enzyme inhibitors normalizes or significantly reduces blood pressure in 40–60% of patients with mild or moderate hypertension. The recently published studies of Corea et al. [18], Wicker et al. [19] and MacInnes et al. [20] on verapamil confirm a similar percentage of success with verapamil monotherapy. According to these authors the association of verapamil with diuretics or beta-blockers significantly increases the percentage of blood pressure normalization.

Nitrendipine, a new dihydropyridine derivative, has been shown in chronic studies by Muller et al. [21] and Ruddel et al [22] to normalize blood pressure levels of patients with mild or moderate hypertension in a percentage similar to or slightly greater than other monotherapy treatments. At variance from what has been claimed by McGregor et al. [23], the association of a diuretic to nitrendipine caused a significant further blood pressure reduction [22]. According to Weber et al. [24] and Nannan et al. [25] the association of nitrendipine and beta-blocker was also very effective clinically.

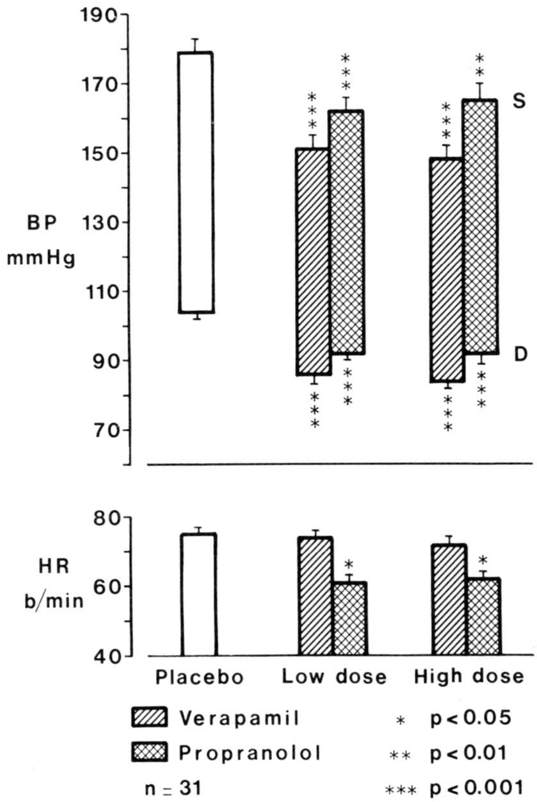

Fig. 3. Comparison on supine blood pressure and heart rate in 31 essential hypertensive patients after low and high doses of verapamil (80 and 160 mg t.i.d.) and propranolol (60 and 120 mg t.i.d.) (means ± SE)

Conclusions

1) Calcium antagonists significantly lower blood pressure in hypertensive patients without clinically relevant signs of reflex sympathetic activation and water and sodium retention, phenomena which have limited the clinical use of previously available direct vasodilators.

2) The frequency by which calcium antagonists can normalize blood pressure during chronic treatment is not different from that observed with the use of other antihypertensive agents.

References

1. Lund-Johansen P (1980) Hemodynamics in essential hypertension. State of art: review. Clin Sci 59:343s
2. Frolich ED, Tarazi RC, Dustan HP (1969) Re-examination of the hemodynamics of hypertension. Am J Med Sci 257:9
3. Conway J (1984) Hemodynamic aspects of essential hypertension in humans. Physiol Rev 64:617
4. Koch-Weser J (1979) Vasodilator drugs in treatment of hypertension. Arch Int Med 113:1017

5. Leonetti G, Bonazzi O, Grazi S, Ligresti A, Romano S, Zanchetti A (1971) Cardiovascular and renal effects of acute administration of a new antihypertensive compound: guancydine. Eur J Pharmacol 4:1
6. Gross F (1977) Drugs acting on arteriolar smooth muscle (vasodilator drugs). In: F. Gross (ed) Antihypertensive agents. Springer Berlin Heidelberg New York, pp 397–476
7. Leonetti G, Cuspidi C, Sampieri L, Terzoli L, Zanchetti A (1982) Comparison of cardiovascular, renal and humoral effects of acute administration of two calcium channel blockers in normotensive and hypertensive subjects. J Cardiovasc Pharmacol 4:319
8. Brown B, Churchill P (1983) Renal effects of methoxy-verapamil in anesthetized rats. J Pharmacol Exp Ther 225:372
9. Dietz IR, Davis JO, Freeman RH, Villareal D, Echtenkamp SF (1983) Effects of intrarenal infusion of calcium entry blockers in anesthetized dogs. Hypertension 5:482
10. Marre M, Misumi R, Raemsch KD, Corvol P, Menard J (1982) Diuretic and natriuretic effects of nifedipine in isolated perfused rat kidneys. J Pharmacol Exp Ther 223:263
11. Di Bona GF, Sawin LL (1984) Renal tubular site of action of felodipine. J Pharmacol Exp Ther 228:420
12. Doyle AE, Anavekar SN, Oliver LE (1980) A clinical trial of verapamil in the treatment of hypertension. In: A. Zanchetti, D.M. Krikler (eds) Calcium antagonism in cardiovascular therapy: experience with verapamil. Excerpta Medica, Amsterdam pp 252–259
13. Lederballe-Pederson O (1983) The experimental use of calcium antagonists in the treatment of arterial hypertension. Postgrad Med J 59 (Suppl 2):84
14. Leonetti G, Sala C, Bianchini C, Terzoli L, Zanchetti A (1980) Antihypertensive and renal effects of orally administered verapamil. Eur J Clin Pharmacol 18:375
15. Olivari MT, Bartorelli C, Polese A, Fiorentini C, Guazzi M (1979) Treatment of hypertension with nifedipine, a calcium antagonist agent. Circulation 59:1056
16. Leonetti G, Pasotti C, Ferrari GP, Zanchetti A (1980) Double blind comparison of the antihypertensive effects of verapamil and propranolol. In: Zanchetti A, Krikler DM (eds) Calcium antagonism in cardiovascular therapy: experience with verapamil. Excerpta Medica, Amsterdam pp 260–269
17. Leonetti G, Pasotti C, Ferrari GP, Zanchetti A (1984) Verapamil and propranolol: a comparison of two antihypertensive agents. Acta Med Scand Suppl 681:137
18. Corea L, Bentivoglio M, Verdecchia P, Providenza M (1984) Calcium antagonists and diuretics in arterial hypertension: a useful combination. J Roy Soc Med 62:23
19. Wicher P, Roudaut R, Gosse P, Dall'Occhio M (1984) Short and long-term treatment of mild to moderate hypertension with verapamil. J Roy Soc Med 62:45
20. MacInnes GF, Findlay I, Murray GD, Dargie HJ (1984) Calcium antagonists and beta-blockers. J Roy Soc Med 62:69
21. Muller FB, Bolli P, Erne P, Block LH, Kiowski W, Bühler FR (1984) Antihypertensive therapy with long-acting calcium antagonist nitrendipine. J Cardiovasc Pharmacol 6 (Suppl 7):1073s
22. Rüddel H, Schmieder R, Lagenwitz W, Neus J, Wagner O, Wilhelm von Eiff A (1984) Efficacy of nitrendipine as baseline antihypertensive therapy. J Cardiovasc Pharmacol 6 (Suppl 7):1049s
23. MacGregor G, Rotellar C, Markandu ND, Smith SJ, Sagnella GA (1982) Contrasting effects of nifedipine, captopril and proranolol in normotensive and hypertensive subjects. J Cardiovasc Pharmacol 4 (Suppl 2):358s
24. Weber MA, Drayer JIM (1984) The calcium channel blocker nitrendipine in single and mulitple-agent antihypertensive regimens: preliminary report of a multicenter study. J Cardiovasc Pharmacol 6 (Suppl 7):1077s
25. Nannan ME, Melin JA, Vanbutsele RJ, Lavenne F, Detry JMR (1984) Acute and long-term effects of nitrendipine on resting and exercise hemodynamics in essential hypertension. J Cardiovasc Pharmacol 6 (Suppl 7):1043s

Discussion

(pp. 437–442)

Garthoff: Have you measured changes in aldosterone in your short-term study with felodipine which could account for the step-wise increase in potassium excretion?

Leonetti: Although, the evaluation of the study is still on the way the preliminary results show a slight increase of plasma aldosterone but this does not justify the increased potassium excretion: serum potassium was unchanged despite the slight kaliuresis.

Bühler: It is interesting to note that one only has to lose some 80–100 mmol of sodium and one does not develop sodium retention. All one needs in terms of diuresis with the Ca^{2+}-antagonist is to get rid of some 6–8 grams of salt.

Kazda: Is there some rebound sodium retention in patients after interruption of the Ca^{2+}-antagonist treatment?

Leonetti: In our study with felodipine there was a follow-up period of 5 days after the withdrawal of felodipine. We have seen no signs of sodium retention, but also the blood pressure rise toward pretreatment values was very slow and only after 5 days the recovery of blood pressure was complete.

Bühler: There is some discussion as to whether the addition of a diuretic adds much to the anti-hypertensive response. Dr. McGregor has not gained much by adding a diuretic to a Ca^{2+}-antagonist. You said the effect is significant, but what does it mean practically?

Leonetti: The data I have presented concerning the effects of adding diuretics or beta-blockers to verapamil or nifedipine, are taken from literature: In the work of Corea et al. I have referred to, there was a further lowering of 10 mm Hg or more of systolic and diastolic blood pressure when a diuretic was added to verapamil and this is also my own clinical experience when a diuretic is added to verapamil to nifedipine.

Bühler: If I interpret your data correctly, there really is not much to choose between verapamil and any of the dihydropyridines, if it comes to antihypertensive efficacy. Is that correct?

Leonetti: Your interpretation of my data is correct: indeed we have not found a significant difference in the antihypertensive efficacy between verapamil and nifedipine. When I select a Ca^{2+}-antagonist for the treatment of hypertension, the choice between verapamil or nifedipine is based on the specific contra-indications and the nature and incidence of side effects of each drug.

Bayer-Symposium IX
Cardiovascular Effects of Dihydropyridine-Type
Calcium Antagonists and Agonists, 445–453

Calcium Antagonists for Identification of Mechanisms and Treatment in Patients with Essential Hypertension*

F. R. Bühler, P. Bolli, W. Kiowski, F. B. Müller, and P. Erne

Summary

The sympathetic nervous activity contributes to the pathophysiology of essential hypertension in an early phase and in younger patients mainly through increased beta-adrenoceptor-mediated functions and in a later phase and in older patients in whom beta-adrenoceptor-mediated functions are blunted, through increased alpha-adrenoceptor-mediated and calcium influx-dependent vasoconstriction. Intracellular free calcium concentration is elevated in platelets of hypertensive patients and relates directly to the height of their blood pressure, likely reflecting increased intracellular calcium concentration in vascular smooth muscle cells. A sympathetic factor is suggested further by the enhanced alpha-1 and alpha-2-adrenoceptor-mediated and calcium influx-dependent vasoconstriction both of which are normalized by antihypertensive treatment in parallel with a normalization of intracellular free calcium and of the increased adrenaline sensitivity of latelets. The higher sensitivity to adrenaline for thrombin-induced calcium increase in platelets of hypertensive patients indicates potentiation of calcium influx (and mobilization from intracellular stores) by adrenaline, a mechanism that is mediated by alpha-2-adrenoceptors. As this effect is more pronounced in younger patients increased adenylate cyclase sensitivity may prevail in the early and alterations in calcium influx-dependent mechanisms in the later phase of essential hypertension. The transition into a hypertensive state with reduced reflex cardiovascular counter-regulation co-determines the antihypertensive effectiveness of calcium antagonists in these patients.

Introduction

The pathophysiology of essential hypertention is characterized by different development phases. In an early stage in offspring of hypertensive patients or in borderline hypertensives beta-adrenoceptor-mediated cardiovascular responses, i.e.

* This work was supported by grant No 3.807.080 from the Swiss National Foundation

heart rate [1, 2], exercise tachycardia [1] and hence cardiac output as well as plasma renin activity [3] and renin responsiveness [4] are augmented. Individuals with borderline hypertension have higher noradrenaline concentrations than normotensive controls when exposed to mental and physical stress and higher noradrenaline concentrations are associated with disturbed aggressive behavior [5, 6].

In the later phase of hypertension beta-adrenoceptor-mediated effects tend to be blunted which relates to a change in beta-adrenoceptors with age. Accordingly, excersise-induced tachycardia and heart rate response to isoproterenol are reduced [1, 7, 8], plasma renin activity is normal or low [3, 9] and hyporesponsive to sympathetic stimuli [4, 10], and peripheral vasodilator response to beta-adrenoceptor stimulation is diminished [11, 12]. With blunting of beta-adrenoceptor-mediated functions alpha-adrenoceptor-mediated vasoconstriction relatively prevails. Hence, the established phase of essential hypertension is characterized by an elevated peripheral vascular resistance to which enhanced postjunctional alpha-1 and alpha-2-adrenoceptor-mediated [13, 14] and calcium influx-dependent vasoconstriction may be operated to a great extent through postjunctional alpha-1 and alpha-2-adrenoceptors and this may lead to increased intracellular free calcium concentration in vascular smooth muscle cell as reflected by an increased calcium concentration in platelets of patients with essential hypertension [16]. Decreased beta-adrenoceptor-mediated functions in the later phase of essential hypertension appear not to be the result of a change in receptor number or their affinity [17, 18] and therefore reduced beta-adrenoceptor responses associated with older age and higher pressure are more likely due to alterations distal to the receptor site. In established essential hypertension plasma adrenaline concentrations are elevated in at least one third of patients [1, 2, 19, 20] at rest as well as during physical excersise [1, 2] or cold pressure test [21] whereas no difference beween normotensives and hypertensives was found for noradrenaline [1, 22] but which in contrast to adrenaline tended to increase with age [1, 22, 23].

The transition from an early phase of essential hypertension where beta-adrenoceptor-mediated functions prevail to a later one where alpha-adrenoceptor-mediated and calcium influx-dependent vasoconstriction dominates determines the pharmacotherapeutic approach to essential hypertension. The former types f patients respond best to beta-adrenoceptor-blockade [20, 24] and in the latter alpha-adrenoceptor-blocking drugs [25] and particularly calcium antagonists are most effective [26], in part because cardiovascular homeostatic reflex counter-regulation is less likely evoked consequent to the fall in blood pressure.

Intracellular Calcium and Blood Pressure

Free calcium concentration determines tension development in the vascular smooth muscle cell [28]. Platelets of patients with essential hypertension have a igher cytosolic free calcium concentration when compared with normotensive subjects and free cytosolic calcium concentration is directly related to the height of blood pressure [16]. As platelets and smooth muscle cells have a number of common features, i.e. an alpha-2-adrenoceptor cyclase system [29] and a calcium-dependent contraction-coupling mechanism [30] platelets may serve as a model or the vascular smooth muscle cell. Elevated intracellular free calcium concentrations were also found in erythrocytes of hypertensive patients [31] but barely in lymphocytes [32]. Calcium overload has also been reported in adipocytes of patients with essential hypertension and spontaneously hypertensive rats [33] suggesting the possibility of a more generalized mishandling of calcium in hypertension.

Elevated cytosolic free calcium concentration in patients with essential hypertension can occur as a consequence of increased calcium influx due to a defect in membrane permeability [34] or in ionic membrane pump mechanism(s) [35, 36]. Accordingly, elevated basal calcium ATPase activity observed in platelets of patients with essential hypertension [37] may counter the elevated intracellular calcium concentration by increased calcium extrusion. On the other hand, a defective calcium extrusion from the cell as found in membranes of vascular smooth muscle cells and erythrocytes of genetically hypertensive rats [38, 39] and patients with essential hypertension [37] could represent a further means of increasing intracellular calcium concentration. Abnormalities in the plasma membrane of vascular smooth muscle [40, 41], cardiomyocytes [41], erythrocytes [42–44], hepatocytes and synaptosomes [42, 45] have been described in spontaneously hypertensive rats. The possibility of a generalized membrane defect linked to calcium transport is suggested by the decreased ability of these cells to bind calcium on the inner surface of the plasma membrane [34].

Adrenoceptor Mechanisms Leading to Eleveated Intracellular Calcium

Elevated plasma adrenaline concentrations as a marker of adrenergic activity have been reported in about one third of patients with essential hypertension [1, 2, 19, 20] and thus increased adrenergic activity could be pathophysiologically important in essential hypertension. Adrenaline by stimulating the alpha-2-adrenoceptor causes vasoconstriction [14, 46] and initiates, mainly by contributing to other platelet activating agents, shape change and aggregation of platelets [29]. Incubation of platelets with adrenaline alone does not induce an immediate change in free calcium concentration but potentiates the thrombin-induced increase in intracellular calcium demonstrating a complex mechanism for adrenaline induced activation of platelets. PGI_2 counteracts the thrombin-induced in free calcium concentration by intracellular calcium sequestration. This antagonizing effect of PGI_2 on thrombin-induced increase in free calcium concentration could be overcome by smaller doses of adrenaline in platelets of patients with essential hypertension than in those from normotensive subjects demonstrating a greater sensitivity to adrenaline of platelets from hypertensive patients [47] and this suggests a potentiation of the thrombin-induced calcium influx and mobilisation from internal stores by adrenaline in patients with essential hypertension. The sensitivity of the intracellular calcium elevation-response to adrenaline and thrombin is greater in younger (below the age of 40) hypertensives while there is no age related difference in platelets from normotensive subjects [47]. Since yohimbine was able to prevent this effect this appears to be a specific action of adrenaline on the alpha-2-adrenoceptors.

Increased sensitivity to adrenaline of platelets from patients with essential hypertension lends support to the contribution of the adrenergic nervous system to the pathophysiology of essential hypertension. As this effect is more pronounced in younger patients this suggests an increased adenylate cyclase sensitivity in the early phase of essential hypertension whereas alterations in calcium influx-dependent mechanisms prevail in older patients. As an increased sensitivity in platelets of hypertensive patients was noted also with thrombin alone supersensitivity is determined distal to the receptor and also involves a potentiation of response arising from the elevated platelet free calcium "per se".

Adrenoceptor-Mediated and Calcium-Influx-Dependent Vasoconstriction is Enhanced in Essential Hypertension

Postjunctional alpha-1 and alpha-2-adrenoceptor-mediated vasoconstrictor tone was quantified in patients with essential hypertension and normotensive subjects by measuring the vasodilation in the forearm following intraarterial infusions of the alpha-1 antagonist prazosin (0.5 μg/min/100 ml tissue) and the alpha-2 antagonist yohimbine (30 μg/min/100 ml tissue), respectively using venous occlusion plethysmography. Calcium influx-dependent vasoconstriction was determined by the intraarterial infusion of the calcium entry blocker nitrendipine (20 μg/min/100 ml tissue). "Non-specific", i.e. neither adrenoceptor-mediated nor calcium influx-dependent vasodilation was assessed by intraarterial infusion of sodium nitroprusside (0.6 μg/min/100 ml tissue) and by measuring forearm blood flow during reperfusion following 10 min forearm ischaemia. As determined in previous dose-response studies the doses infused of these drugs were such as to produce their maximal vasodilator effect in the forearm without inducing systemic haemodynamic changes.

Figure 1 shows a greater increase in forearm blood flow in patients with essential hypertension to postjunctional alpha-1 and alpha-2-blockade as well as to calcium entry blockade while there was no significant difference between hypertensive patients and normotensive subjects to "non-specific" vasodilation with sodium nitroprusside or during reperfusion following forearm ischaemia with an increase in forearm blood flow comparable to alpha-adrenoceptor and calcium entry blockade, respectively. An enhanced postjunctional alpha-1 and alpha-2-adrenoceptor-mediated and calcium influx-dependent vasoconstriction may contribute to the elevated vascular resistance in essential hypertension. Since, as shown in previous studies [13, 15], the increases in forearm blood flow to alpha-1-adrenoceptor-blockade with prazosin and to calcium entry blockade with verapamil relates in hypertensive patients directly to plasma adrenaline concentrations suggests an association between calcium influx-dependent enhanced vasoconstriction and the activity of the sympathetic nervous system.

Enhanced calcium influx-dependent vasoconstriction in the presence of elevated intracellular free calcium concentration in platelets of hypertensive patients

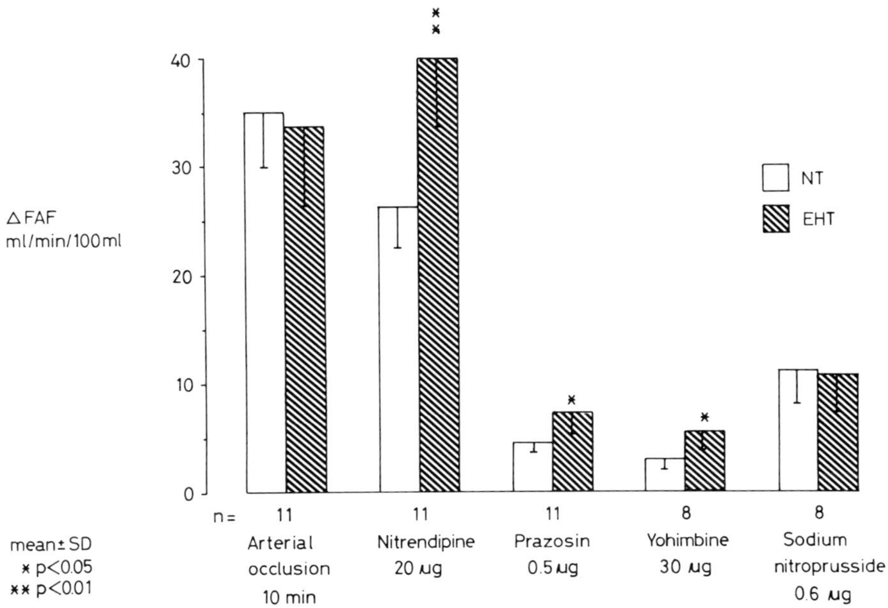

Fig. 1. Mean (±SD) increase in forearm blood flow (△ FAF) to calcium entry blockade with nitrendipine, to alpha-1 and alpha-2-blockade with prazosin and yohimibine, respectively as well as to "non-specific" vasodilation after 10 min forearm ischaemia (arterial occlusion) and to sodium nitroprusside. Drugs were infused into the left brachial artery and doses are indicated in µg/min/100 ml forearm tissue. Patients with essential hypertension are shown in hatched bars and age and sex matched normotensive control subjects in open bars.

indicates a complex cellular mishandling of calcium by the vascular smooth muscle cell in essential hypertension [48]. The contribution of the sympathetic nervous system is suggested by the enhanced alpha-adrenoceptor-mediated vasoconstriction as well as adrenaline's stimulating effect on alpha-2-adrenoceptors resulting in vasoconstriction [14, 46] and increased sensitivity to adrenaline of thrombin-induced increased in platelet free calcium concentration [47].

Antihypertensive Therapy Normalizes Vasoconstriction and Platelet Free Calcium in Parallel

Elevated vascular resistance is the haemodynamic hallmark of essential hypertension and therefore its normalization is the ultimate goal of antihypertensive treatment. Lowering of elevated blood pressure by calcium antagonists, beta-blockers or diuretics resulted in a fall in platelet free calcium concentration [16].

To investigate whether antihypertensive treatment while reducing platelet free calcium concentration would also produce a parallel reduction in the enhanced calcium influx-dependent vasoconstriction five male patients with essential hypertension were treated with the calcium entry blocker nitrendipine and the beta-

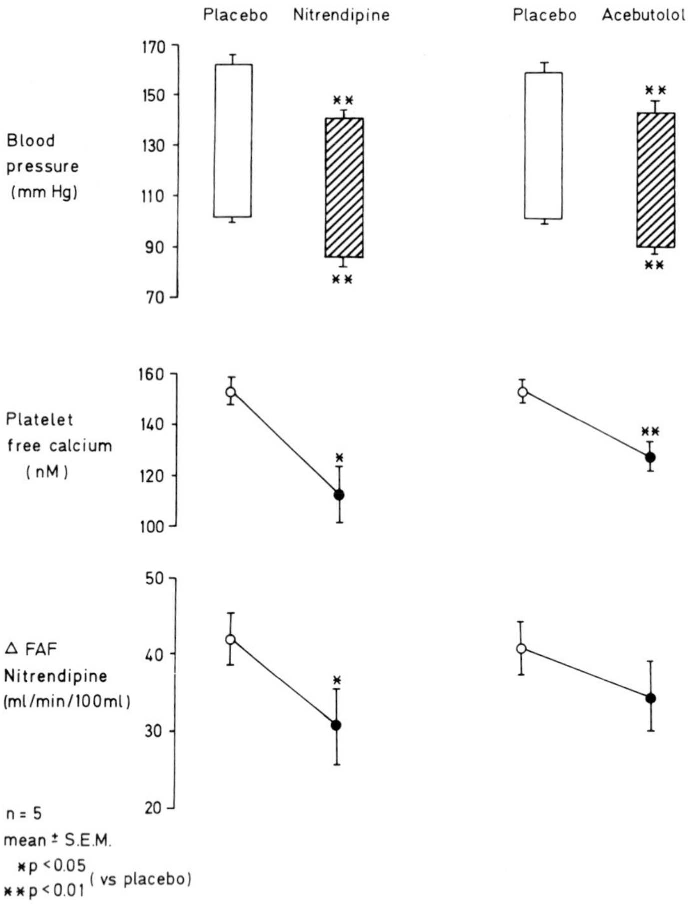

Fig. 2. Blood pressure, platelet-free calcium concentration, and increase in forearm blood flow (Δ FAF) in response to intraarterial nitrendipine (20 μg/100 ml forearm tissue), during placebo (*open symbols*) and after 6 weeks of antihypertensive therapy with nitrendipine or acebutolol (*filled symbols*)

blocker acebutolol. Assignment to calcium entry or beta-blockade was at random, each was given for 6 weeks, and followed by a within patient crossover of medication separated by a 2 weeks' placebo phase.

Figure 2 shows the parallel reduction in blood pressure and platelet free calcium concentration after 6 weeks treatment with nitrendipine or acebutolol. Calcium influx-dependent vascular tone as assessed by the increase in forearm blood flow to intraarterially infused nitrendipine showed before antihypertensive therapy values which were comparable to those of earlier studies in untreated hypertensives and which were found to be significantly greater than in normotensive subjects (Fig. 1). After 6 weeks treatment with nitrendipine or acebutolol the increase in forearm blood flow to intraarterial nitrendipine was greatly reduced to values found in normotensive subjects indicating that in parallel with the reduction in blood pressure and platelet free calcium concentration the enhanced calcium influx-dependent vasoconstrictor component became normalized. The direct relation ($r = 0.791$, $p < 0.01$) between the difference in the increase in forearm blood flow due to treatment and the treatment-induced change in platelet free calcium concentration further suggests that platelet free calcium concentration may reflect intracellular calcium concentration in vascular smooth muscle cells. Reduction of intracellular calcium concentration consequent to antihypertensive therapy induces a decrease in vascular tone and normalization of elevated vascular resistance and blood pressure. Normalization of enhanced sensitivity of platelets to adrenaline and to thrombin-induced increase in free calcium concentration following antihypertensive treatment [47] may reflect normalization of the sympathetic nervous system's contribution to elevated vascular resistance and this could be consistant with the observation that the enhanced alpha-1-adrenoceptor-mediated vasoconstriction found in patients with essential hypertension is normalized by antihypertensive treatment [49].

Both calcium antagonists and beta-adrenoceptor blockers seem to interfere with pathophysiological mechanisms that lead to elevated intracellular calcium. Platelets may serve as an experimental model for the vascular smooth cell to study details of antihypertensive drug interference and thereby may help to obtain more insight into the mode of action of antihypertensive drugs as well as to identify pathophysiological mechanisms in patients with essential hypertension.

References

1. Bertel O, Bühler FR, Kiowski W, Lütold BE (1980) Decreased beta-adrenoreceptor responsiveness as related to age, blood pressure and plasma catecholamines in patients with essential hypertension. Hypertension 2:130–138
2. Bühler FR, Kiowski W, Van Brummelen P, Amann FW, Bertel O, Landmann R, Lütold BE, Bolli P (1980) Plasma adrenoceptor-mediated and cardiac, renal and peripheral vascular adrenoceptor-mediated responses in different age groups of normal and hypertensive subjects. Clinical and Experimental Hypertension 2:409–426
3. Bühler FR, Burkart F, Lütold BE, Küng M, Marbet G, Pfisterer M (1975) Antihypertensive betablocking action as related to renin and age: a pharmacological tool to identify pathogenic mechanisms in essential hypertension. Am J Cardiol 36:653–669
4. Burkart F, Bühler FR, Pfisterer M, Lütold BE, Küng M (1976) Hemodynamic responses to exercise and acute betablockade in renin subtypes of essential hypertension. Clin Sci 51:70
5. Perini C, Müller FB, Bühler FR (1985) Plasma catecholamines in borderline hypertension and subjects with genetic risk for hypertension. Abstract, meeting of the American Federation for Clinical Research, Washington, May 1985
6. Esler M, Julius S, Zweifler A, Randall O, Harburg E, Gardiner H, Quattro V de (1977) Mild high renin essential hypertension: A neurogenic human hypertension? N Engl J Med 296:405–411
7. London GM, Safar ME, Weiss YA, Milliez PL (1976) Isoproterenol sensitivity and total body clearance of propranolol in hypertensive patients. J Clin Pharmacol 16:174
8. Astrand PO, Rodahl K (1970) Textbook of work physiology. MacGraw Hill, New York
9. Brunner HR, Sealey JE, Laragh JH (1973) Renin subgroups in essential hypertension. Circ Res (suppl I) 32:99
10. Lowder SC, Hamet P, Liddle GW (1976) Contrasting effects of hypoglycemia on plasma renin activity and cyclic adenosine 3′,5′-mono-phosphate (cyclic AMP) in low renin and normal renin essential hypertension. Circ Res 38:105–109

11. Fleisch JH (1980) Age-related changes in the sensitivity of blood vessels to drugs. Pharmacol Therap 8:477–487
12. van Brummelen P, Bühler FR, Kiowski W, Amann FW (1981) Age-related decrease in cardiac and peripheral vascular responsiveness to isoproterenol. Clin Sci 60:571–577
13. Amann FW, Bolli P, Kiowski W, Bühler FR (1981) Enhanced alpha-adrenoceptor-mediated vasoconstriction in essential hypertension. Hypertension 3 (suppl I):119–123
14. Bolli P, Erne P, Ji BH, Block LH, Kiowski W, Bühler FR (to be published) Adrenaline induces vasoconstriction through postjunctional alpha-2-adrenoceptors and this response is enhanced in patients with essential hypertension. J Hypertension
15. Hulthén UL, Bolli P, Amann FW, Kiowski W, Bühler FR (1982) Enhanced vasodilatation in essential hypertension by calcium channel blockade with verapamil. Hypertension 4 (suppl II):26–31
16. Erne P, Bolli P, Bürgisser E, Bühler FR (1984) Correlation of platelet calcium with blood pressure. Effect of antihypertensive therapy. N Engl J Med 310:1084–1088
17. Landmann R, Bittiger H, Bühler FR (1981) Characterization of high affinity beta-adrenoceptors on human mononuclear leucocytes. Life Sci 29:1761–1771
18. Landmann R, Hulthén UL, van Brummelen P, Kiowski W, Amann FW, Bühler FR (1982) Increased beta-2-adrenoceptor binding capacity in mononuclear leucocytes is associated with blunted beta-adrenoceptor-mediated cardiovascular responses in essential hypertension. Ninth Scientific Meeting of the International Society of Hypertension, Mexico City, February 21–24, 1982, p 235
19. Franco-Morselli R, Elghozi JL, Joly E, Diginilio S, Meyer P (1977) Increased plasma adrenaline concentration in benign essential hypertension. Brit Med J II:1251–1254
20. De Champlain J (1981) Use of circulating catecholamines for the detection of autonomic abnormalities in human hypertension. In: Laragh JH, Bühler FR, Seldin DW, eds. Frontiers in hypertension research. New York, Springer, 306–311
21. Bolli P, Amann FW, Hulthén L, Kiowski W, Bühler FR (1981) Elevated plasma adrenaline reflects sympathic overactivity and enhanced alpha adrenoceptor-mediated vasoconstriction in essential hypertension. Clin Sci 61 (suppl 7):161–164
22. Sever PS, Owikowska B, Birch M, Turnbridge RDG (1977) Plasma noradrenaline in essential hypertension. Lancet 1:1078–1081
23. Lake CR, Ziegler NG, Coleman MD, Kopin IJ (1977) Age-adjusted plasma norepinephrine levels are similar in normotensive and hypertensive subjects. N Engl J Med 296:208–213
24. Bühler FR, Laragh JH, Baer L, Vaughan ED Jr, Brunner HR (1972) Propranolol inhibition of renin secretion. A specific approach to diagnosis and treatment of renin-dependent hypertensive diseases. N Engl J Med 287:1209–1214
25. Bolli P, Amann FW, Bühler FR (1980) Antihypertensive response to post-synaptic alpha-blockade with prazosin in low- and normal renin hypertension. J Cardiovasc Pharmacol 2:S399–S405
26. Bühler FR, Hulthén UL, Kiowski W, Bolli P (1982) The place of the calcium antagonist verapamil in antihypertensive therapy. J Cardiovasc Pharmacol 4:S350–S357
27. Erne P, Bolli P, Bertel O, Hulthén UL, Kiowski W, Müller FB, Bühler FR (1983) Factors influencing the hypotensive effects of calcium antagonists. Hypertension 5 (suppl II):97–102
28. Kuriyama H, Yto Y, Suzuki H, Kitamura K, Itoh T (1982) Factors modifying contraction relaxation cycle in vascular smooth muscles. Am J Physiol 243:H641–662
29. Owen NE, Feinberg H, Le Breton GC (1980) Epinephrine induces Ca^{2+} uptake in human blood platelets. Am J Physiol 239:H483–488
30. Niedermann R, Pollard TD (1975) Human platelet myosin. II in vitro assembly and structure of myosin filaments. J Cell Biol 67:72–92
31. Ziedek W, Losse H, Dorst KG, Zumkley H, Vetter H (1982) Intracellular sodium and calcium in essential hypertension. Klin Wochenschr 60:859–862
32. Favre L, Lew PD, Vallotton MB (1984) Cytosolic free calcium and intracellular calcium stores are normal in neutrophils from patients with essential hypertension. J Hypertension
33. Postnov YV, Orlov SN (1980) Alteration of membrane control over intracellular calcium in essential hypertension and in spontaneously hypertensive rats. In: Losse H (ed) Intracellular electrolytes and arterial hypertension. Thieme, Stuttgart New York, pp 144–151

34. Postnov YV, Orlov SN (1984) Cell membrane alteration as a source of primary hypertension. J Hypertension 2:1–6
35. Reuter H (1983) Calcium channel modulation by neurotransmitters, enzymes and drugs. Nature 301:569–574
36. Blaustein MP (1974) The interrelationship between sodium and calcium fluxes across cell membranes. Rev Physiol Biochem Pharmacol 70:33–82
37. Resink TJ, Tkachuk VA, Erne P, Bühler FR (submitted for publication) Calmodulin stimulation of platelet membrane Ca^{2+}-ATPase: blunted response in patients with established essential hypertension.
38. Kwan CY, Belbeck L, Daniel EE (1980) Abnormal biochemistry of vascular smooth muscle plasma membrane isolated from hypertensive rats. Mol Pharmacol 17:137–140
39. Devynck MA, Pernolle MG, Nunez AM, Meyer P (1981) Analyses of calcium handling in erythrocyte membranes of genetically hypertensive rats. Hypertension 3:397–403
40. Wei WJ, Janis RA, Daniel EG (1976) Studies of subcellular fractions from mesentric arteries of spontaneously hypertensive rats: alterations in both calcium uptake and enzyme activities. Blood Vessels 13:293–308
41. Orlov SN, Postnov YV (1980) Calcium accumulation and calcium binding by the cell membranes of cardiomyocytes and smooth muscle of aorta in spontaneously hypertensive rats. Clin Sci 59:207s–209s
42. Devynck MA, Pernollet MG, Nunez AM, Meyer P (1981) Calcium binding alteration in plasma membranes from various tissues of spontaneously hypertensive rats. Clin Exp Hyper 3:797–808
43. Postnov YV, Orlov SN, Pokudin NI (1979) Decrease of calcium binding by the red blood cell membrane in spontaneously hypertensive rats and in essential hypertension. Pflügers Archiv 379:191–195
44. Orlov SN, Pokudin NI, Postnov YV (1983) Calmodulin-dependent Ca^{2+}-transport in erythrocytes of spontaneously hypertensive rats. Pflügers Archic 397:54–56
45. Kravtsov GM, Orlov SN, Pokudin NI, Postnov YV (1983) Calcium transport in synaptosomes and subcellular fractions of brain tissue in spontaneously hypertensive rats. Clin Sci 65:127–135
46. van Brummelen P, Jie K, Timmermanns PBMWM, Van Zwieten P (1985) Postjunctional alpha-adrenoceptors and the regulation of arteriolar tone in humans. J Cardiovasc Pharmacol 7 (suppl 6):149–152
47. Erne P, Resink TJ, Bolli P, Hefti A, Ritz R, Bühler FR (to be published) Free calcium response to adrenaline in platelets of normal and hypertensive subjects. J Hypertension
48. Robinson BF (1984) Altered calcium handling as a cause of primary hypertension. J Hypertension 2:453–460
49. Bolli P, Amann FW, Burkart F, Bühler FR (1982) Role of alpha-adrenoceptor-mediated vasoconstriction for antihypertensive beta-blockade. J Cardiovasc Pharmacol 4 (suppl 1):162–167

Discussion

(pp. 445–453)

Van Breemen: Dr. Bühler, what makes the platelets take up extra Ca^{2+} in your hypertensive patients?

Bühler: I wish I knew the complete answer to that. There is an enhanced adrenaline induced increase in cellular Ca^{2+} which is linked to phosphorylation of the contractile proteins and to hypersensitive shape change. But there is also blunting of extrusion mechanisms, such as the calmodulin activatable Ca^{2+}-ATPase.

Kazda: Your finding that Ca^{2+}-antagonists are more effective in patients with low renin and less effective in patients with high renin, can be confirmed also by our observations in rats. There are two forms of experimental hypertension which are extremely sensitive to Ca^{2+}-antagonists, the DOCA salt hypertension and the salt-induced hypertension in Dahl-rats. Both of them have extremely low renin. On the other hand the 2-kidney 1-clip hypertension with high plasma renin activity is rather insensitive to Ca^{2+}-antagonists.

Leonetti: Dr. Bühler, I was surprised of your positioning of the converting enzyme inhibitor, because Italian experience is not in agreement with yours. In a study of more than 1,400 Patients with an age ranging from 35 to more than 70 years the people over 60 years had a blood pressure reduction similar or even greater than the middle age people during treatment with captopril. On which basis do you suggest captopril for younger and not for the older hypertensive patients?

Bühler: Tony Amery's group in Louvain has shown in Clinical Science that there is an inverse relationship between efficacy of captopril with age, indicating that the younger patients are more responsive. The indirect evidence is the fact that there is a direct renin-related efficacy of captopril, and these are more often the younger patients.

Leonetti: Tarazi's and Salvetti's group found a direct correlation between the renin levels and the blood pressure reduction in the acute phase of captopril treatment, but this correlation was no more present under chronic treatment.

Bühler: I do not want to be evangelistic, you can use whatever lowers blood pressure. But if you want to make more sense out of treatment and if you want to have an increased chance of succeeding in lowering blood pressure, this is probably a reasonable approach.

Nayler: Do you know what in fact the blunting of the calmodulin-sensitive ATPases means? You would have to know what the turnover rate of the enzyme is and how far into its capacity it was working. Do you have data on that?

Bühler: The basal activity of the Ca^{2+}-ATPase is slightly increased in patients with essential hypertension but stimulation with calmodulin is blunted. This only holds true for the calmodulin-dependent Ca^{2+}-ATPase, and not for the Ca^{2+}-Mg^{2+}-ATPase.

Nayler: It is intriguing because we find that the extrusion mechanism for Ca^{2+} for cardiac cell membranes is also diminished in the SH-rats at least compared to WKY's so it may be that a general Ca^{2+}-extrusion phenomenon is impaired.

Cauvin: Have you performed any Quinn-2 measurements with epinephrine or another agonist in a Ca^{2+}-free solution? It is possible to interpret that enhanced response in the hypertensive platelets as being an increased release from an intracellular Ca^{2+} store with a subsequent decreased extrusion.

Bühler: Yes, it is possible, that subsurface Ca^{2+}-pools, are being mobilised. There is some indication that adrenaline increases intracellular Ca^{2+} in the thrombin-preincubated platelet.

Lichtlen: What is really the evidence that Ca^{2+} increases in the platelets in the same way as it does in the smooth muscle cells? In man it is very difficult to measure Ca^{2+}-accumulation in smooth muscle cells. Are there any animal studies on the Ca^{2+}-content in vascular smooth muscle cells?

Bühler: There is no evidence that correlates platelet Ca^{2+} with Ca^{2+} in smooth muscle cells. We tried to get it as close as possible: In man there is a correlation between changes in forearm vascular resistance and free Ca^{2+} in platelets.

Lichtlen: The decrease in resistance observed after administration of Ca^{2+}-antagonists does not prove that the Ca^{2+}-content necessarily is increased in smooth muscle cells; there can be many other reasons for smooth muscle relaxation after Ca^{2+}-antagonists.

Bühler: But we got very close to it. We have shown enhanced Ca^{2+}-influx-dependent vasoconstriction, and we can reduce constriction with a parallel reduction in intracellular Ca^{2+}.

Fleckenstein: We have many data indicating that Ca^{2+} is increased in spontaneously hypertensive rats in the vascular wall. If you give the Ca^{2+}-antagonist then not only pressure but the Ca^{2+}-content is normalized. Another observation is an age-related increase of Ca^{2+}-content in vascular smooth muscle. This is true for humans and all animal species we have studied. One part of this Ca^{2+} remains tive, another part is sequestered in the cell.

Lichtlen: Where is the Ca^{2+} located, is it inside the muscle cell or is it in the interstitial space?

Fleckenstein: We know that the Ca^{2+} increases in the media. In elderly patients we have precipitated Ca^{2+} blacks in the interstitium, but also inside the smooth muscle cells there are Ca^{2+}-deposits but also active Ca^{2+}. We have measured this with a specific Ca^{2+}-electrode. With these findings I understand the results of Dr. Bühler in that sense, that the aging patient due to the increase of vascular active Ca^{2+}-content has at least a disposition for high vascular tone. This can be probably more easily decreased by Ca^{2+}-antagonists as compared to younger patients in whom high blood pressure is perhaps more dependent on other mechanisms, e.g. a hyperactive sympathetic system.

Casteels: If you have a decrease of the Ca^{2+}-extrusion of your platelets, wouldn't you expect a decline of their survival?

Bühler: This is a possibility but I am not aware of data on the survival time of platelets.

Casteels: Are there any indications that other enzymes, e.g. the Na^+-K^+-ATPase is depressed, too?

Bühler: We do not have data to answer this question.

Van Breemen: Because the active tension is up in the hypertensive blood vessels therefore you imply that the free Ca^{2+} inside the myoplasm of the smoo muscle cells must be up. Then you look for another cell which is easier to approach experimentally than the smooth muscle cell which has the same expected change in free Ca^{2+}. (You could take a red blood cell or a white blood cell just as well as a model for a smooth muscle cell, but I understand red cell Ca^{2+} does not necessarly go up). So first you made this beautiful step of eliminating the animal for a model, but now you still have the problem of using another cell as a model for a smooth muscle cell. Besides the problems the beauty of the correct analogy is that you can at least study the mechanism that has changed during hypertension.

Bühler: There is more to be said for that model because the platelet has a similar receptor setting, has contractile proteins, which are phosphorylated in the same way and has the same extrusion pumps.

Kadowitz: Was the forearm blood flow response to verapamil and the one to nitroprusside enhanced to the same extent? Have you looked at other vasodilators and looked at the dose-response relationship? Could this enhanced response just be related to the fact that the hypertensive forearm vasculature had a higher tone?

Bühler: The sodium nitroprusside response in fact was not significantly different although there was a trend of an increased response in patients with essential hypertension. In other studies we have shown as you did in the pulmonary circulation and in the cat mesenteric artery that there are postjunctional alpha$_2$-receptor-mediated effect in man and both are enhanced in essential hypertension.

There was no difference in the response to sodium nitroprusside between normotensive and essential hypertensive subjects. This also holds true for different points of the dose response curve.

Garthoff: Having your correlation with plasmarenin activity in mind, I would like you to ask, what happens to aldosterone under treatment with Ca^{2+}-antagonists in your studies? Are there similar correlations between blood pressure and aldosterone level as shown to exist for plasma-renin activity?

Bühler: We have no plasma aldosterone measurements of our own but Waldhäusl in Vienna and Reid in Glasgow have shown that Ca^{2+}-antagonists blunt the angiotensin-II-stimulation of aldosterone biosynthesis and this anti-aldosterone effect may contribute to a diuretic effect of the Ca^{2+}-antagonists.

Groß: I wonder about the meaning of the correlation between an age-dependent decrease in baroreceptor sensitivity and blood pressure decrease, since you showed that in long-term treatment there was a re-setting of the baroreflex. Are there other mechanisms beside this operative, for instance, an age-dependent increase in Ca^{2+} in the smooth muscle as suggested by Dr. Fleckenstein?

Bühler: I tried to make the point that it is not a single mechanism that is decisive for the antihypertensive response to a Ca^{2+}-antagonist in a given patient. It is rather a multitude of reflex mechanisms co-determining the fall in blood pressure: the baroreflex via efferent β-adrenergic transmission in the heart and the kidney forming part of it.

Session VII: Tissue Protection

Chairman: W. G. Nayler

Bayer-Symposium IX
Cardiovascular Effects of Dihydropyridine-Type
Calcium Antagonists and Agonists, 460–471

Dihydropyridines and the Protection of the Ischaemic and Anoxic Myocardium

W. G. NAYLER, J. S. DILLON, and W. J. STURROCK

Introduction

A variety of experimental models have been used to investigate whether the Ca^{2+} antagonists protect the myocardium against the deleterious effects of ischaemia and reperfusion and by now verapamil, nifedipine and diltiazem have all shown to be effective. In the case of verapamil there is clear evidence that its efficacy depends upon its prophylactic use [1]. Precisely why these drugs are effective is unclear. Many mechanisms may be involved, including energy preservation – arising either as a direct consequence of a redcution in afterload or diminished contractility, a reduced rate of loss of the adenosine triphosphate, precursors, inhibition of ischaemia and reperfusion-induced arrhythmias, a reduction in Ca^{2+} overload upon reperfusion and, in the case of diltiazem, an inhibition of mitochondrial $Na^+:Ca^{2+}$ exchange. It has also been noted that ischaemia renders the myocardium hypersensitive to these drugs [2]. Again, the precise reason for this hypersensitivity is unknown. It could be due to an ischaemia-induced change in receptor affinity or density; alternatively some of metabolic consequences of the ischaemic episode could be involved. These consequences could include the accumulation of protons [3] and the overflow of norepinephrine from the cardiac stores [4].

This communication is concerned with experiments which were aimed at answering the following questions:

a) does ischaemia modify the cardiac dihydropyridine binding sites,
b) do the dihydropyridines resemble the phenylalkylamines in reducing the ischaemia-reperfusion induced overflow of norepinephrine, and
c) does the late addition of nifedipine attenuate reperfusion-induced Ca^{2+} overload?

Methods

Adult male Sprague Dawley rats (250–300 gm) were used for these studies. They were maintained on a standard diet, and tail cuff measurements showed them to be normotensive.

Experimental Protocols

1. ^{3}H-nitrendipine Binding Studies

The rats were lightly anaesthetized with a diethylether-O_2 mixture and heparinized. The hearts were then excised, immersed in ice-cold perfusion buffer and perfused in the Langendorff mode, as previously described [5]. The perfusion buffer was a modified Krebs-Henseleit solution containing, in mM/l: NaCl, 119.0; $NaHCO_3$, 25.0; KCl, 4.6; KH_2PO_4, 1.2; $MgSO_4$, 1.2; $CaCl_2$, 1.3 and glucose, 11.0. It was gassed with 95% O_2 + 5% CO_2 (pH 7.4), maintained at 37 °C, and unless otherwise stated, delivered to provide a mean coronary flow of 10–12 ml/min. Spontaneously beating preparations were used to avoid the possibility of electrical stimulation spontaneously releasing the endogenous norepinephrine.

After 15 minute's aerobic perfusion the hearts were randomly divided into two groups. One group were perfused for another 60 min as described above. The other group were made globally ischaemic for 60 minutes, by totally occluding the coronary flow. Irrespective of flow, however, left ventricular wall temperature was maintained at 37 °C. After the required period of aerobic perfusion or ischaemia the hearts were removed, and immersed in ice-cold homogenizing medium containing 250 mM sucrose and 10 mM Tris HCl, (pH 8.1). The ventricles were removed, minced into small pieces (< 1 mm^3), and then homogenized in 15–20 ml of ice-cold homogenizing medium, using two 8–10 s bursts of a Kika Werk Ultra Turrax homogenizer operating at two-thirds maximum speed. The resultant homogenate was diluted 1:10 (wet weight: homogenizing volume) and filtered through 2 layers of gauze. A volume of ice-cold potassium chloride (KCl) and tetrasodium pyrophosphate (Na_4PPi) was then added to the filtrate to give a final concentration of 0.3 M KCl and 25 mM Na_4PPi before it was centrifuged at 177,000 xg for 40 min at 0–4 °C in an International centrifuge B-60 (swing bucket rotor SB 283). The resultant pellet was resuspended in homogenizing medium and layered over a 25% (w/w) sucrose gradient before being recentrifuged at 131,000 xg for 40 min. The interphase was carefully collected, centrifuged at 177,000 xg for 40 min, resuspended in 50 mM Tris (pH 7.4) and used for binding studies.

The isolated sarcolemmal fragments were enzymatically characterized in terms of their Na^+K^+ ATPase and 5′cyclic ATPase activity [6], and used for ^{3}H-nitrendipine binding studies.

^{3}H-nitrendipine binding was carried out using the method described by Belleman et al. [7]. Binding was carried out for 90 minutes in triplicate, using a protein concentration of 0.05–0.1 mg/ml in a final volume of 0.5 ml.

The incubation reaction mixture contained 150 mM NaCl, 1 mM $CaCl_2$, and 50 mM Tris Buffer, pH 7.4. For saturation kinetics the ^{3}H-nitrendipine was varied from 0.05 to 12.0 nM; non-specific binding was defined by the inclusion of 20 μM unlabelled nitrendipine. After 90 minute's incubation bound and free ^{3}H-nitrendipine was separated after dilution with 3.5 ml cold (4 °C) 50 mM Tris buffer. Separation was by rapid vacuum filtration across GF/B filters and was followed by two additional washes with 3.5 ml cold Tris.

The radioactivity of the filters was counted (with 30–40% efficiency) in Filter Count Scintillant, using a Packard Tricarb Spectrometer. The specificity of ^{3}H-nitrendipine binding was checked by using standard displacement techniques, with 10^{-10}-10^{-5} M nifedipine and 10^{-9}-10^{-4} M D 600. Protein was assayed by the Lowry technique [8].

Because of the photolabitity of the dihydropyridines all these binding studies were carried out under a sodium lamp.

Analysis of Data

Initial estimates of equilibrium binding parameters (K_D and Bmax) were obtained from Scatchard, Hill and Hofstee analysis, using the "EBDA" programme [9]. A file was then produced and the data analysed with the aid of a weighted non-linear square computer curve fitting programme, "LIGAND" [10], used to obtain final parameter estimates.

K_D is defined as the concentration of ligand required to occupy 50 percent of the binding sites, and Bmax as the number of binding sites.

2. *Norepinephrine Overflow Studies*

The hearts were initially perfused as described above for 15 minutes and then randomly divided into two groups: *control* and *experimental.*

The *control* hearts were perfused as described above for another 30 or 75 minutes and then assayed for norepinephrine (see below).

The *experimental* hearts were perfused as described above for 15 min, and then made globally ischaemic at 37 °C for 15,30 or 60 min, with global ischaemia being achieved by total occlusion of coronary flow. After the required period of ischaemia the hearts were reperfused at 37 °C for another 15 minutes, and then assayed for norepinephrine (see below). Reperfusion was limited to 15 minutes, preliminary results having shown that the washout of norepinephrine was complete within that time.

Drug Administration

(a) Pretreatment Series. In some experiments either nifedipine, nitrendipine or nisoldipine was added to the perfusion buffer after the first 2 minute's perfusion with drug-free buffer. Thirteen minutes later the hearts were made globally ischaemic (at 37 °C) for 15 or 60 min, and then reperfused for 15 minutes with perfusion buffer containing the appropriate drug. The left ventricles were then isolated and assayed for norepinephrine. Since nifedipine, nisoldipine and nitrendipine are photolabile the entire perfusion apparatus and buffer was protected from light.

To provide appropriate controls hearts which had already been perfused with standard buffer for 15 minutes were perfused for another 30, 45 or 75 minutes with buffer containing either nifedipine, nisoldipine or nitrendipine.

(b) Drug Added Only upon Reperfusion. In other experiments hearts were perfused for 15 minutes, made globally ischemic for 15 minutes and then reperfused, with either nifedipine, diltiazem or verapamil being added only upon reperfusion.

Norepinephrine Assay

At the end of each perfusion sequence the left ventricles were assayed for norepinephrine. The details of this assay procedure have been described elsewhere in detail [11] and therefore will only be summarized here. The general outline of the process is shown in Fig. 1. It involves perchloric acid treatment followed by alumina extraction. Thus, the left ventricles were isolated, frozen in liquid N_2, and weighed. The tissue was then homogenized in perchloric acid (Fig. 1), centrifuged, and the supernatant subjected to alumina extraction as previously described except for the following modification: glass pasteur capillary pipette-polystrene tube systems (Meteor Glass Comp, Vineland, New Jersey, USA, Disposable Products Pty. Ltd., Adelaide, South Australia) were used, instead of the 2.0 ml microfilter tubes (BAS, Bioanalytical Systems Inc., West Lafayette, Indiana, USA) used previously. This modification was introduced because preliminary studies showed that the metabolite 3,4-dihydroxyphenylethylene-glycol interacts with the polyethylene in the BAS microfilter tubes. The final eluate was subjected to high performance liquid chromatography with electrochemical detection. The following compounds were detected:- 3,4-dihydroxyphenylethyleneglycol (DHPG), norepinephrine, epinephrine, dihydroxybenzylamine (DHBA), dopamine (DA) and 3,4-dihydroxyphenylacetic acid, a precursor of dopamine. DHBA served as the internal standard, DHPG as a relatively stable metabolite, and DA as a precursor of norepinephrine. Because these metabolites and precursors were

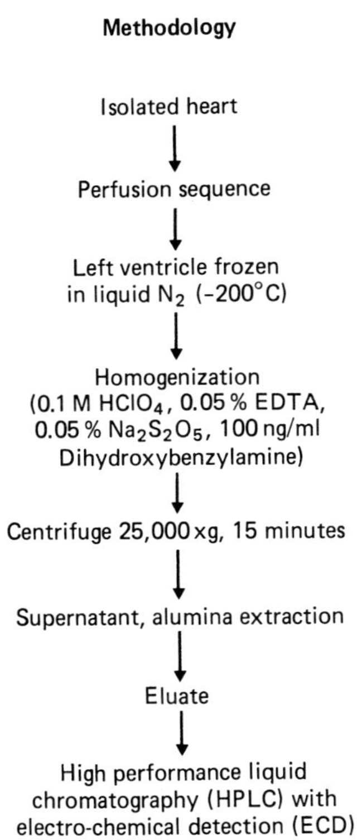

Fig. 1. Schematic summary of the extraction procedure used for norepinephrine and its metabolites and precursors

assayed we could distinguish between an increased rate of norepinephrine turnover and an enhanced rate of displacement.

Dry Weights. These are obtained by drying the weighed remnants of each heart at 100 °C to constant weight. The wet: dry weight ratio was then applied to the left ventricular wet weights.

Chemicals

Nifedipine, nitrendipine and nisoldipine were supplied as a gift from Bayer AG, Germany. Verapamil (as racemate verapamil hydrochloride) and diltiazem (as d-cis diltiazem) were gifts from Knoll AG, Germany and Tanabe Co., Japan, respectively. Verapamil and diltiazem were dissolved in perfusion buffer; the dihydropyridines were dissolved in 1 percent alcohol and then diluted with buffer. Preliminary studies showed that the amount of alcohol used to dissolve the dihydropyridine had no effect on either the norepinephrine content to the heart or the assay.

Tests of Significance

Results are presented as mean ± SEM of n experiments, the estimations for which were made in duplicate. Tests of significance were calculated by Student's "t" test, talking $p=0.05$ as the limit of significance.

3. Does the Late Addition of Nifedipine Prevent the Reperfusion Induced Ca^{2+} Overload?

In another series of experiments rat hearts were perfused as described above, made ischaemic for 30 min at 37 °C and then reperfused. On some occasions nifedipine (10^{-6} M) was added so that it was present before and after the ischaemic episode. On other occasions either nifedipine (10^{-6} M) or Bay K 8644 (10^{-6} M) was added only upon reperfusion. This concentration of Bay K 8644 was used because preliminary studies showed that when added to isolated spontaneously beating hearts it increased peak tension development by 150 percent.

After reperfusion the hearts were dried to constant weight and assayed for cell Ca^{2+}, as described elsewhere [12].

Results

Effects of Ischaemia on Sarcolemmal ^{3}H-nitrendipine Binding

Characterization of Sarcolemmal Membrane Fragments

Table 1 shows that the yield of sarcolemma obtained from the aerobically perfused hearts was not significantly different from that obtained after sixty minute's ischaemia. At the same time there was a significant reduction in the activity of the ouabain sensitive ATPase and cyclic 5′ AMPase activity (Table 1).

Table 1. Sarcolemmal profile

Yield	Aerobic	Ischaemic
(mg protein/gm heart wt)	0.60 ± 0.02	0.58 ± 0.04
Na^+ K^+ ATPase (ouabain sensitive) (μmoles Pi/mg protein/h)	19.0 ± 1.1	11.3 ± 0.5
5′ AMPase (μmoles Pi/mg protein/h)	14.0 ± 0.6	11.5 ± 0.7

Mean ± SEM, n = 6

^{3}H-nitrendipine Binding. Binding studies on sarcolemmal fragments isolated from aerobically perfused hearts confirmed the existence of two populations of ^{3}H-nitrendipine binding sites: *high affinity* sites (Table 2) with a K_D of 0.24 ± 0.04 nM and Bmax of 313 ± 110 fmol/mg protein, and low affinity sites with a K_D of 47.6 ± 8.7 nM and a Bmax of 12.4 ± 1.9 pmol/mg protein. ^{3}H-nitrendipine which was bound to these sites was displaceable by nifedipine, with a K_i value of 1.49 nM for the high affinity sites, and 5.3 μM for the low affinity sites (Table 3). D 600 was also able to displace bound nitrendipine, but with much higher K_i values (0.83 μM for the high affinity and 71 μM for the low affinity sites).

Table 2. Effect of ischaemia on ^{3}H-nitrendipine binding

High affinity sites			Low affinity sites		
K_D (nM)	B_{max} (fmol/mg)	Hill Coefficient	K_D (nM)	B_{max} (pmol/mg)	Hill Coefficient
Aerobic perfusion					
0.24 ± 0.04	313 ± 110	0.993 ± 0.005	47.6 ± 8.7	12.38 ± 1.88	0.985 ± 0.008
60 min ischaemia					
0.22 ± 0.05 N.S.	82.4 ± 14.5 $p < 0.03$	0.993 ± 0.003	15.8 ± 2.9 $p < 0.03$	6.1 ± 1.7 $p < 0.01$	0.994 ± 0.003

Each result is mean ± SEM of six separate experiments. Tests of significance relate to significance of change caused by sixty minute's ischaemia at 37 °C

Table 3. Effect of ischaemia on the K_i of nitrendipine binding sites in isolated sarcolemma

	High affinity		Low affinity	
	Nifedipine	D 600	Nifedipine	D 600
Control (Aerobic perfusion)	1.49 nM	0.83 μM	5.3 μM	71 μM
Ischaemia (60 min)	0.79 nM	0.1 μM	1.1 μ M	11 μM

Effect of Ischaemia on ^{3}H-nitrendipine Binding

Sarcolemmal membranes prepared from hearts which had been made ischaemic for sixty minutes at 37 °C retained two populations of ^{3}H-nitrendipine binding sites (Fig. 2). In the case of the high affinity sites the K_D remained unchanged, but there was a significant reduction ($p<0.03$) in Bmax (Table 2). The Hill coefficient, however, was unchanged. The low affinity sites (Table 2) showed changes in both K_D and Bmax, the K_D being reduced ($p<0.03$) from 47.6 ± 8.7 to 15.8 ± 2.9 nmol, and the Bmax from 12.3 ± 1.9 to 6.1 ± 1.7 pmol/mg protein ($p<10.01$). As Table 3 shows, however, the nitrendipine binding sites still displayed their preferential binding of dihydropyridines, despite a reduction in the K_i values from 1.49 to 0.79 nM for the high affinity sites, and from 5.3 to 1.1 μM for the low affinity sites.

We can conclude, therefore, that sixty minutes ischaemia does affect the binding activity but not the specificity of the dihydropyridine binding sites.

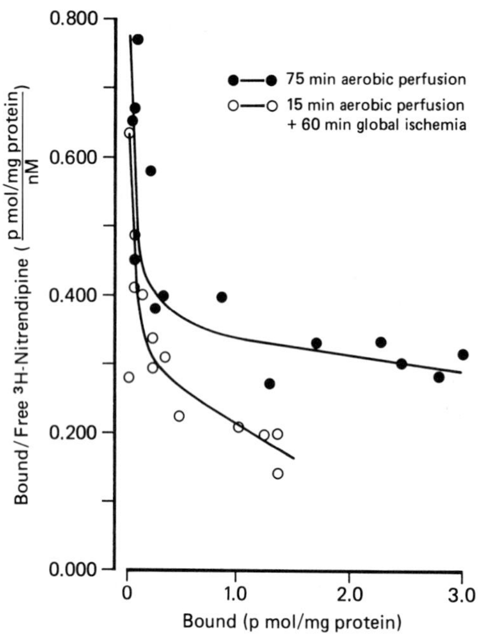

Fig. 2. Scatchard plot of ^{3}H-nitrendipine binding to rat cardiac sarcolemmal fragments isolated after 75 min aerobic perfusion, or 15 minute's aerobic perfusion followed by 60 min ischaemia at 37 °C

Dihydropyridines and the Overflow of Norepinephrine Caused by Ischaemia and Reperfusion

Figure 3 shows that whereas hearts which are perfused under aerobic conditions retain their endogenous reserves of norepinephrine, hearts which are made ischaemic and then reperfused exhibit a loss of norepinephrine, the loss increasing as the duration of the ischaemic episode is extended. Figure 4 shows that nifedipine prevents the overflow of norepinephrine that occurs upon reperfusion after short (15 min) but not long periods of ischaemia. This effect is not peculiar to nifedipine, because, as Fig. 5 shows, nitrendipine and nisoldipine are equally effec-

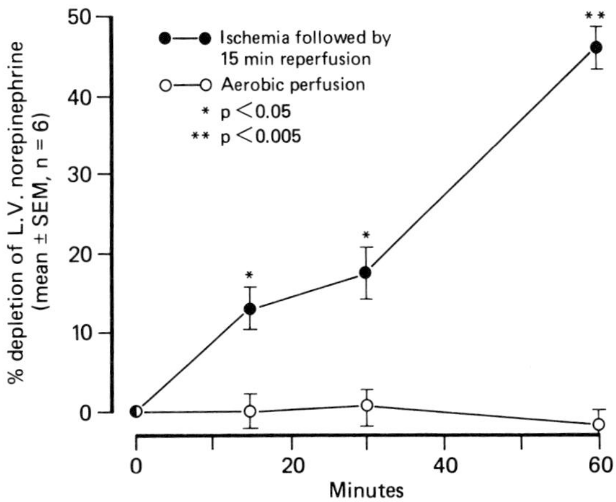

Fig. 3. Percentage depletion of left ventricular norepinephrine during aerobic perfusion (*open circles*), and 15, 30 and 60 min global ischemia followed by 15 minute's reperfusion. Each result is the mean ± SEM of six separate experiments. Percentage depletion was calculated relative to the left ventricular norepinephrine content of hearts perfused under aerobic conditions for an equivalent period of time. The norepinephrine assays were performed in duplicate

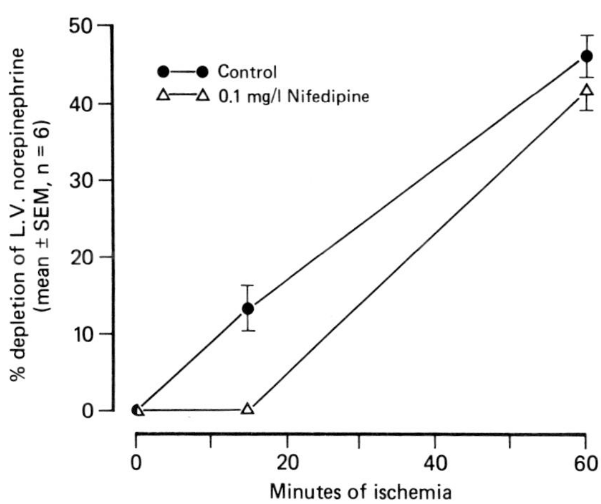

Fig. 4. Effect of 0.1 mg/l nifedipine on the overflow of norepinephrine caused by either 15 or 60 min ischaemia followed by 15 minute's reperfusion. Control refers to untreated hearts which were made ischaemic and reperfused for the same periods of time. Note that nifedipine prevented the displacement of norepinephrine caused by reperfusion after the short but not the prolonged period of ischaemia. Each result refers to six individual experiments in which the norepinephrine content of the left ventricles was determined in duplicate. When nifedipine was present it was added before the hearts were made ischaemic as well as upon reperfusion

tive. Figure 5 also shows that the other Ca^{++} antagonists are effective when added prior to the ischaemic episode and upon reperfusion. A different picture emerges however, when the Ca^{2+} antagonists are added only upon reperfusion, because as Fig. 6 shows under these conditions, and even after only fifteen minute's ischaemia nifedipine, but neither verapamil nor diltiazem, attenuate this overflow of norepinephrine.

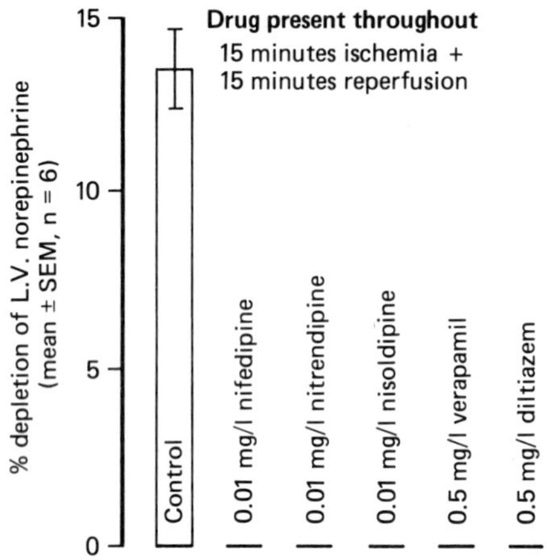

Fig. 5. Effect of a variety of Ca^{2+} antagonists on the ischaemia-reperfusion induced displacement of norepinephrine. Ischaemia was limited to 15 minutes; reperfusion was for 15 minutes. Control refers to untreated hearts. When drugs were present they were added 13 minute's before the hearts were made ischaemic and their presence was continued throughout reperfusion. In each series six separate experiments were made

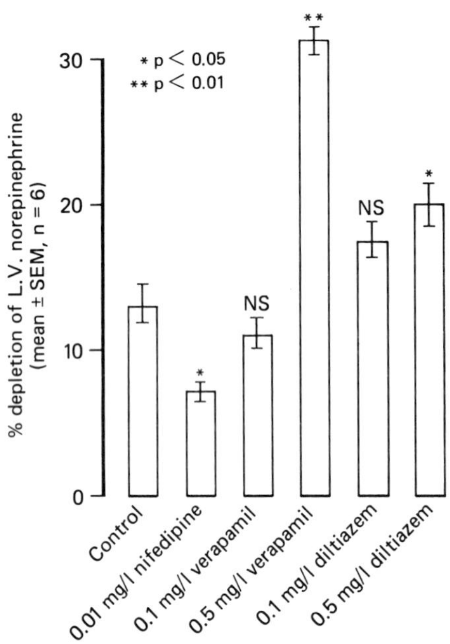

Fig. 6. Effect of Ca^{++} antagonists on ischaemia-reperfusion induced norepinephrine overflow when added only upon reperfusion after 15 minute's ischaemia. Tests of significance relate to the differences in the left ventricular norepinephrine content after the ischaemia-reperfusion episode relative to the control ischaemia-reperfusion

One question which naturally arises with experiments such as these is whether we are dealing with an "overflow" of norepinephrine, or with an altered rate of synthesis or breakdown. However, because we assayed for both the precursor and metabolites of norepinephrine and found no change in either we can be reasonably certain that we are dealing simply with an increased rate of norepinephrine overflow and mobilization. Likewise the inhibitory effect of the dihydropyridines on this ischaemia-reperfusion induced mobilization of norepinephrine was not accompanied by changed levels of precursors or metabolites, and therefore reflects an effect on overflow rather than synthesis or degradation.

Does the Late Addition of Nifedipine Prevent the Reperfusion-Induced Ca^{2+} Overload

Table 4 shows that whereas the addition of nifedipine so that it was present before and after the ischaemic episode reduced ($p<0.01$) the gain in Ca^{2+} caused by reperfusing after 30 min ischaemia, its addition only upon reperfusion failed to reduce Ca^{2+} overload. Under these same conditions adding 10^{-6} M of the Ca^{++} agonist, Bay K 8644 increased the rate of Ca^{++} gain upon reperfusion. Thus whereas untreated hearts increased their cellular Ca^{++} content by only 15% during the first two minutes of reperfusion, hearts which were reperfused with Krebs containing 10^{-6} M Bay K 8644 increased their cellular Ca^{++} content by 18%. Presumably, therefore the dihydropyridine binding sites can still be activated after a prolonged period of ischaemia.

Table 4. Effect of nifedipine on Ca^{2+} gain during reperfusion

Perfusion sequence	Ca_i^{2+} (µmoles/gm dry wt)
60 min control aerobic	3.48 ± 0.16
Control ischaemia and reperfusion	
30 min ischaemia	14.62 ± 0.31
15 min reperfusion	
Nifedipine (10^{-6} M) throughout	
30 min ischaemia,	7.62 ± 1.0
15 min reperfusion	
Nifedipine (10^{-6} M) on reperfusion	
30 min ischaemia	20.32 ± 0.45
15 min reperfusion	

Each result is mean ± SEM, 6 expts. Ischaemia was at 37 °C. Ca_i^{2+} refers to cellular Ca^{2+}

Discussion

These results show that sixty minute's ischaemia does affect the dihydropyridine binding sites in that both the Bmax and K_D of the low affinity sites is reduced, together with the Bmax of the high affinity sites. Since it is the low affinity sites which exhibit K_D values within the range needed for Ca^{2+} antagonism [13] it is possible that the ischaemia-induced decrease in the affinity of these sites that is described here could contribute to the hypersensitivity exhibited by ischaemic heart muscle [2, 14]. Certainly this hypersensitivity cannot be accounted for in terms of an increased number of dihydropyridine binding sites.

Our experiments also indicate that although the dihydropyridine binding sites can be activated after a prolonges period of ischaemia – as indicated by the ability of Bay K 8644 to promote an increased rate of Ca^{2+} gain upon reperfusion, the addition of nifedipine only upon reperfusion failed to attenuate the reperfusion induced gain in Ca^{2+} – a finding which is in agreement with that of Higgins and

Blackburn [15]. Two conclusions can be reached from these observations. Firstly, although pretreatment with Ca^{2+} antagonists reduces the magnitude of the gain in Ca^{2+} which occurs upon reperfusion (Table 4), the primary route of Ca^{2+} entry is probably not through the slow channels. Otherwise we would have expected nifedipine to be effective when added only upon reperfusion. In addition we can probably safely conclude that the beneficial use of nifedipine in the management of ischaemia depends upon their prophylactic use. This conclusion is further supported by other findings described here – mainly the ability of nifedipine (and the other – dihydropyridines) to abolish the ischaemia-reperfusion induced mobilization of norepinephrine when used prophylactically. This ability of the Ca^{2+} antagonists to modulate norepinephrine overflow under these conditions is in marked contrast to their failure to attenuate norepinephrine release caused by electrical stimulation [16] or a raised K^+ [17]. It may, however, contribute to their usefulness in the management of angina and the ischaemic myocardium. Norepinephrine stimulates myocardial oxygen consumption, constricts the coronary vasculature, generates Ca^{2+}-dependent slow action potentials and arrhythmias, accelerates platelet aggregation and, if autoxidized, generates free oxygen radicles. It follows, therefore, that the ability of the dihydropyridines to attenuate or abolish the overflow of norepinephrine during periods of ischaemia and reperfusion is advantageous.

In conclusion, these results establish that despite the complex series of events that are triggered by periods of ischaemia and reperfusion (Fig. 7) the prophylactic use of the dihydropyridines should be beneficial, despite the fact that both the affinity and the density of the dihydropyridine binding sites are affected by the ischaemic episode. Additional experiments are needed now to establish whether reperfusion exacerbates these ischaemia-induced changes in dihydropyridine density and affinity.

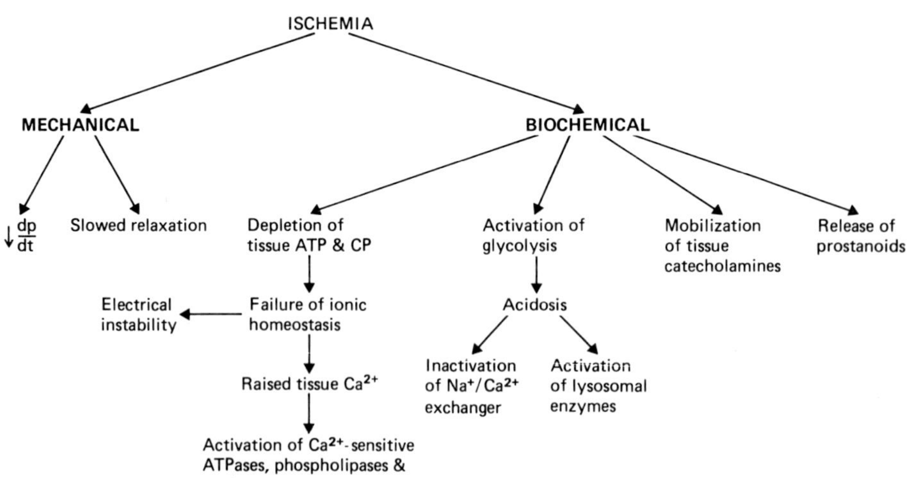

Fig. 7. Schematic representation of some of the consequences of ischaemia

References

1. Bourdillon PD, Poole-Wilson PA (1982) The effects of verapamil, quiescence and cardioplegia on calcium exchange and mechanical function in ischaemic rabbit myocardium. Circ Res 50:360–368
2. Smith HJ, Goldstein RA, Griffin JM, Kent KM, Epstein SE (1976) Regional contractility: selective depression of ischemic myocardium by verapamil. Circ 54:629–35
3. Hondeghem LM, Katzung BG (1984) Antiarrhytmic agents: the modulated receptor mechanism of action of sodium and calcium channel-blocking drugs. Annu Rev Pharmacol Toxicol 24:387–423
4. Smith HJ, Halliday SE, Briscoe MG, Snow HM (1984) Facilitation of calcium blocking and membrane effects by intrinsic sympathomimetic activity. Cardiovasc Res 28:30–36
5. Nayler WG, Scott EM (1982) The effect of chemical sympathectomy on mitochondrial function in the ischaemic and reperfused myocardium. Br J Pharmac 77:707–715
6. Daly MJ, Elz JS, Nayler WG (1984) Sarcolemmal enzymes and Na^+–Ca^{2+} exchange in hypoxic, ischaemic and reperfused rat hearts. Am J Physiol 247:H 237–H 243
7. Bellemann P, Ferry D, Lubbecke F, Glossmann H (1981) [^{3}H]-nitrendipine, a potent calcium antagonist, binds with high affinity to cardiac membranes, Arzneim Forsch/Drug Res 31:2064
8. Lowry OH, Rosebrough NJ, Farr AL, Randall RJ (1951) Protein measurement with the Folin phenol reagent. J Biol Chem 193:265
9. McPherson GA (1983) A practical computer-based approach to the analysis of radioligand binding experiments. Comput Prog in Biomed 17:107
10. Millard RW, Grupp G, Grupp IL, DiSalvo J, DePover A, Schwartz A (1983) Chronotropic, inotropic, and vasodilator actions of diltiazem, nifedipine, and verapamil. A comparative study of physiological responses and membrane receptor activity. Circ Res 52:29
11. Nayler WG, Sturrock WJ (1983) An inhibitory effect of verapamil and diltiazem on the release of noradrenaline from ischaemic and reperfused hearts. J Mol Cell Cardiol 16:331–344
12. Nayler WG, Perry SE, Elz JS, Daly MJ (1984) Calcium, sodium and the calcium paradox. Circ Res 55:227–237
13. Marsh, JD, Loh E, Lachance D, Barry WH, Smith TW (1983) Relationship of binding of a calcium channel blocker to inhibition of contraction in intact cultured embryonic chick ventricular cells. Circ Res 53:539
14. Abrahamsson T, Sjoquist, Per-Ove, Almgren O (1984) Effects of nifedipine on blood flow and segment shortening in normal and ischemic myocardium: potentiation by ischemia of the negative inotropic effect. J Cardiovasc Pharmacol (to be published)
15. Higgins AJ, Blackburn KJ (1984) Prevention of reperfusion damage in working rat hearts by calcium antagonists and calmodulin antagonists. J Mol Cell Cardiol 16:427–438
16. Karaki H, Nakagawa H, Urakawa N (1984) Effects of calcium antagonists on release of [^{3}H] noradrenaline in rabbit aorta. Eur J Pharmacol 101:177–183
17. Borda LJ, Shuchleib R, Henry PD (1980) Hypoxic contraction of isolated canine coronary artery. Mediation by potassium-dependent exocytosis of norepinephrine. Circ Res 46:870–879

Discussion

(pp. 460–471)

Brown: Apparently, released noradrenaline is available for an extracellular action. You have not said how you know that.

Nayler: Because we have also assayed coronary effluent norepinephrine. And the concentrations that we reach are staggering. So it certainly gets out into the extracellular and into the vascular space.

Fleckenstein: Norepinephrine also contributes to the uptake of Ca^{2+}. Have you any idea to what extent this contributes to Ca^{2+} uptake?

Nayler: The only thing I can tell you that in catecholamine-depleted hearts the rate of Ca^{2+} gain is slowed.

Kazda: In preventing the catecholamine release, all the dihydropyridines you investigated i. e. nitrendipine, nisoldipine and nifedipine seemed to be equally effective. On the other hand we know that in the negative inotropic effect, there are differences between these compounds, nifedipine being the most potent in negative inotropic effect and nisoldipine is much less potent.

Nayler: No, I would not like to say that they are equally effective because we have not done full dose response curves.

Kazda: You have also shown that verapamil at the higher dose even potentiates the ischemic loss of catecholamines. What is the explanation for the difference between the low and the high dose of verapamil?

Nayler: I cannot give it yet. But we have seen that situation before. We found that the high dose of verapamil was less effective than the low dose in its effect on Ca^{2+} gain during reperfusion. Verapamil is an extremely complex drug, and I guess that some of its other activities are coming into play.

Hugenholtz: Would you predict from your experiments that we ought to use the combinations of beta-blockers and Ca^{2+}-antagonists because there would be an additive effect?

Nayler: Yes, I would predict it would be an additive effect.

Lichtlen: If I follow up correctly, we should now add nifedipine when reperfusing with streptokinase.

Nayler: Yes, I'd like to see that done regularly.

Hugenholtz: But that is the very point, I think. You are repeating this over and over again, but I don't see anybody believing it or doing it, and yet we reperfuse. As I argued in our trial we may well have not seen a difference in mortality because we in fact are adding to the damage by doing our successful reperfusion without effects of cardioprotection.

Lichtlen: There is one problem which will be encountered when reperfusion is combined with intracoronary administration of Ca^{2+}-antagonists: In the healthy muscle one will get a strong negative inotropic effect if the drug is given into a coronary artery and that again might compromise what you gain in the ischemic area. Normal left ventricular function will be depressed.

Nayler: I think that is why it is so important to know what has happened to those receptors.

Brown: Does it really matter very much what changes occur in the low-affinity binding sites? I am not quite sure what they are doing. Would you actually measure the K_D very accurately with that sort of concentration range? You used 30 nanomolar displacing nitrendipine and yet K_D was in the 60 nanomolar bracket.

Nayler: We can measure it accurately. It doesn't make any difference if we take it up further and further. We ought to be looking at the low affinity nitrendipine binding sites because that are in therapeutic range.

Brown: In that case you really have to measure it very accurately. And I think you'd really have to carry the concentration well up to about ten times the K_D.

Bayer-Symposium IX
Cardiovascular Effects of Dihydropyridine-Type
Calcium Antagonists and Agonists, 474–477

Protection Against Complete Cerebral Ischemia by Nimodipine

P. A. STEEN

It is well established that after a period of complete cerebral ischemia, a brief 10–15 min hyperemia period is followed by a delayed hypoperfusion period lasting probably more than 18 and less than 48 h as described by White et al. (1982) and our own group (Steen et al. 1978).

The hypoperfusion is severe with CBF down to 20–25% of control, but at least until recently there has been no evidence clearly showing that this hypoperfusion has been detrimental. If a no-reflow situation occurs, or the microcirculation is reduced by massive tissue edema, this would obviously explain further damage (Siesjø 1981), but complete cerebral ischemia with very severe brain damage and a dismal outcome has been described with complete and rapid normalization of tissue metabolites including the high energy phosphates and thus apparently without a no-reflow phenomenon (Steen et al. 1978).

To further investigate if this delayed hypoperfusion was indeed deleterious, we infused nimodipine to dogs in an attempt to alleviate this and correlate the neurologic outcome with the post-ischemic CBF in a separate group of dogs (Steen et al. 1983).

The cerebral blood flow was measured by diverting all the blood from the sagittal sinus of the dog through a flow probe after stopping all collateral flow through bone and muscle. By this method we measure the flow from approximately 50% of the brain, mainly cortex.

The dogs were made ischemic by occlusion of the aorta and both venae cavae for 10 minutes. The treated group was given nimodipine 10 μg/kg/min for 2 hours.

Nimodipine nearly doubled cerebral blood flow in the delayed hypoperfusion period compared to untreated dogs (approximately 45% vs. 25% of the pre-ischemic control values).

At the same time there was also an increase in cerebral oxygen consumption possibly indicating that the increase in flow was indeed important for brain function.

Parallel to the improvement in CBF, nimodipine significantly improved the neurologic outcome.

Now it is impossible to start treatment of for instance cardiac arrest before the arrest occurs, and even though nimodipine improved the post-ischemic CBF and outcome, it was possible that the improved outcome was due to protective effects occuring during the period of complete ischemia, and not due to alleviation of the hypoperfusion.

A similar series of experiments was therefore performed with nimodipine given only post-ischemia (Steen et al. 1984). Again nimodipine significantly improved post-ischemic CBF, this time with no significant change in cerebral oxygen consumption or in cerebral metabolite levels 2 hours post-ischemia.

The neurologic results 48 h post-ischemia were this time intermediate, not significantly different from neither controls nor dogs given nimodipine pre-ischemia.

What conclusion could we draw? We knew that nimodipine can increase CBF in the post-ischemic hypoperfusion period both when treatment was started before and after the ischemic episode. This was in agreement with most of the literature. Bayers own laboratory had thus reported that the hypoperfusion was completely abolished with nimodipine after complete cerebral ischemia in cats (Hoffmeister et al. 1982). White et al. (1982, 1983) in Detroit had reported similar results after 20 min of circulatory arrest in dogs for other calcium blockers, flunarizine, lidoflazine, verapamil and $MgSO_4$. Some uncertainly apply to the latter results. White's method for measuring cerebral blood flow has to my knowledge never been properly evaluated and his control CBF values were 2–3 times what is normally reported for dogs.

We therefore repeated the study for flunarizine in the dog using the same method as we had used with nimodipine (Newberg et al. 1984). For flunarizine we were unable to confirm White's results. Flunarizine failed to influence post-ischemic CBF and did not improve the neurologic outcome after 10 minutes of complete cerebral ischemia.

None of these studies reported on regional distribution of CBF, however, and Smith et al. (1983) from Siesjø's laboratory found that although global CBF post-ischemia was improved by nimodipine, there were great regional differences in rat brain. Thus it was possible that the calcium entry blockers only increased blood flow to already well perfused areas of the brain, without improvements in really ischemic areas.

Our neurologic results gave no clear answers. The outcome was improved if the treatment was started pre-ischemia, but this could be due to effects occuring during the ischemic event, and post-ischemic treatment only gave intermediate results. Before possible human application it is furthermore neccessary to do primate studies.

We have therefore recently given nimodipine in a controlled, blind study to pig-tailed monkeys after 17 min of complete cerebral ischemia (Steen et al. 1985). Anesthesia was induced with 0.5% halothane and 66% nitrous oxide in oxygen. Pancuronium was given with controlled ventilation and PEEP to produce moderate hypocarbia, 4,4 kP. Arterial pressure, ECG, EEG, temperature and end-tidal CO_2 were monitored, blood gases, hematocrit, blood glucose, serum electrolytes and the fluid balance were measured. Steady state was obtained and halothane discontinued for 5 minutes before induction of ischemia.

17 min of complete cerebral ischemia was obtained by a combination of hypotension to 50 mmHg with trimetaphan and a neck tourniquet abruptly inflated to 2 atmospheres. Hypotension was maintained with additional doses of trimetaphan and PEEP. Nitrous oxide was discontinued and the monkeys were ventilated with 100% oxygen with the addition of Xe 133. Scintillation counters were placed on the monkeys' heads to evaluate the absence of cerebral blood flow during ischemia and the return of flow immediately post-ischemia.

At the end of the ischemic period, MABP was brought back to normal with a norepinephrine infusion. 5 minutes post-ischemia treatment with either placebo or nimodipine 10 μg/kg over 2 minutes followed by 1 μg/kg/min for 10 hours was given in a randomized, blind fashion.

Optimal life support was then given in our intensive care unit. The blood pressure was kept within normal range, if necessary with either a norepinephrine or trimetaphan infusion. The monkeys were ventilated with 100% oxygen for 2 hours post-ischemia. This was then changed to 50% oxygen – 50% nitrous oxide until extubation to reduce any stress reaction in animals with small brain damage. $PaCO_2$ was maintained at 4 kP and PEEP at 1–3 cm H_2O. Muscle paralysis was maintained with pancuronium, and respiratory care was given with tracheal suctioning, intermittent deep lung inflations, chest physiotherapy and turning every 4 hours.

The monkeys were extubated at 24 hours post-ischemia if spontaneous ventilation was adequate. 5% dextrose in 0,45% NaCl was given as maintainance fluid until adequate oral intake. Lactated Ringers was given to compensate for any abnormal urine output. Penicillin and gentamycin were given prophylactically. Low urinary output despite an adequate fluid balance was treated with furosamide and any seizures with diazepam. When the condition permitted the monkeys were moved to padded open pens or returned to their cages when they behaved close to normal. 27 monkeys were studied. 6 were discarded for various reasons, 3 treated and 3 untreated. One had incomplete ischemia, one received a large glucose load inadvertently, one was too old, and three had severe cardiovascular problems. Of the monkeys that completed the protocol, the treated group had significantly better neurologic outcome than the untreated when judged by an independent observer 96 hours post-ischemia. Four of them were completely normal, but none of the untreated.

The mean histopathology score was also significantly better for the treated monkeys, but the difference was not significant using a Mann-Whitney rank test. However there was a significant correlation between neurologic function rank and histopathology rank.

We conclude that nimodipine significantly improves cerebral blood flow and neurologic outcome after complete cerebral ischemia. Apart from a possible hypotensive response to a bolus injection and a slight tachycardia during continuous infusion, no potentially detrimental cardiovascular effects were apparent.

References

1. White BC, Gadzinski DS, Hoehner PJ, Krome C, Hoehner T, White JD, Trombley JH Jr (1982) Effect of flunarizine on canine cerebral cortical blood flow and vascular resistance post cardiac arrest. Ann Emerg Med 11:119
2. Steen PA, Milde JH, Michenfelder JD (1978) Cerebral metabolic and vascular effects of barbiturate therapy following complete global ischemia. J Neurochem 31:1317
3. Siesjø BK (1981) Cell damage in the brain: A speculative synthesis. J Cereb Blood Flow Metabol 1:155
4. Steen PA, Newberg LA, Milde JH, Michenfelder JD (1983) Nimodipine improves cerebral blood flow and neurologic recovery after complete cerebral ischemia in the dog. J Cereb Blood Flow Metabol 3:38
5. Steen PA, Newberg LA, Milde JH, Michenfelder JD (1984) Cerebral blood flow and neurologic outcome when nimodipine is given after complete cerebral ischemia in the dog. J Cereb Blood Flow Metabol 4:82
6. Hoffmeister F, Benz W, Heise A, Krause HP, Neuser W (1982) Behavioral effects of nimodipine in animals. Arzneim Forsch 4:347
7. White BC, Winegar CD, Wilson RF, Krause GS (1983) Calciumblockers in cerebral resuscitation. J Trauma 23:788
8. Newberg LA, Steen PA, Milde JH, Michenfelder JD (1984) Effect of flunarizine on cerebral blood flow and neurologic recovery after complete cerebral ischemia in the dog. Stroke 15:666
9. Smith M-L, Kågstrøm E, Rosen I, Siesjø BK (1983) Effect of the calcium antagonist nimodipine on the delayed hypoperfusion following incomplete ischemia in the rat. J Cereb Blood Flow Metab 3:543
10. Steen PA, Gisvold SE, Milde JH, Newberg LA, Scheithauer BW, Lanier WL, Michenfelder JD (1985) Nimodipine improves outcome when given after complete cerebral ischemia in primates. Anesthesiology 62:406

Discussion

(pp. 474–477)

Nayler: Have you tried free radical scavengers as compared to nimodipine?

Steen: No, we have not. There are groups at the moment looking at that, but there are no published reports to my knowledge at the moment.

Brown: How was the Mg^{2+} in the American study given?

Steen: Mg^{2+} was given as an i. v. infusion starting a couple of minutes post ischemia.

Scriabine: Dr. Steen, I think you had tried other Ca^{2+}-antagonists, I remember seeing one paper with negative results, was that in dogs or in monkeys and what drug was it?

Steen: That was flunarizine in dogs. It had absolutely no effects.

From the audience: Did you look at the state of the cerebral blood vessels after the post-ischemic period, was the intima intact?

Steen: Our neuropathologists looked only at the neurons, not at the vessels.

Hugenholtz: One keeps hearing about a trial in patients admitted with severe cranial damage after car accidents. Could you tell us how that situation is?

Steen: There are studies on nimodipine with arterial spasm. That has been published in the New England Journal and a second study is coming up. I don't think anybody at the moment would like to study it in car accident patients because that's the patients where you don't want any drugs that give a cerebral vasodilation. Therefore, you have to have other studies and other models first, where you don't have problems with the intracranial pressure. And that is what you probably don't see in savable cardiac arrest patients.

Hess: You used norepinephrine infusions in the dogs. Are you absolutely sure that it is not the case that the Ca^{2+} channel blockers act only in the presence of norepinephrine because that might have an effect of its own on the vessels, which might then be antagonised in the brain by the Ca^{2+} channel blockers.

Steen: You cannot be absolutely sure that it does not do it in these brains where you indeed probably have a lot of damage to the blood-brain barrier, and thus possibly effects of norepinephrine in contrast to the situation with an intact blood-brain barrier.

Bayer-Symposium IX
Cardiovascular Effects of Dihydropyridine-Type
Calcium Antagonists and Agonists, 480–499

Interdependence of Antihypertensive, Anticalcinotic, and Antiarteriosclerotic Effects of Calcium Antagonists – Model Experiments on Spontaneously Hypertensive Rats (SHR)

A. FLECKENSTEIN, M. FREY, J. ZORN, and G. FLECKENSTEIN-GRÜN

Introduction

In vascular smooth muscle (as in myocardial fibres) a transmembrane supply of Ca^{++} ions is required for active tension development: Whereas restriction of Ca^{++} delivery to the contractile system damps mechanical activity, hypercontractile disorders result from a disproportional augmentation of Ca^{++} entry into the intracellular space. Thus excessive intrusion of Ca^{++} into the cytoplasm has to be considered the decisive reason for phasic and tonic hyperactivity of the arterial and arteriolar vasculature, culminating in vasospasm. Conversely, Ca^{++} antagonists which lower transmembrane Ca^{++} uptake not only in myocardial fibres, but also in smooth muscle (see [6–13, 31]), possess a wide scope of action* against practically all types of vasoconstrictor responses of the coronary, pulmonal, cerebral, renal, or mesenteric arteries.

Another important target of Ca^{++} antagonists are the resistance vessels of systemic circulation both in animals and humans. Thus Ca^{++} antagonists are successfully used for the treatment of acute hypertensive crises as well as for antihypertensive long-term therapy. As shown on our previous papers on this subject, spontaneously hypertensive rats (SHR) also responded to suitable Ca^{++} antagonists with a dramatic fall in blood pressure, whereas chronic treatment of SHR kept the blood pressure at a normal height.

However, the most important therapeutic prospects of a long-term therapy with Ca^{++} antagonists seem to arise from their prophylactic efficacy against progressive Ca^{++} overload of the arterial walls which regularly develops in the course of protracted hypertension. Thus in SHR, Ca^{++} antagonists can prevent calcific arterial destruction and sclerotic damage. It is the aim of the present article to depict the interdependence of the functional and histological manifesta-

* For details see Fleckenstein, A. (1983) Calcium Antagonism in Heart and Smooth Muscle – Experimentals Facts and Therapeutic Prospects, John Wiley, New York Chichester Brisbane Toronto Singapore. The experimental studies were supported by grants of the Federal Ministry for Scientific Research and Technology, Bonn/Germany (Fed. Rep.)

Table 1. Highly specific 1,4-dihydropyridine calcium antagonists derived from the prototypical substance nifedipine[a]

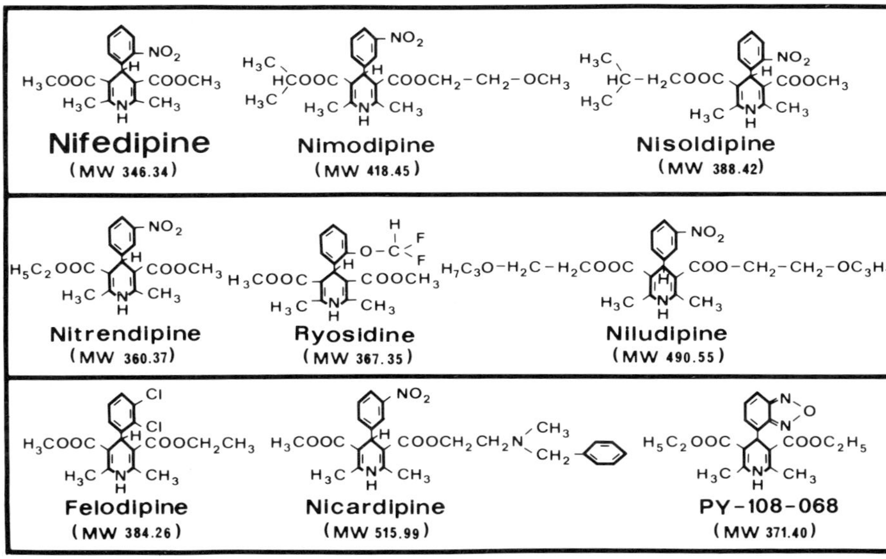

[a] Nifedipine has been identified in our laboratory as a top calcium antagonist in 1969/1970 (see [6–13, 18, 20, 25]). The code name was "Bay a 1040", the usual trade name is "Adalat"

tions of Ca^{++} antagonism in the arteries and arterioles of such spontaneously hypertensive rats, with particular reference to the actions of the Ca^{++} antagonistic 1,4-dihydropyridine compounds listed in Table 1.

I. Experimental Data on Therapeutic Blood Pressure Control with Calcium Antagonists

The long series of investigation on the antihypertensive effects of Ca^{++} antagonists began with the use of verapamil even before the Ca^{++}-antagonistic mechanisms of action of this drug had been generally recognized. Apart from early experimental observations of our laboratory in 1964 [5], four clinical research groups directed by Heidland [27], Brittinger [3], Bender [2], and Belz [1], carried out the first therapeutic trials in different German clinics in the mid and late sixties, quite independently of each other. They were particularly interested in the *acute* antihypertensive effects of verapamil. Brittinger and his colleagues realized the usefulness of verapamil in the treatment of hypertensive crises. Moreover, studies of Japanese workers in the early seventies showed the therapeutic value of verapamil also in chronic hypertension.

A detailed experimental analysis of the Ca^{++} dependency of systemic vascular resistance and its acute attenuation by the Ca^{++} antagonists verapamil, D 600 (gallopamil), and nifedipine was published in 1972 by Grün and Fleckenstein [25],

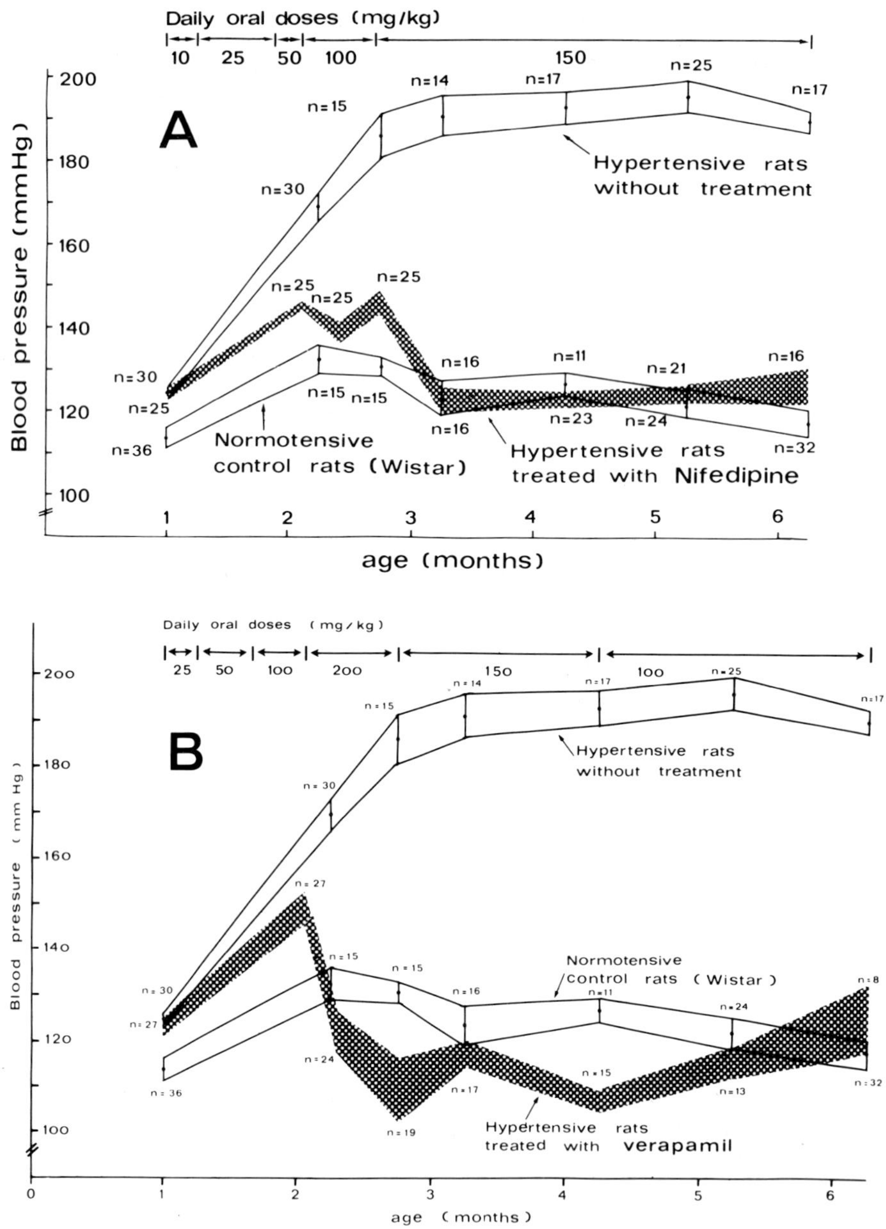

Fig. 1. Normalization of systolic arterial blood pressure of rats suffering from spontaneous hypertension by chronic oral administration of nifedipine (**A**) or verapamil (**B**) during 5 months. Treatment lasted from the end of the first to the end of the 6th month of age. Data from H. v. Witzleben, M. Frey, J. Keidel, and A. Fleckenstein (see [11, 14, 21])

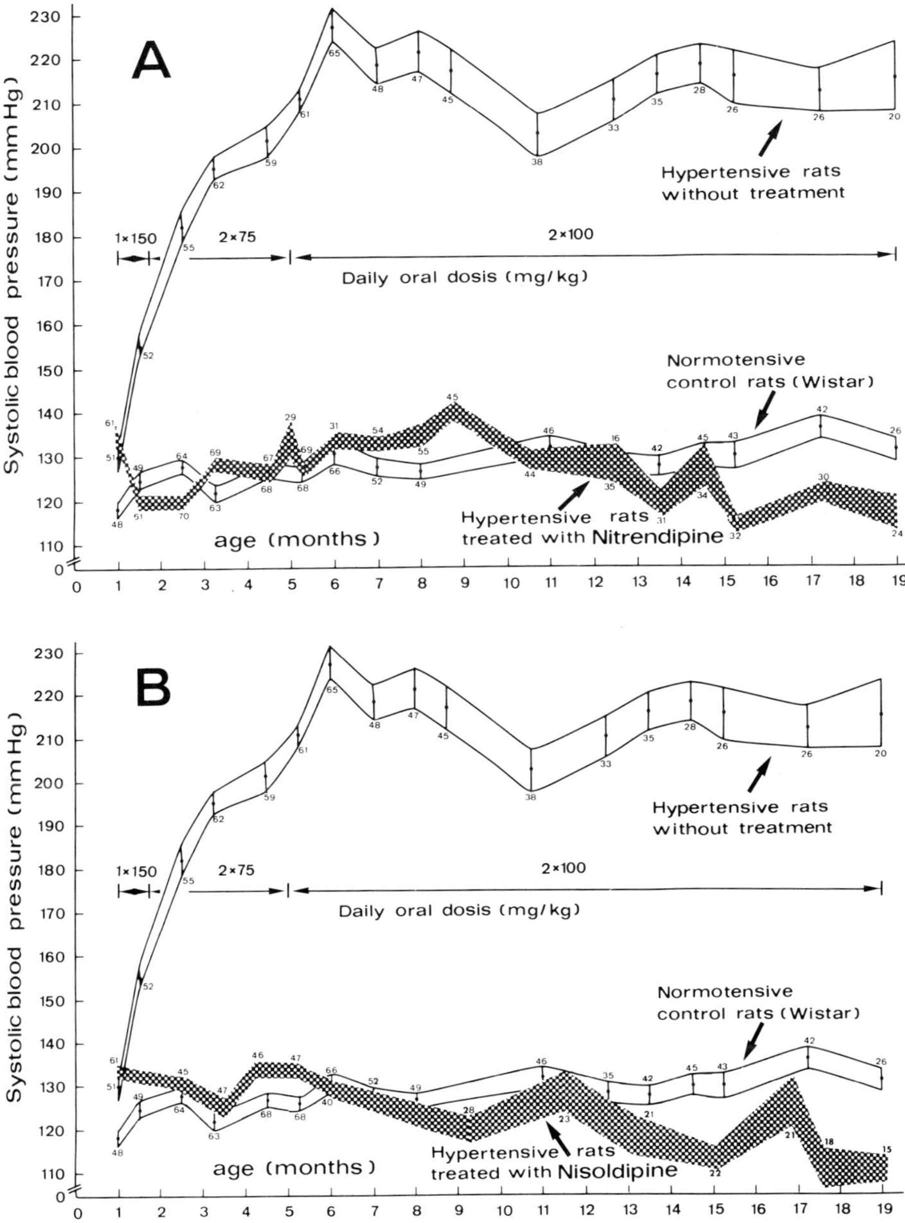

Fig. 2. Normalization of systolic arterial blood pressure of rats suffering from spontaneous hypertension by chronic oral administration of nitrendipine (**A**) or nisoldipine (**B**) over 18 months. Treatment began at an age of 1 month and lasted until the 19th month

followed by some other papers [19, 24, 26]. Furthermore, to vitualize the antihypertensive effects of verapamil and other Ca^{++} antagonists in long-term studies, we treated spontaneously hypertensive rats with daily oral doses during 4 to 18 months. The therapy was always started at an age of 1 month. As can be seen from the upper curves in Fig. 1 A, B, hypertensive rats which were not given a Ca^{++} antagonist, showed an increase of blood pressure of nearly 100% within 5 months up to approx. 200 mm Hg. In contrast, hypertensive rats treated with nifedipine or verapamil, behaved like normotensive control Wistar rats of the same age, because the blood pressure of the Ca^{++}-antagonist-treated rats (represented by the hatched curves) remained at the low level of 110 mm Hg. When, however, the therapy was discontinued, arterial blood pressure rapidly rose within days to the high level of untreated hypertensive rats. Besides nifedipine, other Ca^{++}-antagonistic 1,4-dihydropyridine derivatives have also been shown in our studies to exert antihypertensive actions. This applies – for nimodipine, nisoldipine, nitrendipine, niludipine, ryosidine, felodipine, nicardipine (see Fig. 2 A, B). Diltiazem, a Ca^{++} antagonist discovered in Japan [33], acted similarly.

In recent years, nifedipine and further Ca^{++} antagonists have also been shown to exert antihypertensive actions in other disease models: For instance, normalization of high blood pressure by chronic treatment with nifedipine was also observed in Na^{+}-loaded salt-sensitive Dahl rats [23]. Similarly, conscious renal-hypertensive dogs are rather responsive to Ca^{++} antagonists. As shown by Hiwatari and Taira [28], an acute fall of blood pressure could be obtained in these animals with a single oral dose of 1 to 3 mg niludipine/kg. Diltiazem too proved to be effective in the treatment of spontaneously hypertensive, renal-hypertensive and desoxycorticosterone/saline-loaded hypertensive rats [30].

II. Parallel Suppression of Hypertension and Arterial Calcium Overload with Calcium Antagonists

According to our observations with the Ca^{++} antagonists of group A (nifedipine, nitrendipine, nisoldipine, nimodipine, verapamil, diltiazem), a strong antihypertensive action is a common property of all these agents. Differences in strength can usually be compensated by adjusting the dose. Another effect shared by all antihypertensive Ca^{++} antagonists of group A, is the prevention of excessive Ca^{++} accumulation in the arterial walls [11, 14–17, 21]: In untreated hypertensive rats, the Ca^{++} content of the arterial walls steadily rises until, at an age of 18 to 20 months, it may reach a value which is approx. twice to thrice as high as in normotensive Wistar control rats of the same age (see Fig. 3).

However, with the help of Ca^{++} antagonists, both blood pressure and arterial Ca^{++} content could be kept even in these long-term experiments at normal. Figures 4 and 5 show a series of observations on spontaneously hypertensive rats with or without prophylactic oral administration of the 1,4-dihydropyridine Ca^{++} antagonists nitrendipine, nisoldipine and nimodipine. In fact, corresponding with the complete prevention of hypertension over on observation period of

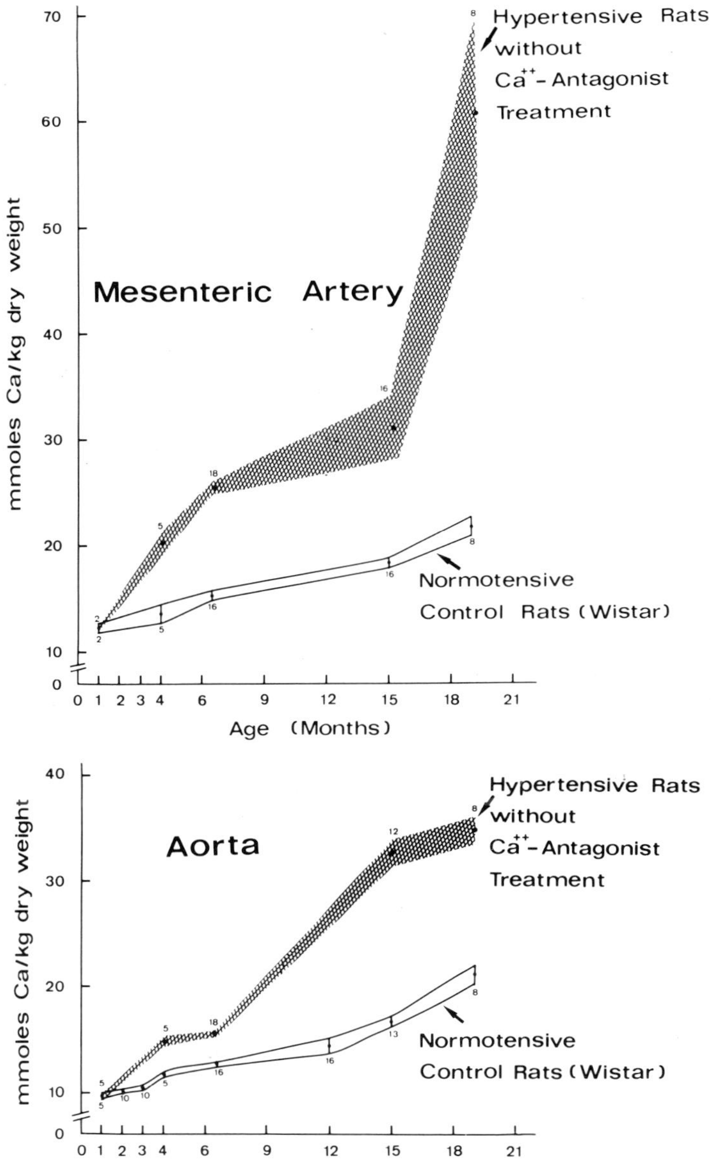

Fig. 3. Age-dependent progressive elevation of the Ca^{++} contents of the rat arterial walls (mesenteric artery and aorta) over on observation period of 18 months in normotensive Wistar control rats, and in SHR not receiving treatment with Ca^{++} antagonists. Spontaneously hypertensive rats consistently exhibited much higher degrees of Ca^{++} accumulation in the arterial tissues than normotensive control rats

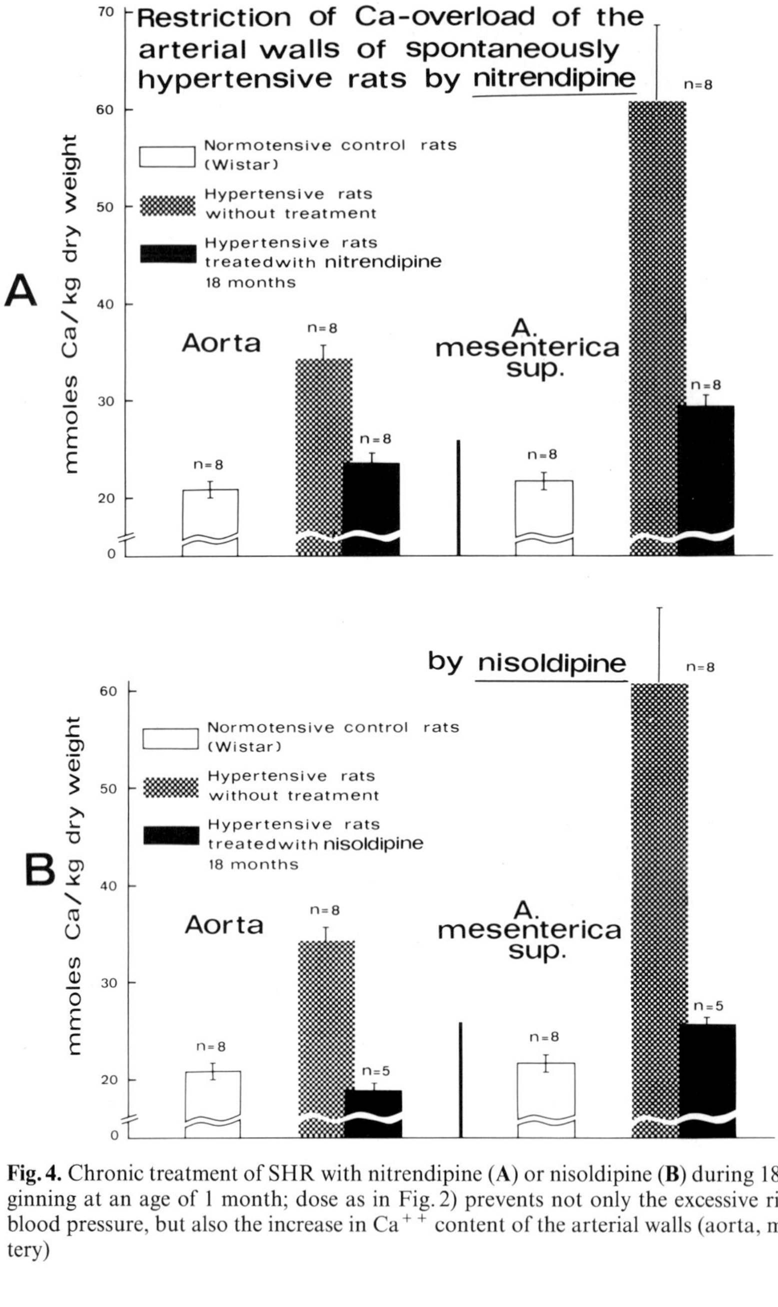

Fig. 4. Chronic treatment of SHR with nitrendipine (**A**) or nisoldipine (**B**) during 18 months (beginning at an age of 1 month; dose as in Fig. 2) prevents not only the excessive rise in arterial blood pressure, but also the increase in Ca^{++} content of the arterial walls (aorta, mesenteric artery)

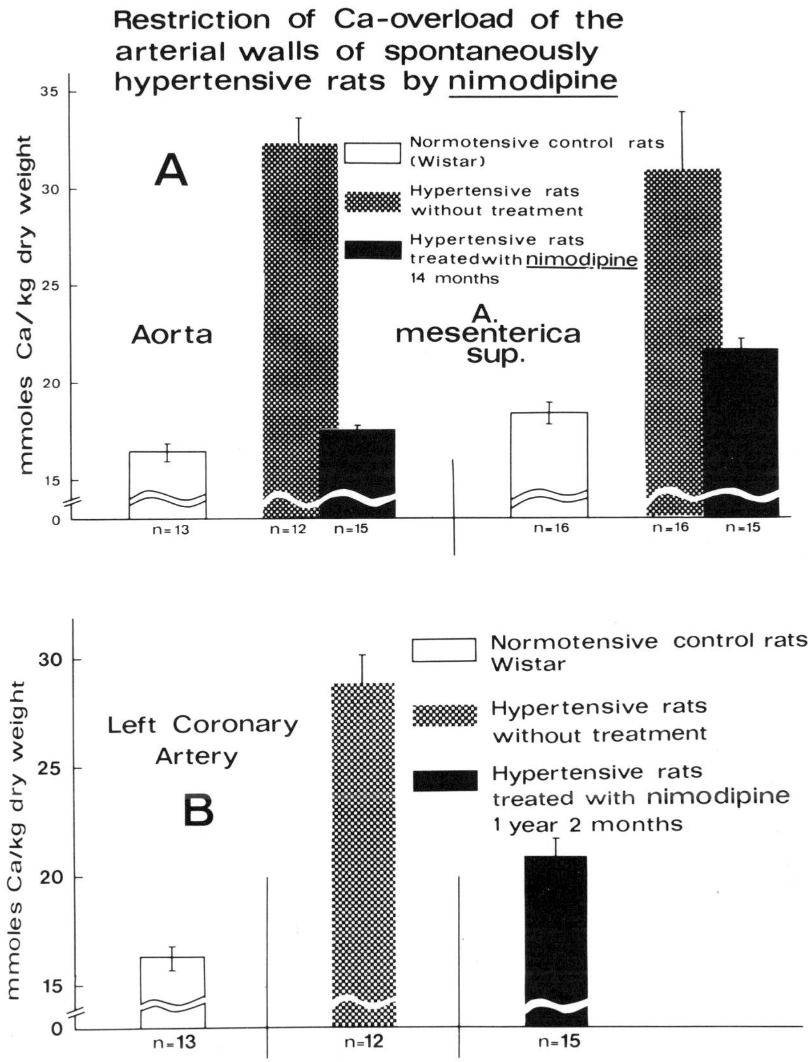

Fig. 5. Long-term oral treatment of SHR with nimodipine (2 × 100 mg/kg daily) over 14 months beginning at an age of 1 month. Again the aortic and mesenteric arterial walls (**A**) and the coronary wall tissue (**B**) respond to the prophylactic Ca^{++}-antagonist therapy with a stop of abundant Ca^{++} accumulation

14 to 18 months, there was also *no* abnormal increase in the Ca^{++} content of the aortic and mesenteric arterial walls. The same is true of the coronary vasculature (Fig. 5B). We have never found in these experiments with Ca^{++} antagonist of group A, any dissociation between their antihypertensive and their anticalcinotic actions.

A

B

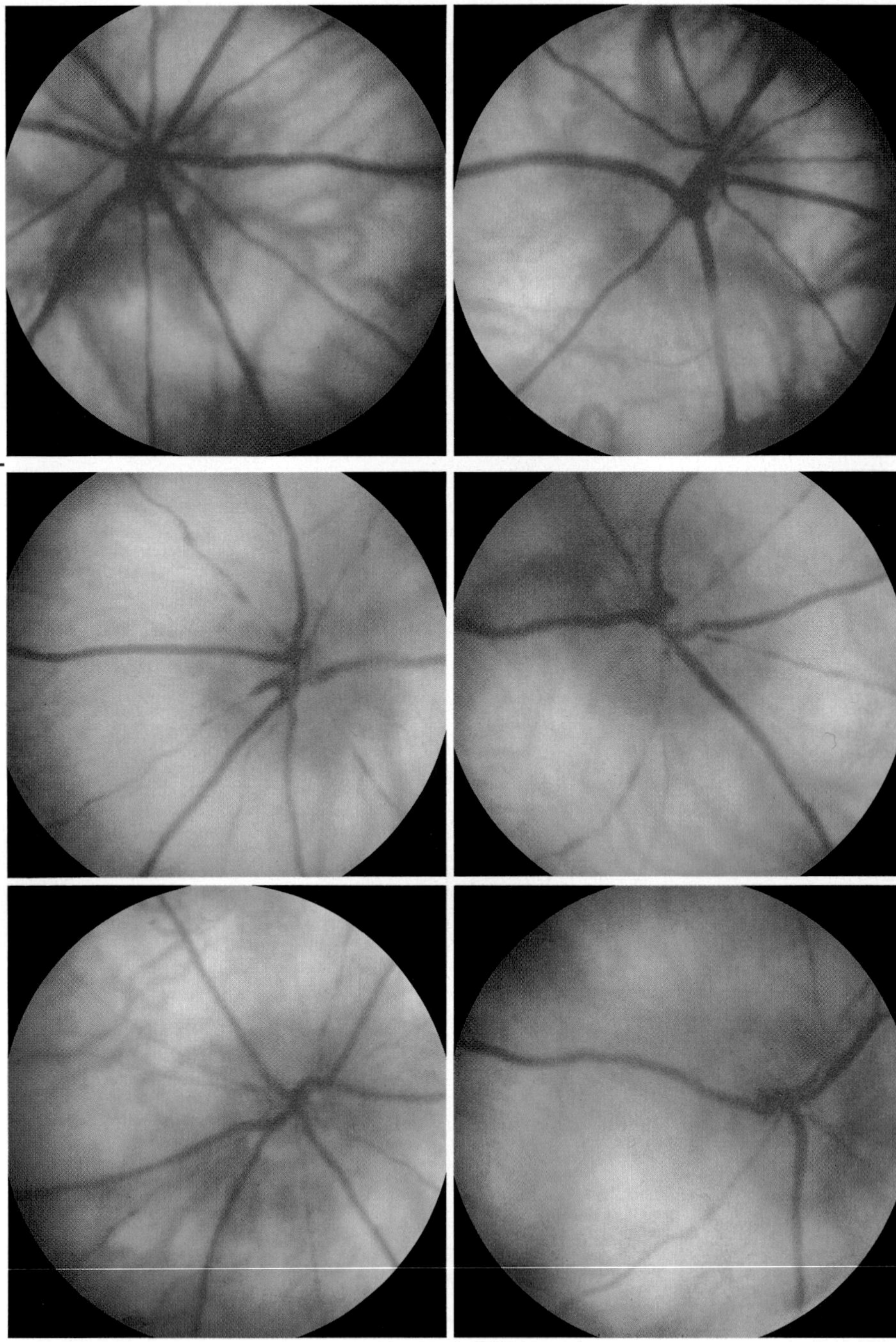

Fig. 6. A Normal ocular fundus of non-hypertensive Wistar control rats. **B** Severe arteriolar vasoconstriction and development of aneurysm-like caliber irregularities in untreated 19-month-old SHR. The diameter of the venoles, characterized by a larger width, is not significantly altered in SHR

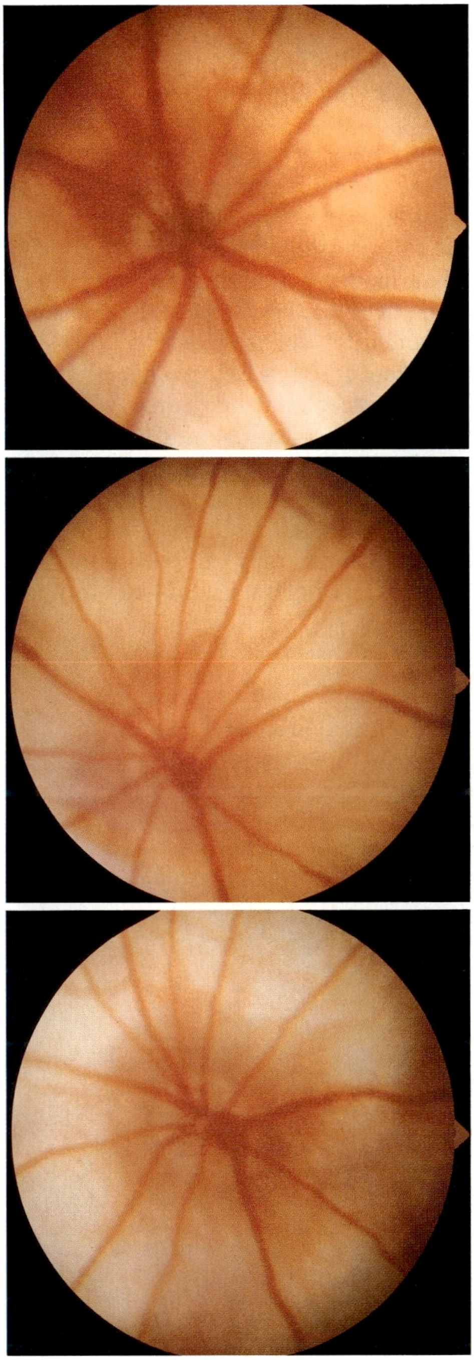

Verapamil (Daily oral dose 100–150 mg/kg contained in diet calculated from food consumption)

Nitrendipine (Daily dose 2 × 100 mg/kg given with stomach tube)

Nisoldipine (Daily dose 2 × 100 mg/kg given with stomach tube)

Fig. 6. C Complete prevention of arteriolar spasm and aneurysm-like caliber irregularities in 19-month-old SHR by long-term treatment with Ca^{++} antagonists over 18 months

III. Prevention of Severe Arteriolar Constriction and Structural Damage by Long-Term Treatment of Spontaneously Hypertensive Rats with Calcium Antagonists

In spontaneously hypertensive rats, which are generally regarded to resemble human patients with essential hypertension, the increase in systemic arteriolar tone can directly be visualized by examination of the ocular fundus. As already known from observations of Takahashi [34], the caliber of the retinal arterioles diminishes in spontaneously hypertensive rats during the period of progressive blood pressure elevation. In consequence, the ratio between the caliber of the retinal arterioles and the veins, which is normally around 1:2, changes considerably. Thus in our studies, the arteriolar diameter in the state of fully developed hypertension, was only about one fourth of that of the accompanying retinal veins (see Fig. 6A, B). However, apart from uniform spastic constriction, irregularities of the arteriolar diameter appear in the form of indentations, aneurysmal dilations or rosary-like alternations of extremely narrowed and expanded sections. There is a clear time-dependent progression of these luminal irregularities in that the ocular arterioles of three-month-old hypertensive rats only exhibited a uniform contriction, whereas at a later stage, the occurrence of aneurysm-like protuber-

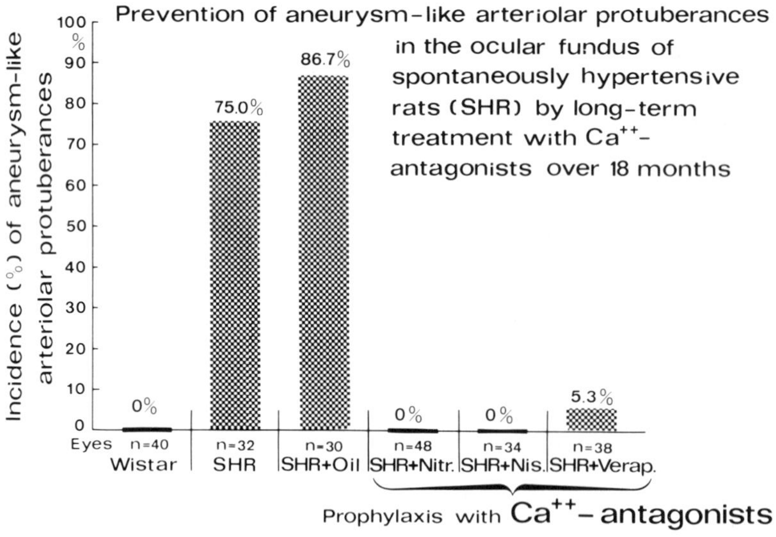

Fig. 7. Ophthalmoscopic assessment of aneurysm-like luminal irregularities of the retinal arteriles in 19-month-old normotensive control Wistar rats, in 19-month-old SHR without Ca^{++} antagonist treatment, and in 19-month-old SHR at the end of prophylactic administration of nitrendipine (*Nitr.*), nisoldipine (*Nis.*), or verapamil (*Verap.*) over 18 months. Incidence (%) means the number of eyes with arteriolar protuberances in the ocular fundus in relation to the total number of eyes in each group. Since the SHR were given nitrendipine and nisoldipine in an oil solution, an additional control group of 30 SHR was formed in which the animals received corresponding quantities of pure oil withouth nitrendipine and nisoldipine ("oil blanks") over 18 months

ances became more and more frequent. Accordingly, our ophthalmoscopic photographs of the ocular fundus of several series of untreated 19-month-old hypertensive rats revealed an incidence of aneurysm-like caliber irregularities of about 75 to 87%. However, with the use of Ca^{++} antagonists, all these severe arteriolar changes could be totally prevented in the overwhelming majority of hypertensive rats (see Fig. 6C). In fact, the ocular arterioles of 60 spontaneously hypertensive Ca^{++}-antagonist-treated rats, which were kept in the physiological blood pressure range over 18 months, showed no constriction and in only a few cases minor luminal irregularities. The order of protective potency of the Ca^{++} antagonists tested as yet over 18 months was nitrendipine = nisoldipine > verapamil (see Fig. 7).

It is interesting to note that, even in the late stage of untreated hypertension, the 19-month-old animals still responded to single oral doses of Ca^{++} antagonists (100 mg/kg of nifedipine, nitrendipine) not only with a steep fall of blood pressure, but also with a rapid dilation of the constricted ocular arterioles (see Fig. 8 and Fig. 9). However, the aneurysms-like luminal protuberances did not acutely disappear. This indicates that a great part of the arteriolar narrowing in the ocular fundus is of spastic rather than sclerotic nature, whereas the aneurysms probably reflect a more pronounced structural alteration of the arteriolar walls.

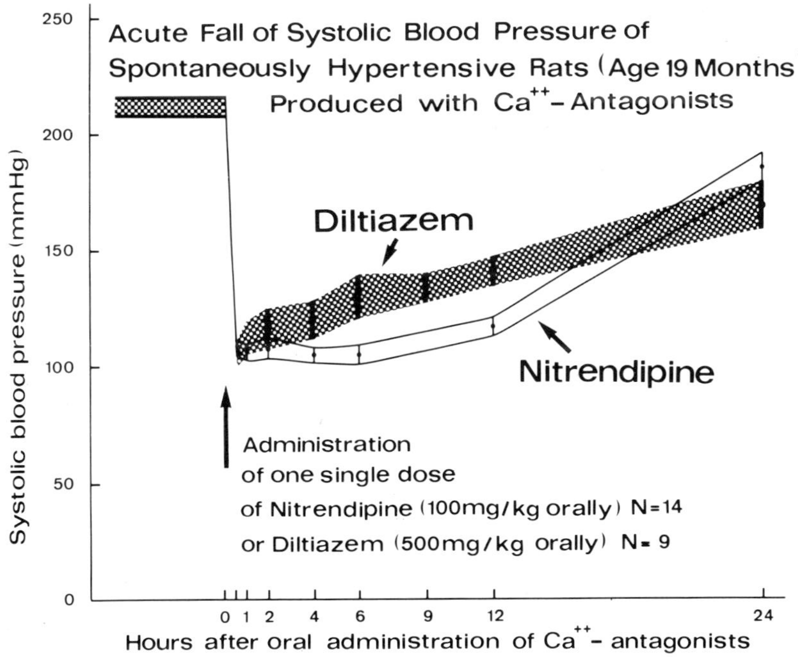

Fig. 8. Instantaneous normalization of arterial blood pressure of 19-month-old spontaneously hypertensive rats (SHR) following oral administration of one single dose of nitrendipine (N = 14) or diltiazem (N = 9). Before administration of nitrendipine or diltiazem, the SHR had maintained a blood pressure level of more than 200 mg Hg for at least 14 months (see Fig. 2, upper curves)

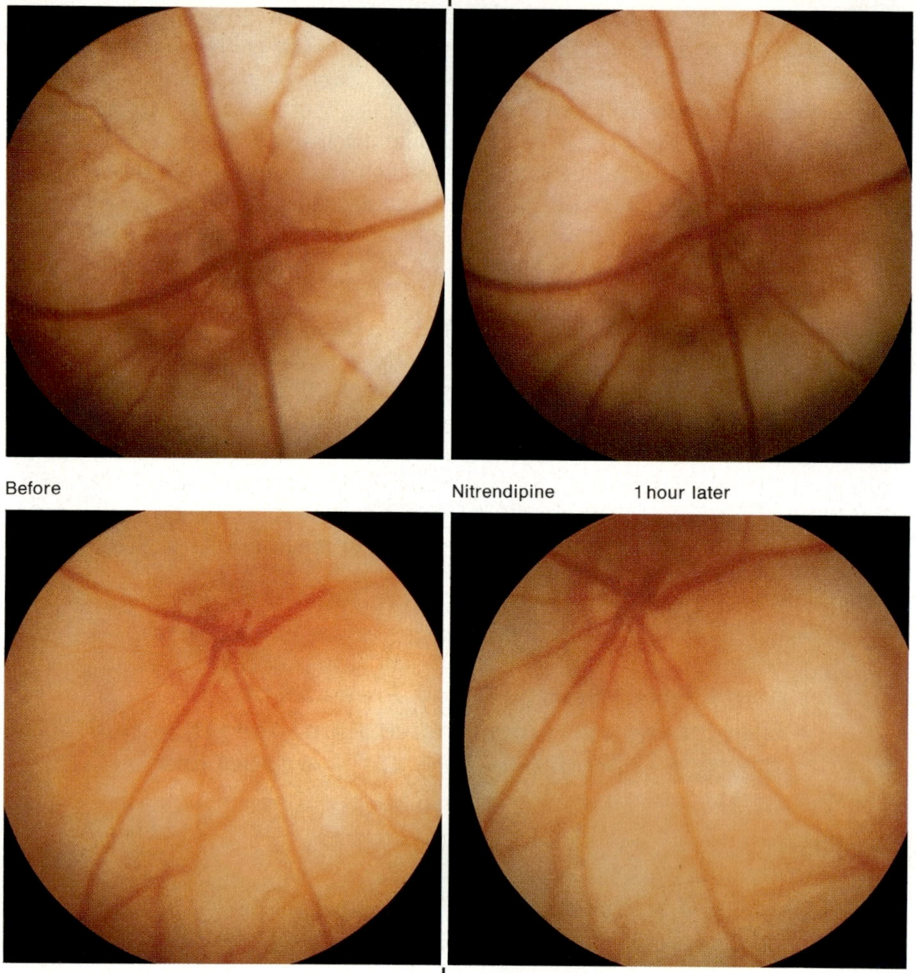

Fig. 9. In response to the Ca^{++} antagonists, the arteriolar spasm in the ocular fundus disappears simultaneously, i.e. within one hour, with the acute fall in blood pressure, whereas the aneurysms persist. SHR, at an age of less than 12 months, tolerated the acute lowering of blood pressure without undesired side effects. Two heavily arteriosclerotic 19-month-old SHR (out of 23) died within 24 hours after administration of the Ca^{++} antagonists

Fig. 10 A–C. Antiarteriosclerotic long-term protection of spontaneously hypertensive rats, evidenced on the mesenteric artery and its branches. **A, B** Spontaneously hypertensive rats *without* Ca^{++} antagonist treatment over 19 months: Without prophylaxis, complete or partial obliteration of the arterial lumen occurs in the majority of the mesenteric vessels. Simultaneously, calcific incrustations and enormous thickening of the arterial walls regularly develop

IV. Antiarteriosclerotic Arterial Protection of Spontaneously Hypertensive Rats (SHR) with Calcium Antagonists

In untreated SHR, larger arteries with a thicker media always undergo still more spectacular changes than the ocular arterioles do. Or more precisely: Approximately at the same time at which the arterioles develop aneurysms, the larger ar-

A

B

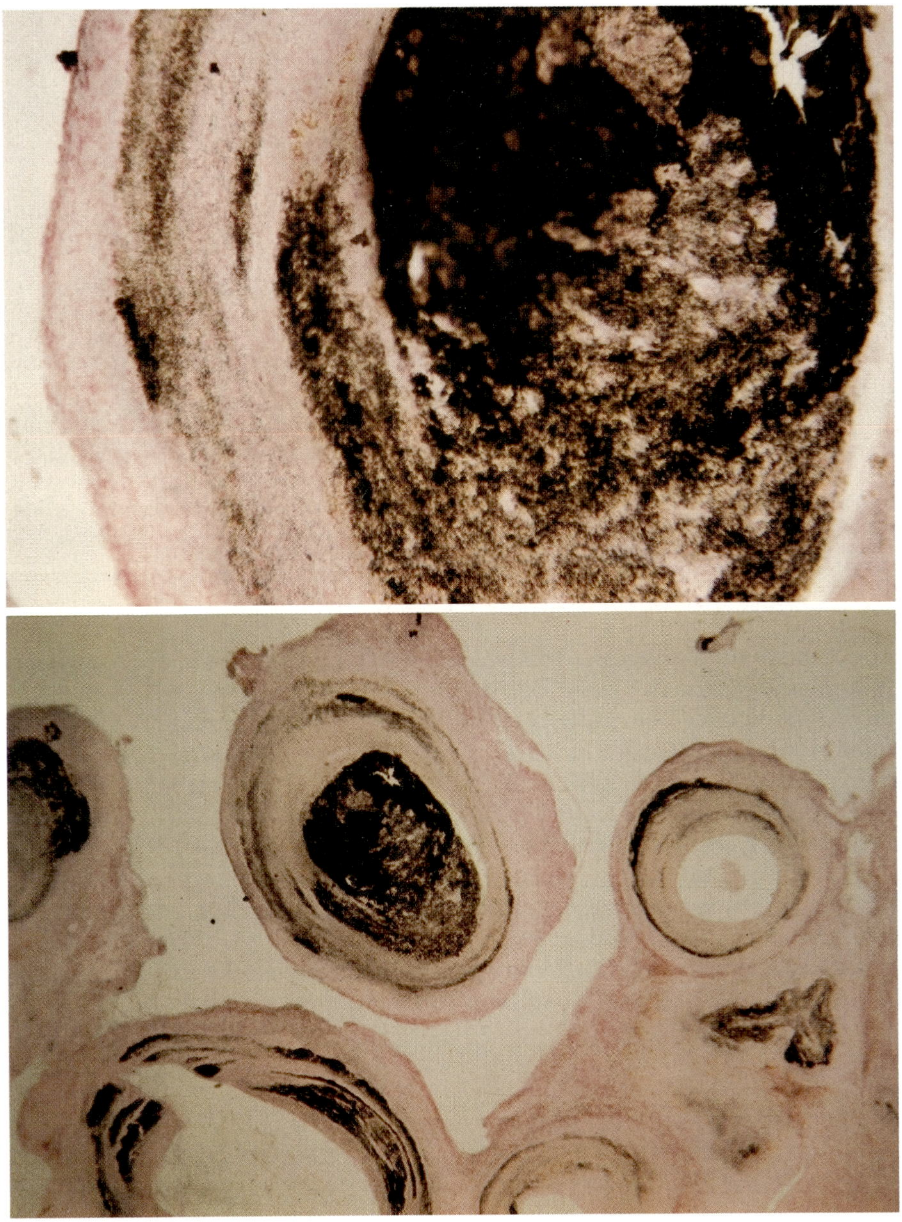

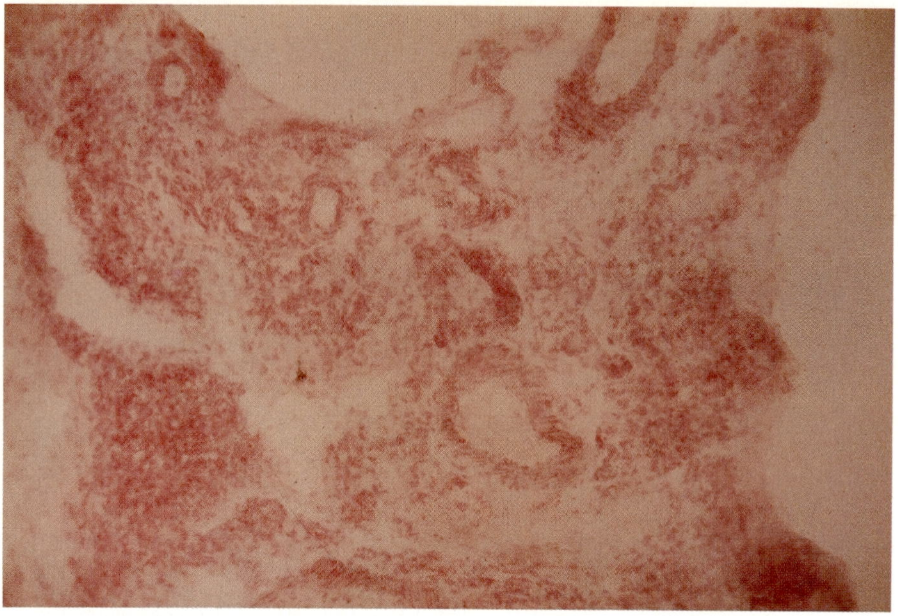

Fig. 10C. Spontaneously hypertensive rat after prophylactic long-term treatment with nitrendipine (2 × 100 mg/kg orally per day) over an observation period of 18 months. Complete preservation of structural integrity, i.e. no calcification, luminal narrowing or wall thickening of the mesenteric artery and its branches. Among a total of 60 Ca-antagonist-protected SHR, there was in no case a significant arterial damage. For visualization of tissue calcium as black areas, v. Kossa's technique was applied in the histological sections **A–C,** followed by additional staining with "Nuclear Fast Red", Merck Inc.

teries exhibit arteriosclerosis. This is most dramatic in the mesenteric artery and its branches. Here severe media calcification with enormous wall thickening, partial or total luminal obliteration, and ischemic damage of the gut were common findings (see Figs. 10 A, B). However, again all these pathological changes of the arterial wall structure could be totally prevented by our Ca^{++}-antagonistic long-term prophylaxis over 18 months (see Fig. 10 C). Interestingly, the mesenteric arterial walls which always accumulate particularly great amounts of Ca^{++} during untreated hypertension, also underwent the most dramatic morphological alterations ever seen in our studies on hypertensive rats. The histological sections of these arteries often exhibited striking similarities with the well-known "Periarteritis nodosa" in humans. Conversely, the antiarteriosclerotic prophylaxis with Ca^{++} antagonists was most perspicuous in this particular section of systemic circulation.

V. Discussion

There is ample evidence that the anticalcinotic or antiarteriosclerotic efficacy of Ca^{++} antagonists is not necessarily a simple consequence of their antihypertensive action, but may also manifest itself independently of any appreciable blood pressure change. Our first results [29] on "Inhibition of arteriosclerotic vascular lesions by prophylactic treatment with $MgCl_2$, KCl, and organic Ca^{++} antagonists. Quantitative studies with ^{45}Ca in rats" were presented at a satellite symposium of the 25th Congress of the International Union of Physiological Sciences in Tübingen (July 1971). Since that time, we have incessantly called attention to the vasoprotective effects which Ca^{++} antagonists can exert experimentally against various types of Ca^{++}-induced arterial damage. As it has turned out in these studies [11, 15–17, 22, 29], excessive Ca^{++} incorporation into the arterial walls is a primary causative factor in the pathogenesis of arteriosclerosis rather than merely a concomitant or subsequent phenomenon. Thus we have found, that all major risk factors that favour human arteriosclerosis (advanced age, diabetes, hypertension, excessive doses of dihydrotachysterol, vitamin D_3, nicotine) are capable of enhancing arterial Ca^{++} uptake in healthy rats, and thereby facilitate or produce severe calcific alterations of the arterial walls. Conversely, suitable Ca^{++} antagonists proved to be able to protect the arterial walls against calcinosis and structural damage. If such risk factors are acting in combination (for instance nicotine plus vitamin D_3), tremendous degrees of deleterious arterial Ca^{++} accumulation can be attained within a few days inspite of the fact that the increase in blood pressure is nil or modest. Table 2 summarizes our studies on rats in which the anticalcinotic efficacy of various Ca^{++} antagonists was established under different experimental conditions. The particular references are given in brackets.

Table 2. Types of arterial calcinosis studied in experiments on rats

Types	Effective Ca-antagonists examined
1. Intoxication with dihydrotachysterol (AT 10) or vitamin D_3 [11, 12, 15–17, 22, 29]	Verapamil, diltiazem
2. Hereditary spontaneous hypertension [11, 12, 14–17, 21]	Nifedipine, nisoldipine, nitrendipine, nimodipine, verapamil
3. Advanced age [15, 16]	Verapamil
4. Alloxan diabetes [11, 12, 15, 16]	Verapamil
5. Chronic oral administration of nicotine[a]	Nifedipine, verapamil, diltiazem
6. Combined administration of vitamin D_3 plus nicotine[a]	Diltiazem, verapamil

[a] See the abstracts: Naunyn-Schmiedebergs Arch. Path. Pharmacol. *325*, R 43 (1984); Pflügers Arch. ges. Physiol. *400*, R 25 (1984); and J. Mol. Cell. Cardiol. *16* (Suppl. 2), 64 (1984)

Ca^{++} antagonists were hitherto used in vascular therapy for *acute* functional vasodilation and spasmolytic purposes. The primary aim was to improve as quickly as possible the blood supply to heart and other organs by removal of purely functional obstacles (spasms) or by enlargement of collaterals and partially obliterated arteriosclerotic vessels. However in the present context, it is a question of much greater medical significance as to whether these drugs are also capable of exerting long-term anticalcinotic and antiarteriosclerotic effects, and in this way, counteract vascular damage just at the roots. This would mean that the Ca^{++} antagonists do not only afford symptomatic improvement, but also interfere with the fundamental pathogenic process of excessive arterial Ca^{++} engulfment and its destructive consequences. Spontaneous hypertension of rats represents a particularly interesting model on which the complexity of the arterial protection by Ca^{++} antagonists can be visualized. Obviously, *chronic hypertension* maintained over 18 months is closely linked with the development of severe arteriosclerotic lesion of systemic arteries (particularly mesenteric artery). Suitable Ca^{++} antagonists prevent both essential hypertension and associated arterial damage. However, the situation is complicated by the fact that

(a) progressive arterial Ca^{++} overload (of milder degree) also occurs in ageing *normotensive* rats, and can be experimentally enhanced at a constant normal blood pressure by the well-known "coronary risk factors" (high doses of nicotine, dihydrotachysterol, vitamin D_3, or alloxan-induced diabetes), and

(b) Ca^{++} antagonists interfere even in these cases with destructive Ca^{++} overload of the arterial walls and other organs. In other words: Vascular protection of SHR by Ca^{++} antagonists seems to be exerted in a double way, namely by a superposition of antihypertensive and anticalcinotic effects.

Needless to say: All these experimental observations encourage a broader use of Ca^{++} antagonists in human antihypertensive therapy, particularly at an advanced age as proposed by Bühler [4] and by Laragh [32]. Clinical evidence of antiarteriosclerotic properties of Ca^{++} antagonists is still missing. However, a further spread of the long-term treatment of hypertension with Ca^{++} antagonists will certainly create favorable conditions for parallel studies on human arteriosclerosis too.

Summary

In spontaneously hypertensive rats, which are commonly regarded as models of human essential hypertension, general arteriolar spasm and sclerosis of the arterial walls are the most spectacular vascular alterations. Particularly interesting in SHR is an easily discernible constriction of the retinal arterioles and the appearance of aneurysm-like luminal protuberances. While spastic caliber-narrowing can be instantaneously neutralized with a single suitable dose of Ca^{++} antagonists even after 19 months of untreated hypertension, the aneurysms do not disappear acutely. In untreated SHR, larger arteries, as for instance the mesenteric artery and its branches, undergo still more dramatic changes than the arterioles of the ocular fundus do. In histological sections of the intestinal arteries, the pathological changes consisted of severe calcification, enormous wall-thickening, partial or total luminal obliteration, and in consequence, ischemic tissue damage. The arterial alterations often exhibited striking similarities with the well-known "Periarteritis nodosa" in humans. Conversely, with suitable Ca^{++} antagonists (group A = nifedipine, nitrendipine, nisoldipine, nimodipine, verapamil, diltiazem), SHR were completely protected against arteriolar spasm, hypertension, and every histologic impairment of arterial integrity.

References

1. Belz GG (1970) Die Wirkung des α-Isopropyl-α((N-methyl-N-homoveratril)-γ-aminopropyl)-3,4,5-trimethoxyphenyl-acetonitril auf den Blutdruck des Menschen bei oraler Medikation im akuten Versuch. Arzneim Forsch (Drug Res) 20:799–802
2. Bender F (1970) Die Behandlung der tachykarden Arrhythmien und der arteriellen Hypertonie mit Verapamil. Arzneim Forsch (Drug Res) 20:1310–1316
3. Brittinger WD, Schwarzbeck A, Wittenmeier KW, Twittenhoff WD, Stegaru B, Huber W, Ewald RW, v. Henning GE, Fabricius M, Strauch, M (1970) Klinisch-experimentelle Untersuchungen über die blutdrucksenkende Wirkung von Verapamil. Dtsch Med Wschr 95:1871–1877
4. Bühler FR (1983) Age and cardiovascular response adaptation: determinants of an antihypertensive treatment concept primarily based on betablockers and calcium entry blockers. Hypertension 5, Suppl 2:94–100
5. Fleckenstein A (1964) Die Bedeutung der energiereichen Phosphate für Kontraktilität und Tonus des Myokards. Verh d Dtschen Gesell f Innere Med 70. Kongreß, S 81–99
6. Fleckenstein A (1970/71) Specific inhibitors and promoters of calcium action in the excitation-contraction coupling of heart muscle and their role in the prevention or production of myocardial lesions. In: Harris P, Opie L (eds) Calcium and the heart. Proceed. of the Meeting of the Europ Section of the Internat Study Group for Research in Cardiac Metabolism, London, Sept. 1970. Academic Press, London New York, pp 135–188
7. Fleckenstein A (1977) Specific pharmacology of calcium in myocardium, cardiac pacemakers, and vascular smooth muscle. Ann Rev Pharmacol Toxicol 17:149–166
8. Fleckenstein A (1981) Fundamental actions of calcium antagonists on myocardial and cardiac pacemaker cell membranes. In: Weiss GB (ed) New perspectives on calcium antagonists. Clin Physiol Series, American Physiological Society, pp 59–81
9. Fleckenstein A (1982) Basic membrane actions of calcium antagonists with special reference to verapamil. In: Godfraind T, Albertini A, Paoletti R (eds) Calcium modulators. Proceed. of an Internat. Symp. on Calcium Modulators, Venice, June 1982. Elsevier Biomedical Press, Amsterdam New York Oxford, pp 297–310
10. Fleckenstein A (1983) History of calcium antagonists. In: Schwartz A, Taira N (eds) Calcium channel-blocking drugs: A novel intervention for the treatment of cardiac disease. Monograph Nr. 95 of the American Heart Association, Circ Research, Part II, Vol. 52, No. 2, pp 3–16
11. Fleckenstein A (1983) Calcium antagonism in heart and smooth muscle – Experimental facts and therapeutic prospects. John Wiley, New York Chichester Brisbane Toronto Singapore
12. Fleckenstein A (1984) Calcium antagonism: History and prospects for a multifaceted pharmacodynamic principle. In: Opie LH (ed) Calcium antagonists and cardiovascular disease. Raven Press, New York, pp 9–28
13. Fleckenstein A, Döring HJ, Janke J, Byon YK (1975) Basic actions of ions and drugs on myocardial high-energy phosphate metabolism and contractility. In: Handbook of experimental pharmacology, Vol. XVI/3. Springer Berlin Heidelberg New York, pp 345–405
14. Fleckenstein A, Fleckenstein-Grün G (1980) Cardiovascular protection by Ca antagonists. Europ Heart J 1:15–21

15. Fleckenstein A, Frey M, Fleckenstein-Grün G (1983) Protection by calcium antagonists against experimental arterial calcinosis. In: Pyörälä K, Rapaport E, König K, Schettler G, Diehm C (eds) Secondary prevention of coronary heart disease. Workshop of the Internat Soc and Federation of Cardiology, Titisee, Oct. 1983. Thieme, Stuttgart New York, pp 109–122
16. Fleckenstein A, Frey M, Leder O (1982/83) Prevention by calcium antagonists of arterial calcinosis. In: Fleckenstein A, Hashimoto K, Herrmann M, Schwartz A, Seipel L (eds) Drug development and evaluation – New calcium antagonists – Recent developments and prospects, Diltiazem Workshop, Freiburg/Germany, May 1982. Fischer, Stuttgart New York, pp 15–31
17. Fleckenstein A, Frey M, v. Witzleben H (1982/83) Vascular calcium overload – a pathogenetic factor in arteriosclerosis and its neutralization by calcium antagonists. In: Kaltenbach M, Neufeld, HN (eds) New therapy of ischemic heart disease and hypertension. Proceed. of the 5th Internat Adalat Symp, Berlin, May 1982. Excerpta Medica, Amsterdam Oxford Princeton, pp 36–52
18. Fleckenstein A, Grün G, Byon YK, Döring HJ, Tritthart H (1975) The basic Ca antagonistic actions of nifedipine on cardiac energy metabolism and vascular smooth muscle tone. In: Hashimoto K, Kimura E, Kobayashi T (eds) New therapy of ischemic heart disease. 1st Internat Adalat Symposium, Tokyo, 1975. University of Tokyo Press, pp 31–44
19. Fleckenstein A, Nakayama K, Fleckenstein-Grün G, Byon YK (1975) Interactions of vasoactive ions and drugs with Ca-dependent excitation contraction coupling of vascular smooth muscle. In: Carafoli E, Clementi F, Drabikowski W, Margreth A (eds) Calcium transport in contraction and secretion. Proceed. of an Internat Symp in Bressanone/Italy, Mai 1975. North Holland, Amsterdam Oxford; American Elsevier, New York, pp 555–566
20. Fleckenstein A, Tritthart H, Döring HJ, Byon YK (1972) Bay a 1040 – ein hochaktiver Ca^{++}-antagonistischer Inhibitor der elektro-mechanischen Koppelungsprozesse im Warmblüter-Myokard. Arzneim Forsch (Drug Res) 22:22–33
21. Fleckenstein-Grün G, Fleckenstein A (1980/81) Calcium antagonism, a basic principle in vasodilation. In: Zanchetti A, Krikler DM (eds) Calcium antagonism in cardiovascular therapy: Experience with verapamil. Internat Symp, Florence/Italy, Oct. 1980. Excerpta Medica, Amsterdam Oxford Princeton, pp 30–48
22. Frey M, Keidel J, Fleckenstein A (1978/80) Verhütung experimenteller Gefäßverkalkungen (Mönckebergs Typ der Arteriosklerose) durch Calcium-Antagonisten bei Ratten. In: Fleckenstein A, Roskamm H (eds) Calcium-Antagonismus Proceed Internat Symp, Frankfurt, 1978. Springer, Berlin Heidelberg New York, pp 258–264
23. Garthoff B, Kazda S (1981) Calcium antagonist nifedipine normalizes high blood pressure and prevents mortality in salt-loaded DS substrain of Dahl rats. Eur J Pharmacol 74:111–112
24. Grün G, Bayer M, Fleckenstein A (1972) Der Einfluß des pH auf den Ca^{++}-abhängigen Tonus der Coronar-Gefäßmuskulatur. Naunyn-Schmiedebergs Arch Pharmakol, Suppl to vol 274, R 43
25. Grün G, Fleckenstein A (1972) Die elektro-mechanische Entkoppelung der glatten Gefäßmuskulatur als Grundprinzip der Coronardilatation durch 4-(2′-Nitrophenyl)-2,6-dimethyl-1,4-dihydropyridin-3,5-dicarbonsäure-dimethylester (Bay a 1040, Nifedipin). Arzneim Forsch (Drug Res) 22:334–344
26. Grün G, Weder U, Fleckenstein A (1972) The mutual antagonism between H and Ca ions in the control of vascular tone and autoregulation. Pflügers Arch ges Physiol Suppl to Vol. 335, R 10
27. Heidland A, Klütsch K, Öbek A (1962) Myogenbedingte Vasodilatation bei Nierenischämie. Münch Med Wschr 104:1636–1637
28. Hiwatari M, Taira N (1979) Antihypertensive effect of niludipine (Bay a 7168) on conscious renal-hypertensive dogs. Arzneim Forsch (Drug Res) 29:1373–1376
29. Janke J, Hein B, Pachinger O, Leder O, Fleckenstein A (1972) Hemmung arteriosklerotischer Gefäßprozesse durch prophylaktische Behandlung mit $MgCl_2$, KCl und organischen Ca^{++}-Antagonisten (quantitative Studien mit Ca^{45} bei Ratten). In: Betz E (ed) Vascular smooth muscle. Proc. Satellit Symp XXV. Internat Congr Physiol Sciences, Tübingen, Juli 1971. Springer, Berlin Heidelberg New York, pp 71–72

30. Kiyomoto A (1978/79) Antihypertensive effects of diltiazem in rats. In: Bing RJ (ed) New drug therapy with a calcium antagonist, Diltiazem. Hakone Symp, 1978. Excerpta Medica, Amsterdam Princeton, pp 112–125
31. Kohlhardt M, Bauer B, Krause H, Fleckenstein A (1972) Differentiation of the transmembrane Na and Ca channels in mammalian cardiac fibres by the use of specific inhibitors. Pflügers Arch ges Physiol 335:309–322
32. Laragh JH (1984) Proceed. of a Symp. on "Calcium Metabolism and Calcium Channel Blockers for Understanding and Treating Hypertension". Amer J Med 77 (Suppl 6 B) 1–23
33. Nakajima H, Hoshiyama M, Yamashita K, Kiyomoto A (1975) Effect of diltiazem on electrical and mechanical activity of isolated cardiac ventricular muscle of guinea pig. Jpn J Pharmacol 25:383–392
34. Takahashi S (1972) On the fundus of spontaneously hypertensive rats. In: Okamoto K (ed) Spontaneous hypertension. Its pathogenesis and complications, Igaku Shoin, Tokyo; Springer, Berlin Heidelberg New York, pp 160–165

Discussion

(pp. 480–499)

Kazda: You have shown in this very extensive experiment that different pathogenic stimulation induces vascular calcinosis and independently of the kind of this stimulation the calcinosis can be prevented by one or other calcium antagonist. Additionally you have shown that also an accumulation of calcium in extracellular space can be also prevented by the calcium antagonist. Finishing this symposium a very simple question: Do we know what is the mechanism of action of the Ca^{2+}-antagonist at all? Are we able to formulate now a theory of mechanism of their action? Two days ago we had a lot of discussions about membrane channels and the specificity of Ca^{2+}-antagonist regarding these channels but these cannot explain your results and our findings as well. At the moment I do not understand really what is the way for the Ca^{2+} going into the cell through the membrane producing the deleterious calcium overload.

Fleckenstein: I was always not in favour of the term "slow channel blocker": As we have shown there are not only effects on the physiological entry mechanism of Ca^{2+}, but also other protective effects of certain Ca^{2+}-antagonists. It is conceivable that under pathological conditions other channels are opened, for instance by anoxic stimuli. Probably, with vitamin D 3 a channel distinct from the "slow channel" is opened. Even the effects on the elastic fibers, I have demonstrated, can thus be explained. With verapamil, e. g. the formation of eye cataracts and Ca^{2+}-overload in the lens can be inhibited. The lens is a non-excitable tissue and nevertheless it can be protected against Ca^{2+}-overload. Therefore, the term Ca^{2+}-antagonists seems to be more suitable to cover all these Ca^{2+}-antagonistic actions.

Nayler: Can I just take this argument one step further? I think we agree now that there are many properties of the Ca^{2+}-antagonists which are not yet recognised. We have been extremely puzzled by the presence of a huge number of low affinity binding sites for verapamil. At first we thought this was just an experimental novelty. But now we realize that if there are in the cell membrane such a large number of sites which are capable or accumulating the drugs specifically, then we surely may alter many other aspects of membrane function, not just the slow channel. I think we have to come around the full circle and look at these drugs again very clearly in a dose dependent manner and see what particular aspect of calcium channel transport or membrane function are being altered. I think we can be reasonably sure that none of these drugs has any effect on the sodium calcium exchange at the sarcolemma. But there are membrane perturbations other than an including slow channel function which are being effected. That is where our future work must go particularly when considering the use of these very high doses.

Fleckenstein: Thank you. I agree completely.

Scriabine: Can we exclude the possibility that the efflux of Ca^{2+} out of vascular smooth muscle cell is not enhanced by dihydropyridines and can we exclude their possible effect on the Ca^{2+} absorption from the intestinal tract?

Nayler: I do not know about Ca^{2+} absorption in the intestinal tract. There is an effect on the extrusion mechanism, there is an effect of some of the slow channel blockers on the membrane-located ATPase which is Ca^{2+} sensitive.

Fleckenstein: An influence on the absorption of Ca^{2+} from the gut is not likely since we have no decrease of the plasma Ca^{2+} level even if we apply high doses of this Ca^{2+}-antagonist. The only effect which we could find in our experiments is blockade of the uptake of Ca^{2+} into the vascular smooth muscle. The increase in plasma Ca^{2+} in the rats fed with dihydrotachysterol or injected with vitamin D 3 was the same as in animals which had no Ca^{2+}-antagonists.

Lichtlen: What is the lowest effective antisclerotic dose? You always show us experiments done with high doses. Did you ever look onto lower doses, which are closer to these doses we use clinically?

Fleckenstein: In order to shorten our experiments we have given enormous doses of vitamin D 3 and dihydrotachysterol. In order to antagonize these doses one has also to use high doses of Ca^{2+}-antagonists. In other experiments, when we injected vitamin D 3 over 2 months we reduced considerably the dose of vitamin D 3 and got practically the same results as far as Ca^{2+}-accumulation is concerned. In these cases we could influence the calcinotic process with a fraction of these doses. The dosage in rats of these drugs is always considerably higher per kg body weight than in humans.

Nayler: Looking not at Ca^{2+} but at atheroma formation in the thoracic aorta and abdominal aorta of cholesterol-fed rabbits we have been able to block with a dose of 5 mg per kg twice daily. So, low doses can be protective. I agree with Prof. Lichtlen's point that patients could not be put on such huge doses. Do we need them?

Groß: In some of your experiments you showed that the high doses needed for preventing Ca^{2+}-overload of the vessels lowered blood pressure only back to control. Therefore, one should not relate the doses needed just to body weight but more to the pharmacological effect of the drug in these animals.

Wettke: Did you have a look at the cerebral vessels after your experiments?

Fleckenstein: In contrast to the reports in literature we found calcification in cerebral vessels with these relatively high doses of vitamin D 3. There was a quantitative difference in the degree of calcification: In the aorta, renal artery and the coronary artery it was always more intense than in the basilar artery.

Wettke: Is there an effect of dihydropyridines on these vessels, too?

Fleckenstein: It depends certainly on the type of calcinosis. If you produce calcinosis with vitamin D 3 the 1,4-dihydropyridines were not very efficient; this type of calcinosis is better influenced by verapamil and diltiazem. But if the Ca^{2+}-accumulation is due to hypertension, the efficacy of the 1,4-dihydropyridines in our experiments was always by far the best.

Schattenberg: Morphologically, diabetics have a thickening of the basement membrane at the capillaries. Did you see in diabetic rats under longtime treatment with nifedipine a change in thickness of the basement membrane?

Fleckenstein: In these experiments we did not use nifedipine.

Hess: I had some problems taking all this discussion about all kinds of possible mechanism. One mechanism of those drugs has been demonstrated and that is on the Ca^{2+}-channel. Besides a lot of observation – that are subject to interpretation – no other mechanism has clearly been demonstrated. Is it surprising that we have all these observations – that we cannot explain – as these drugs interfere with one of the most important regulatory mechanisms in living cells that we know of? And I challenge those who say that they have observations that clearly point to some other mechanism, to show it.

Fleckenstein: I am surprised that you have to address me since we have found that the Ca^{2+}-influx is specifically blocked. There are other effects too which are not identical with slow channel blockade which we have described first and we cannot neglet these effects. They are perhaps therapeutically important.

Scriabine: There is still one additional observation which always puzzled me in relation to the mechanism of action of Ca^{2+}-antagonisms: Why is the Ca^{2+} entry induced by the ionophore A 23187 also antagonised by Ca^{2+}-antagonists, 1,4-dihydroparidines and verapamil?

Van Breemen: Just because you use another mechanism to introduce Ca^{2+} into the cells does not mean that the inhibitor acts on that mechanism because contraction as well as calcinosis is probably a threshold phenomenon. If you can reduce Ca^{2+} entry below that threshold by any means – no matter on what mechanism – you are going to have beneficial effect.

Subject Index